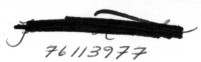

THE ANATOMY OF THE EYE
AND ORBIT

First Edition	.	.	.	.	.	1933
Reprinted .	.	.	.	.	.	1936
Reprinted .	.	.	.	.	.	1938
Reprinted .	.	.	.	.	.	1939
Second Edition	.	.	.	.	.	1940
Reprinted .	.	.	.	.	.	1942
Reprinted .	.	.	.	.	.	1945
Third Edition	.	.	.	.	.	1948
Reprinted .	.	.	.	.	.	1949
Reprinted .	.	.	.	.	.	1951
Fourth Edition	.	.	.	.	.	1954
Reprinted .	.	.	.	.	.	1958
Fifth Edition	.	.	.	.	.	1961
Reprinted .	.	.	.	.	.	1964
Reprinted .	.	.	.	.	.	1966
Sixth Edition	.	.	.	.	.	1968
Reprinted .	.	.	.	.	.	1969

EUGENE WOLFF'S

ANATOMY OF THE EYE AND ORBIT

Including the central connections, development, and comparative anatomy of the visual apparatus

SIXTH EDITION

Revised by

R. J. LAST

M.B., B.S.(Adelaide), F.R.C.S.(Eng.)

PROFESSOR OF APPLIED ANATOMY AND WARDEN
ROYAL COLLEGE OF SURGEONS OF ENGLAND

WITH 465 ILLUSTRATIONS, INCLUDING
56 IN COLOUR

W. B. SAUNDERS COMPANY

Philadelphia and Toronto

PRINTED IN GREAT BRITAIN

PREFACE TO THE SIXTH EDITION

SINCE the appearance of the last edition of *Wolff's Anatomy of the Eye and Orbit* there has been a vast increase of published work. This is particularly so in electron microscopy, where to publish a book, or even a paper, is to risk being out of date before being in print. Those who know previous editions of this book, and the readers of the following pages, will be aware of the doubts and uncertainties left by photomicroscopy of the eye. Electron microscopy has elucidated a few of these, but has itself introduced still more uncertainties. Much remains to be known. Progress is continuous and exciting prospects open up as, for example, with the new scanning electron microscope.

In this edition I have preserved the photomicroscopic findings as they already existed, to retain a full perspective. There are now added some electron microscopic findings and for this I must thank Dr. C. Pedler, of the Institute of Ophthalmology in London, and his very skilful assistant Mrs. R. Tilly for the excellent electron micrographs in the following pages. Mr. P. V. Rycroft F.R.C.S. has provided me with three electron micrographs of human cornea.

There are many other additions to current understanding of ocular anatomy. The work of Niels Ehlers on the precorneal film is very noteworthy. The constitution of the third nerve nucleus *in man* is still speculative. After consultation with Professor R. Warwick an amended account of this nucleus *in the monkey* is now included. For the rest there are countless alterations and additions that I hope will make this edition up to date while at the same time keeping the original pattern and character of Wolff's own work.

There are many additions to the bibliography, but no removals; original references are retained if only for their historical interest.

R. J. LAST

ROYAL COLLEGE OF SURGEONS,
LONDON

EXTRACTS FROM
PREFACE TO THE FIRST EDITION

THIS *Anatomy of the Eye and Orbit* is based mainly on lectures and demonstrations which I have had the honour to give during ten years as Demonstrator of Anatomy at University College, and for the last three years as Pathologist and Lecturer in Anatomy to the Royal Westminster Ophthalmic Hospital.

It is an attempt to present to the Student and Ophthalmic Surgeon the essentials of the structure, development, and comparative anatomy of the visual apparatus in conjunction with some of their clinical applications. The motor nerves to the eye muscles have received special attention, as have also the illustrations, many of which are from my own preparations.

EUGENE WOLFF.

HARLEY STREET,
LONDON, W.1.

CONTENTS

ANATOMY OF THE EYE AND ORBIT

CHAPTER I

THE BONY ORBIT AND PARANASAL SINUSES

THE BONY ORBIT

THE two orbital cavities are placed on either side of the sagittal plane of the skull between the cranium and the skeleton of the face. Thus situated they encroach about equally on these two regions (Winckler).

Above each orbit is the anterior cranial fossa, medially are the nasal cavity and air sinuses, below is the maxillary sinus (antrum of Highmore), while laterally from behind forwards are the middle cranial and the temporal fossæ.

The orbit is essentially intended as a socket for the eyeball and also contains the muscles, nerves, and vessels, which are essential for its proper functioning. Moreover, it serves to transmit certain vessels and nerves destined to supply the areas of the face around the orbital aperture.

Seven bones take part in the formation of the orbit, namely : the maxilla and palatine, the frontal, the sphenoid and zygomatic bone, the ethmoid and the lacrimal bone.

The orbit has *roughly* the shape of a quadrilateral pyramid whose base, directed forwards, laterally, and slightly downwards, corresponds to the orbital margin, and whose apex is the optic foramen or, as some hold, the medial end of the superior orbital fissure ; or the bar of bone between these two apertures (Whitnall).

As stated above, the comparison with a quadrilateral pyramid is a rough one only, for since the floor (which is the shortest orbital wall) does not reach the apex, the cavity is triangular on section in this region.

Also, since the orbit is developed around the eye, and is bulged out by the lacrimal gland, it has a tendency towards being spheroidal in form, and its widest part is not at the orbital margin but about 1·5 cm. behind this. Moreover, this results in the fact that its four walls are for the most part separated from each other by ill-defined rounded borders, so that Whitnall compares the shape of the orbit to a pear whose stalk is the optic canal. It is important to note that the medial walls of the orbits are almost parallel, whereas the lateral walls make an angle of about 90° with each other. The direction of each orbit is given by its axis which runs from behind forwards, laterally and slightly downwards.

The roof or vault of the orbit is triangular in shape. It is formed in great part by the triangular orbital plate of the frontal bone and behind this by the lesser

A.E.—1

wing of the sphenoid. It does not look directly downwards but slightly forwards as well. It is markedly concave anteriorly and more or less flat posteriorly. The anterior concavity is greatest about 1·5 cm. from the orbital margin and corresponds to the equator of the globe.

It presents :

(a) *The fossa* for the lacrimal gland. This lies behind the zygomatic process of the frontal bone. It is simply a slight increase in the general concavity of the anterior and lateral part of the roof, and is better appreciated by touch than by sight. It contains not only the lacrimal gland but also some orbital fat found principally at its posterior part (accessory fossa of Rochon-Duvigneaud). It is bounded below by the ridge corresponding to the zygomatico-frontal suture, at the junction of roof and lateral wall of the orbit. It is usually quite smooth, but may be pitted by the attachment of the suspensory ligament of the lacrimal gland when this is well developed.

(b) *The fovea* for the pulley of the superior oblique is a small depression situated close to the fronto-lacrimal suture some 4 mm. from the orbital margin (Figs. 1 and 2). Sometimes (10 per cent.) the ligaments which attach the U-shaped cartilage of the pulley to it are ossified. Then the fossa is surmounted most often posteriorly by a spicule of bone (the *Spina trochlearis*). Extremely rarely a ring of bone, representing the trochlea completely ossified, may be seen (Winckler). Above the fovea the frontal sinus separates the two plates of the frontal bone ; the cavity extends lateral and posterior from the fovea to a very variable extent.

(c) *The fronto-sphenoidal suture*, which is usually obliterated in the adult, lies here between the orbital plate of the frontal bone and the lesser wing of the sphenoid.

The roof of the orbit is separated from the medial wall by fine sutures between the frontal bone above and the ethmoid, lacrimal, and frontal process and those of the maxilla below. In or just above the fronto-ethmoidal suture are the anterior and posterior ethmoidal canals (Figs. 1 and 2) (see later). The roof is separated from the lateral wall posteriorly by the superior orbital fissure, anteriorly by the slight ridge that marks the fronto-zygomatic suture. The orbital aspect of the roof is usually quite smooth, but may be marked by certain small apertures and depressions. The apertures known as the *Cribra orbitalia of Welcker* are found most commonly to the medial side of the anterior portion of the lacrimal fossa. They are not always present and are best marked in the foetus and infant (Winckler). They give the bone a porous appearance, and, according to Toldt, are for veins which pass from the diploe to the orbit.

In the posterior part of the orbit, in or around the lateral part of the lesser wing of the sphenoid, small orifices may also be found which serve as communications between the orbit and the cranial dura mater and contain vessels during life.

Numerous small grooves may be seen in the roof of the orbit. These lead to the above orifices and are made by vessels or nerves.

Very rarely one may find an antero-posterior fissure up to 14 mm. long filled with periorbita and dura mater.

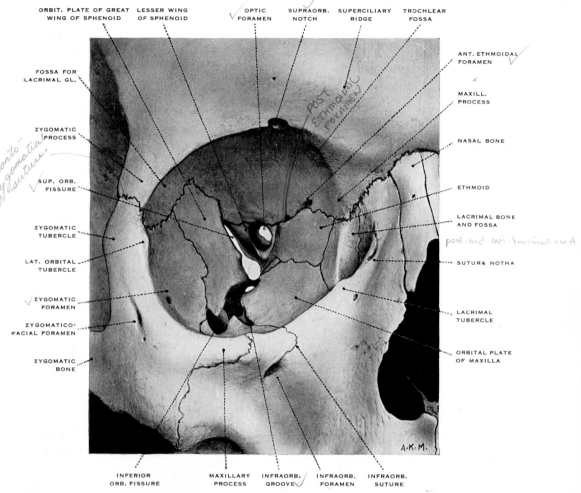

FIG. 1.—THE RIGHT ORBIT VIEWED ALONG ITS AXIS.

Structure.—The roof of the orbit is very thin, translucent, and fragile except where it is formed by the lesser wing of the sphenoid, which is 3 mm. thick. If the bone be held up to the light, one can make out the ridges and depressions on the cranial aspect formed by the sulci and gyri of the frontal lobe of the brain. This is especially true of the posterior two-thirds. The translucency of the anterior third enables the outline of the orbital extension of the frontal sinus to be seen.

Occasionally in old age portions of the bone may be absorbed, and then the periorbita is in direct contact with the dura mater of the anterior cranial fossa.

It is quite easy, in the disarticulated skull, to break the roof of the orbit by slight pressure with the finger.

Also punctured wounds through the lids are sometimes inflicted with the points of umbrellas or walking-sticks, and the roof of the orbit may easily be fractured by direct violence (Fisher).

The roof of the orbit is invaded to a varying extent by the frontal sinus and sometimes by the ethmoidal air-cells. The frontal sinus may extend laterally to the zygomatic process and backwards close to the optic foramen. The sphenoidal sinus or the posterior ethmoidal air-cells not infrequently invade the lesser wing of the sphenoid.

Relations.—The frontal nerve lies in direct contact with the periorbita for the whole extent of the roof (Figs. 276 and 277). The supraorbital artery accompanies it only in the anterior half. Beneath the nerve is the levator palpebræ, and deep to this again is the superior rectus.

The trochlear nerve lies medially, in contact with the periorbita, on its way to the superior oblique muscle.

The lacrimal gland occupies the lacrimal fossa, and the superior oblique lies at the junction of the roof and the medial walls.

Invading the roof to a variable extent, as seen above, are the frontal sinus and the ethmoidal air-cells.

Above the roof are the meninges covering the frontal lobe of the brain (Fig. 280).

The medial wall of the orbit (Fig. 2) is the only wall which is not obviously triangular. It is roughly oblong, either quite flat or slightly convex towards the orbital cavity. It runs parallel with the sagittal plane, and consists from before backwards of four bones united by vertical sutures.

(*a*) The frontal process of the maxilla.

(*b*) The lacrimal bone.

(*c*) The orbital plate of the ethmoid.

(*d*) A small part of the body of the sphenoid.

Of these the orbital plate of the ethmoid takes by far the largest portion. It often shows a characteristic mosaic of light and dark areas. The dark areas correspond to the ethmoidal air-cells, while the light lines between them correspond to the partitions between the cells (Fig. 19).

In the anterior part of this wall is the *lacrimal fossa*, formed by the frontal process of the maxilla and the lacrimal bone. It is bounded in front and behind by the *anterior* and *posterior lacrimal crests*. Above there is no definite boundary, while below the fossa is continuous with the bony naso-lacrimal canal. At their point of junction the hamulus of the lacrimal bone curves round from the posterior to the anterior lacrimal crest and bounds the fossa to the lateral side (Fig. 2). At this point the fossa is some 5 mm. deep, while it gradually gets shallower as we trace it upwards. It is about 14 mm. in height. The lacrimal bone and frontal process of the maxilla take varying parts in the formation of the fossa ; and so the position of the vertical suture between them varies also.

The anterior lacrimal crest on the frontal process of the maxilla is ill-defined above but well marked below, where it becomes continuous with the lower orbital margin and here often presents a *lacrimal tubercle* (Fig. 1).

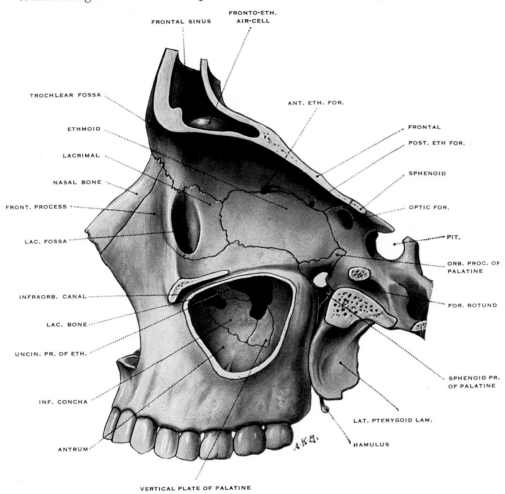

FIG. 2.—THE MEDIAL WALL OF THE ORBIT.

The lacrimal bone separates the upper half of the fossa from the anterior ethmoidal air-cells, and the lower part from the middle meatus of the nose (see also p. 231).

The Structure of the Medial Wall.—The medial is by far the thinnest orbital wall (0·2–0·4 mm.). It is translucent, so that if held up to the light, the ethmoidal air-cells can be plainly seen.

The orbital plate of the ethmoid, as its former name (lamina papyracea) implies, is, in fact, as thin as paper, and infection from the ethmoidal air-cells can easily get into the orbit. *This is the reason why ethmoiditis is the commonest cause of orbital cellulitis.*

Despite its thinness, however, the orbital plate but rarely shows senile absorptive changes, whereas the thicker lacrimal bone, especially that portion which enters into the formation of the lacrimal fossa, is often absorbed.

VARIETIES.—The lacrimal bone may be divided by accessory sutures into several parts (Schwegel, Henle, Hyrtl).

A Wormian bone may be developed in its upper and fore part.

An accessory lacrimal bone, such as is found in many lower animals, may be split off the front of the ethmoid.

The hamulus may be absent, may exist as a separate bone, or may be double.

Relations.—Through the medial wall lie, from before backwards (Fig. 3), the lateral wall of the nose, the infundibulum and ethmoidal air-cells, and the sphenoidal air sinus. The optic foramen lies at the posterior end of the medial wall (Fig. 2).

The superior oblique occupies the angle between the roof and medial wall, and the medial rectus runs along this wall, while between the two muscles are the anterior and posterior ethmoidal and the infratrochlear nerves and the termination of the ophthalmic artery (Fig. 277).

Anteriorly the lacrimal sac lies in its fossa, surrounded by the lacrimal fascia, while just behind it is the attachment of the lacrimal fibres of orbicularis oculi (Horner's muscle), the septum orbitale, and the check ligament of the medial rectus (Figs. 224 and 225).

The floor of the orbit is roughly triangular, corresponding to the shape of the roof. It is not quite horizontal, but slopes slightly downwards from the medial to the lateral side. The lowest part of the floor of the orbit is found in a concavity some 3 mm. deep at the lateral and anterior part. The floor (47·6 mm. long), the shortest of the orbital boundaries, is formed by three bones :

    (1) The orbital plate of the *maxilla.*
    (2) The orbital surface of the *zygomatic.*
    (3) The orbital process of the *palatine bone.*

Of these the *maxilla* takes by far the largest portion. The *zygomatic* forms the antero-lateral part, while the *palatine bone* occupies a small area behind the maxilla.

The floor of the orbit is traversed by the *infraorbital sulcus*, which runs almost straight forwards from the inferior orbital (spheno-maxillary) fissure. At a variable distance (usually about half-way) it is converted into a *canal* by a plate of bone which grows over it from its *lateral* side to meet the medial in a suture (the infraorbital suture), which is but rarely obliterated (Fig. 3). This suture can be traced over the lower orbital margin to the medial side of, and into, the infra-orbital foramen (Fig. 1). It sometimes cuts across the zygomatico-maxillary suture.

The infraorbital canal, formed as described above, sinks anteriorly into the orbital floor and opens at the infraorbital foramen some 4 mm. from the orbital

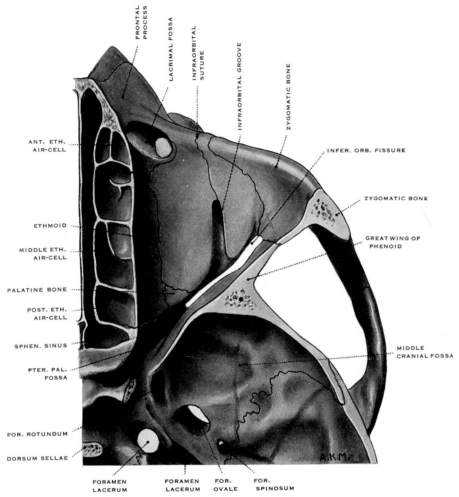

FIG. 3.—THE FLOOR OF THE ORBIT.

margin. It transmits the infraorbital vessels and nerve. Along its course it gives off the *middle* and *anterior superior alveolar* (*dental*) *canals*, for the corresponding nerves and vessels.

Lateral to the opening of the naso-lacrimal canal a small pit or roughness marking the origin of the inferior oblique muscle may (rarely) be found.

The floor of the orbit is separated from the medial wall only by a fine suture ;

the lateral wall is separated from it posteriorly by the inferior orbital (spheno-maxillary) fissure, while anteriorly it is continuous with it (Fig. 3).

VARIETIES.—Not infrequently the roof of the infraorbital canal and sometimes its floor may be incomplete, but otherwise only very rarely does the floor of the orbit show holes, the result of senile absorption. Langer has seen three cases where the infraorbital canal ran in the suture between the maxilla and the zygomatic bone.

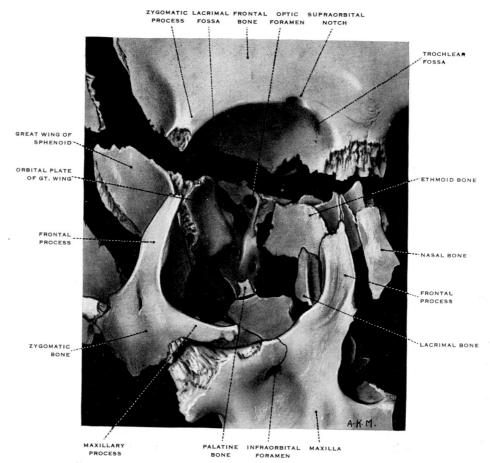

FIG. 4.—THE BONES OF THE RIGHT ORBIT IN SITU BUT SEPARATED.

Relations and Structure.—*Below* the floor of the orbit for nearly its whole extent is the maxillary sinus, a most important practical relation. *For as the bone between them is only 0·5–1 mm. thick, tumours of the antrum can easily invade the orbit, causing proptosis.* It is in fact thinnest at the inferior orbital groove and canal (see Fig. 14).

More posteriorly is the air-cell inside the orbital process of the palatine bone, and sometimes extensions from the ethmoidal air-cells may invade the floor.

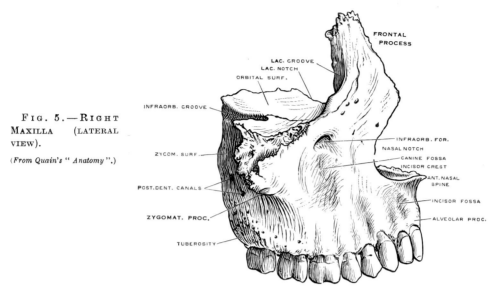

FRONTAL
PROCESS

LAC. GROOVE
LAC. NOTCH
ORBITAL SURF.

INFRAORB. GROOVE

INFRAORB. FOR.
NASAL NOTCH
ZYCOM. SURF.
CANINE FOSSA
INCISOR CREST
ANT. NASAL
SPINE

POST. DENT. CANALS

INCISOR FOSSA

ZYGOMAT. PROC.

ALVEOLAR PROC.

TUBEROSITY

Fig. 5.—Right
Maxilla (lateral
view).

(From Quain's " Anatomy ".)

The inferior rectus is in contact with the floor near the apex of the orbit, but anteriorly it is some distance away, being separated from it by the inferior oblique muscle and some fat. Lateral to the inferior rectus and lying on its lateral edge or between it and the lateral rectus is the nerve to the inferior oblique (Fig. 281).

The inferior oblique arises just lateral to the opening of the naso-lacrimal canal and passes backwards, laterally, and upwards for the most part near the floor (Fig. 275).

The infraorbital vessels and nerve lie in the infraorbital sulcus and canal.

The lateral wall of the orbit is triangular in shape, the base being anterior. It makes an angle of 45° with the median sagittal plane and faces medially, forwards and slightly upwards in its lower part. It is slightly convex posteriorly, flat at its centre, while anteriorly the orbital surface of the zygomatic bone 1 cm. behind the orbital margin is concave.

The lateral wall of the orbit is formed by two bones :

(*a*) Posteriorly by the orbital surface of the greater wing of the sphenoid.

(*b*) Anteriorly by the orbital surface of the zygomatic (malar) bone.

The sphenoidal portion is sharply separated from the roof and floor by the superior and inferior orbital fissures respectively.

The zygomatic portion passes imperceptibly into the floor, and is separated from the roof by the fronto-zygomatic suture, which is roughly horizontal and often marked by a slight ridge. The suture between the two portions of the lateral wall is vertical (Fig. 1).

The lateral wall presents :

(1) *The Spina recti lateralis.*—This is a small bony projection situated on the inferior margin of the superior orbital fissure at the junction of its wide and

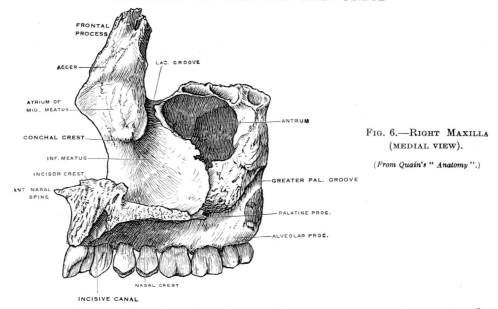

FIG. 6.—RIGHT MAXILLA (MEDIAL VIEW).

(*From Quain's " Anatomy ".*)

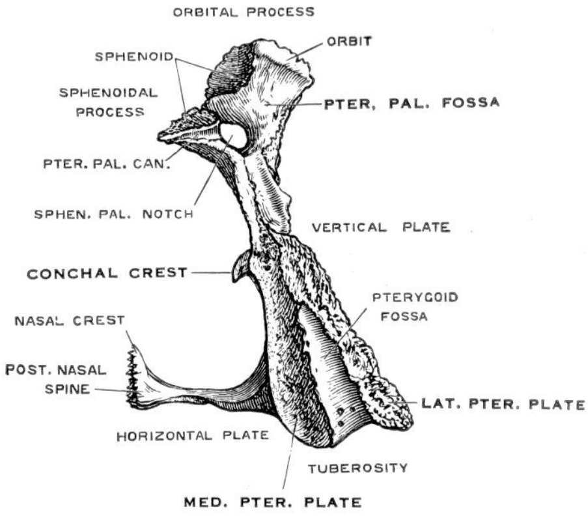

FIG. 7.—RIGHT PALATINE BONE (FROM BEHIND).

(*From Quain's " Anatomy ".*)

narrow portions. It may be pointed, rounded, or grooved, and gives origin to a part of the lateral rectus muscle, but it is produced mainly by a groove which lodges the superior ophthalmic vein. This groove is prolonged upwards, then runs anterior to the spine. Not infrequently the spine is duplicated.

(2) *The Zygomatic Groove and Foramen.*—The groove which lodges the nerve and vessels of the same name runs from the anterior end of the inferior orbital fissure to a foramen in the zygomatic bone. This leads into a canal which divides into two, one branch opening on the cheek, the other in the temporal fossa. Thus the branches of the zygomatic nerve reach their destination. If the nerve divides before entering its canal, there may be two or even three grooves and foramina in the orbit.

(3) *The Lateral Orbital Tubercle* (Whitnall).—This is a small elevation on the orbital surface of the zygomatic bone just within the lateral orbital margin and about 11 mm. below the fronto-zygomatic suture. It gives attachment to :

(*a*) The check ligament of the lateral rectus muscle.

(*b*) The suspensory ligament of the eyeball.

(*c*) The aponeurosis of the levator palpebræ superioris (Fig. 275).

(4) Not infrequently there is a foramen in or near the suture between the greater wing of the sphenoid with the frontal, near the lateral end of the superior orbital fissure. This leads from the orbit to the middle cranial fossa, and transmits a branch of the meningeal artery and a small vein (Testut).

Structure.—Being the one most exposed to injury, the lateral is the thickest of the orbital walls, and is especially strong at the orbital margin. Behind this is a relatively weaker part, then comes a thicker portion, and the most posterior portion, walling in the middle cranial fossa, is thinner again (Fig. 3). The most posterior is, in fact, the feeblest portion. Here on either side of the spheno-zygomatic suture it is only 1 mm. thick and its lamellar structure makes it translucent. In 30 per cent. of cases, according to Nippert, there exist in this area supplementary fissures which represent the extensive primitive communication between the orbit and the temporal fossa.

Relations.—The lateral wall separates the orbit *anteriorly* from the temporal fossa containing the temporal muscle ; posteriorly from the middle cranial fossa and the temporal lobe of the brain (Figs. 3 and 280).

Inside the orbit the lateral rectus muscle is in contact with this wall all the way. Above it are the lacrimal nerve and artery.

The spina recti lateralis and the *orbital tubercle* with their attachments have already been described, as has the zygomatic canal and its contents.

The lacrimal gland reaches down on to the lateral wall, and the *lacrimal nerve* receives a parasympathetic branch from the zygomatic (Fig. 281).

The following **fissures** and **canals** lie between the various orbital walls :

The superior orbital (sphenoidal) fissure.

The inferior orbital (spheno-maxillary) fissure.

The anterior and posterior ethmoidal canals.

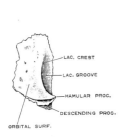

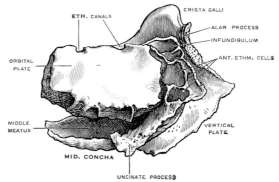

Fig. 8.—Right Lacrimal Bone (lateral view).

(*From Quain's " Anatomy ".*)

Fig. 9.—The Ethmoid Bone (from the right side).

(*From Quain's " Anatomy ".*)

The superior orbital (sphenoidal) **fissure** lies between the roof and lateral wall of the orbit. It is the gap between the lesser and greater wings of the sphenoid, and is closed laterally by the frontal bone.

It is wider at the medial end, where it lies below the optic foramen, and is often described as comma- or retort-shaped. Sometimes there is gradual reduction in size towards the lateral extremity, but usually it is composed of two limbs, a narrow *lateral* portion and a wider *medial* part. At the junction of the two limbs is the *Spina recti lateralis* (Fig. 1).

The superior orbital fissure is some 22 mm. long, and is the largest communication between the orbit and the middle cranial fossa. Its tip is 30 to 40 mm. from the fronto-zygomatic suture. Its medial end is separated from the optic foramen by the posterior root of the lesser wing of the sphenoid on which is found the infra-optic tubercle. This lies below and lateral to the optic foramen on the middle of the vertical part of the medial border of the wide part of the superior orbital fissure (Fig. 1).

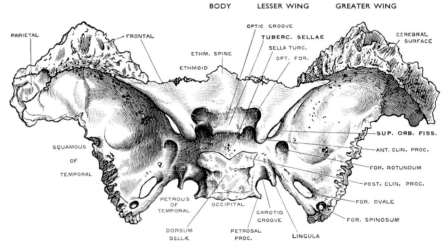

FIG. 10.—THE SPHENOID BONE (FROM ABOVE).
(*From Quain's " Anatomy ".*)

The common tendinous ring (*anulus tendineus communis*) spans the superior orbital fissure between the wide medial and narrow lateral parts. The lateral rectus arises here, from both margins of the fissure.

One or more fronto-sphenoidal foramina may be present in the fronto-sphenoidal suture and transmit an anastomosis between the middle meningeal and the lacrimal arteries.

According to Hovelacque *the lateral limb is closed by dura mater and nothing passes through it*. This is not the usual teaching, but it is borne out by my own (Eugene Wolff) dissections (see Figs. 259 and 260). Passing above the anulus are the fourth, frontal, and lacrimal nerves, the superior ophthalmic vein, and the recurrent lacrimal artery.

Passing within the anulus or between the two heads of the lateral rectus are the superior division of the 3rd nerve, the naso-ciliary and sympathetic root of the ciliary ganglion, the inferior division of the 3rd, then the 6th (and then some-times the ophthalmic vein or veins)—in that order from above downwards.   The 6th nerve is actually passing from below the inferior division of the 3rd to lie lateral and between the two divisions (Fig. 261).

As a rule nothing passes below the anulus, rarely the inferior ophthalmic vein.

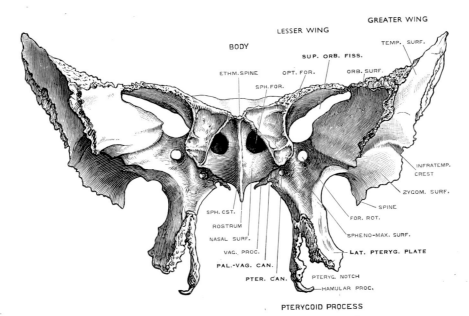

FIG. 11.—THE SPHENOID BONE (FROM IN FRONT).
(From Quain's " Anatomy ".)

The inferior orbital (spheno-maxillary) fissure lies between the lateral wall and floor of the orbit.   Through it the orbit communicates with the pterygo-palatine and infratemporal fossæ.   It commences below and lateral to the optic foramen, close to the medial end of the superior orbital fissure.   It runs forwards and laterally for some 20 mm., its anterior extremity reaching to about 2 cm. from the inferior orbital margin (Figs. 1 and 3).

The inferior orbital fissure is bounded anteriorly by the maxilla and the orbital process of the palatine bone ; posteriorly by the whole of the lower margin of the orbital surface of the greater wing of the sphenoid.

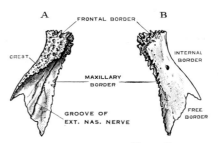

FIG. 12.—THE RIGHT NASAL BONE
(A, MEDIAL VIEW ; B, LATERAL VIEW).
(From Quain's " Anatomy ".)

In the majority of cases it is closed anteriorly by the zygomatic (malar) bone.

The fissure is narrower at its centre than at its two extremities, the anterior end sometimes being markedly expanded.

The width of the inferior orbital fissure depends on the development of the maxillary sinus and thus is relatively wide in the fœtus and infant.

The lateral border is sharp and may have grooves above and below it ; it is higher than the medial border anteriorly, but lower posteriorly. It is closed in the living by periorbita and the muscle of Müller.

The inferior orbital fissure is near the openings of the foramen rotundum and the spheno-palatine foramen (Figs. 1 and 2).

The inferior orbital fissure transmits the infraorbital nerve, the zygomatic nerve, branches to the orbital periosteum from the pterygo-palatine ganglion, and a communication between the inferior ophthalmic vein and the pterygoid plexus (Fig. 280).

The ethmoidal foramina lie between the roof and medial wall of the orbit either in the fronto-ethmoidal suture *or actually in the frontal bone*. They are the openings of canals which are formed in greater part by the frontal but are completed by the ethmoid (Figs. 1, 2, 9 and 19).

The anterior ethmoidal canal looks backwards as well as laterally. Its posterior border is ill-defined and continuous with a groove on the orbital plate of the ethmoid. It opens in the anterior cranial fossa at the side of the cribriform plate of the ethmoid, and transmits the anterior ethmoidal nerve and artery.

The posterior ethmoidal canal transmits the posterior ethmoidal nerve and artery. Supplementary foramina are common.

The optic foramen, or rather the **optic canal,** leads from the middle cranial fossa to the apex of the orbit, and it is formed by the two roots of the lesser wing of the sphenoid. It is directed forwards, laterally, and somewhat downwards, its axis making an angle of about 36° with the median sagittal plane. If produced forwards, the axis passes approximately through the middle of the infero-lateral quadrant of the orbital opening. Hence it is neither in the axis of the orbit nor of its lateral wall (Winckler). If produced backwards it would meet its fellow at the dorsum sellæ of the sphenoid. The canal is funnel-shaped, the mouth of the funnel being the anterior opening. This is oval in shape, with the greatest diameter vertical. The cranial opening, on the other hand, is flattened from above down, while in its middle portion the canal is circular on section. With regard to the intracranial opening, the upper and lower borders are sharp, the medial and lateral rounded. The inter-optic groove is thus continuous with the medial wall without line of demarcation (Fig. 10).

The lateral border of the orbital opening is more or less well defined. It is formed by the anterior border of the posterior root of the lesser wing of the sphenoid. The medial border is less well defined.

The distance between the intracranial openings of the two canals is 25 mm. The distance between the orbital openings is 30 mm.

The roof of the canal reaches farther forwards than the floor, while posteriorly the floor projects beyond the roof. This gap in the roof is filled in by a fold of dura mater with a free posterior edge (the falciform fold) (Fig. 272).

The optic canal is close to the sphenoidal air sinus, sometimes to a posterior ethmoidal air-cell. According to Fazakas, the longer the optic canal, the thinner its medial wall and the more likely it is to encroach on a posterior ethmoidal air-cell. Often only a very thin plate of bone separates the optic canal from these. At times the canal makes a ridge inside the sinus. Not infrequently the sinus or a posterior ethmoidal air-cell may invade the lesser wing to a greater or smaller

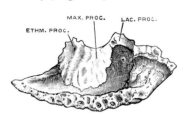

Fig. 13.—The Right Inferior Concha (lateral view).
(From Quain's " Anatomy".)

degree, and they have been known to surround the canal completely.

Above the canal is the posterior part of the gyrus rectus and olfactory tract.

The optic canal is separated from the medial end of the superior orbital fissure by a bar of bone, on which there is a tubercle or roughness for the anulus tendineus (Fig. 1).

The optic canal transmits the optic nerve and its coverings of dura, arachnoid, and pia (Figs. 291, 292) (see p. 323) ; the ophthalmic artery which lies here below then lateral to the nerve and embedded in its dural sheath (Figs. 292, 293) ; and a few twigs from the sympathetic which accompany the artery. Separating artery and nerve is a layer of fibrous tissue which may (rarely) be ossified.

The measurements of the optic canal are as follows (Winckler) :

The orbital opening is 6 to 6·5 mm. by 4·5 to 5 mm.

The cranial opening is 5 to 6 mm. by 4 to 5 mm.

In the middle portion it is 5 by 5 mm.

The canal is further narrowed by the periosteum.

The lateral wall is 5 to 7 mm. long, which is the width of the posterior root of the lesser wing of the sphenoid.

The roof, 10 to 12 mm. in length, varies with the development of the lesser wing of the sphenoid between the anterior clinoid process and the body of the sphenoid.

The upper and medial walls are longer than the others. The longer the optic canal, the narrower it is, and vice versa (Fazakas).

A thorough investigation of the optic canal shows that variations in contour, as seen radiologically, are produced by the development of the lower root of the lesser wing of the sphenoid (E. Leon Kier, *Invest. Radiol.* **I,** 5, pp. 346–362, Sept. 1966).

The orbital margin has the form of a quadrilateral with rounded corners. The orbital margin usually has the form of a spiral ; the inferior orbital margin

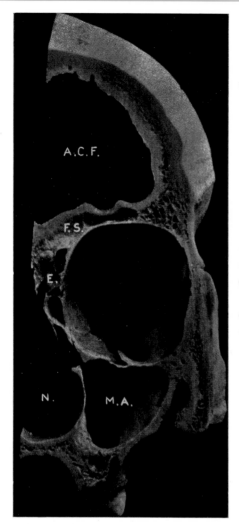

FIG. 14.—FRONTAL SECTION OF THE LEFT
HALF OF SKULL JUST BEHIND ORBITAL
MARGIN AND PASSING THROUGH LARGEST
PART OF CAVITY (GREATEST ORBITAL HEIGHT
= 37·5 MM.); SEEN FROM IN FRONT.
NATURAL SIZE.

The floor of the orbit is deeply grooved
by the infra-orbital sulcus.

A.C.F. = Anterior cranial fossa.
F.S.　= Frontal sinus.
E.　　= Ethmoidal air cells.
N.　　= Nasal cavity.
M.A.　= Maxillary sinus (showing
　　　　the ostium maxillare).
(From Whitnall, 1932.)

is continuous with the anterior lacrimal
crest, while the superior is continued down
into the posterior lacrimal crest. The
lacrimal fossa thus lies in the orbital margin (Poirier).

Each side measures some 40 mm., but
usually the width is greater than the
height ; the relation between the two is
given by the *orbital index*,[1] which varies
in the different races of mankind. The
opening is directed forwards and slightly
laterally, and is tilted so that the upper
and lower margins slope gently downwards from the medial to the lateral side.

The orbital margin is made up of
three bones, the frontal, zygomatic, and
maxilla.

The superior orbital margin is formed
entirely of the frontal bone, i.e. by its
orbital arch.

It is generally concave downwards,
convex forwards, sharp in its lateral two-
thirds, and rounded in the medial third.
At the junction of the two portions, some
25 mm. from the mid-line and situated
at the highest part of the arch, is the
supraorbital notch, whose lateral border is
usually sharper than the medial. Not infrequently it is converted into a foramen

---

[1] The orbital index (of Broca)—

$$= \frac{\text{Height of Orbit} \times 100}{\text{Width of Orbit}}$$

Taking the orbital index as the standard, three
classes of orbit are recognised :

1. *Megaseme (large)*.—The orbital index is 89 or
over. This type is characteristic of the yellow races,
except the Esquimaux. The orbital opening is
round.

2. *Mesoseme (intermediate)*.—Orbital index between 89 and 83. This type is found in the white
races (European 87, English 88·4, according to
Flower).

3. *Microseme (small)*.—Orbital index 83 or less.
This type is characteristic of the black races. The
orbital opening is rectangular.

by the ossification of the ligament which closes it below.   The posterior opening then is 3 to 6 mm. from the orbital margin.   It transmits the supraorbital nerve and vessels.   Notch and foramen are easily palpable in the living.

Sometimes medial to this a second notch (of Arnold) or foramen is found. This transmits the medial branches of the supraorbital nerves and vessels where these have divided inside the orbit.

Supraorbital grooves leading from these notches or foramina are sometimes seen.

A groove may also be present some 10 mm. medial to the supraorbital notch for the supratrochlear nerve and artery.

A supraciliary canal (Ward) is found in about half the cases (Fig. 1).   It is a small opening near the supraorbital notch, and transmits a nutrient artery and a branch of the supraorbital nerve to the frontal air sinus.

The lateral orbital margin, being the most exposed to injury, is the strongest portion of the orbital outlet.   It is formed by the zygomatic process of the frontal and by the zygomatic bone.   If looked at from the side it appears to be concave forwards and not to reach as far forward as the medial margin.

In the spheno-zygomatic suture there are not infrequently ossicles resembling the Wormian bones of the cranium.

Another suture occurs in 21·1 per cent. of Japanese skulls, in which the zygomatic bone may be in two parts (*Os Japonicum*).

The inferior orbital margin is raised slightly above the floor of the orbit.   It is formed by the zygomatic bone and the maxilla, usually in equal portions.

The zygomatic portion forms a long thin spur (the maxillary or marginal process) which lies on the maxilla (Figs. 1 and 4).

The suture between the two, which is not infrequently marked by a tubercle, can be felt lying usually about half-way along the margin just above the infraorbital foramen (Fig. 1).

Sometimes, however, the zygomatic (malar) may reach the anterior lacrimal crest, thus excluding the maxilla, or may take only a very small part itself in the formation of this margin.

The medial margin is formed by the anterior lacrimal crest on the frontal process of the maxilla and the posterior lacrimal crest on the lacrimal bone.   These crests overlap ; the medial margin is thus not a continuous ridge, but runs up from the anterior lacrimal crest across the frontal process of the maxilla to the superior margin (Fig. 1).

AGE AND SEX CHANGES

The changes in the orbit during the period of growth depend partly on the development of the cranium and skeleton of the face, between which the orbit is placed, and also on the growth of the neighbouring air sinuses.

A.E.—2

The orbital margin is sharp and well ossified at birth. As Fisher points out : " The eyeball is therefore well protected from stress and injury during parturition. When we recollect the relatively large size and the advanced stage of development of the eye at birth, it is clearly specially desirable that such protection should be afforded ; that it is efficacious, the rarity of birth injuries of the globe in cases of unassisted labour can testify."

The orbital margin is sharp at birth ; at seven years, except at its upper part, it is less sharp, and as the supero-medial and infero-lateral angles are better marked than the others the orbital opening tends to be triangular.

The form of the orbit on coronal section behind the orbital margin is that of a quadrilateral with rounded corners. In the newborn it has the form of an ellipse higher on the lateral than on the medial side.

The infantile orbits look much more laterally than the adult, i.e. their axes, or the lines drawn from the middle of the orbital opening to the optic foramen, make an angle of 115°, and, if produced backwards, meet in the middle at the nasal septum. In the adult the axes make an angle of 40°–45° with each other, and, if produced backwards, meet at the upper part of the clivus of the sphenoid. These axes, too, lie in the horizontal plane in the infant, whereas in the adult they slope downwards from 15° to 20°.

The orbital fissures are relatively large in the child owing to the narrowness of the orbital surface of the greater wing of the sphenoid, and the wide and narrow portions are not well differentiated.

The orbital index is high in the child, the vertical diameter of the orbital opening being practically the same as the horizontal, but later the transverse increases more than the vertical (see table below). The size of the orbits is relatively great ; thus they do not grow much after seven years.

The interorbital distance is small. This is of some practical importance. *Children are not infrequently brought to the ophthalmic surgeon because they are thought to squint when the strabismus is apparent only. This appearance is due to the narrow interorbital distance, which makes the eyes look too close together. With the growth of the frontal and ethmoidal air-cells the interorbital distance increases, and so causes the " squint " to disappear.*

The infraorbital foramen is usually present at birth ; but at times it may be represented by the terminal notch of an infraorbital groove whose roof has not grown over to convert it into a canal and which thus reaches to the orbital margin.

The orbital process of the zygomatic (malar) bone may almost reach the lacrimal fossa, and this condition may persist to ten years.

The roof of the orbit is relatively much larger than the floor at birth compared with the adult proportions. The foetal skull has a large cranium (orbital roof) and a small face (orbital floor). The fossa for the lacrimal gland is shallow, but the accessory fossa (p. 2) is well marked.

The optic canal has no length at birth, *so that it is actually a foramen* ; at one year it measures 4 mm. The axis also changes with age ; essentially while facing forwards and laterally it looks much more downwards at birth than in the adult.

The periosteum or periorbita is much thicker and stronger at birth than in the adult.

The following table gives a résumé of the changes in the orbital opening (Winckler).

	Form	Height	Width	Index
Fœtus (8 months) . .	Oval	14 mm.	18 mm.	77·7
New-born (6 months) .	Rounded	27 mm.	27 mm.	100
Child (7 years) . .	Quadrilat.	28 mm.	33 mm.	84·8
Adult	Quadrilat.	35 mm.	39 mm.	89·7

Senile Changes.—Here the changes are those due to absorption of the bony walls. Thus in the skulls of old people holes are sometimes found in the *roof* of the orbit. In such cases the periorbita is in direct contact with the dura mater.

The medial wall, although normally very thin, rarely shows senile holes in its ethmoidal portion. Parts of the lacrimal bone are, however, commonly absorbed.

The lateral wall not uncommonly shows holes or such marked thinning that it becomes very fragile in these places.

As regards the *floor*, senile changes very rarely produce holes apart from those in the roof or floor of the infraorbital canal.

In old people, too, the orbital fissures, especially the inferior, become wider owing to absorption of their margins.

In longheaded (dolichocephalic) skulls the orbits tend to look more laterally than in the shortheaded (brachycephalic) (Mannhardt, *Archiv für Ophth.*, 1871, Bd. 17, Abt. 11).

Mensuration.—There is a great difference between the measurements given by different authorities. The following is a useful average :

Depth of orbit . . . ·. .	40 mm.
Height of orbital opening	35 mm.
Width of orbital opening	40 mm.
Interorbital distance	25 mm.
Volume	30 c.c.

Volume of orbit : Vol. of eye = 4·5 : 1 (Ovio)

Sex Differences.—Up to puberty there is little difference between the orbits and, in fact, the skulls of male and female.

After this the male skull takes on its secondary sexual characters, seen especially in the formation of the lower jaw and in the forehead region.

The female remains more infantile in form. The orbits tend to be rounder and the upper margin sharper than in the male. The glabella and superciliary ridges are less marked or almost absent.   The forehead is more vertical and the frontal eminences more marked.   The contours of the region are rounder and the bones smoother.   The zygomatic process of the frontal bone is more slender and pointed.

The female orbit is more elongated and relatively larger than the male (Merkel).

THE PERIORBITA (Figs. 15, 16, 276)

The periorbita or orbital periosteum lines the bones of the orbit.   Generally it adheres but loosely to the bones which it covers, so that for the most part it may be lifted from them by blood or pus or during the course of certain operations.

At various points, however, it is firmly fixed :

(1) At the orbital margin, where it is thickened to form the arcus marginale and becomes continuous with the periosteum covering the bones of the face.

(2) At the sutures.

(3) At the various fissures and foramina ; and

(4) At the lacrimal fossa.

Through the superior orbital fissure, the optic foramen, and anterior ethmoidal canal (Fig. 276) it becomes continuous with the endosteal layer of the dura mater.

In the superior orbital fissure it becomes a dense membrane, which just allows sufficient room for the various structures to pass through.

In the optic foramen the fibrous (dura mater) sheath of the optic nerve is closely adherent to the periosteum of the canal (see p. 323).

At the optic foramen, also, the periorbita splits, a portion becoming continuous with the dural covering of the optic nerve ; here also it gives origin to the muscles and sends processes which are continuous with the muscle sheaths. Fine lamellar processes also pass from the periorbita, which divide the fat into lobules and form coverings for the vessels and nerves.

Through the inferior orbital fissure it is continuous with the periosteum covering the bones of the infratemporal and pterygo-palatine fossæ, through the temporal canal with that of the temporal fossa and via the zygomatic canal with that on the front of the zygomatic bone.

It is adherent to the posterior lacrimal crest, and here gives off a layer to enclose the lacrimal fossa, being separated from the sac by some loose areolar tissue, and then passes down the duct to become continuous with the periosteum of the inferior meatus.

These facts can be made out and should be remembered in doing an exenteration of the orbit.   Having divided the periosteum at the orbital margin, one finds little difficulty in removing the periosteal cone except at the above places, where bands of varying strength have to be divided.

The periorbita consists of two layers.   In the outer, next the bone, oblique fibres are well seen.   These cannot be made out in the inner, which is much weaker than the outer.   It is this inner layer which gives a covering to the

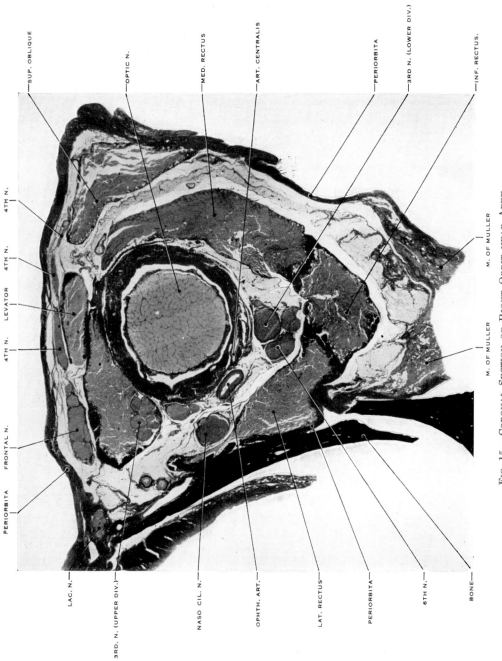

SUP. OBLIQUE

OPTIC N.

MED. RECTUS

ART. CENTRALIS

PERIORBITA

3RD N. (LOWER DIV.)

INF. RECTUS.

4TH N.

4TH N.

LEVATOR

4TH N.

4TH N.

FRONTAL N.

PERIORBITA

M. OF MULLER

M. OF MULLER

LAC. N.

3RD. N. (UPPER DIV.)

NASO CIL. N.

OPHTH. ART.

LAT. RECTUS

PERIORBITA

6TH N.

BONE

Fig. 15.—Coronal Section of Right Orbit near Apex.

21

frontal and lacrimal nerves and forms the space in which the lacrimal gland is lodged.

The periorbita is liable to become ossified, especially where it roofs over the infraorbital canal and where it is attached to the posterior lacrimal crest.

Orbital periosteum, like that elsewhere, is sensitive. It is supplied by those 5th nerve branches which lie in contact with it—frontal, lacrimal, zygomatic, infraorbital and ethmoidal.

The Muscle of Müller (*Musculus orbitalis*).—In the region of the inferior orbital (spheno-maxillary) fissure some plain muscle fibres are found with the periorbita, which give the latter in this region a rosy tint. This is the muscle of Müller. It is more extensive than one would imagine. It not only spans the inferior orbital fissure but extends backwards, deep to the anulus tendineus, to the front of the cavernous sinus, while anteriorly it gradually gets lost in the periorbita. It has a width of 12 mm. Its action in the human is very doubtful. In certain mammals, where there is no long lateral wall to separate the orbit from the temporal fossa, the muscle of Müller is large and takes the place of this wall (see also pp. 196, 267, 500).

Relations.—Above is orbital fat in which are the inferior ophthalmic vein and its tributaries. The inferior surface lies on the fatty tissue of the pterygo-palatine fossa in which are found the infraorbital nerve, the pterygo-palatine ganglion with the arteries and veins surrounding it. Through the muscle pass anastomotic branches between the ophthalmic and veins of the pterygoid plexus.

Nerve supply.—Branch from the pterygo-palatine ganglion (sympathetic) (Fig. 17).

Function.—The muscle was held by some to be the cause of the proptosis in exophthalmic goitre, either directly, or indirectly through pressure on the veins which pass through it. But while the muscle acts as a protruder in some of the lower animals, it does not act in this way in man, in whom it is vestigial. The free venous anastomosis, moreover, negatives any effect which a compression of the veins might have had. True proptosis in exophthalmic goitre is due to increased volume of the infraorbital fibro-fatty tissue produced by a myxomatous type of œdema. Apparent exophthalmos is a widening of the palpebral fissure due to overaction of the smooth muscle component of levator palpebræ superioris.

Certain Points of Importance in the Neighbourhood of the Orbital Margin

The Superciliary Ridges are elevations above the orbital margins which meet in the mid-line in the *glabella* which forms the prominence above the nose. The prominence of the ridges and of the glabella has nothing to do with the size of the frontal sinuses. They are larger in the male than in the female and absent in the infant.

The Frontal Eminences are rounded elevations on the vertical plate of the

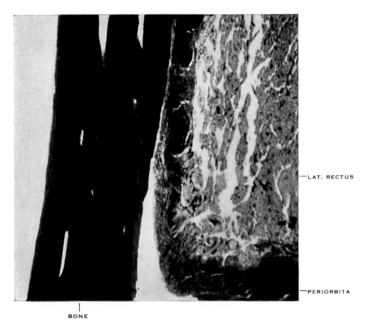

—LAT. RECTUS

—PERIORBITA

BONE

FIG. 16.—DETAIL OF FIGURE 15.

Note how loosely attached periorbita is to the bone.

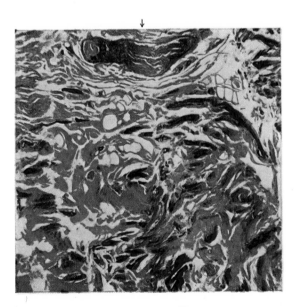

↓

FIG. 17.—DETAIL OF FIGURE 15.

To show fibres of muscles of Müller.   Arrow points to nerve of supply.

frontal bone some 2 in. above the orbit ; they are more prominent in the female and even more so in the infant.

The Infraorbital Foramen lies 4–5 mm. below the tubercle on the lower orbital margin which marks the suture between the zygomatic bone and the maxilla. It is usually oval, and looks downwards as well as forwards. Its upper margin is sharp and crescentic, while the lower border is ill-defined. The foramen may be double—indeed, up to five have been described.

The supraorbital notch, the infraorbital foramen, and the mental foramen are on the same vertical line, which passes between the two bicuspid teeth.

The Temporal Crest runs from the zygomatic process of the frontal bone upwards and backwards to become continuous with the temporal lines on the parietal bones.

The Sutura Notha (Fig. 1) is a groove on the frontal process of the maxilla, and runs parallel with the anterior lacrimal crest. It lodges a branch of the infraorbital artery.

Surface Anatomy

The Upper Orbital Margin forms a well-marked prominence, more so in the lateral sharp portion than in the medial more rounded part. Its form can be made out easily by touch.

It should be noted carefully that the eyebrow corresponds in position only in part to the upper orbital margin.

The head of the eyebrow lies for the most part *under* the medial part of the margin, to palpate which the finger must press *upwards*.

The body lies *along* the margin, while the tail runs well above the lateral part of the margin, which can be felt and usually seen below it.

The zygomatic process of the frontal bone often forms a marked prominence under the skin.

The Supraorbital Notch can be felt at the junction of the lateral two-thirds with the medial third, and not infrequently the supraorbital nerve can be rolled under the finger.

The Lateral Orbital Margin is only visible down to the level of the lateral canthus, but can easily be felt in its whole extent.

The Lower Orbital Margin, as opposed to the upper, forms no prominence, since the skin of the lower lid passes without sudden change of plane into that of the cheek. Just beyond it, especially in the old, lie the naso-jugal and malar furrows.

It is easily palpable as a sharp ridge beyond which the finger can pass into the orbit. On the lower and lateral side the little finger can pass between the eye and the orbital margin for about ½ in. (1·25 cm.).

The Lacrimal Tubercle can be felt in the sharp anterior lacrimal crest, as can the **tubercle** at the middle of the lower margin which marks the suture between the zygomatic bone and maxilla.

The pulley of the superior oblique is easily felt with the tip of the thumb, just within the supero-medial angle of the orbital margin.

The Lateral Orbital Tubercle (Whitnall's) can be felt just within the lateral orbital margin at its middle by passing the finger into the orbit and rubbing it up and down against the margin.

The Infraorbital Foramen, or rather its sharp crescentic upper margin, can,

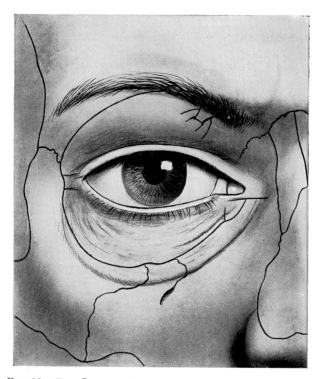

FIG. 18.—THE SURFACE ANATOMY OF THE ORBITAL OPENING.

not infrequently, be made out 4–5 mm. below the tubercle on the lower orbital margin which marks the zygomatico-maxillary suture.

The Zygomatic (Malar) Tubercle can be felt below and behind the zygomatic process of the frontal bone, and between the two is a V-shaped interval, at the bottom of which is the fronto-zygomatic suture.

The Anterior Lacrimal Crest is easily defined. Behind it the finger passes into the lacrimal fossa, and behind this again the posterior lacrimal crest can be felt.

It should be noted carefully that the finger in the lacrimal fossa lies below the medial angle of the eye and not under the ridge made by the medial palpebral ligament.

The Temporal Crest can be felt arching backwards from the zygomatic process of the frontal bone.

The Nasal Bone, sitting on the frontal process of the maxilla, can be seen and palpated down to its lower end, where it joins the mobile cartilage of the nose.

THE PARANASAL SINUSES

The Maxillary Sinus.—The maxillary sinus (antrum of Highmore) is a pyramidal cavity situated in the maxilla (Figs. 2, 19).

Its base forms part of the lateral wall of the nose ; its apex lies under the zygomatic bone. In the disarticulated skull the base presents a large opening, which is, however, partly closed in the articulated skull by the uncinate process of the ethmoid above, the inferior concha below, the palatine behind, and the

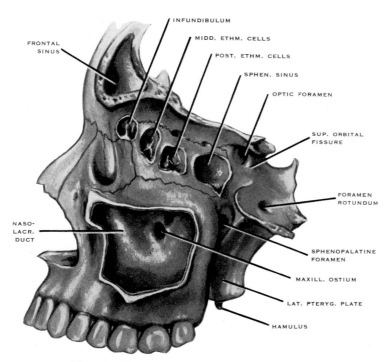

FIG. 19.—THE ACCESSORY SINUSES OF THE NOSE.

lacrimal in front (Fig. 2). The mucous membrane covers this in still further, so that finally there is only one small opening (sometimes two) situated near the roof of the antrum, and therefore bad for gravitational drainage if the antrum contains excess fluid. The ostium opens into the middle meatus of the nose in the hiatus semilunaris (Fig. 20). The naso-lacrimal duct forms a ridge in the anterior part of this wall (Fig. 19).

The antero-lateral wall looks on to the face, and may be reached by everting the upper lip. In it are the canals containing the anterior and middle superior alveolar (dental) nerves (Fig. 286).

The posterior wall faces the infratemporal fossa, of which it forms the anterior wall. In it are the canals for the posterior superior alveolar (dental) nerves.

The roof of the antrum is formed by the orbital plate of the maxilla, which constitutes the floor of the orbit. In it is the infraorbital canal containing the infraorbital nerve and vessels. The canal raises a ridge in the front part of the roof.

The floor is formed by the alveolar process, and is about $\frac{1}{2}$ in. (1·25 cm.) below the nose. The sinus lies above the posterior five teeth (i.e. the two premolars and the three molars). The roots of these teeth occasionally produce elevations on the floor of the sinus. With advancing years the floor descends by resorption of alveolar bone ; sometimes as a result of this the roots, especially of the first molar, may actually project into the sinus, covered only by mucous membrane.

The Frontal Sinuses.—The frontal sinuses are cavities of variable extent situated anteriorly between the two plates of the frontal bone (Figs. 2, 276, 278). They are separated by a septum, which is often deviated to one or other side. In the peripheral parts of the sinus there are also small partitions forming loculi. In some cases a frontal sinus may extend laterally to the zygomatic process ; in others, especially if the septum is much to one side, it may be reduced to a mere slit.

On an average (Logan Turner) the height is $1\frac{1}{4}$ in. (3 cm.), the breadth 1 in. (2·5 cm.), and depth $\frac{3}{4}$ in. (2 cm.).

The posterior wall of the sinus is thin, contains few diploë, and separates it from the meninges and frontal convolutions.

The anterior wall looks on to the forehead. It contains diploë, hence osteomyelitis spreads more readily in this than in the posterior wall.

The floor of the frontal sinus separates it from the orbit and nose.

Behind and below the ethmoidal air-cells are only separated from the sinus by a thin plate of bone. Not infrequently a *fronto-ethmoidal air-cell* forms a prominence in the floor of the sinus (Fig. 2).

The frontal sinus opens into the nose by the infundibulum. This narrow canal passes between the anterior ethmoidal air-cells and opens into the hiatus semilunaris in the middle meatus, in front of the openings of the anterior ethmoidal air-cells and the maxillary sinus (Fig. 20).

Hence infection in one sinus can and does easily spread to the others.

The Ethmoidal Air-cells.—The ethmoidal air-cells are situated for the most part in the lateral mass of the ethmoid, but are completed by the frontal, palatine, sphenoid, maxilla, and lacrimal.

Above them are the meninges and frontal convolutions in the anterior cranial fossa.

In front is the infundibulum of the frontal sinus, behind is the sphenoidal sinus.

Below is the nose, laterally the orbit and lacrimal fossa. (See Figs. 3 and 276.)

The air-cells are separated from these structures by very thin plates of bone, which are not good barriers to the spread of infection. Thus the orbital plate is not much thicker than paper : hence the reason why ethmoiditis is the commonest cause of orbital cellulitis.

The ethmoidal air-cells are divided by irregular septa into anterior, middle, and posterior (Fig. 19).

The anterior and middle open into the middle meatus of the nose ; the anterior in the hiatus semilunaris, the middle on the bulla ethmoidalis (Fig. 20).

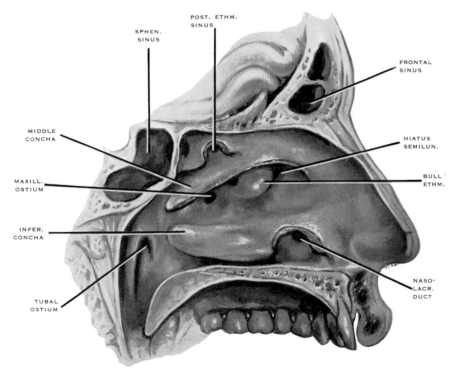

POST. ETHM. SINUS

SPHEN. SINUS

FRONTAL SINUS

MIDDLE CONCHA

HIATUS SEMILUN.

MAXILL. OSTIUM

BULL ETHM.

INFER. CONCHA

NASO- LACR. DUCT

TUBAL OSTIUM

Fig. 20.—The Lateral Wall of the Nose to show the Openings of the Accessory Sinuses and Naso-lacrimal Duct.

The posterior lie antero-medial to the optic canal and open into the superior meatus.

The Sphenoidal Air Sinus.—The sphenoidal sinus lies in the body of the sphenoid bone (Figs. 20, 315, 366).

There is a vertical median septum often deviated to one or other side of the mid-line. A variable amount of a transverse septum is also usually present, and runs most often from above downwards and forwards. It is known as the " carotid buttress " (Cushing), because it is used as a landmark for protecting the internal carotid artery when approaching the pituitary body by the nasal route. According to Cope it can be seen in a fourth of the X-rays of the region. The sphenoidal sinus lies in front of the pituitary fossa. The sinus gradually enlarges by resorption of bone. As age advances the sinus extends below the pituitary fossa and into the root of the lesser wing. It may excavate the basi-sphenoid and basi-occiput till close to the anterior margin of the foramen magnum.

Above the sphenoidal sinus are the pituitary body and the optic nerve, which often makes a ridge inside the sinus. It is this close relation which causes the optic nerve to be involved at times in sinusitis, giving rise to a sudden loss of vision (retro-bulbar neuritis) (Fig. 292).

Below is the nose, and in the floor of the sinus is the pterygoid canal which may make a ridge in the sinus.

In front are the ethmoidal air-cells, the posterior of which often bulges into the sinus.

Laterally are the cavernous sinuses, containing the internal carotid artery and the 6th nerve. In front of this the body of the sphenoid bone forms the medial wall of the orbit.

The sphenoidal sinus opens into the highest meatus, or spheno-ethmoidal recess.

When the sphenoidal sinus is very large it may send a prolongation between the foramen rotundum and the foramen ovale. Such an extension of the sinus may explain certain cases of involvement of the nerves in sinus disease.

Nerve Supply

The *maxillary sinus* is supplied by multiple branches of the maxillary nerve. The infra-orbital nerve supplies the roof by perforating branches. The superior alveolar nerves on their way to the teeth supply the posterior, lateral and anterior walls. The anterior superior alveolar nerve supplies the nasal wall alongside the naso-lacrimal duct, and behind this the anterior (greater) palatine nerve supplies the nasal wall and ostium.

The *frontal sinus* is supplied by the supra-orbital nerve. The *anterior* and *middle ethmoidal air cells* are supplied by the anterior ethmoidal nerve, while the *posterior ethmoidal air cells* and the *sphenoidal sinus* are supplied by the posterior ethmoidal nerve.

Lymph Drainage

The sphenoidal sinus and posterior ethmoidal air cells drain back to retro-pharyngeal lymph glands. The remainder (i.e. middle and anterior ethmoidal air cells, frontal and maxillary sinuses) drain to the submandibular lymph glands.

DEVELOPMENT

The accessory sinuses of the nose all arise as out-buddings from the nasal mucosa.

The bud which is to form the frontal sinus passes up from the ethmoid bone, and at one year is just present in the frontal bone.   The stalk remains as the infundibulum.   At 7 years it is about the size of a pea.   Then it starts growing rapidly, but does not reach its full size till about 25 years.

Similarly, the ethmoidal air-cells are just present at birth as small depressions, and grow rapidly after 7 years.

At 2 years the sphenoid bone is still spongy, the sphenoidal sinus being represented by a slight depression at its future opening.   It really only starts growing at 8 years.

The maxillary sinus is a groove in the lateral nasal wall at birth.   At 1 year it has just reached the infraorbital canal.   It grows rapidly with the second dentition, so that at 12 years it is nearly like the adult, whose form, however, it does not acquire till 18 years.

BIBLIOGRAPHY

Cope, V. Z. (1916–17): *Brit. J. Surg.*, **4**, 107.

Eisler, P. (1930), *in* : Kurzes Handbuch der Ophthalmologie, *Berlin*, **1**, 1.

Fazakas, S. (1933): *Zbl. ges. Ophthal.*, **28**, 494.

Fisher, J. H. (1904): Ophthalmological Anatomy, *London*.

Hoeve, J. Van Der (1922) : *Ann. Otol., etc., St. Louis*, **31**, 297.

Nippert, O. (1931): *Z. Morph. Anthr.*, **29**, 1–82.

Onodi, A. (1903) : *Arch. Laryng., Rhin.*, **14**, 360.

—— (1907) : Der Sehnerv und die Nebenhöhlen der Nase, *Wien*.

—— (1913) : The Relations of the Lachrymal Organs to the Nose and Nasal Accessory Sinuses (English trans. by D. Mackenzie), *London*.

Turner, A. L. (1901) : The Accessory Sinuses of the Nose, *Edinburgh*.

—— (1908): *Lancet*, **2**, 396 ; (1908), *Brit. med. J.*, **2**, 730.

Ward, F. O. (1858) : Outlines of Human Osteology, 2nd edition, *London*.

Welcker, H. (1887) : *Arch. Anthrop., Braunschw.*, **17**, 1.

Whitnall, S. E. (1911): *J. Anat. Physiol.*, **46**, 36.

—— (1932) : Anatomy of the Human Orbit, second edition, *Oxford*. A very detailed study and the most comprehensive in the English language.

CHAPTER II

THE EYEBALL

The eye is a cyst which is kept distended by the pressure inside it : it is, as it were, moulded on the fluid which it contains.

It is in this way and by the use of glass-like membranes kept taut by the internal pressure that the regularity of its transparent surfaces has been brought about and an accurate optical instrument made from soft tissues (Rochon-Duvigneaud).

ALTHOUGH we speak of the globe of the eye, it is not a true sphere, but consists of the segments of two somewhat modified spheres placed one in front of the other. The anterior of these two segments is the smaller, more curved than the posterior, and called the cornea.

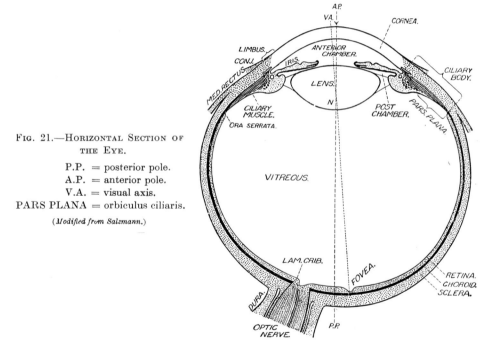

FIG. 21.—HORIZONTAL SECTION OF
THE EYE.

P.P. = posterior pole.
A.P. = anterior pole.
V.A. = visual axis.
PARS PLANA = orbiculus ciliaris.

(*Modified from Salzmann.*)

It is for this reason that the antero-posterior diameter of the globe is greatest (24 mm.). Also the eyeball is slightly flattened from above down, hence the vertical diameter (23 mm.) is slightly less than the horizontal (23·5 mm.).

So constituted, the eyeball is placed in the anterior part of the orbit, nearer the roof than the floor, and slightly closer to the lateral than the medial wall.

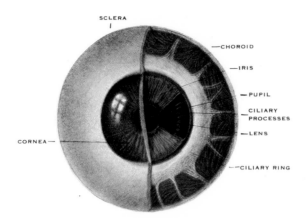

FIG. 23.—ANTERIOR VIEW OF THE EYE.

Portions of the cornea, sclera, and iris have been removed to show the deeper structures.

(From Hirschfeld and Leveillé, 1853.)

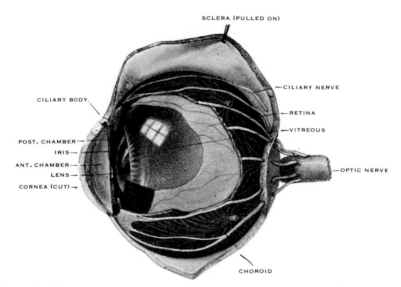

FIG. 24.—PREPARATION TO SHOW THE COATS AND CONTENTS OF THE EYE.

Portions of the sclera, cornea, choroid, ciliary body, iris, and retina have been removed.

(From Hirschfeld and Leveillé 1853.)

As regards the depth that it normally occupies in its socket, a straight-edge placed against the superior and inferior orbital margins will just touch or just miss the front of the cornea.

But a line joining the medial and lateral margins will have nearly one-third of the globe in front of it.

The eyeball is, in fact, least protected on the lateral side, and it is therefore from this side that the surgeon finds his easiest approach.

For this reason, too, rupture of the globe takes place most frequently up and medially from blows which come from the lower and lateral side.

The globe of the eye consists of three concentric coverings or tunics enclosing the various transparent media through which the light must pass before reaching the sensitive retina :

1. The outermost coat is fibrous, protective in function, and made up of a

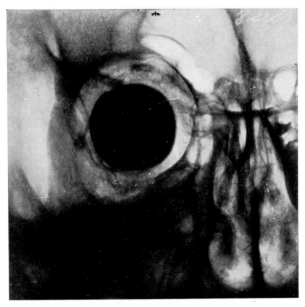

FIG. 22.—TO SHOW THE POSITION OF THE EYE IN THE ORBIT.
The eye was injected with a saturated solution of lead nitrate before the X-ray was taken.
The actual injection fluid was kindly suggested by Professor H. A. Harris.

posterior five-sixths, which is white and opaque and called the *sclera,* and an anterior part which is transparent, the *cornea.*

2. The middle coat is mainly vascular and nutritive in its function. It is made up from behind forwards of choroid, ciliary body, and iris.

3. The innermost tunic is the retina, consisting essentially of nerve elements and forming the true receptive portion for visual impressions.

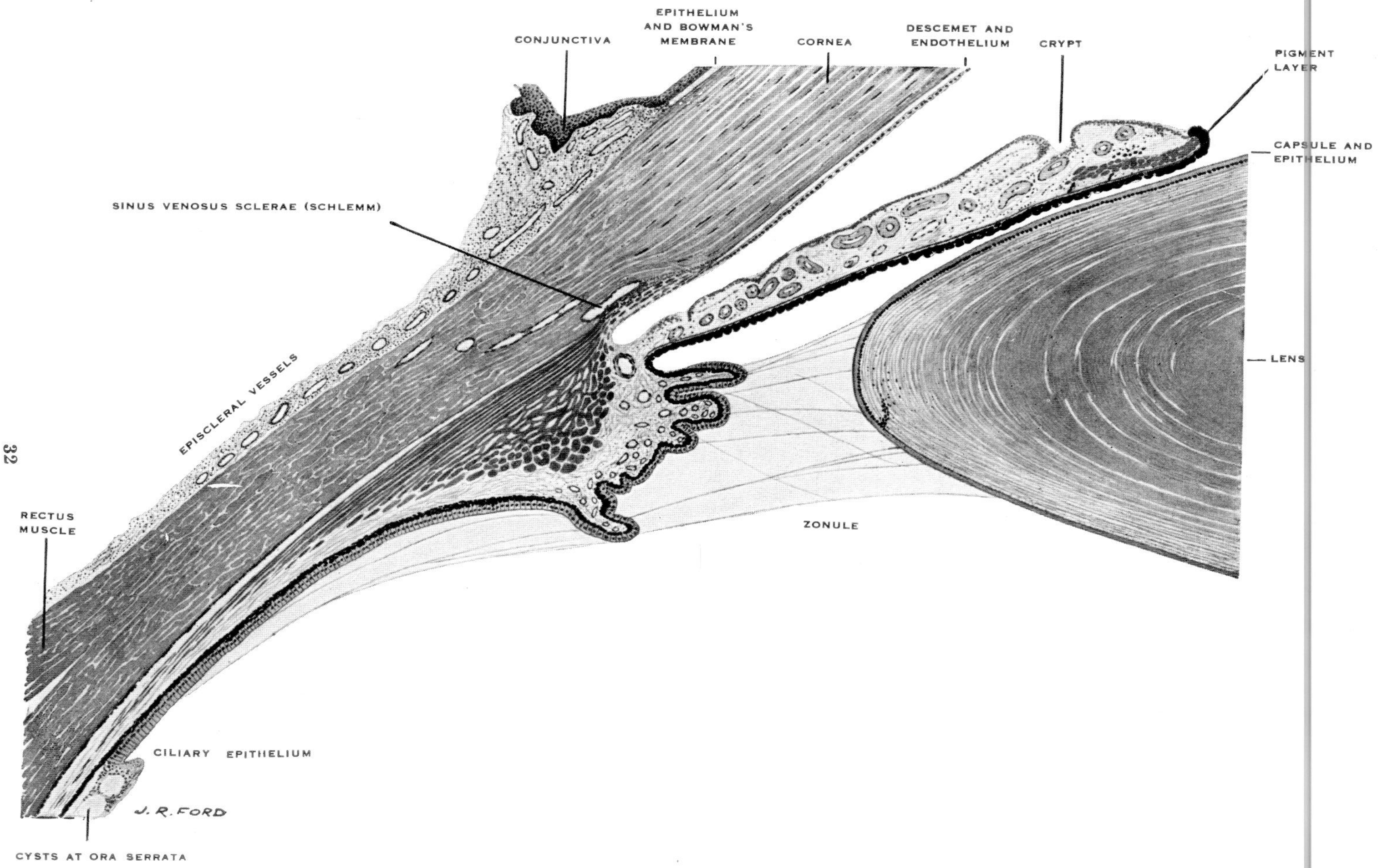

PIGMENT LAYER

CAPSULE AND EPITHELIUM

LENS

CRYPT

DESCEMET AND ENDOTHELIUM

CORNEA

ZONULE

EPITHELIUM AND BOWMAN'S MEMBRANE

CONJUNCTIVA

SINUS VENOSUS SCLERAE (SCHLEMM)

EPISCLERAL VESSELS

CILIARY EPITHELIUM

J. R. FORD

CYSTS AT ORA SERRATA

RECTUS MUSCLE

32

FIG. 25.—ANTERO-POSTERIOR SECTION THROUGH THE ANTERIOR PORTION OF THE EYE.

THE CORNEA

The cornea is transparent, and resembles a little watch-glass. Its curvature is somewhat greater than the rest of the globe, and so a slight furrow (the sulcus scleræ) separates it from the sclera.

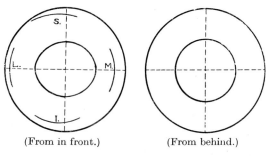

FIG. 26.—TO SHOW THE CORNEA—OVAL FROM IN FRONT; CIRCULAR FROM BEHIND.

(From in front.)　　　(From behind.)

This furrow is best demonstrated in the living by making the image reflected from a mirror pass from the cornea to the sclera. The image is first narrowed horizontally (Tscherning), then may divide into two.

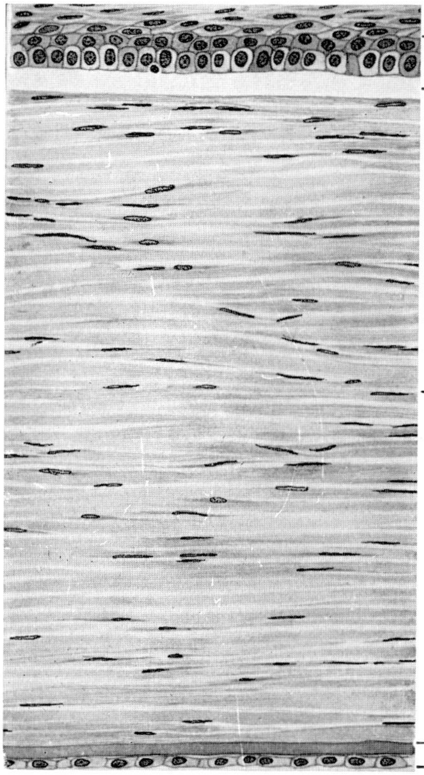

The cornea and sclera are structurally continuous, and even histologically it is very difficult to tell where one ends and the other begins. The line of junction between the two is best seen (with the naked eye) when an eye which has just been removed from the living is divided by a meridional section. Looked at from in front, the cornea is elliptical, being 12 mm. in the horizontal meridian and 11 mm. in the vertical.

From behind, the circumference of the cornea appears circular. This difference is due to the fact that the sclera and conjunctiva overlap the cornea anteriorly more above and below than laterally.

Ideally the cornea forms part of the surface of a sphere, but very often it is curved more

EPITHELIUM

BOWMAN'S MEMBRANE

STROMA

DESCEMET'S MEMBRANE
ENDOTHELIUM

FIG. 27.—TRANSVERSE SECTION OF CORNEA.

A.E.—3

in one meridian than another, *giving rise to the condition of astigmatism.* Usually it is more curved in the vertical than in the horizontal meridian, i.e. astigmatism with the rule.

The radius of curvature of the anterior surface is 7·84 mm. (Steiger), that of the posterior 7 mm. (Merkel and Kallius). These radii only hold good for the central third, or optical zone, the peripheral portions being more flattened. *Hence a higher convex glass is often necessary when looking at the periphery of the fundus with the ophthalmoscope.*

The cornea is thicker at the periphery (1 mm.) than at the centre, where it is 0·58 mm.[1]

Contrary to popular opinion, most of the refraction of the eye takes place, not in the lens, but at the surface of the cornea. Maintenance of transparency is an obvious essential ; this is a function mainly of the epithelial cells on its surfaces. The living cells are rich in glycogen, enzymes and acetylcholine ; their activity regulates that of the corneal corpuscles and controls the transport of water and electrolytes through the lamellæ of the substantia propria (see *The Cornea World Congress, London,* 1965).

Structure.—Behind the precorneal film (p. 243) there are the following five layers:

1. *Layer of Stratified Squamous Epithelium.*—This may be regarded as the continuation of the conjunctival epithelium forwards. But unlike the limbal epithelium its two surfaces are, as near as matters, parallel to each other.

This layer is some 50–100 μ in thickness and consists of five layers of cells (Virchow). The deepest of these, the *Basal* cells, stand in a palisade-like manner, in perfect alignment, on a basement membrane. These basal cells are columnar with rounded heads and flat bases, which often present processes which spread out on the basement membrane. Each has a slightly oval nucleus whose long axis is that of the cell and placed near the head of the cell. The cells are connected with the membrane by fine denticulations which are not very strong.

Actually there are two kinds of basal cells : the shorter ones are clear cells, the longer ones dark often club-shaped and appear to be making their way into the next layer (Fig. 29). The basal layer is the germinal layer, and some of the cells show mitoses. The daughter cells are gradually pushed up into the more superficial layers.

The next layer (the *Wing* [or umbrella] cells) consists of polyhedral cells whose rounded heads are directed anteriorly and whose concave bases fit over the heads of the basal cells and send processes, the wings, between them. Each contains an oval nucleus whose long axis is parallel with the surface of the cornea (Fig. 30).

The next two or three layers are also polyhedral, and the most superficial are flattened but do not lose their nuclei, *nor do they normally show keratinisation.* The flattened nuclei of the surface cells project backwards leaving the surface perfectly smooth, which makes it the most brilliant in the body.

[1] According to Koby (*Rev. gén. d'Ophtal*, 1930, **44**, 222), using the slit-lamp.

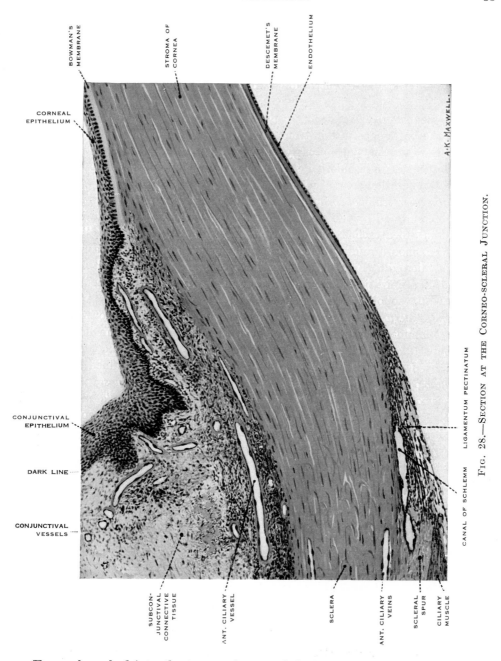

FIG. 28.—SECTION AT THE CORNEO-SCLERAL JUNCTION.

Even when shed into the tears, where each looks like a tile, the most superficial cells keep their nuclei (Rochon-Duvigneaud). Knüsel, however, says that
with vital staining the cells appear to lose their nuclei at times.

As in the epidermis, the various cells appear to be united by cell bridges forming prickle-cells. The spaces between the cells, which are difficult to make out in the normal eye, form a lymph space which can be injected, and *which may be greatly distended pathologically, for instance in glaucoma.* These spaces are best seen between the basal cells, and gradually disappear in the more superficial ones.

A few leucocytes (wandering cells) may be found normally in the spaces between the basal cells just in front of Bowman's membrane (Fig. 27). Pathologically they may increase greatly in number.

In spite of its avascularity the corneal epithelium possesses a very active power of regeneration after abrasion.

Electron microscopy of corneal epithelium. These conclusions from light microscopy are confirmed by the electron microscope. The irregular and interlocking cell borders are attached by formations known as " desmosomes ". The cell borders are smooth and regular on the free surface, and there is a regular projection of microvilli (Fig. 31). The surface cells are nucleated, vital, and show no sign of keratinization ; they seem to be filled with what histochemical studies show to be phospholipids (Ehlers, 1965).

2. *The Anterior Limiting Membrane* (*Bowman's Membrane*) or the anterior "elastic" lamina does not consist of elastic tissue. It is a thin homogeneous sheet about 12 μ in thickness between the basement membrane and the substantia propria. It is separated from the epithelium by a sharply defined border, *and under pathological conditions as well as after death the epithelium separates readily from Bowman's membrane.* The anterior surface of Bowman's membrane is absolutely parallel with the surface of the cornea. Hence the difficulty often of seeing abrasions which have removed the whole thickness of the epithelium. Posteriorly the line of demarcation from the stroma is ill-defined. In fact, it may be regarded as a modified portion of the stroma. Peripherally it ends abruptly in a rounded border (Figs. 25 and 28).

Bowman's membrane is not a true elastic membrane nor does it regenerate when once it has been destroyed. It, however, shows a good deal of resistance to injury or infection.

Electron Microscopy of Bowman's Membrane.—An acellular mass of collagen fibrils are disposed irregularly. They are much finer than the fibres of the underlying substantia propria (Figs. 29, 32).

3. *The Substantia propria* of the cornea is composed of a modified connective tissue of which the constituents have very nearly the same refractive index so that in the perfectly fresh condition it is difficult to make out any indications of structure. After death, and with the aid of certain reagents, the cornea may be ascertained to consist of alternating lamellæ of fibrous tissue (about 60 in number according to Bowman) the planes of which are parallel to the surfaces of the cornea (Quain).

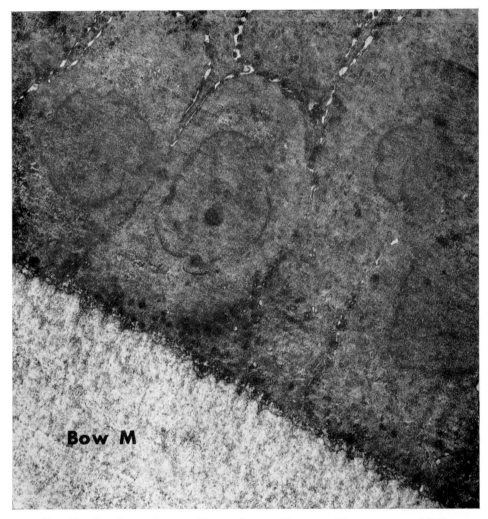

FIG. 29.—THE BASAL CELLS OF HUMAN CORNEA (ELECTRON MICROGRAPH, × 4,000).

The cells lie on a basement membrane. Deep to this are the irregularly arranged fine collagen fibrils of Bowman's membrane (Bow M).

(*By courtesy of Dr. C. Pedler, Institute of Ophthalmology, London. Preparation by Mrs. R. Tilly.*)

The lamellæ are made of bands and each tape-like band is itself composed of fibrils, so fine that according to Virchow they can be only made out individually by previous interstitial injection of the cornea with a substance like chromic acid and subsequent staining with special stains such as Lyon blue. Individual fibrils can therefore not be made out in ordinary microscopic section. Moreover, the fibrils in each band are so closely united to each other and with those of

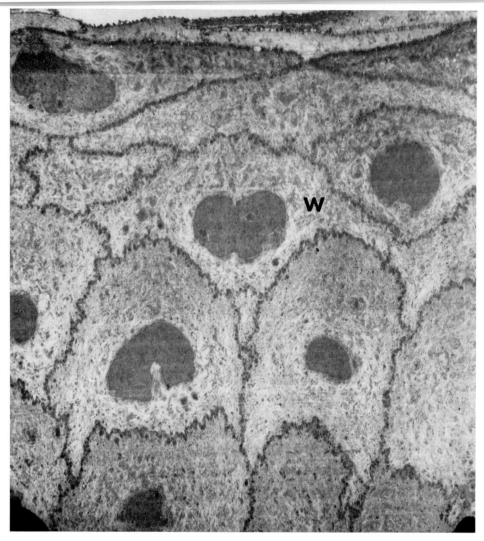

FIG. 30.—THE SURFACE CELLS OF HUMAN CORNEA (ELECTRON MICROGRAPH, × 4,000).

Blunt microvilli project from the flat surface cells.   The wing cells (W) fit over the rounded heads of the deeper cells.

(*Courtesy of Mr. P. V. Rycroft F.R.C.S.*)

neighbouring bands that it is impossible to separate the cornea into lamellæ or bands without much tearing taking place.

The bands of each lamella are parallel to each other but those of alternate layers make a right angle or near this with each other.

We would expect, in any antero-posterior section, to find bands cut along their length and transversely in alternate layers as is shown in Waldeyer's well-known picture.   But

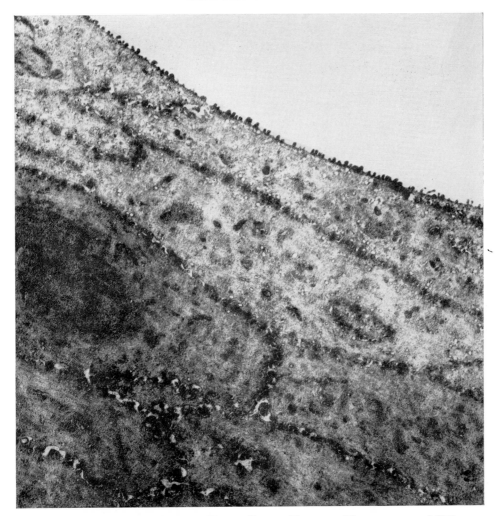

FIG. 31.—THE SURFACE CELLS OF HUMAN CORNEA (ELECTRON MICROGRAPH, × 6,500).

These flattened cells are vital and show no sign of keratinization. Microvilli project from the free surface.

(*By courtesy of Dr. C. Pedler, Institute of Ophthalmology, London. Preparation by Mrs. R. Tilly.*)

since we cannot make out the fibrils nor the union between the bands, it is a striking fact that in any section at right angles to the surfaces the bands appear to be cut along their length. This effect is heightened by the spaces in which the corneal corpuscles lie being parallel to the surface.

While most corneal fibres are parallel to the surface some *oblique* ones are found, especially anteriorly near Bowman's membrane. They probably run along the perforating corneal nerves.

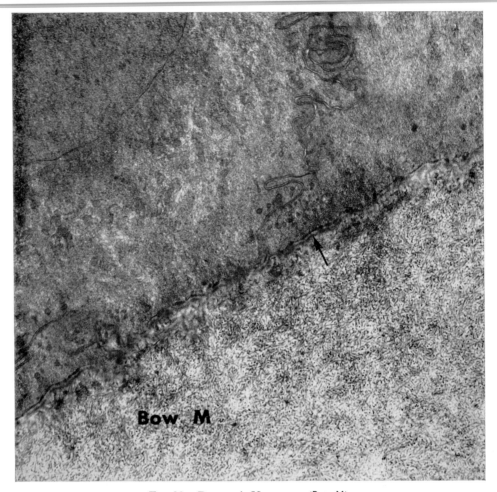

FIG. 32.—BOWMAN'S MEMBRANE (Bow M).

The irregular arrangement of an acellular feltwork of very fine fibrils is typical. Note the inter-locking of the surfaces of the two basal cells shown. The cells of the basal layer of epithelium lie on a basement membrane (arrow). Human cornea, × 16,000.

(By courtesy of Mr. P. V. Rycroft, F.R.C.S.)

Between the lamellæ (*v. inf.*) are found :

    (*a*) Fixed cells.
    (*b*) Wandering cells.

Fixed cells are connective tissue cells, called here corneal corpuscles, which resemble the corpuscles (osteocytes) of bone. Each consists of a flattened cell with a large flattened nucleus and having branching processes which communicate with those of neighbouring corpuscles.

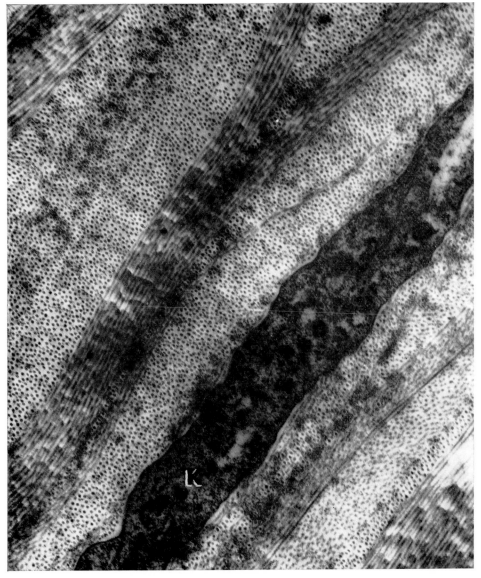

Fig. 33.—The Substantia Propria of Human Cornea (Electron Micrograph, × 29,000).

The layers of collagen fibres, lying alternately at right angles, are well shown. Portion of a corneal corpuscle (K—keratocyte) lies within a lamella.

(*By courtesy of Dr. C. Pedler, Institute of Ophthalmology, London. Preparation by Mrs. R. Tilly.*)

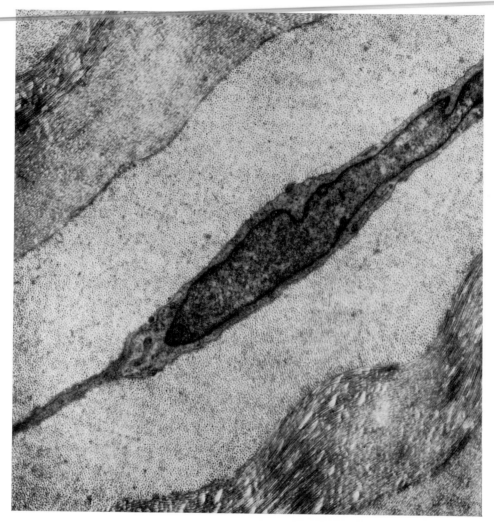

FIG. 34.—A HUMAN CORNEAL CORPUSCLE (ELECTRON MICROGRAPH, × 13,500).

It lies centrally in a lamella, whose fibres are here cut transversely.

(*By courtesy of Dr. C. Pedler, Institute of Ophthalmology, London. Preparation by Mrs. R. Tilly.*)

Wandering white cells may also be seen. They escape from the marginal loops of the corneal blood-vessels, are few in number normally, but play an important part in inflammation.

Electron Microscopy of Substantia Propria.—This confirms the alternating direction of the fibres ; in each layer they are parallel, and in alternate layers they lie at right angles. The presence of elastic fibres has not been confirmed. In man the corneal corpuscles commonly lie *within*, and not between, the collagen lamellæ (Figs. 33, 34).

4. *The Posterior Limiting (Descemet's) Membrane* (or posterior elastic membrane) is a strong, homogeneous, and very resistant membrane. It is some 6 μ thick. Unlike Bowman's membrane, it is sharply defined from the corneal stroma. There is in fact a plane of separation between them which is made use of in lamellar keratoplasty. It is very resistant to chemical reagents and likewise to pathological processes going on in the cornea. When the entire cornea has broken down into pus, we often see the thin Descemet's membrane offering resistance and remaining unimpaired for days (Fuchs).

Descemet's membrane is normally in a state of tension: if wounded it gapes slightly and tends to assume a curve which is the opposite of the normal, i.e. it tends to curl up and roll out (Salzmann). While showing this type of elasticity it does not stain with all elastic stains although it does with some and does not therefore consist of true elastic tissue. In fact, it agrees very much in its staining reactions with those of the capsule of the lens.

Unlike Bowman's membrane, which never regenerates, Descemet's membrane can be re-formed.

Descemet's membrane often tapers at its edge, but although it appears to end here, it can be traced into a *portion* of the Ligamentum pectinatum iridis (see p. 60).

Thus this ligament is not formed of a fibrillation of Descemet as often stated, for it contains other structures besides it (p. 60).

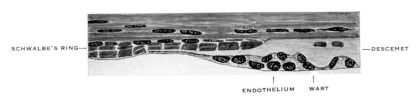

FIG. 35.—THE EDGE OF DESCEMET'S MEMBRANE.

Note the oval nuclei (black) in single file in front of Schwalbe's ring.

At the periphery of the cornea the posterior surface of the membrane presents rounded wart-like elevations, the Hassal-Henle bodies, which tend to increase with age (see p. 242, and Fig. 39).

Electron Microscopy of Descemet's Membrane.—Very fine collagen fibres are arranged with the utmost regularity in an almost crystalline pattern. In man they are disposed in two layers, an outer " banded " layer against the corneal substantia propria and an inner stroma against the endothelium (Figs. 36, 37). Although Descemet's membrane displays the physical property of elasticity there is no evidence that the fibres themselves are composed of elastin.

5. *The Endothelium* is the most posterior layer of the cornea, and consists of a single layer of flattened *epithelial-like* cells, continuous round the angle of the anterior chamber with those on the front of the iris (see p. 82). The cells at

the back of the cornea with their nuclei can be seen by means of the slit-lamp in the living eye—the only place in the body where this is possible (see p. 241).

Electron Microscopy of the Endothelium.—There is no basement membrane. Adjacent cells interlock by reciprocal tortuous surfaces. Abundant cellular organelles (Fig. 38) indicate a high degree of metabolic activity.

Embryologically the cornea is the continuation forwards of three structures :

(*a*) The epithelium and Bowman's membrane of the conjunctiva.

(*b*) The substantia propria of the sclera.

(*c*) Descemet's membrane and the posterior endothelium of the uveal tract.

Pathologically, too, this is of importance, for the epithelium is liable to be affected in diseases of the conjunctiva, the stroma in diseases of the sclera and Descemet and the endothelium in diseases of the uveal tract.

THE LIMBUS

The limbus is the transition zone between the conjunctiva and sclera on the one hand and the cornea on the other. The transparent corneal tissue ends just behind a line which joins the ends of Bowman and Descemet.

Owing mainly to the overlap of conjunctiva and subconjunctival tissue, Bowman is 1 mm. shorter than Descemet, which also approaches nearer to the angle of the anterior chamber, but is still separated from it by the whole of the corneo-scleral trabecular system, i.e. by about $1\frac{1}{2}$ mm.

(*a*) *The Conjunctivo-corneal Junction.*—The conjunctiva is a thin and transparent skin ; i.e. a fibrous membrane surfaced with epithelium. It is rather loosely attached to the sclera by a tenuous subconjunctival connective tissue. *The conjunctiva ends at the limbus, and only the epithelium passes centrally to surface the cornea* (Figs. 28, 49). The overlap of conjunctival and subconjunctival tissue forms a translucent membrane over the extreme margin of transparent cornea (Fig. 59). The width of this film when studied with the naked eye is seen to vary greatly. At times the white sclera ends sharply without any film.

Bowman's membrane, which usually ends suddenly in a rounded border but may be bevelled, gives place to a thin layer of conjunctival fibrous tissue which is here closely adherent to the sclera.

The basal layer of the corneal epithelium which has been kept rigidly aligned by Bowman becomes wavy and may even become papillary as soon as it loses the support of this membrane. The five-layered corneal epithelium gives place to one of ten to twelve layers. The cells of the basal layer become smaller and poorer in protoplasm and the nuclei more densely staining. This causes the basal layer to appear under the low power of the microscope as a *dark line.*

The marginal vessels (superficial marginal plexus) occupy a triangular area whose apex lies where Bowman ends and whose base is formed by episcleral tissue and sclera.

The Sclero-corneal Junction.—If, in a preparation of the anterior segment of

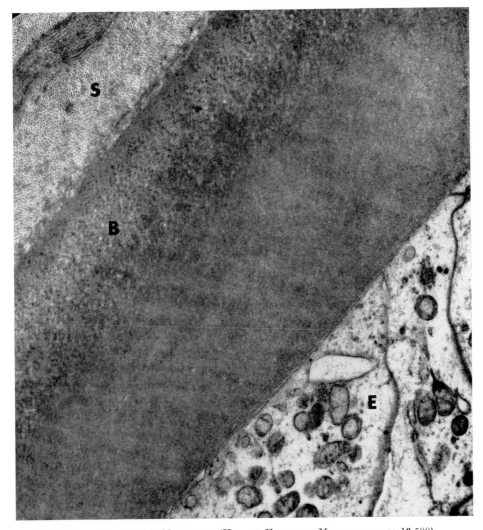

FIG. 36.—DESCEMET'S MEMBRANE (HUMAN, ELECTRON MICROGRAPH, × 13,500).

Lying against the substantia propria of the cornea (S) is the banded layer (B) of Descemet's membrane. Deep to this is the stroma of Descemet's membrane, lined by the endothelium (E).

(By courtesy of Dr. C. Pedler, Institute of Ophthalmology, London. Preparation by Mrs. R. Tilly.)

the eye which has been fixed in formalin or alcohol, we make two incisions through the centre of the cornea at right angles to each other, we obtain four segments. If now we pick up at the apex of one segment some corneal tissue with forceps, we can strip the laminæ quite easily till we come to the white sclera, where we are stopped abruptly. Under the microscope this point corresponds to the place where the regular corneal lamellæ give place to the oblique and circular fibres of

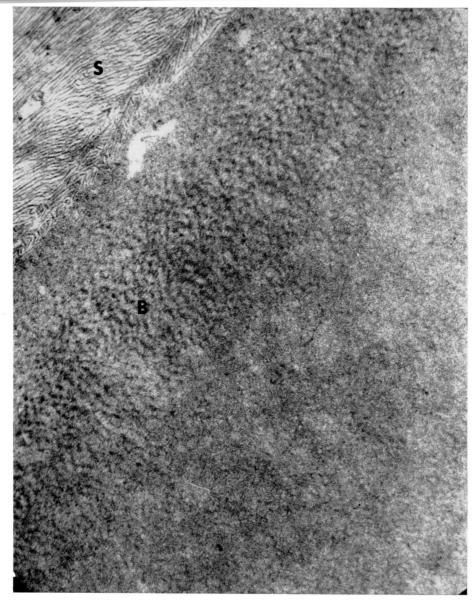

Fig. 37.—Descemet's Membrane (Human, Electron Micrograph, × 20,000).

The banded layer (B) lies near the substantia propria (S) of the cornea.
(*By courtesy of Mr. P. V. Rycroft, F.R.C.S.*)

the sclera which, as it were, form a frame to the cornea (Rochon-Duvigneaud). The regular corneal lamellæ continue a little beyond the line joining Bowman and Descement. The oblique fibres and star-shaped cells characteristic of the

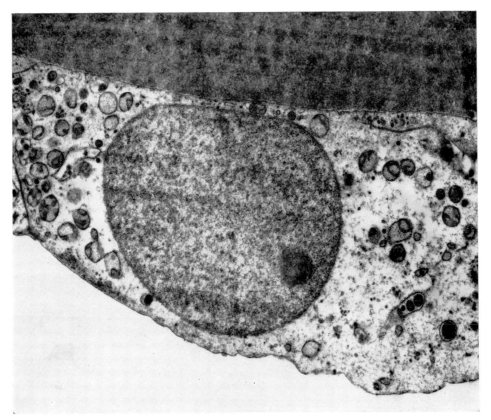

FIG. 38.—THE ENDOTHELIUM (HUMAN, ELECTRON MICROGRAPH, × 10,000).

The cell lining Descemet's membrane has a large nucleus and multiple organelles.
(By courtesy of Dr. C. Pedler, Institute of Ophthalmology, London.   Preparation by Mrs. R. Tilly.)

sclera commence a little sooner anteriorly than posteriorly ; but the main over-lap of the cornea is by conjunctiva and subconjunctival tissue rather than by sclera as usually stated (Rochon-Duvigneaud).   Neither does the cornea fit into the groove in the sclera like a watch-glass, as generally described (and in previous editions of this anatomy).   In fact, the fibres of the corneal lamellæ (transparent and regular) run directly into the fibres of the sclera (opaque and less regularly arranged).

THE VESSELS AND NERVES OF THE CORNEA

The cornea is avascular.   It is generally stated, however, that small loops derived from the anterior ciliary vessels invade the periphery for about 1 mm. But these vessels are not in the cornea.   They are in the subconjunctival connective tissue which overlaps it.   The termination of these vessels, which can of course be seen in the living, marks the end of Bowman's membrane. The nourishment is obtained by lymphatic permeation through the spaces between the lamellæ. No actual lymphatic vessels lined by endothelium are found.

Nerves.—The cornea is supplied by the ophthalmic division of the 5th cranial, via the ciliary nerves and those of the surrounding conjunctiva. *The first division of the 5th nerve, in fact, supplies almost the whole of the eye and its appendages, giving warning of injury, for instance, of a foreign body, and hence may well be called the sentinel of the eye.* The anterior ciliary nerves enter the sclera from the

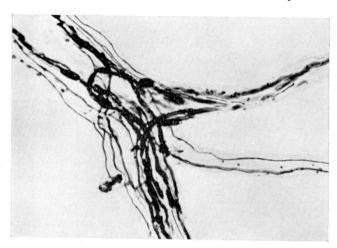

FIG. 39.—FLAT SECTION OF NERVES AT LIMBUS (STAINED BIELCHOWSKY).

perichoroidal space a short distance behind the limbus. They inosculate with each other and with the conjunctival nerves, forming pericorneal plexuses at various levels. The nerves pass into the cornea as 60–80 myelinated trunks at its junction with the sclera. After having gone about 2–4 mm., they usually lose their myelin sheaths (Fig. 234) and divide into two groups —anterior and posterior. The anterior (40–50) pass through the substance of the cornea and then form a plexus under Bowman's membrane. Having traversed this, the fibres inosculate again to form a subepithelial plexus, and lastly actually in amongst the epithelial cells an intraepithelial plexus [1] is found.

In the plexuses, however, the nerves seem to maintain their individuality, since peripheral incisions, as for iridectomy, leave a *sector* of anæsthesia (Rochon-Duvigneaud).

The posterior (40 or 50) pass to the posterior part of the cornea. But there are no nerves in the central posterior part of the cornea, nor in Descemet or the endothelium. According to Dogiel, the nerves in the stroma at the periphery of the cornea end in small plates with serrated edges. Krause's end-bulbs are found beneath the epithelium at the limbus (Fig. 217), and in the epithelium of the cornea itself the nerves end in rounded or pear-shaped end-bulbs (see also p. 243).

[1] While this is the classical description, it would appear that in man the three plexuses cannot be demonstrated as they can in the lower animals.

THE SCLERA (FROM σκληρός = HARD)

The sclera forms the posterior opaque five-sixths of the fibrous protective coat of the eye. Its anterior portion is visible, and constitutes the " white " of the eye.

In childhood (or pathologically) when the sclera is thin it appears bluish owing to the uvea showing through. In old age it may become yellowish owing to a deposition of fat. The inner surface of the sclera is brown owing to adherent suprachoroidal pigment and is marked by grooves in which the ciliary nerves and vessels lie.

The sclera is thickest behind (about 1 mm.), and gradually becomes thinner when traced forwards. It is very thin at the insertion of the recti muscles (0·3 mm.), but the thickness of tendon and muscle = 0·6 mm. (Fig. 25). At the site of attachment of the optic nerve 3 mm. to the medial side of and just *above* the posterior pole of the eye, the sclera becomes a thin sieve-like membrane—the *lamina cribrosa*, through the holes of which the axons of the ganglion cells of the retina pass.

The lamina cribrosa forms the weakest spot in the outer fibrous tunic of the eye. In glaucoma, therefore, it is here that the eye will give, and result in the cupped disc—characteristic of the *chronic* form of the disease when the intraocular pressure has been raised for some time.

Moreover, as the fibres of

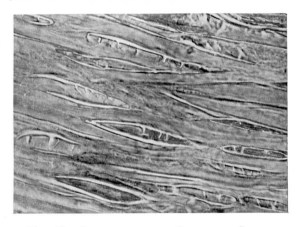

FIG. 40.—ANTERO-POSTERIOR SECTION OF SCLERA.

the optic nerve pass through the lamina cribrosa they lie in canals whose walls are little distensible and hence are easily strangulated by inflammatory swelling.

The outer surface of the sclera is received into the fascia bulbi, to which it is connected by fine trabeculæ (see also p. 265).

The sclera is pierced by three sets of apertures—posterior, middle, and anterior.

The Posterior apertures are situated round the optic nerve, and through them pass the long and short ciliary vessels and nerves.

The Middle apertures, 4 mm. behind the equator of the eye, give exit to the venæ vorticosæ, which come from the choroid, and some lymphatics.

The Anterior apertures are for the anterior ciliary vessels (which come from the muscular branches to the recti), perivascular lymphatics, and sometimes nerves which may have ganglia on them (see also p. 52).

The sclera contains the sinus venosus scleræ (canal of Schlemm), which indents its deep surface at the corneo-scleral junction. A circular flange of sclera thus lies deep to the outer circumference of the sinus venosus scleræ. Wedge-shaped in section, it is known as the *scleral spur* (Figs. 28, 44, 45, 48, 52, 60, 66).

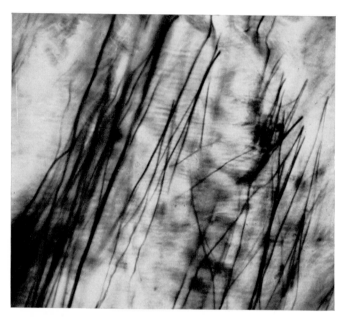

FIG. 41.—ELASTIC FIBRES IN SCLERA IN POSTERIOR PORTION OF THE EYE.

Structure.—The sclera consists of dense bands of fibrous tissue some 10–16 μ in thickness and 100–140 μ in width. The bands are mostly parallel with the surface and cross each other in all directions. They may divide dichotomously and then reunite. The imbrication of the fibres is so dense, especially in its posterior part, that it is almost impossible to separate them by dissection. The deeper bands are stronger than those next the episclera. The tendons of insertion of the recti muscles run into the sclera as parallel fibres and then spread out in a fan-shaped manner to become lost among the meridional fibres of the sclera. The tendons of the oblique muscles behave similarly but here they lose themselves among the oblique or equatorial fibres of the sclera.

Just as the direction and strength of the trabeculæ of bone are determined by the stresses and strains to which they are subject, so the plan of the scleral fibres is determined by the intraocular tension and the pull of the various muscles.

The adaptation of the sclera to these stresses and strains is effected by the disposition of the fibrous bands, by the wavy course of the connective tissue fibres, and by the great abundance of the elastic fibres (Redslob).

The different parts of the sclera have different functions to perform. This is recognised by the orientation of the fibres. In the posterior portion the external fibres are arranged like the net around a balloon, while the internal fibres spread out fanwise. Thus they will give gradually in a case of increased intraocular tension. Moreover, the wavy fibres become straight due to the tension of the elastic fibres. When the tension diminishes, the elastic fibres are relaxed and the connective tissue fibres become wavy again. Everything takes place as if the sclera were a spring (Redslob).

The anterior portion has a different function. It forms a rigid skeleton for the insertion of the ocular muscles. This rigidity is brought about by the strictly circular direction of the scleral fibres.

With age the connective tissue fibres tend to become sclerosed. This condensation is seen especially around the canals of the venæ vorticosæ.

The sclera is very rich in elastic fibres (Fig. 41) placed on the surface of the fibrous bands. They are especially abundant at the equator, around the optic nerve and at the limbus.

Elastic fibres are not present in the embryo. They only develop after birth and increase up to adult life. In old age they diminish again.

The fixed cells of the scleral tissue resemble those of the cornea, but the nuclei are more irregular, and the syncytium formed by the processes not so closed (Salzmann).

Pigmented cells of various shapes are met with, especially in the deeper layers near the choroid, and on the vessels and nerves which pass through the sclera. Also at the points where the anterior ciliary vessels enter there is often a collection of pigment, especially in dark people.

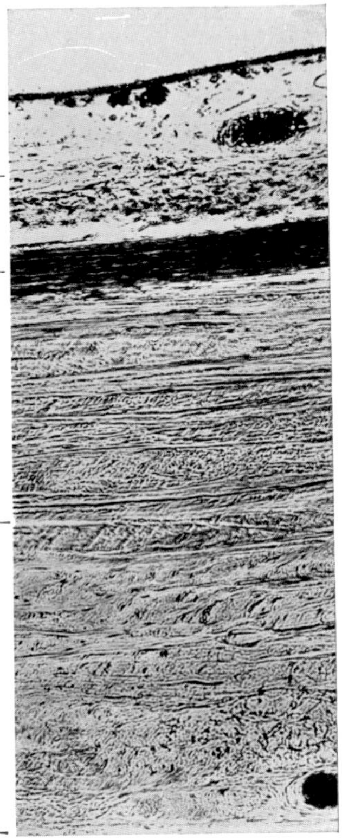

FIG. 42.—TO SHOW THE STRUCTURE OF THE SCLERA AND THE LONG CILIARY NERVE IN THE SUPRACHOROIDAL SPACE. (ZENKER. MALLORY'S PHOSPHOTUNG. HÆM.)
(Wolff's preparation.)

These pigment cells have obviously migrated from the uvea, and point the way by which malignant disease of the interior of the eye often makes its way to the outside.

If a section be taken passing through the cornea and sclera, no line of demarcation can be made out, the fibres of one being continuous with those of the other. At their junction, however, we find the sinus venosus scleræ (canal of Schlemm).

The sclera is almost avascular except for the vessels which pass through it to and from the interior of the eye.

Posteriorly around the optic nerve we find the vascular circle of Zinn or Haller.

The episcleral tissue is the loose connective and elastic tissue which covers the sclera and anteriorly connects the conjunctiva to it. It is for the most part continuous superficially with the loose tissue of Tenon's space, while its deeper layers become more and more dense and gradually give place to sclera proper. It differs both from the loose tissue of Tenon's space and the sclera, both of which are relatively avascular, by containing quite a fair number of vessels.

Behind the insertion of the recti muscles the episcleral tissue is thin and the vessels, two veins to each artery, form a wide-meshed net. The arteries here come from the posterior ciliaries.

In front of the attachment of the muscles the episclera is much thicker and much richer in vessels. The meshes of the vascular net, too, are much smaller. A capillary net exists only in this anterior zone of the sclera. It is a marked filling of this net which is called " ciliary injection " (Salzmann).

Nerves of the Sclera.—The ciliary nerves pierce the sclera around the optic nerve. The long ciliary nerves accompany the long posterior ciliary arteries and so reach the ciliary body. At the level of the orbiculus ciliaris the nerves divide into branches. Some go to the ciliary body, some accompanied by vessels penetrate the sclera, most commonly at the equator or some 2–4 mm. from the limbus (Fig. 39). When they reach the surface, the branches inosculate, forming loops around the limbus, from the convexity of which branches pass into the cornea. Nerves also pass from the episcleral tissue inwards into the sclera.

Some scleral nerves have a curious course. They enter the sclera and may even reach its outer surface. They then bend round sharply and turn back to the point of entrance. The extremity of the loop sometimes presents a mushroom-like thickening. These scleral loops are found most commonly about 1·6 mm. from the limbus. In their intrascleral course the nerves are often accompanied by pigment and appear under the conjunctiva as hyaline elevations surrounded by a ring of pigment, which are very sensitive (Redslob).

SINUS VENOSUS SCLERÆ (THE CANAL OF SCHLEMM)

Position and Form.—The sinus venosus scleræ is a circular channel placed at the corneo-scleral junction at the bottom of the so-called scleral furrow. For most part of its course it is single (with perhaps a very small vas comes) but there may be two or more canals. It has been likened to a river which divides into branches and then unites again. According to Leber, there may be a plexiform arrangement of these branches, which may number up to seven, especially in the region where the canal is joined by branches from the ciliary muscle.

The canal is flattened from without inwards and tends to be wider posteriorly. It may be oval or triangular with the apex towards Descemet. It occupies

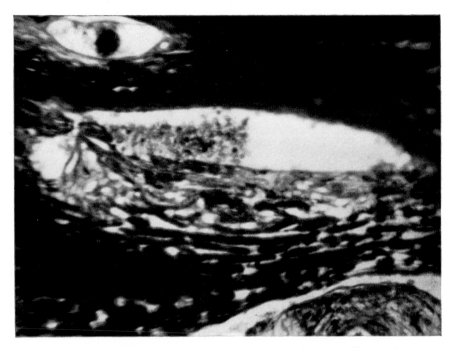

Fig. 43.—Section of Sinus Venosus Scleræ (Canal of Schlemm).
Note multinuclear cap in projection of inner wall, and fine fibrils beneath endothelium. The canal contains blood.

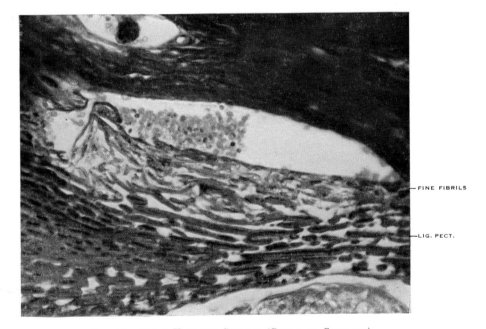

FINE FIBRILS

LIG. PECT.

Fig. 44.—Sinus Venosus Scleræ (Canal of Schlemm).
Inner wall juts into canal. Fine fibres beneath endothelium. In trabeculæ of ligamentum pectinatum denser core can be made out.

A.E.—52]

approximately the posterior half of the distance between the scleral spur and Descemet, and thus its length on cross-section is about half a millimetre. Its width on cross-section is always less than that of the ligamentum pectinatum.

Structure and Relations.—The canal of Schlemm is lined by endothelium whose nuclei project in towards the lumen ; but, apart from this, it has no proper wall of its own : its bed is, as it were, gouged out of the sclera. It may be directly on the sclera but more usually it is separated from it by a compact layer of varying thickness containing much elastic tissue and a varying number of nuclei. In any case, its relations with the sclera are quite different from those of the venæ

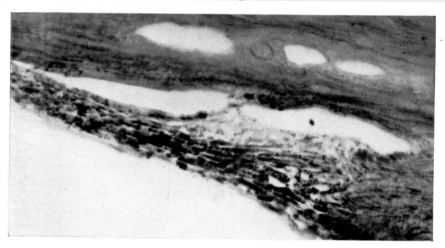

Fig. 45.—Section of Sinus Venosus Scleræ (Weigert's Elastic Stain).

Note that the fine fibrils next to the canal contain no, or practically no, elastic tissue, whereas the ligamentum pectinatum stains well.

vorticosæ, where these vessels pass through the sclera : they have walls of their own and are separated from the sclera by loose connective tissue.

Here and there partly and more rarely completely crossing the lumen of the canal are partitions of sclera resembling those of the dural venous sinuses. The anterior ciliary veins have in general the same structure as the canal. The canal is bounded posteriorly by the scleral spur which also overlaps it somewhat to the inner side.

The inner wall of the sinus venosus scleræ is usually flat but it may project into the lumen like a villus (Figs. 43, 44, 45), and may indeed reach the outer wall. It is usually lined by a single layer of cells, which are like those covering an arachnoid granulation, and may be in two or more layers and may even form a multi-layered cap (Figs. 43, 44).

The inner wall of the sinus venosus scleræ, also, is usually described as being formed by the trabeculæ of the ligamentum pectinatum iridis and, although both Salzmann and Rochon-Duvigneaud have noted a different type of tissue directly under the endothelium, their descriptions are no doubt the result of noting the appearance seen when hæmatoxylin and eosin or van Gieson has been used as the stain. For Salzmann says it resembles the tissue under the endothelium of the outer wall of the canal, while Rochon-Duvigneaud describes it as compact or dense. With Mallory's triple stain after Zenker fixation this tissue is seen to consist of a reticulum of very fine fibrils. This layer probably has the consistence

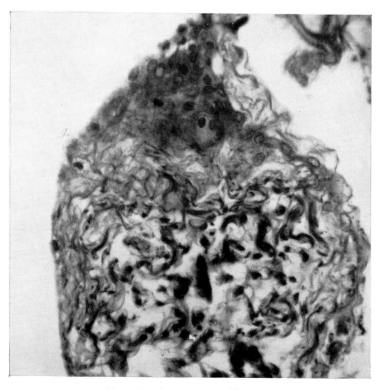

Fig. 46.—Arachnoidal Villus.
Note multi-nuclear cap. Also fine fibrils below endothelium and coarse subarachnoid trabeculæ forming core.

of cotton wool and I[1] would suggest is homologous with the tissue under the endothelium of a Pacchionian body or arachnoidal villus, that is with the protruded arachnoid (Fig. 46). Deep to this are some fibres which resemble those of the main mass of the ligamentum, but are frailer and contain no core of connective and elastic tissue. These no doubt represent the subarachnoid trabeculæ. Then and then only come the fibres of the ligamentum pectinatum iridis with their well-marked core of connective and elastic tissue ; they have the characteristics of scleral tissue and doubtless represent the dura through which the villus

[1] Eugene Wolff.

makes its way. Thus it would appear that the inner wall of the canal of Schlemm has essentially the same basic structure as a Pacchionian body or arachnoidal villus.

Not infrequently one may see conical extensions (Sondermann's canals) of the lumen of the canal into the inner wall of the canal. They have been described as opening into the spaces between the trabeculæ. But this is probably not so.

The Normal Content of the Canal.—It is generally stated that on section the canal usually contains no blood and that Schlemm (1830) found it full of blood because he examined the eye of a man who had been hanged and in whom therefore the veins of the head were engorged.

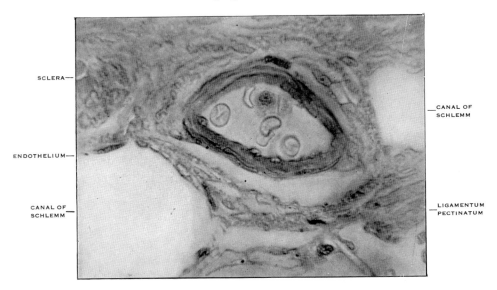

FIG. 47.—PORTION OF THE SINUS VENOSUS SCLERÆ (CANAL OF SCHLEMM) WITH AN ANTERIOR CILIARY ARTERY ACTUALLY IN THE CANAL.

But Leber in sections of normal eyes (or eyes which were affected with cataract only) found blood in the canal of fifteen out of seventeen eyes. It is true in some there was very little blood, but this does not alter the argument. Also in favour of the canal normally containing some blood is the fact that Fuchs found that in individuals with a thin sclera a dark line concentric with the limbus can be made out by focal illumination.

The evidence derived from gonioscopy is equivocal. With the gonioscope the canal may appear grey, that is without blood, or pink, that is with blood ; the pink staining may affect a section only. It seems to depend largely on whether the gonio-glass presses on the limbus or the cornea (see Busacca, 1945).

Summing up this evidence, Wolff thought it would be fair to say that the canal of Schlemm contains aqueous and blood in varying proportions ; but normally almost entirely aqueous, since the aqueous veins are clear or almost so.

Communication with the Anterior Chamber.—Although the dispute, originally started between Schwalbe and Leber, has not been quite settled, it is generally held that particulate matter (red blood corpuscles, etc.) can get into the spaces between the trabeculæ, but not into the canal of Schlemm. Aqueous of course does, and can leave the canal by the aqueous and anterior ciliary veins.

Communicating and Neighbouring Vessels.—The intrascleral plexus (*vid. inf.*) receives junctional branches from the canal of Schlemm which form very characteristic collecting trunks. They run from the convex anterior aspect of the canal into a vein of the plexus, as a straight vessel or after having made a hook-shaped bend. They are minute, flattened, and have an oblique course. They may thus act as valves, the usual type of which are absent (Maggiore).

There may be some thirty collector channels leaving the canal at irregular intervals, but mostly near the horizontal meridian (Theobald).

Some fourteen or more branches from the ciliary muscle pass through the sclera to join the plexus of veins in the neighbourhood of the canal (Leber).

The arteries near the canal probably form a circular vessel which runs close to and parallel with the canal. It is so figured by Maggiore. Sometimes the artery may actually be found in the canal (Wolff) (Fig. 47).

Also Friedenwald has described fine arterial branches actually opening into the canal. These he holds are important in explaining the draining of aqueous from the canal. This work, however, has not been confirmed.

According to Maggiore, the canal of Schlemm receives junctional branches from a vascular plexus situated in the depths of the limbus and composed of a reticulum mainly venous with which are constantly associated some fine arterial branches and capillary loops. The arterial branches which had not been described before are branches of the anterior ciliaries. These vessels, which are generally very fine, run into the deep layers of the sclera and, giving off successive anastomosing branches, form a net with large and irregular meshes which accompanies the venous plexus and is joined to this by means of fine loops of very characteristic aspect, which insinuate themselves radially into the periphery of the cornea and running up to the commencement of the canal of Schlemm not infrequently pass beyond it in a centripetal direction.

This vascular plexus, unlike the episcleral, is hidden from clinical observation, but is responsible for the violet colouring which the limbus assumes in inflammation of the uveal tract.

Maggiore describes four plexuses in the region of the limbus:

1. Conjunctival (see p. 219).
2. The plexus of the fascia bulbi.
3. Episcleral plexus (see p. 219).
4. The intrascleral plexus.

Aqueous Veins.[1]—The aqueous veins of Ascher are vessels varying in size from 0·01 to 0·1 mm. in diameter. Thus while a slit-lamp is usually necessary to see them, the largest can just be made out with a loupe.

[1] See Ascher, K. W. (1942), *Amer. J. Ophthal.*, **25**, 31; (1949) *Archiv. Ophthal.*, *Chicago*, **42**, 66; Goldmann H. (1946), *Ophthalmologica, Basel*, **11**, 146; Ashton, N. (1952), *Brit. J. Ophthal.*, **36**, 265.

They are found near the limbus (about 2 mm. from it), most often infero-nasally and often commencing in a hook-shaped bend where they come out of the sclera. They contain a clear fluid or very diluted blood and run a short course from 0·1 to just over a centimetre.

They join an episcleral vein, the blood of which may become more diluted, or clear fluid and blood may run side by side unmixed. Thus is formed a laminated vein of Goldmann. Sometimes a clear central stream is flanked by a blood column on either side.

Aqueous veins are exit channels of the aqueous, hence the name.

Indeed, Norman Ashton has traced one of these vessels, seen during life, into the canal of Schlemm after the removal of the eye. An aqueous vein is therefore an efferent from the canal of Schlemm which remains separate or nearly so until it has passed through the sclera.

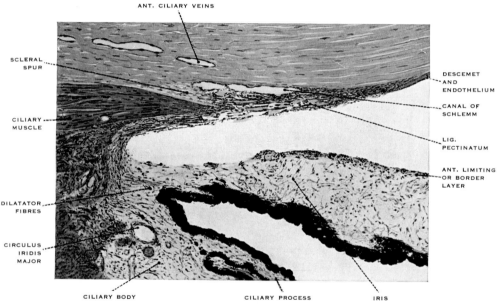

FIG. 48.—SECTION OF THE ANGLE OF THE ANTERIOR CHAMBER. (Same slide as Fig. 28.)

COMPARATIVE ANATOMY OF THE ANGLE OF THE ANTERIOR CHAMBER (THE IRIDO-SCLERAL OR CILIO-SCLERAL ANGLE)

In the quadruped mammals (and also in birds and reptiles) the ciliary body of the adult is divided into two layers by a fissure (the intra-ciliary sinus or the cilio-scleral space or space of Fontana) which passes more or less deeply from before backwards between the ciliary processes and the ciliary muscle always placed directly against the sclera.

In the primates the ciliary body is, on the contrary, compact and has no fissure or sinus, because the ciliary processes throughout their length are adherent by their line of insertion to the ciliary muscle.

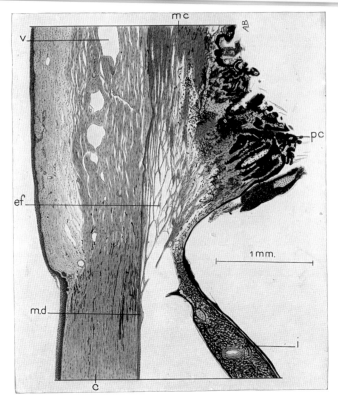

Fig. 49.—Meridional Section of Angle of Anterior Chamber of Hyena.

mc, the ciliary muscle of which the deep portion goes with the ciliary processes while the superficial portion is adherent to the sclera ; pc, ciliary processes ; i, iris and pectinate ligament ; ef, the cilio-scleral space or space of Fontana ; c, cornea with an interstitial pigmentary zone ; md, membrane of Descemet ; v, sinus venosus scleræ.

(*From Rochon-Duvigneaud.*)

This is fundamentally the difference which exists between the angle of the anterior chamber of the primates and that of the other mammals (Rochon-Duvigneaud).

The intra-ciliary space or sinus of the latter is filled by the trabeculæ of the true pectinate ligament, of which the most superficial attach the ciliary processes and the root of the iris (which otherwise would hang loose) to the sclera from the region of the canal of Schlemm to the end of Descemet. It will thus be seen why Hueck described the ligament as iridis, i.e. of the iris.

The obliteration of the ciliary sinus in the primates necessarily does away with the necessity of cilio-scleral trabeculæ and further causes an attachment of the iris to the tendon of the ciliary muscle (Fig. 48), thus forming a cilio-iridial arcade which makes the fibres of the true pectinate ligament unnecessary. These fibres present in the human fœtus (see p. 443 and Fig. 397) have largely disappeared in the adult.

Hence, in the human the cilio-iridial arcade limits the anterior chamber while in quadrupeds this is prolonged through the meshes of the true pectinate ligament or space of Fontana to the bottom of the cilio-scleral sinus, well beyond the scleral attachment of the tendon of the ciliary muscle.

The adherence of the ciliary processes to a strong ciliary muscle which is characteristic of the primates, assures the direct action of the muscle on the lens through the Zonule. It thus makes for an improved mechanism of accommodation. In other words, the necessity of a more extensive power of accommodation has brought about the adherence of the surface of origin of the Zonular fibres, represented by the ciliary epithelium to the ciliary muscle. This adhesion makes for the obliteration of the ciliary sinus and the disappearance of the trabeculæ of the pectinate ligament, which partition its cavity. The more central fibres which form arcades and which attach the iris to the end of Descemet's membrane (that is the true pectinate ligament) become unnecessary when the iris gains attachment to the tendon of the ciliary muscle (to form the cilio-iridial arcade). Their almost complete disappearance in the primates and more especially in man practically clears the angle of all trabeculæ and hence the anterior chamber is limited by the cilio-iridial arcade and the space of Fontana is obliterated (Rochon-Duvigneaud).

NORMAL APPEARANCES AS SEEN WITH THE GONIOSCOPE[1]

The structures which may be made out with the gonioscope are :

(1) The root of the iris.

(2) A portion of the anterior surface of the ciliary body.

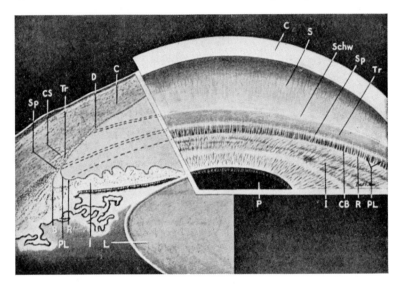

FIG. 50.—SECTION OF THE ANGLE OF THE ANTERIOR CHAMBER WITH THE CORRESPONDING PARTS AS SEEN BY THE GONIOSCOPE.

P, pupil ; I, iris ; R, ciliary border of iris ; CB, ciliary body ; Sp, scleral spur ; PL, iris processes ; Tr, corneo-scleral trabeculæ covering canal of Schlemm, CS ; Schw, Schwalbe's ring ; S, dome of cornea with limbal vessels ; D, termination of Descemet's membrane ; C, cornea ; L, lens.

(From François, after Troncoso.)

(3) The iris processes.

(4) The ligamentum pectinatum (scleral trabeculæ) with the scleral spur behind it, Schwalbe's ring in front of it, and the canal of Schlemm deep to it.

(5) The posterior aspect of the cornea.

(1) The most prominent portion here is the last ridge.

(2) The anterior surface of the ciliary body which is responsible for the ciliary

[1] See Uribe Troncoso (1947), A Treatise of Gonioscopy, *Philadelphia*. Busacca (1945), Éléments de Gonioscopis, *São Paulo*. François (1948), *Bull. Soc. Belge Ophtal.*, 3.

band forms a concave recess or sinus. It has the same colour as the iris, but is much darker (Troncoso).

(3) The iris processes, that is the remains of the fœtal or true ligamentum pectinatum, bridge over the angle and are usually visible as thin yellowish semi-transparent lines which run vertically from the edge of the iris upwards to disappear in the line formed by the scleral trabeculæ (Troncoso). The iris processes vary in number and so the amount that the angle is hidden varies also.

(4) The ligamentum pectinatum (scleral trabeculæ) forms a band which in young persons is bluish or grey, but in older people is yellowish, possibly with pigment deposits. Behind this the scleral spur forms a narrow whitish line (the posterior annular line) while anterior to it Schwalbe's ring also forms a whitish line which may or may not project (the anterior annular line).

When the canal of Schlemm contains blood, it forms a narrow but well-marked reddish line just in front of the line formed by the scleral spur and taking in about half the band formed by the ligamentum. When empty, the canal of course is invisible. Whether it contains blood or not appears to depend largely on the fit of the contact glass : where this presses on the limbus the canal appears empty ; while opposite this point it tends to be full of blood (see Busacca 1945).

THE LIGAMENTUM PECTINATUM IRIDIS.[1] (CORNEO-SCLERAL TRABECULAR SYSTEM OF ROCHON-DUVIGNEAUD) (CRIBRIFORM LIGAMENT OF HENDERSON.)

The so-called ligamentum pectinatum iridis is a circular band or zone consisting essentially of reticulated tissue and placed in the scleral furrow between the sinus venosus sclerae and the anterior chamber. It reaches from the scleral spur to the end of Descemet, a distance of about 1 mm. On examination after teasing of a stained preparation it may be shown that superficially (i.e. next the anterior chamber) near the scleral spur the meshes of the ligament are wide, irregular, and bounded by fine trabeculæ. Deeper, the trabeculæ are wider, flattened, and surround meshes which are much narrower. Posteriorly there are some twelve to fifteen planes. As we go anteriorly the planes tend to fuse, so that near Descemet there are only three or fewer of what have now become perforated plaques.

Microscopically. On meridional section the ligamentum pectinatum is triangular. The apex of the triangle is attached to Descemet's membrane and

---

[1] The name ligamentum pectinatum iridis is misleading, for, as Fuchs points out, Hueck introduced it because he found that in ungulates, on stripping the iris from the sclera, the tissue that unites these parts projects in a series of ridges resembling the teeth of a comb (pecten). In mammals and birds the ridges are formed by large pigmented trabeculæ which cross the angle of the anterior chamber from the corneo-scleral junction to the front of the iris (see Rochon-Duvigneaud). In man similar ridges occur up to the sixth month of fœtal life, but after that largely disappear. They occur, however, in the adult human eye much more frequently than is commonly supposed (Fig. 65). Thus Fritz showed that some can be seen in most eyes if the angle is opened up and examined with a binocular microscope. In eyes with dark irides they are pigmented and easily seen, while in blue eyes they are non-pigmented, very fine, and easily missed. With the introduction of the gonioscope, they can be found in most eyes (see iris processes, above).

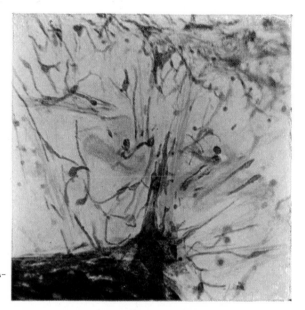

IRIS⁻

FIG. 51.- SECTION ALONG IRIS PROCESS (REMAINS OF TRUE LIGAMENTUM).
It consists of fine connective tissue and pigment cells.

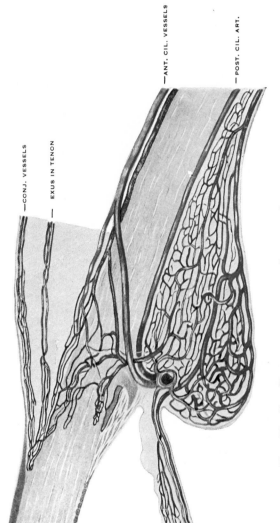

CONJ. VESSELS

EXUS IN TENON

ANT. CIL. VESSELS

POST. CIL. ART.

FIG. 52.—THE BLOOD-SUPPLY TO THE ANTERIOR SEGMENT.

(*From Lauber, after Maggiori.*)

the posterior layers of the cornea or as Schwalbe has it to the " anterior limiting ring " (Fig. 48). The inner side of the triangle lies in the anterior chamber. The outer side is in contact anteriorly with the sclera ; farther back for half to two-thirds of its length it lies in the inner wall of Schlemm's canal.

The base of the triangle is formed by the scleral spur and the ciliary muscle, while the postero-central angle is, as it were, continued in front of the ciliary body into the iris. The triangle is filled with the segments of the trabeculæ which run in straight lines from the apex to the base, diverging slightly. They appear as a rule as little rods of different lengths with rounded and slightly tapering ends, placed end to end. Each represents a distinct plane. Sometimes a segment is oval or, where the section is perpendicular to its length, round.

According to Ranvier, each trabecula consists of a core and a peripheral portion, the whole being covered by endothelium. The endothelium consists of large flat cells whose nuclei usually lie at the bifurcation of a trabecula. These cells are obviously the continuation of Descemet's endothelium but are flatter and larger. The nuclei also instead of being round are slightly flattened.

FIG. 53. — DETAIL OF LIGAMENTUM PECTINATUM (in Figs. 28, 48) UNDER HIGHER MAGNIFICATION (ABOUT 800) TO SHOW THE FOUR LAYERS OF WHICH EACH TRABECULA CONSISTS. (INSET, CROSS-SECTION.)

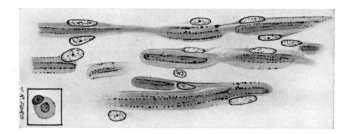

The peripheral portion is hyaline and is the continuation of Descemet itself. The core which takes in a little more than a third of the whole thickness consists of elastic and connective tissue. According to Salzmann (and Fig. 53), the elastic fibres lie on the connective tissue (Salzmann thus described four layers : endothelial, hyaline, elastic, and collagenous). At the apex of the triangle the nuclei of the ligamentum arrange themselves in single file in front of the anterior limiting ring or termination of Descemet (Fig. 35).

The trabeculæ of that portion which lies next the anterior chamber and passes into the root of the iris (uveal part of lig. pect. iridis) are much finer than the remainder (scleral part of lig. pect. iridis), and in them the elastic fibres are absent.

Electron Microscopy on the whole confirms these appearances of the fibres and their endothelial covering.

The holes in the sponge are known as the spaces of Fontana, and on the outer side lie near the canal of Schlemm and on the inner communicate with the anterior chamber.

The anterior limiting ring of Schwalbe (Fig. 35) is a bundle of connective tissue and elastic fibres placed in front of or in the termination of Descemet's membrane. Histologically it consists of the same tissue as the ligamentum pectinatum (scleral trabeculæ) but the fibrils have a different direction : from being meridional they have become circular. The ring varies in position and size not only from eye to eye but in different portions of the same eye. It may form a projection into the anterior chamber (Fig. 50B), in which case it can be seen with the gonioscope.

The scleral furrow of Schwalbe. It should be carefully noted that this furrow is not present normally. It is only formed as an artefact after the inner wall of the canal of Schlemm and the ligamentum pectinatum have been torn away. It is limited anteriorly by the anterior limiting ring and posteriorly by the scleral spur which is the *posterior limiting ring*. The furrow obviously contains the canal of Schlemm and the ligamentum pectinatum.

THE VASCULAR TUNIC OR UVEAL TRACT

The vascular tunic consists from behind forwards of the choroid, ciliary body, and iris, all continuous with each other.

This continuity can easily be made out if the cornea and sclera be carefully dissected off the underlying structures. Such a dissection would show a dark brown sphere attached to the optic nerve behind and having a central hole, the pupil, in front.

On account of the similarity to a grape (uva) of the dark sphere hanging on the optic nerve as on a stalk, the middle coat of the eye has received the name of uvea or uveal tract (Fuchs).

THE CHOROID

The choroid is the most posterior part of the vascular coat of the eye. It is the homologue of the pia-arachnoid, and just as the latter serves to nourish the brain, so the choroid nourishes the outer part of the retina. It is a thin membrane, extending from the optic nerve to the ora serrata, that is, the jagged line where the retina ends. It is very difficult to estimate the thickness of the choroid, for it consists largely of vessels—it has been compared to the corpus cavernosum— and hence diminishes in thickness on enucleation and as the result of fixation. But it is thicker posteriorly (about 0·22 mm.) than anteriorly (about 0·1 mm.), and is especially thick in the macular region (Fig. 151).

Its inner surface, which can be examined by removing the vitreous and retina after opening the eye, is smooth and brown. On separating the choroid from the sclera, on the other hand, the outer surface of the former is found to be rough and shaggy.

The choroid is firmly attached to the margin of the optic nerve, and slightly at the points where vessels and nerves enter it. It is more firmly attached to the sclera behind the coronal equator than in front of this (Moses).

Moses[1] (1965) has measured in the excised eye the strength of the suprachoroidal

---

[1] Moses, R. A. (1965) : *Invest. Ophth.* **4**, 5, 935.

lamellæ and of their attachments to the sclera.   The lamellæ withstood a breaking force of 6 Gm. per centimetre strip width.

Structure.—The choroid consists mainly of blood-vessels, but on either side of these is a non-vascular layer.   On the outer side, i.e. nearest the sclera, is the *lamina suprachoroidea*, and on its inner side the homogeneous *basal lamina (membrane of Bruch)*.   The vessels of the choroid are classically described as being arranged in three superimposed strata—the largest being nearest the sclera and the smallest, the capillaries, called the *chorio-capillaris*, towards the retina.

Thus we may divide the choroid into five layers, which from without inwards are as follows :

1. *The suprachoroid lamina* or lamina fusca is some 10–34 μ in thickness.   It

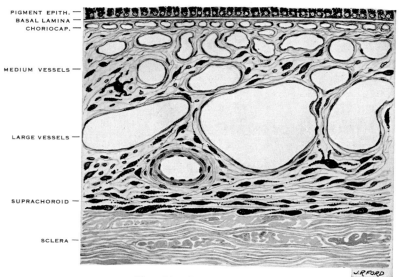

FIG. 54.—CHOROID, TRANSVERSE SECTION.
(After Fuchs and Wolff's preparation.)

consists of flattened laminæ closely applied to each other which limit potential spaces.   These become evident pathologically when the suprachoroid is distended with fluid.   It is then seen that the laminæ join each other at acute angles at certain points and then separate again, giving the whole the appearance of a grill.

The laminæ consist of a delicate mesh of elastic fibres.   They always run from the sclera anteriorly to the choroid and are shorter posteriorly.   Schwalbe taught that these were covered by an endothelial layer limiting lymphatic spaces ; but this is now held to be very doubtful (Redslob).   The laminæ are surfaced by nucleated plaques of protoplasm forming syncytial masses, and there are many fibrocytes containing pigment (chromatophores).[1]   The laminæ are tightly

[1] Wolf-Heidegger in Amsler's *Lehrbuch der Augenheilkunde*, Basel, 1948.

adherent to each other around the places where the vessels pass through them. They are also more tightly adherent to each other posteriorly than anteriorly. Hence it is in the anterior portion that a detachment of the choroid usually takes place.

The chromatophores here are more stunted, with shorter processes than those in the vessel layer. They are more pigmented posteriorly and may be poor in pigment anteriorly. The nucleus is always non-pigmented (Figs. 55, 56). The chromatophores spread out in the plane of the surface of the choroid and are thus seen properly only in a flat section (compare Figs. 54 and 55).

BRANCH OF NERVE
AND GANGLION CELL

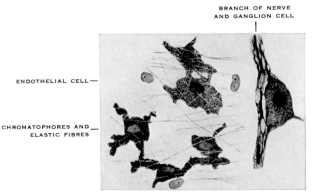

ENDOTHELIAL CELL—

CHROMATOPHORES AND
ELASTIC FIBRES

Fig. 55.—Elements of the Suprachoroid, Teased Preparation; Stained with Mallory's Phospho-molybdic-Acid Hæma-toxylin. × 300.

(*From Salzmann.*)

Unstriped muscle fibres are also found. These are more numerous in front of the equator, where they tend to form star-shaped figures or *muscle stars* (see p. 71).

They have also been described around the optic nerve (Fuchs).

On separating the choroid from the sclera this layer divides, part of it adhering to the former, part to the latter. It is this fact that gives the outer surface of the choroid its shaggy appearance.

The suprachoroidal space contains the long and short posterior ciliary arteries and nerves.

The nerves break up into smaller and smaller branches, which eventually supply the choroid. At the points of division of the nerves are placed multipolar ganglia, which are probably vasomotor in function (Fig. 55).

2 and 3. *The Layer of Vessels.*—Classically this layer is divided into two :

(*a*) The layer of large vessels (Haller's layer).

(*b*) The layer of medium-sized vessels (Sattler's layer).

But, while it is possible in places so to separate them, usually one cannot do so owing to the irregularity of their distribution.

The larger vessels are external and tend to diminish in size as we go towards the chorio-capillaris. The innermost of them are arterioles which join the capillaries by oblique branches and veins that receive oblique venules from them.

As regards the large vessels, the arteries are deep posteriorly but more anter-

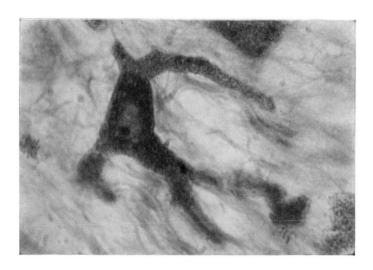

Fig. 56.—Chromatophore of Choroid (flat section).
Nucleus visible (Mallory's triple stain).

iorly they are superficial. In fact, in the greater part of the choroid only veins are found next to the suprachoroid lamina.

The veins are largest posteriorly, especially in the macular region and where they join the venæ vorticosæ after undergoing an ampullary dilatation. No choroidal vein is supplied with valves.

The Stroma consists of loose collagenous tissue containing numerous elastic fibres. The presence of the elastic fibres is one of the great differences between the choroid and the iris. The stroma is especially characterised by the presence of *pigment cells* or chromatophores. These are variable in number depending on the part of the choroid, the age of the individual, his race and general pigmentation. The region round the optic nerve is richest in these cells. The chromatophore consists of a body and processes. The body may be stumpy or elongated and the process long or short, or the whole may be star-shaped. The cells spread out for the most part in a plane parallel to the surface of the choroid and are, therefore, best seen in a flat section. Hence one only infrequently comes across a whole pigment cell in a vertical section. This is especially true of the suprachoroid; in the choroid itself the processes may be three-dimensional.

The cells usually anastomose with each other so as to form a syncytium but may be found isolated. The nuclei are most often round or oval, rarely kidney-shaped. They contain no pigment and their chromatin is evenly spread, there being no nucleolus. The size of the cells and their pigmentation varies; usually the more pigmented, the plumper they are. The pigment granules, *which are of the same size in any particular cell*, are very fine and evenly distributed in the cell body and processes. It is only in the embryo that the region round the nucleus is less or non-pigmented. The granules are light yellowish brown to dark brown; but never so dark as the retinal pigment. The size of the pigment granule is the same for the same individual, but differs from race to race; but always much smaller than those of the pigment epithelium. The cells are melanoblasts.

The connective tissue cells have a very fine and evenly granular cytoplasm which is difficult to make out with ordinary stains. The nucleus is usually oval, but may be round or kidney-shaped. The achromatic ground work is very fine. The chromatin is evenly divided and finely granular. Nucleoli are very rare.

4. *The Chorio-capillaris* consists of capillaries of wide bore (Figs. 91, 102), packed closely together. *They nourish the outer part of the retina.* Unlike the other vascular layers, the chorio-capillaris contains no pigment. Indeed, it is obvious, on looking at any section of the normal choroid, *that it is more pigmented towards its outer than its inner side.*

The chorio-capillaris ends at the ora serrata, whereas the other layers continue on into the ciliary body.

The capillaries of the chorio-capillaris are much wider than elsewhere and show many sac-like dilatations. They form a net which is densest, i.e. with the

A.E.—5

smallest meshes, at the macula. Also here the capillaries have the widest bore and so ensure the richest blood-supply to the cones of the area centralis. Towards the periphery the meshes are larger and tend to be more and more elongated.

5. *The Basal Lamina* (membrane of Bruch ; lamina vitrea ; hyaloid membrane) is a thin almost structureless membrane, 1·5 μ in thickness, placed next the pigment layer of the retina, which indeed used to be regarded as belonging

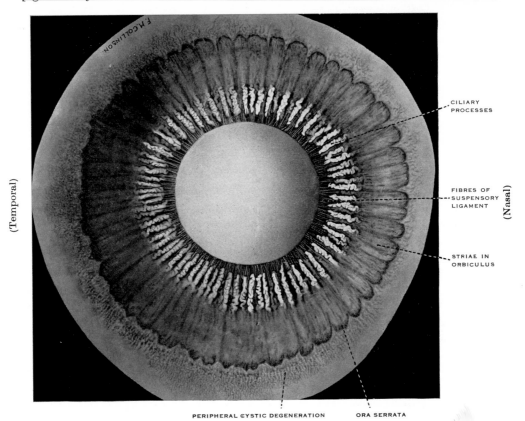

(Temporal)

(Nasal)

CILIARY
PROCESSES

FIBRES OF
SUSPENSORY
LIGAMENT

STRIAE IN
ORBICULUS

PERIPHERAL CYSTIC DEGENERATION   ORA SERRATA

FIG. 57.—CILIARY BODY, SUSPENSORY LIGAMENT, LENS, AND ORA SERRATA (SEEN FROM BEHIND).

Note that the teeth of the ora serrata are worst marked on the temporal side where cystic degeneration (shown by the mottled appearance) is best developed.

to the choroid, since it remains adherent to the membrane when the rest of the retina is removed or detached. It is normally smooth and regular in the visual region.

The basal lamina really consists of two sheets (Coats), the outer (elastic lamina) faintly fibrillated belonging to the choroid, being mesodermal in origin, while the inner (cuticular lamina) is secreted by the retinal epithelium and thus ectodermal. Normally this division is difficult to make out, but pathologically and by special stains it can be demonstrated (Fig. 102). The outer layer of Bruch's membrane gives firm attachment to the fibres which bind together the whole thickness of the choroid. The inner layer of Bruch's membrane consists of a dense network of extremely delicate fibres. When the two portions separate, either pathologically or as an artefact, fine fibrils can be seen traversing the potential space between them. As will be seen later, the layers do separate at the ora serrata, and in the ciliary body a well-marked layer of connective tissue is interposed between them (Figs. 69, 70).

The elastic mesodermal portion when cut, folds up and becomes wavy. It consists of densely matted connective and elastic tissue. This is continuous with the choroidal stroma between the capillaries of the chorio-capillaris (Fig. 102).

It thus comes about that in a flat section of the region the blood of chorio-capillaris appears to run in channels separated by " islands " of connective tissue (Fig. 91). It also follows from the above that the elastic portion of the lamina vitrea may be regarded not as an isolated membrane but as the terminal expansion of the choroidal stroma (Redslob).

Posteriorly the retinal (cuticular or protoplasmic) portion ends[1] with the pigment epithelium while the mesodermal portion continues inwards to reach the neuroglial border tissue of the optic nerve (Fig. 298), or the actual nerve fibres themselves (Salzmann). Here it terminates in a recurved end.

The Ciliary Body

If the eyeball is bisected antero-posteriorly and the vitreous, lens and retina removed, we see the choroid, ciliary body and iris in continuity.

The choroid, as we have seen, extends up to the ora serrata—that is, the rough jagged line where the retina has been torn away anteriorly. Beyond this the ciliary body starts, and can be easily recognised by the fact that it is black, whereas the choroid is brown. If we examine the inner surface of the ciliary body, we see that usually the part just beyond the ora serrata is smooth *to the naked eye* and hence is known as the *pars plana* or *orbiculus ciliaris.*

Under low magnification, however, one sees the striæ ciliaris (of Oscar Schultze) in the orbiculus. These are slight dark ridges which run parallel with each other from the teeth of the ora serrata to the valleys between the ciliary processes (Fig. 57).

Also there is often a dark band just in front, and following the indentations of the ora serrata (Fig. 57). This marks the posterior attachment of the suspensory ligament of the lens.

Farther forward the inner surface presents about seventy radiating ridges of various sizes. These ridges are the *ciliary processes*, and are lighter in colour

---

[1] Where it may present hemispherical excrescences (Fig. 301). These may press upon and even destroy the pigment cells which gave them origin.

than the valleys between them. The region in which they occur is called the *corona ciliaris* [1] (Fig. 57).

The whole ciliary body forms a ring whose width is 5·9 mm. on the nasal side and 6·7 mm. on the temporal : of this the corona ciliaris takes about 2 mm.

On sagittal section (Fig. 25) the ciliary body is triangular in form, with its shortest side anterior. The anterior side of the triangle in its outer part usually

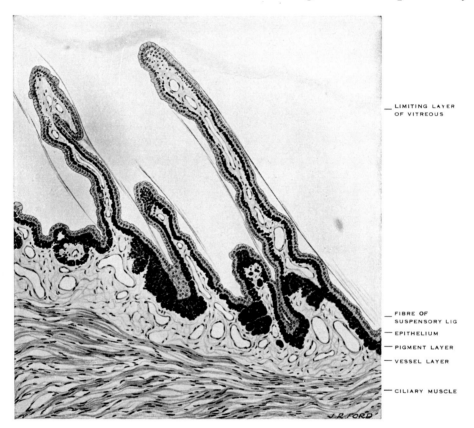

FIG. 58.—OBLIQUE SECTION OF THE CILIARY BODY.
Note that the pigment does not go to the apex of the main ciliary processes. Hence they are white in the living. The ones in between, however, appear black, as the pigment reaches to the apex. (*Wolff's preparation.*)

enters into the formation of the angle of the anterior chamber, but may be covered by the mesh-work of the angle. From about its middle the iris takes origin, and makes, with the remaining part of the anterior surface, an angle, usually quite acute, which opens in the posterior chamber (Fig. 25).

The outer side of the triangle corresponds to the ciliary muscle, and lies

[1] From cilia (lashes), because of the fine radiating folds (Fuchs).

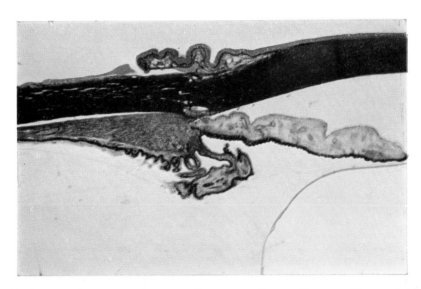

Fig. 59.—Meridional Section of Anterior Segment of Eye. (Zenker. Mallory's Triple Stain.)

This section is from an eye with a small malignant melanoma at the macula. The narrowness of the angle of the anterior chamber is an artefact.

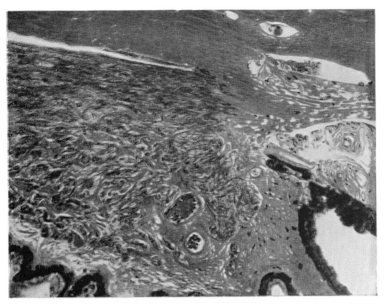

Fig. 60.—Detail of Figure 59.

To show differential staining of muscle (red) and connective tissue (blue) of ciliary body. Note that meridional fibres have very little connective tissue. (Zenker. Mallory's triple stain.)

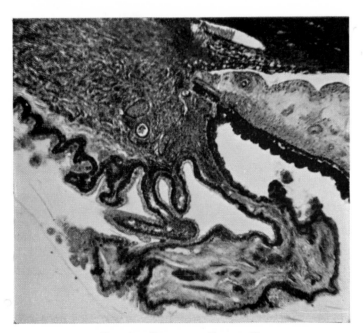

Fig. 61.—Detail of Figure 59

Note large first ciliary process.

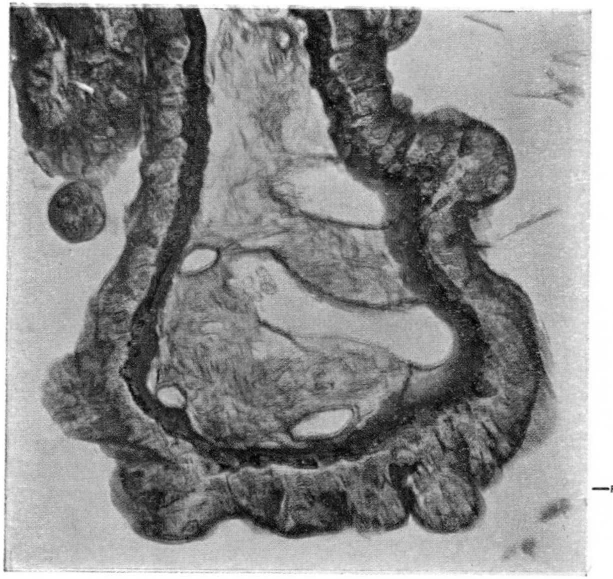

CILIARY PROCESSES
AND VALLEYS WITH
ZONULAR FIBRES

VESSEL LAYER

CILIARY MUSCLE

(a)

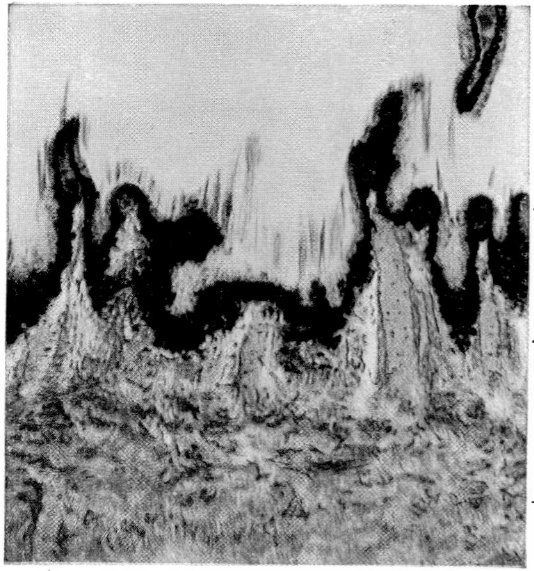

FIG. 63.—CORONAL SECTION OF POSTERIOR POR-
TION OF THE CORONA CILIARIS. (ZENKER. MALLORY'S
TRIPLE STAIN.)

(a) = Artery passing through ciliary muscle.

(*Photomicrograph by Dufay-Chromex.*)

PAPILLARY
PROLIFERATIONS

CLEAR CELLS

PIGMENT CELLS

FIG. 62.—CORONAL SECTION OF CILIARY PROCESS.
(ZENKER. MALLORY'S TRIPLE STAIN.)

Note presence of blue staining, basal lamina and proliferation of clear cells to form papillae.

(*Photomicrograph.*)

against the sclera, the suprachoroidal space, however, coming between them. The inner side corresponds to the ciliary processes, and is in relation anteriorly with the fibres of the suspensory ligament which are bathed in aqueous, and posteriorly with the vitreous. The equator of the lens is about 0·5 mm. from the ciliary processes.

Structure.—From without inwards we find the following layers : (1) Suprachoroidal lamina or space ; (2) ciliary muscle ; (3) layer of vessels and the ciliary processes ; (4) basal lamina ; (5) epithelium ; (6) internal limiting membrane (Membrana limitans interna ciliaris).

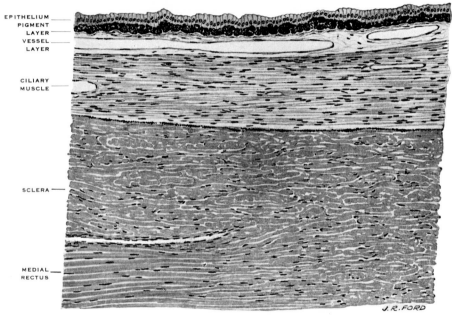

FIG. 64.—CILIARY BODY (ORBICULUS). ANTERO-POSTERIOR SECTION.
(*Wolff's preparation.*)

1. *The Suprachoroid Lamina* resembles that of the choroid in its posterior part, but anteriorly, according to Rochon-Duvigneaud, is more of a serous space.

This is due to the fact that the lamellæ of the choroid and muscle stars gradually lose themselves in the ciliary muscle, so that beyond the middle of the muscle the space usually contains neither of these. At times, however, a band does cross this anterior portion and prevents it being involved in the common detachment of the ciliary body, which may occur pathologically or as an artefact.

2. *The Ciliary Muscle* in an antero-posterior section has the form of a right-angled triangle, the right angle being internal and facing the ciliary processes. The posterior angle is acute and points to the choroid, the hypotenuse runs parallel with the sclera. The form of the whole ciliary body depends on that

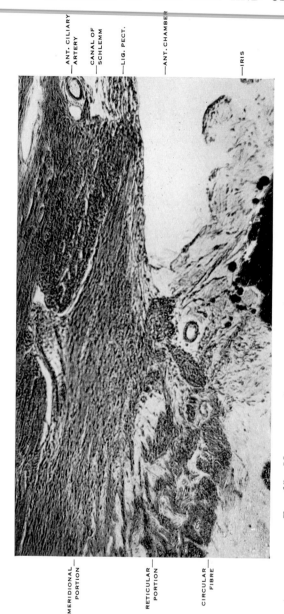

ANT. CILIARY ARTERY

CANAL OF SCHLEMM

LIG. PECT.

ANT. CHAMBER

IRIS

MERIDIONAL PORTION

RETICULAR PORTION

CIRCULAR FIBRE

FIG. 65.—MERIDIONAL SECTION OF THE ANGLE OF THE ANTERIOR CHAMBER.

Note how the deepest fibres of the ligamentum pectinatum pass outwards to give attachment to circular fibres and also to some radial fibres of the ciliary muscle. Also anterior ciliary artery entering muscle. An iris process crosses the angle. (Zenker. Mallory's triple stain.)

of the muscle which consists of flat bundles of unstriped fibres, the outermost running antero-posteriorly, the inner circularly (Figs. 25, 65).

The Longitudinal Fibres, also called Brücke's muscle, take origin largely by tendinous fibres from the scleral spur and the ligamentum pectinatum. Sometimes, however, actual muscle fibres reach the sclera. It is this attachment to the cornea-sclera which is the main union between the uveal tract and the fibrous coat of the eye. The origin from the scleral spur (Figs. 65, 66, 67) is by a narrow tendinous ring the fibres of which pass between the circularly running fibres of the spur and can at times be traced to that portion of the ligamentum pectinatum which bounds the chamber aspect of the canal, with which in fact they are developmentally continuous (see p. 447). The muscle fibres can be traced posteriorly into the suprachoroid lamina to the equator or even beyond. They end usually in branched stellate figures known as muscle stars with three or more rays to each.

The muscle stars are flattened in keeping with the lamellar structure of the suprachoroid lamina and, therefore, appear as very slender spindles in meridional

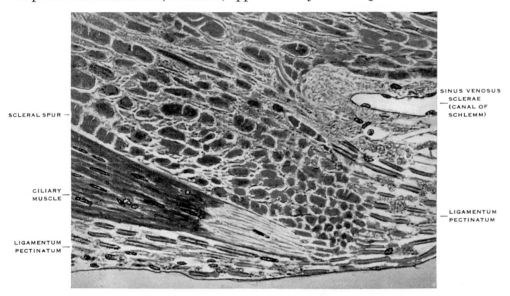

FIG. 66.—MERIDIONAL SECTION TO SHOW RELATIONS OF SCLERAL SPUR.
Note tendon of ciliary muscle and circular fibres of scleral spur.

sections (Salzmann). Their true form can only be studied in teased preparations. They occur on both surfaces of the suprachoroidal lamellæ and become continuous with or are inserted into fine radiating elastic fibres which run into the elastic plexus of neighbouring lamellæ (Salzmann).

Some of the longitudinal fibres appear to bend round and are said to become continuous with the circular fibres. These oblique junctional fibres have been described as the *radial portion* of the muscle. The radial portion lies within the longitudinal fibres. It is distinguished from these by the reticular character of its stroma, but is very often difficult to separate from the circular fibres (see Figs. 25, 65).

The Circular Fibres (or Müller's muscle) occupy the anterior and inner portion of the ciliary body. They lie within Brücke's muscle, and run parallel with the

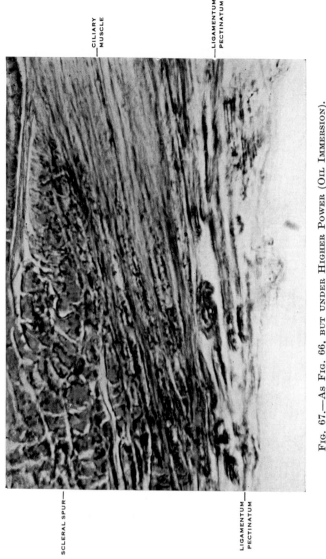

CILIARY MUSCLE

LIGAMENTUM PECTINATUM

SCLERAL SPUR

LIGAMENTUM PECTINATUM

Fig. 67.—As Fig. 66, but under Higher Power (Oil Immersion).

The tendinous fibres of origin of the ciliary muscle are seen running into the scleral spur and the ligamentum pectinatum. (Zenker. Weigert's elastic stain.)

margin of the cornea. The fibres are thus cut transversely in an antero-posterior section (Fig. 65). In many cases those fibres of the ligamentum pectinatum which lie next the inner border of the ciliary muscle pass outwards to give a tendinous attachment to some of the circular fibres and also often to some of the radial fibres of the muscle. As a whole these tendinous fibres of origin form a ring. Passing through the muscle are branches of the long posterior ciliary and the anterior ciliary arteries which supply it. The venous return is viâ the ciliary processes to the choroidal veins and partly viâ the anterior ciliary veins. *The circulus arteriosus iridis major* lies in the ciliary body in front of the circular portion of the muscle (Figs. 25, 48, 65).

The Stroma of the Ciliary Muscle.—In the longitudinal portion the stroma forms thin longitudinal lamellæ which are continuous with those of the supra-choroidal lamina, from which pigment cells can often be traced into the muscle.

In the radial portion the stroma has a reticular structure, and consists of dense connective tissue in which are found blood-vessels, nerves, and, in deeply pigmented eyes, a few chromatophores.

In the circular portion the stroma is looser, and resembles that of the root of the iris, with which it is continuous.

The differentiation between stroma and muscle fibres comes out very well with van Gieson's stain, the former being coloured pink, the latter yellowish green. With Mallory's triple stain muscle fibres are red and connective tissue blue (Fig. 60). The stroma is little apparent in the new-born and increases with age. In the old it tends to become sclerosed and may undergo a hyaline degeneration which indeed is the fate of all the connective tissue of the ciliary body.

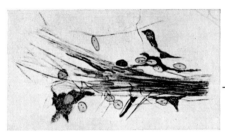

FIG. 68.—A SMALL BUNDLE OF SMOOTH MUSCLE FIBRES IN THE LAMINA SUPRA-CHOROIDEA (SURFACE VIEW). TEASED PREPARATION; STAINING WITH MALLORY'S PHOSPHO-MOLYBDIC-ACID HÆMATOXYLIN. × 200.

(From Salzmann.)

FIBRES OF —CILIARY MUSCLE

The action of both portions of the ciliary muscle is to slacken the suspensory ligament of the lens. This results in decreased tension on the capsule of the lens, which therefore becomes more convex (see Fincham, p. 74)—as in looking at near objects. The circular fibres act directly as a sphincter diminishing the circumference of the ring formed by the ciliary body. This probably also applies to the radial portion of the muscle (Fincham). Now while all are agreed about the sphincteric action of the circular fibres and this probably also applies to the radial fibres, there is still a great deal of dispute as to how the longitudinal portion of the muscle slackens the suspensory ligament of the lens.

Most authors state that it acts by drawing the choroid forwards. When we remember, however, that the insertion of the muscle is into the very delicate tissue of the suprachoroid lamina which also lies to the outer side of the choroid proper, it becomes very difficult to see how it can draw forward the ciliary epithelium to which the suspensory ligament is attached. Even if this were possible it would entail the retina moving forward, which is hardly likely.

Also the posterior attachments of the ciliary muscle consisting largely of delicate elastic tissue seem to be admirably adapted to allow the posterior ends of the muscle to pass forwards during contraction and to guide them back to their original positions on relaxation. They appear, in fact, so constituted that the action of the ciliary muscle far from pulling the choroid forward shall disturb this structure as little as possible.

Now it must be remembered that all fibres of the muscle, no matter of what part, will get thicker during contraction. The effect of this will be to increase the cross-sectional diameter of the whole muscle and make the inner border of the muscle move inwards towards the inner edge of the ciliary body. Thus the whole muscle, including the longitudinal fibres, will in effect act as a sphincter to the ciliary ring. In this connection it should be noted that the ciliary muscle is thickest approximately opposite the equator of the lens. It will therefore presumably bulge inwards most just where one would expect it to have the greatest slackening effect on the zonular fibres.

According to Fincham the general mechanism of accommodation is as follows :

When the eye is in its passive state with the ciliary muscle at rest, the lens-capsule is held under tension by the elastic zonule and vitreous by which it is suspended from the wall of the eyeball, and the zonule is then stretched. Under these conditions the lens-substance is in its normal undistorted form, the capsule exerting no influence upon it. When the muscle contracts the ciliary ring is reduced in diameter, thus reducing the tension of the lens suspensions. The zonule gives up some of its stretch and the elastic capsule, under the freedom now given to it, presses upon the soft lens-substance and moulds it into the accommodated form by compressing it at the equator and in those regions where the capsule is thickest, allowing it to bulge in the thinner parts (see Fig. 175).

Thus, the normal state of the crystalline lens is the passive state : the accommodated form is impressed upon it by the capsule when it is freed to do so by the contraction of the ciliary muscle.

According to Thompson (1912) the longitudinal part of the muscle *takes origin* in the epichoroid, and is *inserted* into the scleral spur. He holds that it exerts a *pumping action* on the canal of Schlemm, which is responsible for the drainage of the aqueous from the anterior chamber. The pull of the muscle on the spur opens the canal and sucks in the aqueous, while the elastic tissue around will pull the spur to its normal position and thus tend to empty the canal.

But thousands of children every year have their ciliary muscles paralysed with atropine, often for long periods, without any increase of tension. This pumping action then, if it does exist, can be of no real importance.

According to Iwanoff the circular fibres of Müller are much better developed in the hypermetropic than in the myopic eye. This accords with the fact that the hypermetropic eye has to accommodate more than the myopic. He also pointed out that normal eyes may show great differences in the relative amounts of the two portions of the muscle.

But Heine showed that if the eye of a monkey, which had been atropised before death, be sectioned its ciliary muscle has the form of the hypermetropic type, whereas an eye similarly treated with eserine has a " myopic " ciliary muscle.

It is probable that the differences in form of the ciliary muscle (which are present at birth) depend simply on the length of the eye, e.g. the long myopic eye has a long ciliary muscle.

The Effect of the Sympathetic on Accommodation.—In the human, as is well known, atropin which acts on the post-ganglionic fibres of the third nerve produces a hypermetropia of 1 dioptre in the emmetrope. This is no doubt the result of abolishing the tone of the ciliary muscle, a state of slight contraction present in all muscles when at rest. Hence, presumably, the third nerve can not only bring the ciliary muscle to a state of rest when the lens is in focus for distance, but can actually make the eye hypermetropic. Hence there is no real need for help from the sympathetic. But that the sympathetic does help is suggested by the following.

(*a*) Cocaine, which stimulates the sympathetic while it does not paralyse the accommodation, does weaken it slightly (Fuchs).

(*b*) In Horner's syndrome it has been found that the near point is closer to the eye on the affected side.

(*c*) Graves showed that in a patient whose lens had been absorbed after an injury, looking in the distance make the capsule relatively taut and cocaine made it quite taut.

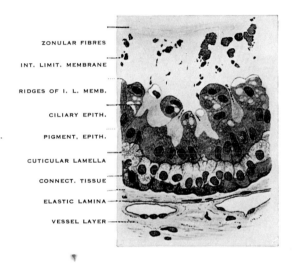

ZONULAR FIBRES

INT. LIMIT. MEMBRANE

RIDGES OF I. L. MEMB.

Fig. 69.—Bleached Transverse Section of the Orbiculus Ciliaris near the Corona Ciliaris. × 380.

CILIARY EPITH.

PIGMENT, EPITH.

(*From Salzmann.*)

CUTICULAR LAMELLA

CONNECT. TISSUE

ELASTIC LAMINA

VESSEL LAYER

(*d*) In dogs and rabbits stimulation of the sympathetic has been shown by some observers (although not by all) to cause flattening of the lens.

This action of the sympathetic is probably brought about by inhibition of the same fibres as the third nerve stimulates and not by stimulation of the meridional fibres.

Accommodation for Distance.—Latterly the idea that there is an active accommodation for distance as well as for near has again been brought forward.

It is said that it is effected by the meridional fibres of the ciliary muscle which are held to be supplied by the sympathetic, thus bringing it (the ciliary muscle) into line with the reciprocal innervation of unstriped muscle elsewhere in the body.

In the human, however, atropin which paralyses the endings of the third nerve, causes a hypermetropia of 1 dioptre in an emmetrope. It would appear, then, that paralysis of the parasympathetic can not only bring the lens to a state where it focuses for distance, but can make the eye hypermetropic.

It is of course possible that stimulation of the sympathetic may diminish the blood supply to the ciliary body and thus reduce its size, which might cause a pull on the suspensory ligament. But, as stated above, it is quite unnecessary to invoke the aid of the sympathetic and, indeed, it is difficult to see how the meridional fibres could in any case affect the suspensory ligament in the manner suggested above.

Lyle,[1] however, states that the radial fibres of the ciliary muscle are innervated by the sympathetic. Knowledge on this point remains incomplete. The evidence is largely pharmacological, and the presence of adrenergic fibres in the parasympathetic could explain the apparent double innervation of the ciliary muscle.[2]

Nerve Supply.—The ciliary muscle is supplied by the short ciliary nerves. These form a plexus containing ganglion cells on the surface of the muscle.[3] The actual nerve endings are, according to Agababow, motor-nerve endings, vaso-motor endings on the vessel walls, reticular plates for ordinary sensation, and arborisations for proprioceptive sense.

3. *The Ciliary Processes.*—Each ciliary process is a ridge some 2 mm. long and 0·5 mm. high, which becomes wider as we trace it anteriorly, where it ends in an expansion known as the head of the process. Its colour is almost white, which makes it stand out in strong contrast to the deep pigmentation of the valleys between the processes (see Fig. 72).

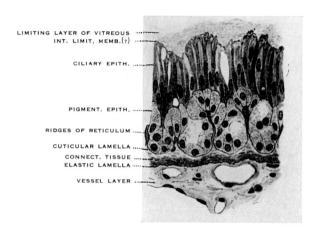

LIMITING LAYER OF VITREOUS
INT. LIMIT. MEMB.(7)

CILIARY EPITH.

PIGMENT. EPITH.

RIDGES OF RETICULUM

CUTICULAR LAMELLA
CONNECT. TISSUE
ELASTIC LAMELLA

VESSEL LAYER

FIG. 70.—BLEACHED TRANS-
VERSE SECTION OF THE ORBI-
CULUS CILIARIS (PARS PLANA)
NEAR THE ORA SERRATA. × 320.

(*From Salzmann.*)

If we separate two ciliary processes, we see smaller dark ridges of various sizes between them.

The ciliary processes consist essentially of blood-vessels (for the most part veins), the continuation forwards of those of the choroid with the exception of the chorio-capillaris. This is the most vascular region of the whole eye, and the ciliary muscle takes no part in its formation (Figs. 58, 62, 63).

In the orbiculus of the ciliary body the vascular layer is much like that of the choroid, with which, indeed, it is directly continuous ; but it is not so wide *and there is no chorio-capillaris* (Figs. 64 and 69). Since also the artery of supply to the whole region passes through the ciliary muscle, the vessels consist

[1] T. Keith Lyle (1958). *Applied Physiology of the Eye* London.
[2] Kuntz (1953). *The Autonomic Nervous System.*
[3] The existence of ganglion cells in the ciliary body and iris of mammals is highly improbable—but they are present in birds (Kuntz).

almost entirely of veins which run backwards parallel with each other.

The ciliary processes are essentially a great thickening of the vascular layer.

4. *The Basal Lamina.*—To the inner side of these vessels is the forward continuation of the basal lamina of the choroid, which, however, has quite a different structure here. For as we trace the choroidal lamina towards the ora serrata we find that it splits into two laminæ, the outer elastic and inner cuticular, and by the time we reach the ciliary body a layer of avascular connective tissue is found between the two. Also the surface of the inner of the two laminæ is raised into ridges which surround slight depressions and are called the reticulum of Heinrich Müller. The depressions form shallow sockets for the cells of the epithelium, which thus get a firmer hold and are better able to withstand the pull of the zonule (Figs. 69, 70 and 74).

The Stroma of the vascular portion of the ciliary body resembles that of the choroid. But the chromatophores are not so plentiful, and indeed may disappear entirely in the anterior portion and in the ciliary processes ; also the connective tissue, in which are found some elastic fibres, is denser and shows up exceedingly well with van Gieson's stain.

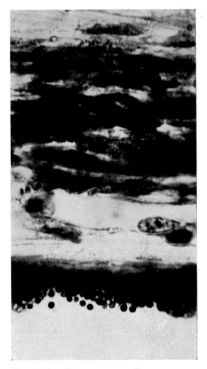

FIG. 71.—SECTION OF RETINA AND CHOROID NEAR ORA SERRATA.

Only rounded pigment granules are seen. But spindle forms also occur here.

5. *The Epithelium* (Pars ciliaris retinæ).—Lining the basal lamina are two layers of cells, the outer of which consists of pigment cells and represents the forward continuation of the pigment layer of the retina. But where the rods and cones cease the cells of the pigment epithelium diminish in height and lose their pigment processes. The cells become much more pigmented so that the nucleus is usually entirely masked.

The pigment consists of rounded granules, which are larger and darker than those of the choroid (and retina). Hence the ciliary body (except the corona ciliaris) is darker than the choroid.

In certain parts, especially in the anterior portion of the ciliary processes, this layer of cells becomes invaginated to form structures which may resemble tubular glands (Fig. 70). Treacher Collins,[1] who first described them, believed that they secreted the aqueous.

[1] E. T. Collins (1890–91), *Trans. Ophthal. Soc. U.K.*, **11**, 55.

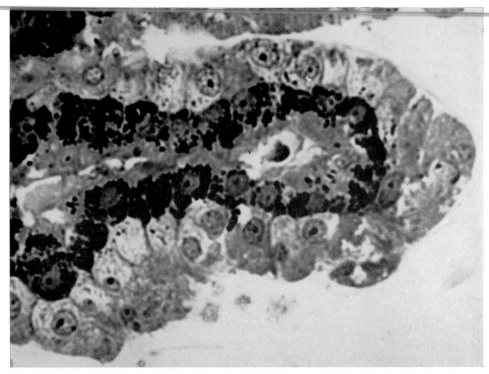

Fig. 72.—The Two Layers of Ciliary Epithelium of Rhesus (Photomicrograph, × 1,500).

(*By courtesy of Dr. C. Pedler, Institute of Ophthalmology, London. Preparation by Mrs. R. Tilly.*)

Electron Microscopy. There is a dense stroma, beneath which the capillaries have characteristically thin walls (Fig. 73). Processes of the pigment cells indent the stroma. There is an elaborate interdigitation between adjacent surfaces of the cells of both layers. The internal limiting membrane, a meshwork of fibres, is indented between adjacent cells of the inner layer. The junctional complexes between cells are minutely described by Bairati and Orzalesi (1966, *Zeit. für Zellforsch.*, 69, 635) but functional interpretations are still largely guess-work.

The *striæ ciliares* and the *dark band* in front of the ora serrata are formed by the pigment epithelium being evaginated into hollows formed by particularly wide meshes of the reticulum of Heinrich Müller. The pigmentation is much less over the ridges of the ciliary processes (Fig. 58), resulting in the whitish appearance of this region. The innermost layer of the ciliary body, i.e. that next the vitreous, consists of non-pigmented cells, and is continuous at the ora serrata with the nervous layer of the retina. It should be noted, however, that these non-pigmented cells are much more firmly united to the pigmented ones than is

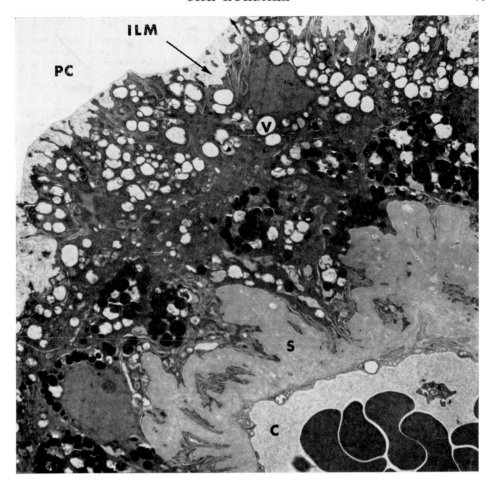

FIG. 73.—CILIARY PROCESS OF RHESUS MONKEY (ELECTRON MICROGRAPH FROM FIG. 72, GLUTARALDE-
HYDE AND OSMIUM TETROXIDE FIXATION, × 4,000).

The capillary (C), with its contained erythrocytes, has an extremely thin wall ; this is characteristic of the ciliary body. Two layers of cells lie on the stroma (S). Pigment granules are seen in the
cells of the outer (i.e. the deeper) layer. The cells of the inner layer show great irregularity at adjacent
surfaces, with infolding (called β-cytomembranes) of the cell membrane ; this is a characteristic feature
of cells engaged in water transport. The pale areas (V) are interpreted as vesicles or, perhaps, sheets
of tubules cut across ; they *may* be secreting or transporting aqueous humour, but this is not certain
(Tormey, 1966, *Trans. Amer. Acad. Ophth. Otolaryng.*, p. 761, believes they are osmium fixation
artefacts). The pale surfaces of the cells of the inner layer are a meshwork that forms the internal
limiting membrane (ILM). The human membrane is almost identical, but in many other animals
it is quite different. PC—posterior chamber.

(*By courtesy of Dr. C. Pedler, Institute of Ophthalmology, London. Preparation by Mrs. R. Tilly.*)

the retina with its pigment epithelium. *Hence (pathological) detachment of the
retina stops at the ora serrata.* The non-pigmented cells are flattened just in front of
the ora serrata. Farther forwards they are cylindrical and over the ridges of

ciliary processes cubical. They may proliferate to form papillæ (Fig. 62). It will be seen later on that these two layers are continued forwards behind the iris, and represent the anterior part of the optic cup.

The transition from the non-pigmented layer of the ciliary body to the pigmented cells on the posterior aspect of the iris takes place *near*, and not *at*, the root of this membrane (Fig. 25).

The cytoplasm of the ciliary epithelium has attracted much attention. Mawas (according to Redslob) has found in the cell refractile granules, mitochondrial formations most marked in the apical portions of the cell, vacuoles containing crystalloids and lipoid vesicles. He has seen changes in the position of the nucleus, changes in its form and chromatin content, all characteristics of secretory cells. After depigmentation he finds the same formations in the pigment epithelium. The mitochondria increase after puncture of the anterior chamber. Diamico has found iron-containing granules in the pigment epithelium which makes the melanin here unique and probably points to a special function of the epithelium. Apart from the mitochondria, Schmeltzer has discovered, in the cytoplasm of the non-pigmented cells, granules which stain blue with indo-phenol. All these facts appear to point to a secretory function of the ciliary epithelium. However this may be, the formation of the aqueous humour is still much disputed. It would seem that the tissue fluid of the ciliary processes, which comes from the capillaries, has the same composition as the tissue fluid elsewhere in the body. It is changed into aqueous in its passage through the ciliary epithelium which takes up certain of its constituents. This is borne out by recent electron microscope studies of the ciliary epithelium (Å. Holmberg, 1959). After paracentesis some of the aqueous appears to be formed by transudation through the vitreous (de Vicentiis [1]), but there is no evidence that this is the normal means of production.

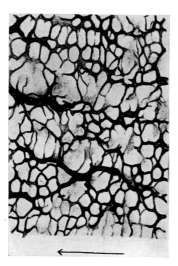

FIG. 74.—SURFACE VIEW OF THE RETICULUM OF H. MÜLLER IN THE ANTERIOR PART OF THE ORBICULUS CILIARIS STAINED BY MALLORY'S HÆMATOXYLIN. × 285. THE ARROW POINTS FORWARDS.

(From Salzmann.)

"A primary fluid whose composition differs widely from that of the blood is elaborated somewhere in the ciliary processes. The composition of this fluid becomes progressively more like that of the blood through diffusional exchange as it courses through the posterior chamber into and through the anterior chamber, and finally out of the eye via the angle and into the blood." [2]

6. *The Internal Limiting Membrane* (Membrana limitans interna ciliaris).— On the inner side of the non-pigmented epithelium is the membrana limitans interna ciliaris, the continuation forwards of the internal limiting membrane of the retina (Figs. 62, 73, 144). It is a very thin membrane which is said to be absent over the posterior part of the orbiculus ciliaris.

[1] de Vicentiis (1959), *J. Physiol.*, **146**, 252.
[2] Kinsey (1959), *Documenta Ophthalmologica*, **XIII**, 40.

THE IRIS

The iris is the most anterior portion of the vascular tunic of the eye. It differs from the choroid and ciliary body in being placed in a more or less frontal plane. It is a thin circular disc, corresponding to the diaphragm of a camera, and is perforated near its centre, usually slightly to the nasal side, by a circular aperture called the pupil.

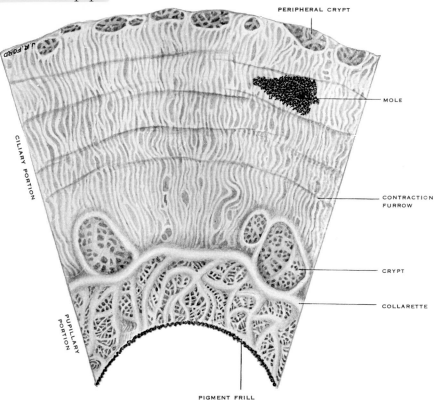

FIG. 75.—THE SURFACE ANATOMY OF THE FRONT OF THE IRIS.

This varies greatly in size under different conditions, being, for instance, pinpoint in bright sunlight and widely dilated in the dark. It thus regulates the amount of light which reaches the retina. It contracts also to accommodation; this has nothing to do with regulating light entry, but serves to sharpen the focus by diminishing spherical aberration.

The iris is attached at its periphery or root to the middle of the anterior surface of the ciliary body. It will be noted that it does not arise from the corneo-scleral junction but farther back, and that, therefore, *not only does part of the sclera* ACTUALLY COME INTO THE ANTERIOR CHAMBER OF THE EYE (see p. 159) BUT AS A RULE PART OF THE CILIARY BODY AS WELL.

A.E.—6

The root is relatively thin and explains the frequency with which it tears away from the ciliary body (irido-dialysis) as the result of contusion injuries.

The iris gets thicker towards the collarette, which is at the thickest part, and then thins again to the pupil.

The pupillary margin rests and is supported on the front of the lens, which is farther forwards than the origin of the iris from the ciliary body. The iris therefore inclines forwards from its attached to its free margin (Fig. 21).

The iris thus has the shape of a cone whose apex is cut off at the pupil. *When the lens is absent, the cone is flattened and the iris becomes tremulous.*

The iris forms a curtain dividing the space between the cornea and the lens into the *anterior* and *posterior* chambers of the eye.

MACROSCOPIC APPEARANCE OF THE IRIS

The anterior surface of the iris. (Figs. 75, 90.)

The ciliary zone presents a series of radial streaks running parallel to each other. These are straight when the pupil is small and wavy when it is dilated.

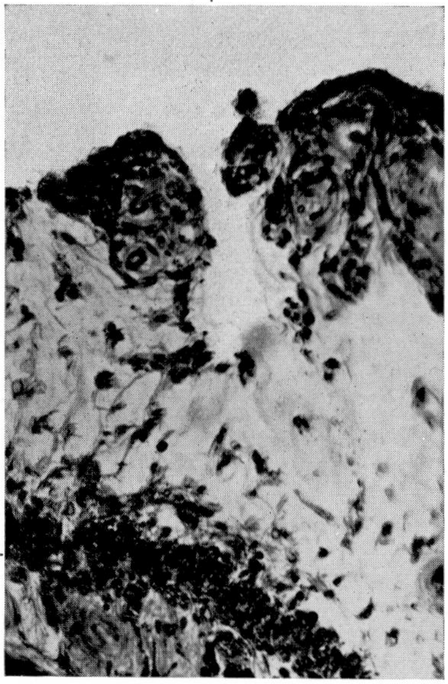

FIG. 76.—MERIDIONAL SECTION OF CRYPT OF FUCHS.

If the iris is stuffed with pigment, as in the dark races of mankind, the anterior surface appears smooth, homogeneous, velvety, the structure being masked by the melanin.

Near the pupillary margin we find a series of ridges, which roughly form a circle, also formed by vessels (namely, the circulus vasculosus iridis minor [1]).

The surface of the ridges is marked by a zigzag line which represents the attachment of the pupillary membrane. This line, called the collarette, divides the anterior surface of the iris into two zones—the outer, the *ciliary zone* and the inner, the *pupillary zone*, which often differ in colour (Fig. 90).

In the region of the circulus minor are many pit-like depressions called the crypts of Fuchs. At these points, as will be seen later, the anterior endothelium and border layer of the iris are deficient so that fluid can get quickly in and out of the iris—for instance, during contraction and dilatation of the pupil.

[1] See Slit-lamp Appearances, p. 245.

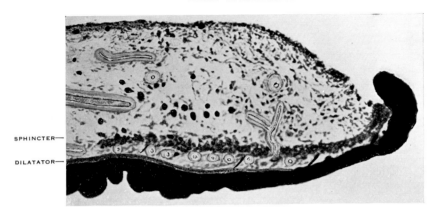

FIG. 77.—THE PUPILLARY MARGIN. ANTERO-POSTERIOR SECTION. (ZENKER. MALLORY'S TRIPLE STAIN.)

Similar crypts are present near the root of the iris, but are small and not seen in the living eye. This is due partly to their size and partly because they are concealed by the margin of the sclera, which projects in front of them. It is only in blue eyes, especially in children, that the peripheral perforated zone becomes apparent as a dark, almost black, circle, close to the root of the iris (Fuchs).

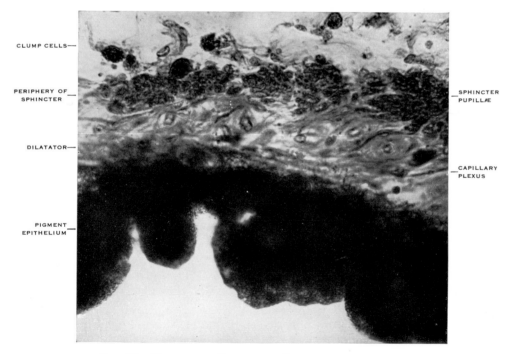

FIG. 78.—MERIDIONAL SECTION OF POSTERIOR LAYERS OF IRIS.

In the new-born neither collarette nor crypts are present. They develop later.

At the pupillary margin there is a fringe of black pigment, better marked when the pupil is small or is thrown into relief by the white of an opaque lens. Under the magnification of a loupe it is seen to have a beaded appearance. It represents the anterior edge of the optic cup (Figs. 75, 90).

At times when the pupillary zone has an especially delicate structure the sphincter pupillæ can be seen as a whitish band about 1 mm. in width close to the pupillary border (Salzmann).

The inner part of the ciliary zone is fairly smooth, but near the outer part one sees several concentric lines which become deeper as the pupil dilates. They are, in fact, *contraction* furrows corresponding to the folds in the palm of the hand.

At the bottom of the furrow there is less pigment than elsewhere in the stroma, so that they are best seen in a dark iris with a contracted pupil (Fuchs).

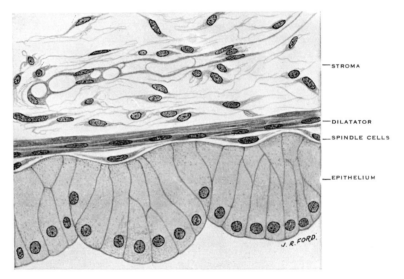

FIG. 79.—BLEACHED SECTION OF IRIS (POSTERIOR PORTION).
(*Wolff's preparation.*)

The posterior surface of the iris appears dark brown and smooth to the naked eye. With the loupe, however, the following fine radial and circular furrows can be made out :

Schwalbe's Contraction Folds are numerous little radial furrows which commence 1 mm. from the pupillary border, wind round this, notching it, and giving it its crenated appearance.

Schwalbe's Structural Furrows—so called because they are present in the vessel layer as well—start about 1·5 mm. from the pupillary margin and, narrow and deep at first, become broader and shallower as they approach the ciliary margin.

The Circular Furrows are finer than the radial. They cross the structural furrows at regular intervals, and are due to the difference in thickness of the pigment epithelium.

Structure.—The iris consists from before backwards of the following five layers :

> 1. The anterior endothelium.
> 2. The anterior limiting (border) layer.
> 3. The stroma.
> 4. The posterior membrane.
> 5. The posterior epithelium.

1. *The Anterior Endothelium.*—While it is present as a continuous layer in certain animals, it is still disputed whether an anterior endothelium exists in the human. Wolfrum believes that it does not, or at any rate only as islands. It is extremely difficult to demonstrate and is certainly not present in the diagrammatic way illustrated in many textbooks of anatomy. In animals it has been demonstrated on surface view by means of silver nitrate.

My own (Eugene Wolff) preparations, stained with Mallory's triple stain, appear to indicate that an anterior endothelium is present in the human (Fig. 60).

2. *The Anterior Limiting Layer* (Figs. 25, 48) is really a condensation of the anterior part of the stroma. It consists of a dense matting produced by anastomosing and intertwining processes of connective tissue and pigment cells. In it are found *obliterated* blood-vessels and numerous nerve endings. The connective tissue cells are star-shaped, have the characteristics of primitive mesenchyme cells, and spread out mostly parallel to the surface. The anterior limiting layer is deficient at the crypts and much thinned at the contraction furrows. On it depends the definitive colour of the iris. In the blue iris the anterior limiting layer is thin, and has only a few pigment cells ; in the brown iris it is thick and densely pigmented.

3. *The Stroma* consists of loose [1] connective tissue containing pigment cells in which are embedded the following structures :

> (*a*) The sphincter pupillæ muscle.
> (*b*) The vessels and nerves of the iris.
> (*c*) The pigment cells.

It is curious that, although the iris gapes readily when cut, it contains very few elastic fibres. Lieto Vollaro has shown that they are situated for the most

---

[1] The stroma, according to Fuchs, may be divided into three portions—anterior (including the anterior limiting layer), posterior denser layers, and a middle layer, the cleft of Fuchs, consisting of very loose tissue. This spongy tissue forms the floor of the crypts. It enables the anterior layer to glide on the posterior in dilatation and contraction of the pupil. The vessels tend to run either anterior or posterior to the cleft of Fuchs. The posterior layer is less dense than the anterior. Here the connective tissue and pigment cells are attached vertically or obliquely to the dilatator ; they also surround the sphincter and are placed radially along the blood-vessels.

part in the posterior part of the stroma and have a radial direction.   Some elastic fibres are also found between the sphincter and dilatator pupillæ.

(*a*) *The Sphincter pupillæ* consists of a flat bar of intertwining plain muscle fibres whose predominant direction is circular, separated by connective tissue containing vessels.   It is 1 mm. broad, forming a ring all round the pupillary margin near the posterior surface of the iris.   It is derived from ectoderm, and its inner edge comes close to the pupillary zone of pigment cells which gave it origin.   When it contracts it constricts the pupil, and tends to pull the edge of the pigment on to the anterior surface of the iris.   It is supplied by the 3rd cranial nerve viâ the short ciliaries (p. 309).

The sphincter muscle does not lie loose in the stroma tissue.   Each portion adheres firmly to surrounding structures by vessels and by radial bundles of connective tissue.   Hence *after an iridectomy the portion of the sphincter remaining does not contract up and the pupil can still react to light.*

There are also two or more definite junctional fibres between the dilatator and sphincter (see below).

(*b*) *The Vessels* form the bulk of the iris : they run radially for the most part, giving rise to the streaks which can be seen on the anterior surface.   Their course is sinuous to allow for movements of the iris.   They straighten out as the pupil constricts and become more wavy as it dilates.

At the root of the iris and near the pupillary margin, however, there are circular anastomoses, known as the circulus vasculosus iridis major and minor.

The former is arterial, and lies actually in the ciliary body in front of the circular portion of the ciliary muscle (Figs. 25 and 48).   The latter is arterial and venous, hence the name circulus *arteriosus* is not correct.

As regards the origin of these vessels, they are derived from the long and anterior ciliary arteries in the following way :

The long ciliary arteries—two in number—pierce the sclera on the lateral and medial sides of the optic nerve.   They run in the suprachoroidal space between choroid and sclera, often grooving the latter.   Just behind the attached margin of the iris each divides.   The branches so formed anastomose with each other and the anterior ciliary arteries (which come from the muscular vessels and pierce the sclera) to form a ring known as the circulus iridis major (see also pp. 91, 93).

From here radial branches run towards the pupil, but near its edge arterial and venous anastomoses take place to form the circulus *vasculosus* iridis minor.

The *nerves* are derived from the long and short ciliaries.   These follow the course of the corresponding arteries, piercing the sclera around the optic nerve and running in the space between choroid and sclera.   Some end in the vessels of the uveal tract, others supply the various intrinsic muscles of the eye.   They are curious in having many gangliform enlargements.

(*c*) *The Pigment Cells* (chromatophores) are of two kinds :

The one type of chromatophore is a slender cell with delicate processes which anastomose with those of neighbouring cells (Fig. 80). They are filled with rounded pigment granules which may be honey-coloured or brown. The oval nucleus is always non-pigmented. Apart from being found in the anterior and posterior layers, around the vessels and sphincter, the chromatophores form at the ciliary margin a close chain uniting the dilatator to the surface of the iris (Redslob).

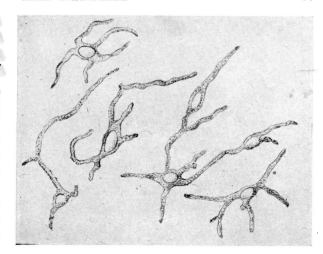

FIG. 80.—CHROMATOPHORES OF IRIS.
(*From Poirier.*)

(*d*) In the neighbourhood of the sphincter pupillæ and rarely near the ciliary border (Fig. 65) one finds the so-called clump cells (Figs. 25, 81, 82). They are rounded pigment cells without processes. Their pigment consists of large, round,

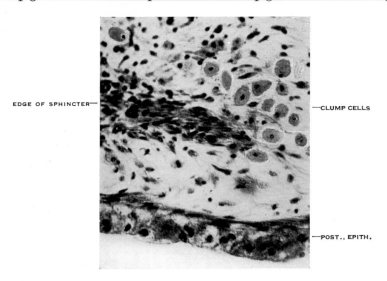

EDGE OF SPHINCTER—

—CLUMP CELLS

—POST., EPITH.

FIG. 81.—BLEACHED SECTION OF PORTION OF IRIS TO SHOW CLUMP CELLS.
(*By courtesy of Dr. N. Ashton.*)

and very dark granules, which resemble those of the cells of the posterior surface of the iris, from which, in fact, they are derived (Elschnig, Lauber) (Figs. 25, 81). They often retain their pigment in blue and partially albinotic irides, and in these

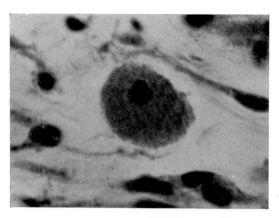

FIG. 82.—ENLARGED VIEW OF BLEACHED CLUMP CELL.

cases can be seen easily with the slit-lamp. When depigmented they are seen to be large rounded cells with slightly granular protoplasm and a relatively small nucleus like that of the pigment epithelium. On cursory examination they might easily be taken for ganglion cells.

4. *The Posterior Membrane*, or membrane of Bruch, consists of a thin layer of plain muscle fibres which, like the sphincter, are derived from the anterior layer of the optic cup and hence ectodermal in origin. They constitute the dilatator pupillæ muscle, and are really the processes of the spindle cells belonging to the next layer (Figs. 79 and 84).

Close to the edge of the pupil the dilatator fuses with the sphincter; also about midway along the length of the sphincter the dilatator sends a few junctional fibres accompanied by pigment (Fuchs' spur).

Von Michel's spur is a similar bundle of dilatator fibres, accompanied by pigment which is attached to the peripheral border of the sphincter. At the iris root a third spoke of dilatator fibres (Grünert's spur) runs into the iris stroma. The dilatator is continued into the ciliary body (Fig. 48), where it takes origin.

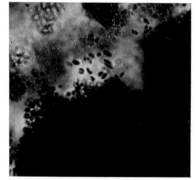

FIG. 83.—PIGMENT CRYSTALS OF POS-TERIOR EPITHELIUM OF IRIS.
Spindles are still present.

When it contracts it draws the pupillary margin towards its origin, and thus dilates the pupil. The dilatator is poorly developed in the new-born, in whom it is difficult to dilate the pupil fully with a mydriatic. It is supplied by the sympathetic via the long ciliary nerves.

It should be mentioned here that the presence of these dilatator fibres is denied by many. As Grynfelt and others have shown, they can only be demonstrated when the iris is bleached. These observations, together with the experiments of Langley and Anderson, put the existence of the dilatator beyond dispute.

5. *The Posterior Epithelium* consists of two layers of cells which are derived from the most anterior part of the optic cup. Being highly pigmented, they are difficult to make out except in albinotic eyes, or in preparations which have been decolorised. The anterior layer consists of flat spindle-cells; the posterior layer

of large polyhedral or cubical cells, with relatively small, round nuclei.

Dilatator fibres are the processes of the spindle-cells which have thus only partially developed into muscle. In the other ectodermal muscle, the sphincter, on the other hand the cell has undergone complete differentiation.

The pigment granules are dark brown, and for the most part round, but some are spindle-shaped (Fig. 83).

After lining the back of the iris the pigment epithelium curls round the pupillary margin, where it gives rise to the black fringe which can be seen with the naked eye (Figs. 75 and 90).

Just as the pigment epithelium of the retina adheres firmly to the basal

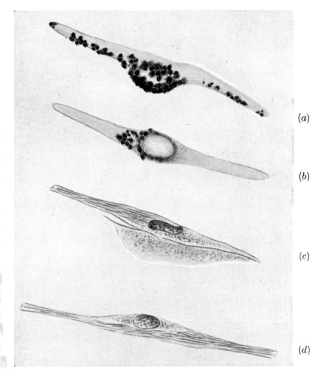

(a)

(b)

(c)

(d)

FIG. 84.—CELLS OF DILATATOR PUPILLÆ.

(a) and (b) after Heerfordt ; (c) and (d) after Wolfrum ; (c) is unipolar.

lamina of the choroid in a detachment of the retina, so, when the posterior of the two layers at the back of the iris remains adherent to the lens in the rupture of a posterior synechia, the anterior remains attached to the posterior membrane.

Thus it will be seen that the iris has fundamentally the same structure as the ciliary body. It consists of uveal and retinal portions. The uveal portion is anterior. The retinal portion is represented, as in the ciliary body, by two layers of cells, but here both are pigmented. Here also the ectodermal cells have become metamorphosed into muscle fibres.

The Colour of the Iris.—Most babies belonging to the white [1] races of mankind are born with blue eyes (Fuchs). The reason for this is that the dark pigment on the posterior aspect of the iris seen through the translucent stroma (which as yet has no pigment of its own) appears blue, just as the veins (although the blood in them is of a port-wine colour) look blue through the skin. As time goes on, pigment is deposited in the anterior limiting layer and the stroma, and, varying

[1] In the dark races the iris stroma contains pigment at birth, and hence in the new-born the iris is not blue (Usher).

with the amount so laid down, the colour changes. If little is deposited, the eye remains blue or grey—if there is much, the eye becomes brown.

The Ciliary Arteries

The ciliary arteries comprise :

    (1) The short posterior ciliary arteries.
    (2) The long posterior ciliary arteries.
    (3) The anterior ciliary arteries.

These supply the whole of the uveal tract, the sclera and the edge of the cornea with its neighbouring conjunctiva.

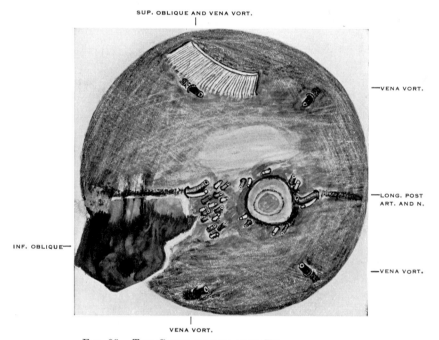

FIG. 85.—THE GLOBE OF THE LEFT EYE FROM BEHIND.

To show the attachment of the oblique muscles and optic nerve. Also the points of entry of the posterior ciliary arteries and nerves and exit of the venæ vorticosæ. Note that the inferior oblique is fleshy almost up to its insertion and that the venæ vorticosæ *appear* to converge towards a common trunk.

(1) **The Short Posterior Ciliary Arteries.**—The posterior ciliary arteries usually come off the ophthalmic as two trunks while the artery is still below the optic nerve. These divide into some 10–20 branches which, running forwards, surround the nerve and pierce the eyeball around it. The majority of these constitute the short posterior ciliary arteries, while the two which pierce the sclera to the medial and lateral side of the nerve respectively are called the *long ciliary arteries* (Fig. 85).

The majority and largest of the short posterior ciliaries, after giving branches to the sclera, pierce it (the sclera) in the region of the posterior pole of the eye (and macular region), i.e. lateral to the optic nerve (Fig. 85). A smaller number and of smaller size pierce the sclera all round but closer to the optic nerve. The canals in the sclera through which they pass are almost directly antero-posterior. The space left free is filled with loose tissue which is a prolongation of the suprachoroid. Some of the short ciliaries anastomose with each other to form the circle of Zinn (see p. 149), which goes to supply the optic nerve, the papilla, and the neighbouring retina. The short ciliary arteries are distributed to the choroid.

(2) **The Two Long Posterior Ciliary Arteries.**—The two long posterior ciliary arteries (nasal and temporal) pierce the sclera on either side of the optic nerve somewhat farther anteriorly than the short ciliaries. Each passes through the sclera in a canal some 4 mm. long. This canal runs outwards, at first very obliquely, then bends forwards at 45° to reach the interior of the eye more rapidly (Redslob). Each artery is accompanied by a ciliary nerve. The mouth of the canal is very wide and may contain in addition to the above a few short ciliary arteries, and arteries, nerves, and veins to the sclera (Leber and Figs. 85, 151). The space left free in the canal is filled with loose connective tissue. The canal gets narrower when traced forwards, but widens again slightly at its anterior end where it terminates in a sharp border. The arteries reach the suprachoroidal space and in it run forwards in the horizontal meridian on either side. Their course here can be followed quite easily from the outside because, owing to the translucency of the sclera, they appear as dark lines (Fig. 85). Without having given off any branches they reach the ciliary muscle, where they divide into two branches which enter the substance of the muscle and

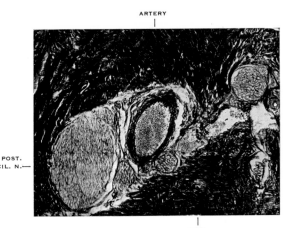

ARTERY

LONG POST. CIL. N.—

VEIN

FIG. 86.—TRANSVERSE SECTION OF THE CANAL FOR THE LONG POSTERIOR CILIARY ARTERY AND NERVE.

Note the accompanying nerves and vessels. The veins are scleral veins and do not correspond to the long ciliary artery.

at its anterior end anastomose with each other and with the anterior ciliary arteries to form the circulus iridis major.

(3) **The Anterior Ciliary Arteries.**—The anterior ciliary arteries do not come directly from the ophthalmic but are derived from the arteries to the four recti muscles from whose tendons they emerge. Usually two arteries emerge from

each tendon, except that of the lateral rectus from which only one comes.   These arteries pass anteriorly in the episclera, give branches to the sclera, limbus, and conjunctiva, and pierce the sclera not far from the corneo-scleral junction, the spot being not infrequently marked by pigment.

The canals through which they pass run almost directly inwards.

The anterior ciliary arteries enter the ciliary muscle (Fig. 65), then anastomose with the long posterior ciliaries to form the circulus iridis major (see also below).

THE VEINS OF THE CILIARY SYSTEM OF VESSELS

(1) **The Venæ Vorticosæ** (or posterior ciliary veins), usually four in number (two superior and two inferior), pierce the sclera obliquely on either side of the superior and inferior recti muscles some 6 mm. behind the equator of the globe. The superior veins leave the eye farther back than the inferior, while the lateral veins tend to be nearer the mid-vertical plane than the medial.   The superior lateral vein is the most posterior (8 mm. behind the equator), and is close to the tendon of the superior oblique (Fig. 85).   The inferior lateral vein is the most anterior (5·5 mm. behind the equator).   Often there are more than four veins.

At times, especially in myopic eyes, they may leave the globe much farther back, even close to the optic nerve.

Their passage though the sclera is as oblique as that of the long posterior ciliary arteries.   The canal, some 4 mm. long, is directed posteriorly and towards the mid-vertical plane of the eye, so that the four veins *appear* to converge towards a common parent trunk (Leber and Figs. 85 and 86).   Their course in the canals can be followed from outside, for, owing to the translucency of the sclera, they appear as dark lines.   The veins may divide in the canals so that the emerging vessels may number six or more.   At its choroidal end the vein has an ampulliform dilatation.

The two superior venæ vorticosæ open into the superior ophthalmic vein either directly or viâ its muscular or lacrimal branches.

The two inferior veins open into the inferior ophthalmic vein, or into the anastomotic branch this gives to the superior ophthalmic vein.

[1] The recti muscles are not in contact with the exit of the venæ vorticosæ, but according to Fuchs and Weichelbaum it is quite possible that the two oblique muscles may at times compress the two lateral veins, especially the lower of these. This is especially liable to occur when the eyes are looking downwards and during convergence.   The stasis so produced may play some part in the increase in myopia, as the result of near work.

Between the vein and the sclera is a lymphatic space which is filled with a prolongation of the suprachoroid.   After its exit from its canal, the walls of the vena vorticosæ become much thicker and develop a well-marked muscularis.

(2) **Small branches from the sclera** correspond to the scleral branches of the

[1] See Leber in Graefe-Saemisch, Handbuch der gesamten Augenheilkunde, 2nd edit., **2**, pt. 2, chap. 11.

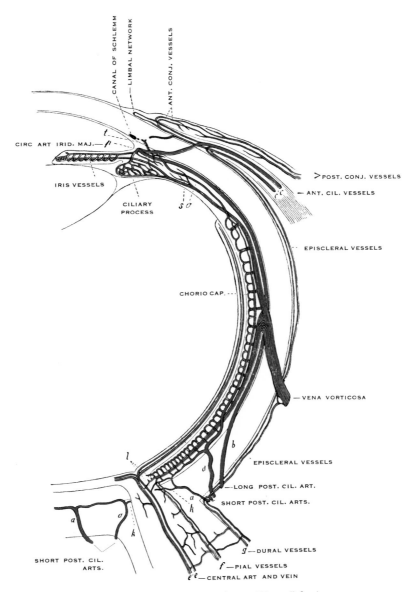

FIG. 87.—THE BLOOD-SUPPLY OF THE EYE. (*From Leber.*)

k = branch of short posterior ciliary artery to the optic nerve.

l = anastomoses between choroidal and central vessels. In the case of the artery this is capillary only.

s = vein from ciliary muscle to vena vorticosa.

t = branch of anterior ciliary vein from ciliary muscle.

o = recurrent artery.

short ciliary arteries. They only carry blood from the sclera—none from the choroid—and are therefore smaller than the corresponding arteries.

(3) **The anterior ciliary veins** are, like the arteries, tributaries of the muscular veins. Since they carry blood only from the ciliary muscle, they are smaller than the corresponding arteries.

Thus it will be seen that the arteries and veins of the ciliary system of vessels do not correspond either in their number, in their course, or in their method of branching. Moreover, very often the arteries are larger than the veins, which is unusual elsewhere in the body. Also the veins, like those of the retina, have no valves.

The Blood-supply to the Uveal Tract

With regard to its arterial supply, the uveal tract is divided into two more or less distinct parts :

(1) The short posterior ciliaries supply the choroid.

(2) The long posterior ciliaries and the anterior ciliaries supply the iris and ciliary body. But the anterior part of the choroid is supplied by the recurrent arteries and these anastomose with the short ciliaries.

The venous return is quite different, being viâ the vena vorticosæ for practically the whole uveal tract. The anterior ciliary veins carry off only the blood of the ciliary muscle. These two systems of veins do communicate. This is seen in the compensatory changes in disturbances of circulation. Thus, for instance, in glaucoma, in which the outflow of venous blood through the venæ vorticosæ is impeded, we see the anterior ciliary veins taking on their work and carrying off larger quantities of blood than usual.

The Arterial Supply of the Choroid.—The short ciliary arteries, after piercing the sclera, lie at first in the suprachoroid, surrounded by pigmented tissue. They pass forwards in a wavy manner and then gradually penetrate the choroid. They divide dichotomously and eventually break up into the capillary network or chorio-capillaris. The larger branches reach to the ora serrata. The arteries in their course forwards are much

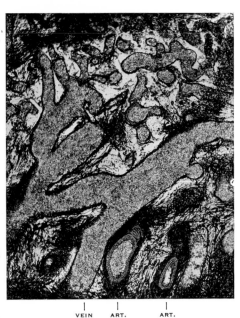

VEIN   ART.   ART.

Fig. 88.—Flat Section of the Choroid at the Macula (Zenker. Mallory's Triple Stain) to show Anastomosing Choroidal Veins.

Note that the arteries have a well-developed muscularis and generally thicker walls than the veins.

(*Wolff's preparation.*)

straighter than the veins, which are very wavy and hence are cut more often in sections, which makes them appear much more numerous than they really are.

The number of vessels in the macular region is much greater than elsewhere, so that here, in a well-injected specimen, an almost inextricable mass of vessels of various sizes is seen which much resembles the corpora cavernosa. The veins certainly do anastomose freely, but the arteries rarely, so that the apparent anastomoses of arteries that one sees with the ophthalmoscope are usually due to the crossings of the vessels, since the walls of the latter are invisible.

The anterior part of the choroid is supplied by the *recurrent ciliary arteries* (Fig. 87). These arise in the ciliary body from the circulus iridis major and from the long posterior ciliary and anterior ciliary arteries before these have been joined to form the circle. Of varying number (10–20) and size, they run backwards between the numerous parallel veins of the orbiculus ciliaris. They divide dichotomously and break up into the chorio-capillaris of the anterior part of the choroid and also anastomose with the short posterior ciliaries. The junction of the two arterial systems may be marked by an intervening capillary network but it is not uncommon for the two systems to be directly continuous, and the equatorial region is not an area of lesser blood-supply as commonly stated. (Wybar (1954) *J. Anat., Lond.,* **88**, 94.) These anastomoses are the only ones between the arteries of the choroid on the one hand and the ciliary body and iris on the other (Fig. 86).

The chorio-capillaris extends, as does the choroid, from the optic nerve to the ora serrata.

The Arterial Supply of the Ciliary Body and Iris.

The recurrent arteries and the arteries to the ciliary muscle arise from the circulus major and from the long posterior ciliaries and anterior ciliaries before these have united to form the circle. They may form a second arterial circle in the ciliary muscle called the circulus arteriosus musculus ciliaris (Leber).

The circulus iridis major lies not, as its name implies, in the iris but in the ciliary body in front of the circular portion of the ciliary muscle (Figs. 25, 48, and 52). The arteries of the ciliary muscle consist of a great number of arteries which divide dichotomously and break up into a fairly dense capillary net which differs markedly in appearance from that of the ciliary processes.

The arteries of the ciliary processes come from the circulus iridis major, often in common with those of the iris. Each ciliary process usually receives one artery, but a larger branch may supply two, or even three, neighbouring processes (Fig. 63). These arteries, like those of the iris, pierce the ciliary muscle. They enter the ciliary process anteriorly and soon break up into numerous branches which anastomose with each other and break up into a dense network of wide capillaries which form the main mass of the ciliary processes. From these come the veins which, constantly anastomosing with each other, pass backwards to the vena vorticosæ, being placed to the inner side of the ciliary muscle (Figs. 64, 87).

The arteries of the iris (Figs. 52, 87) come from the circulus major as num-

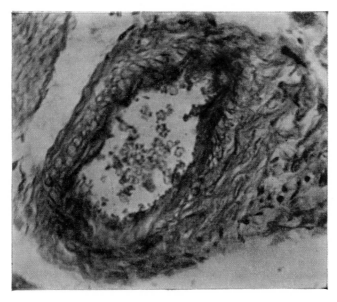

Fig. 89.—Posterior Ciliary Artery in Suprachoroid.
Note well-marked muscularis.

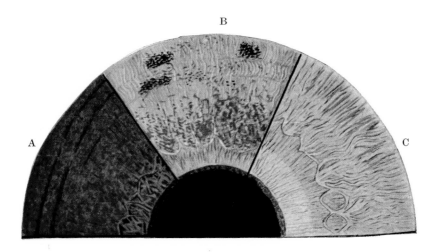

Fig. 90.—Varieties of Human Iris.

A. Deeply pigmented type (Bengali).
B. Medium European.
C. Blonde European.

(*From Mann: Developmental Abnormalities of the Eye, 2nd edition, British Medical Association.*)

erous branches, often in company with those of the ciliary processes. They enter the iris at the site of attachment of a ciliary process, usually several to each process (Leber), and in the intervals between the peripheral crypts. They run with occasional anastomosis radially from the ciliary to the pupillary margin. With the pupil small their course is more or less straight, but becomes more and more wavy as the pupil dilates. They have, like the veins, thick walls in comparison with their calibre (Figs. 25, 92, 93).

During life the branches of the vessels are seen as radial streaks united here and there with each other; more visible in the blue iris, less so in the brown where they can only be made out in the ciliary portion and not at all in the densely pigmented irides of the coloured races. Only in albinotic eyes is the blood column visible and even here only very slightly. At the collarette, which marks the place where the fœtal papillary membrane was attached, a few anastomoses take place. (These, with the corresponding venous anastomoses, make an incomplete circle. A circulus arteriosus iridis minor therefore does not exist. An attempt at a circulus vasculosus only is present.) The majority of the vessels pass directly to the pupillary margin where, after breaking up into capillaries, they bend round into the commencement of the veins.

There is a dense **capillary plexus** around the sphincter and another less dense in front of the dilatator. The capillaries form a loose network in the ciliary region and are but little in evidence, or absent, in the anterior limiting layer.

THE VEINS OF THE UVEAL TRACT

The venæ vorticosæ drain the blood from all parts of the choroid. No veins leave the eye in the region where the posterior ciliary arteries enter (except very rarely in myopic eyes). The small veins from the optic nerve-head, and sometimes from the retina, also join the choroidal veins. The stems of the venæ vorticosæ undergo ampulliform dilatation just before they enter the sclera. They are joined by radial and curved branches which give the whole a whorl-like appearance—apparent on the outer surface of the choroid even in uninjected specimens. It is this appearance which is responsible for the name venæ vorticosæ (Fig. 24). Of the branches which drain the posterior part of the choroid, those that come from the region of the optic nerve are longest and run more or less directly to the venæ vorticosæ. The more they enter the vein from the sides, the shorter and the more bent are they. It is obvious that here the veins do not follow the course of the corresponding arteries.

The anterior tributaries of the vorticose veins come from the iris, the ciliary processes, the ciliary muscle, and the anterior portion of the choroid.

The veins run parallel with each other in the orbiculus ciliaris and then at the ora serrata turn obliquely towards the corresponding vena vorticosa, taking up branches from the choroid as they do so.

The veins of the ciliary muscle mostly pass backwards to join the parallel veins coming from the ciliary processes.   A few, however, pass forwards, and pierce the sclera to join the anterior ciliary veins.

The veins of the ciliary processes pass backwards as a series of parallel anastomosing vessels in the orbiculus to the inner side of the ciliary muscle to reach the choroid and join the venæ vorticosæ (Figs. 52 and 87).

The veins of the iris run like the arteries, anastomosing with each other. Arrived at the ciliary border they enter the ciliary body and join the veins of the ciliary processes, so passing to the venæ vorticosæ.

Structure of the Choroidal Vessels.—*The arteries* show a well-developed muscularis with an adventitia made up of fibrillar collagenous tissue containing thick elastic fibres (Fig. 89).

According to Wolfrum the arterioles possess muscular fibrils with long processes which surround the vessels like the tentacles of an octopus.

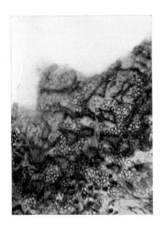

FIG. 91.—FLAT SECTION OF THE CHORIO-CAPILLARIS.

Note the areas of connective tissue (staining denser at the periphery than at the centre) between the streams of corpuscles in the capillaries.

The adventitia of the vessels is more or less continuous with the stroma.

The veins have a perivascular sheath, outside which there is an adventitia of connective tissue.

The *capillaries* of the chorio-capillaris are characterised by their size.   Whereas in an ordinary capillary there is hardly room for one red-blood corpuscle to pass at a time, here there is room for several (Figs. 91 and 102).   They consist of tubes whose walls are formed of endothelial cells.   According to Wolfrum their nuclei are never found towards the side of the retina, i.e. not to interfere with their permeability in this direction ; but this has been denied.

Schaly describes cells of Rouget (pericytes) around the capillaries.   These cells have contractile powers and may help to regulate the blood-supply, especially to the fovea where they are particularly numerous.

Towards the retina the capillaries are bounded by the basal lamina, on either side by connective and elastic tissue continuous with it and so also towards the outer side.   In this tissue endothelial cells but no pigment are found.

Although " bulbiculi ", that is localised dilatations of the vortex veins, were found, Norman Ashton (1952, *Brit. J. Ophthal.*, **26,** 465) could not confirm the presence of glomus cells or arterio-venous anastomoses in the normal choroid.

The Structure of the Vessels of the Iris.—The vessels of the iris are classically described as having an unusually thick adventitia of almost hyaline appearance. This is only partly true and is the appearance given by stains such as hæmatoxylin and eosin, etc.   The adventitia is certainly thick, but if Mallory's connective tissue stain is used a much more accurate idea of the real structure is obtained. The adventitia may be more or less uniform or may be thinner in its inner portion. Most typically, however, the vessel appears to consist of two tubes, one within the other. The outer is the adventitia proper, staining deep blue, and made up of very fine connective tissue fibres, while the inner consists of the essential blood channel that is the endothelial lining, to which are added, in the case of the arteries, muscle cells and elastic fibres. Between these is a relatively large space (Figs. 92, 93) filled with a gossamer-like tissue to which one would call especial attention. A space of this size in this position is, one thinks, unique, for it is absent in the vessels of the ciliary body and choroid, and so far as one is aware has not been described elsewhere in the body.

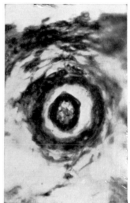

The space is, in the first instance, no doubt associated with the constant concertina-like movement of the iris in dilatation and constriction of the pupil, and thus with the repeated straightening and wrinkling of the iris vessels.

The outer adventitial coat is continuous with the iris stroma, and as Wolfrum points out is really part of, and therefore anchored to it. Such an arrangement, by which the inner tube is separated from the outer by a space, and where the outer is anchored to the loose tissue of the iris stroma, makes for the greatest freedom of movement of the blood current and the least likelihood of its becoming blocked through kinking.

Fig. 92.—Transverse Section of an Artery of the Iris. (Zenker. Mallory's Triple Stain.)

To show the two tubes and the space between them.

(*Wolff's preparation.*)

The arteries and veins are distinguished, not by the thickness of the adventitia which is proportional to the size of the vessels, but by the structure of the inner tube. This is much thicker in the case of the arteries. As opposed to a very current view, the arteries are provided with a media consisting of circular muscle fibres cells), which according to Wolfrum can be followed to the capillaries and elastic fibres in the intima which reach almost as far. In the arterial wall proper one recognises three layers of cells : (1) the endothelial cells lining the vessel, with nuclei whose long axis is that of the vessel itself ; (2) the muscle cells with nuclei at right angles to these ; and (3) outside these again and lining the space between the inner and outer tubes are pale-staining endothelial cells (Fig. 93). (In the case of the capillaries Schaly has demonstrated darker staining cells of Rouget alternating with these endothelial cells.)

As stated above, the space between the inner and outer tubes is unique in its size and width, but it corresponds in position to the perivascular lymphatic spaces of the retinal vessels and to the Virchow-Robin spaces of the cranial vessels. These also are lined on their inner side by endothelial cells. It seems, there-(ore, that the space described above in the iris vessels also probably acts as a lymphatic space.

A.E.—7

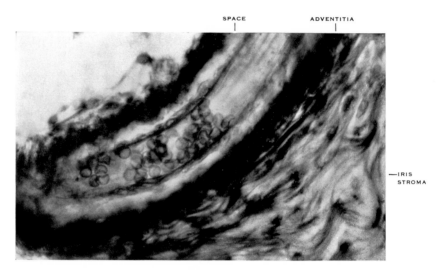

SPACE ADVENTITIA

—IRIS STROMA

FIG. 93.—LONGITUDINAL SECTION OF AN ARTERY OF THE IRIS TO SHOW THE SPACE BETWEEN THE INNER AND OUTER WALLS. ALSO THAT THE ADVENTITIA IS CONTINUOUS WITH THE IRIS STROMA.

THE NERVES OF THE CILIARY BODY (Fig. 94)

These come from the long and short ciliary nerves which accompany the long and short ciliary arteries. They form a plexus in the ciliary muscle. The fibres, which are at first medullated, lie between the muscle fibres. At each bifurcation is a triangular thickening from which innumerable fibrils pass.

Sensory fibres are found and recognised by their club-shaped endings. Vaso-motor nerves are also seen. They are not medullated and surround the vessels of the ciliary processes.

THE NERVES OF THE IRIS

The nerves, which are very numerous, come from the ciliary plexus. Almost all are non-myelinated, but possess cells of Schwann. They form various net-works. There is one in the anterior limiting layer which may be sensory in function. Another forms around the vessels. A third is seen in front of the dilatator. From this plexus the nerve fibrils which emanate are so numerous that each myo-epithelial fibre is thought to receive its own nerve fibre. The fibrils terminate at the muscle fibre by end feet which are often endowed with little refractile spherules from which in turn numerous very fine fibrillæ pass (Redslob). There is also a network around the sphincter. The nerve fibrils penetrate the sarcoplasm and end in a loop or ring (Boeke).

The innervation of the sphincter seems to be in sectors, which explains the vermiform movements of the pupil.

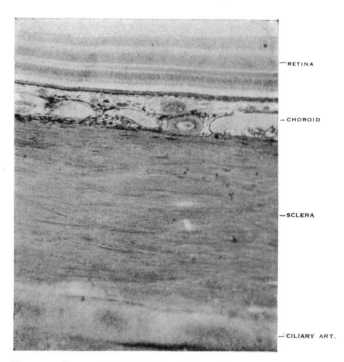

RETINA

CHOROID

SCLERA

CILIARY ART.

FIG. 95.—VERTICAL SECTION OF THREE COATS OF EYE AT THE MACULA.

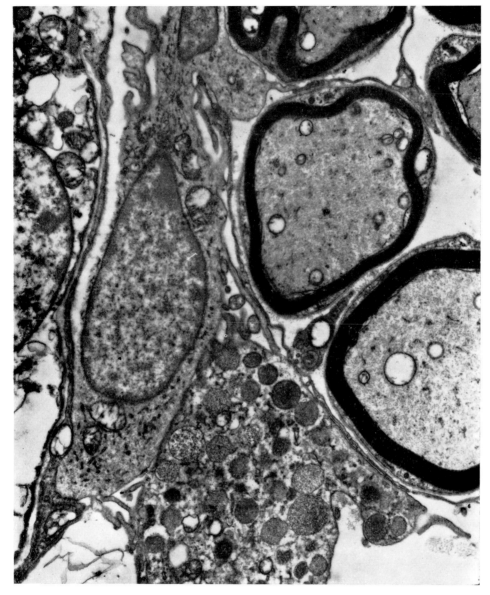

Fig. 94.—The Ciliary Body and a Medullated Nerve (Rhesus Monkey, Electron Micrograph, × 12,000).

Each nerve fibre is medullated. The cells nearby show multiple organelles, indicating considerable activity, but their significance is still unknown.

(By courtesy of Dr. C. Pedler, Institute of Ophthalmology, London. Preparation by Mrs. R. Tilly.)

THE RETINA

The retina is the innermost or nervous tunic of the eye. It is a thin membrane which in the living is quite transparent and of a purplish-red colour, due to the visual purple of the rods. Soon after death, however, the retina becomes white and opaque, and the visual purple disappears under the action of light.

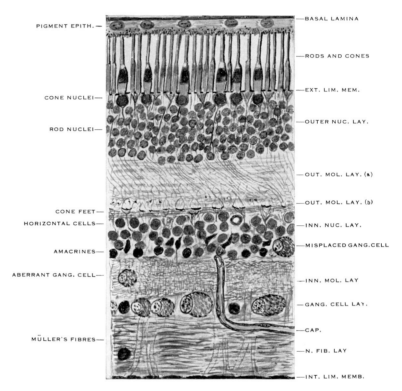

PIGMENT EPITH. —
CONE NUCLEI—
ROD NUCLEI—
CONE FEET—
HORIZONTAL CELLS—
AMACRINES—
ABERRANT GANG. CELL—
MÜLLER'S FIBRES—

—BASAL LAMINA
—RODS AND CONES
—EXT. LIM. MEM.
—OUTER NUC. LAY.
—OUT. MOL. LAY. (a)
—OUT. MOL. LAY. (b)
—INN. NUC. LAY.
—MISPLACED GANG. CELL
—INN. MOL. LAY
—GANG. CELL LAY.
—CAP.
—N. FIB. LAY
—INT. LIM. MEMB.

FIG. 96.—VERTICAL SECTION OF RETINA.
(*Wolff's preparation.*)

If an eye removed during life be sectioned at the equator and the vitreous removed, the dark choroid is seen through the transparent retina. The optic disc appears as a white circular area 1·5 mm. in diameter. It appears white not because of the nerve fibres which compose it, for these are non-medullated and therefore transparent, but because of the lamina cribrosa and the medullated fibres behind it. It also appears white and not pink because its blood supply has been cut off. It is the place where the nerve fibres of the retina pass through the lamina cribrosa to run into the optic nerve and also the site of entry of the central artery and vein of the retina. Some of the branches of the vein will still be carrying blood, while the arteries will be seen as threads or not at all.

A depression is seen in the disc which varies somewhat in position, size, and depth. It is known as the physiological cup. It will be noted that normally the nerve head is quite flat and in a plane with the rest of the retina. It does not form a projection inwards towards the vitreous, and so the name " Papilla "

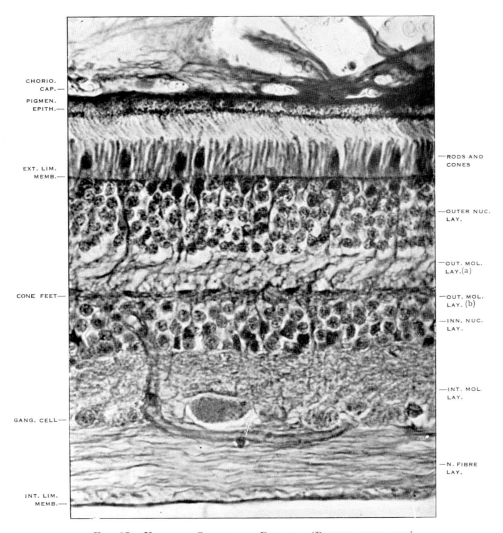

FIG. 97.—VERTICAL SECTION OF RETINA. (PHOTOMICROGRAPH.)

is a misnomer. Briggs, who gave it this name in 1686, was no doubt describing post-mortem material (see below) in which a swelling of the disc is normally present. Some fixatives, too, for instance Zenker acetic, may produce a swelling of the disc as an artefact.

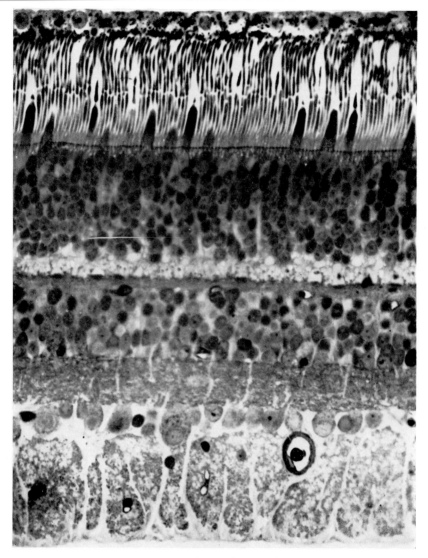

FIG. 98.—THE RETINA OF A BABOON, FROM WHICH ELECTRON MICROGRAPHS (FIGS. 103, 122, 138, 139, 146) WERE MADE. PHOTOMICROGRAPH, × 260.

(*By courtesy of Dr. C. Pedler, Institute of Ophthalmology, London. Preparation by Mrs. R. Tilly.*)

The macula at the posterior pole of the eye appears as a dark-brown area, darker than the surrounding fundus ; and having at its centre a black spot. This appearance is due to the fact that the retina being transparent, the brownish colour of the pigment epithelium and choroid show through. It is darker than the surrounding fundus because the cells of the pigment epithelium are higher and more pigmented than elsewhere. The central dark spot is due to this and to the extreme thinness of the retina at the fovea.

If we attempt to separate the retina from the choroid, we find that the retina proper is attached only at two regions, namely, around the optic disc and in front at its dentate termination, the ora serrata, which extends farther forwards on the nasal than on the temporal side and above than below.

The pigment layer of the retina remains adherent to the choroid all the way.

STRUCTURE

The retina derived from the optic cup is really part of the brain arising as a hollow outgrowth from the fore-brain. The optic nerve, therefore, is not a true nerve, but a fibre tract connecting as it were one part of the brain with another. The outer wall of the cup forms the pigment layer of the retina, the inner wall giving rise to the remainder.

This is the reason why disease in the brain so often runs parallel with that of the retina ; a good example of this being seen in arteriosclerosis, which so often affects both almost equally.

The retina is 100 μ thick at the ora and 350 μ around the macula. At the equator it is 150 μ and at the centre of the fovea 90 μ.

The retina proper consists essentially of the nuclei and processes of three layers of nervous elements placed one on the other, and forming synapses at the so-called molecular zones.

They are :
1. The visual cells (rods and cones).
2. The bipolar cells.
3. The ganglion cells.

The visual cell with its nucleus and process is homologous with a sensory receptor in the skin or elsewhere.

The bipolar cell is the first sensory neurone, and corresponds to the cell body in a posterior root ganglion, its distal process to the peripheral nerve, while its central process corresponds to the fibre in the posterior columns of the spinal cord. The ganglion cells are the second sensory neurones, and are the homologues of cells in the gracile and cuneate nuclei of Goll and Burdach, the first cerebro-spinal cells in the pathway of the sense of touch and sense of position. Their central processes pass to the thalamus (lateral geniculate body) for relay by the third sensory neurone to the cortex.

The whole retina is usually described as having ten layers, which from without inwards are :
1. The pigment epithelium.
2. The layer of rods and cones.
3. The external limiting membrane.
4. The outer nuclear layer.
5. The outer molecular (plexiform) layer.
6. The inner nuclear layer.

7. The inner molecular (plexiform) layer.
8. The ganglion cell layer.
9. The stratum opticum, or nerve fibre layer.
10. The internal limiting membrane.

1. **The Pigment Epithelium of the Retina.**—If the eyeball be divided antero-posteriorly and the vitreous and retina removed, the pigment epithelium is seen as a continuous brown sheet extending from the optic nerve to the ora serrata, contrasting markedly in colour with the black of the orbiculus of the ciliary body. In the macular region, however, a darker area about the size of the disc is seen.

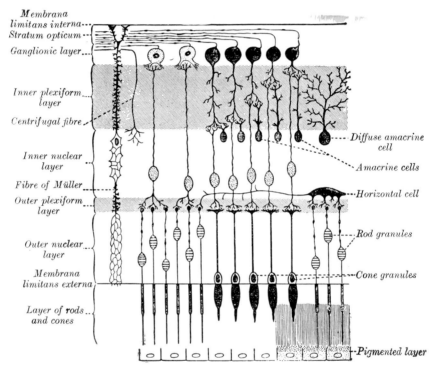

FIG. 99.—PLAN OF THE RETINAL NEURONES.
(From Gray's " Anatomy," after Cajal.)

Note.—The cones ought to reach the pigment epithelium. This simple plan is not confirmed by electron micrographic studies (see p. 125).

Even under low magnification it is seen that the colour of the pigment epithelium is not uniform : there is a fine mottling due to the fact that the cells are not equally pigmented. This is responsible for the granular appearance of the fundus as seen with the ophthalmoscope (Salzmann).

With the ophthalmoscope also, that is under a magnification of 15 times, often a finer mottling still can be made out, due to the pigment in *each* pigment cell tending to collect at the periphery of the cell, leaving the central nuclear portion relatively free (see Figs. 100, 101, and p. 156).

The pigment epithelium consists of a single layer of cells which is firmly attached to the basal lamina of the choroid, but only loosely to the rods and cones. So, in a detachment of the retina, it remains adherent to the choroid with which, therefore, it is often described. Embryologically, however, it belongs to the retina, being developed from the outer portion of the optic cup. Viewed from the side each pigment cell is oblong, some 12–18 μ long and some 5 μ high. Viewed on the flat the cells are placed together like flagstones. They are most often six-sided. Hence the layer is often referred to as the hexagonal epithelium, but one finds cells having anything from four to eight sides. Also, looked at in this way the cell margins appear as clear stripes, due to the cement substance between the cells (Fig. 100).

This cement substance not only separates [1] the cells from each other but also caps the dome of the cell, which is the part adherent to the basal lamina. It thus comes about that, taken as a whole, the cement substance of all the pigment cells has the form of a mould used for making bricks. This is open

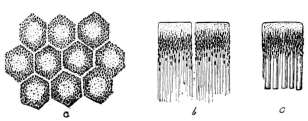

FIG. 100.—PIGMENT EPITHELIUM OF THE HUMAN RETINA.

(Max Schultze, from Quain's *Anatomy*, **3,** pt. iii, 49.) (*a*) Surface view. (*b*) Two cells seen in profile with fine offsets extending inwards. (*c*) A cell still in connection with the outer ends of the rods.

towards the rods and cones. The bricks themselves are represented by the proto-plasm, etc., of the cells. The free edges of the partitions between the various compartments of the mould consist of a denser layer than the remainder and form the membrane which Verhoeff described in 1903 as being homologous to and having the same staining reactions as the external limiting membrane of the retina. This membrane, in sections stained with Mallory's phosphotungstic acid hæma-toxylin, is seen as a broken line thickened at the points of junction of the cell boundaries. In a flat section it forms a net, the holes of which, much larger than those of the external limiting membrane, are naturally hexagonal and of the same size as the pigment cell (Figs. 101, 104).

Following Angelucci we may divide each pigment cell into the dome, the base, and the pigment processes.

[1] Some hold that the cement substance is deficient at the sides towards the dome, and that, there-fore, the pigment epithelial cells form a syncytium.

The Dome is the portion towards the choroid.   It is almost clear of pigment, contains the nucleus, and probably also small droplets of lipoid substances. The nucleus is oval, some 7 μ in length, with its long axis parallel to the basal lamina.   It is poor in chromatin.   The nuclei appear to be of two kinds since some stain blue with Unna's epithelial stain, while others stain red (Oguchi).

The Base of the cell contains pigment and from it the processes project like bristles from a brush.

The Pigment Processes lie in the interstices between the rods and cones. Long in some animals, reaching to the external limiting membrane in frogs for instance, the processes are short in the human, being only 5 μ in length, and do not extend farther than the junction between the inner and outer portions of the rods and cones.   Moreover, the contractile properties seen in amphibia have not been definitely proved for mammalia.   The pigment, called *Fuscin* by Kühne, is brown in colour.   It is present in two forms: rounded granules and spindles about 1·5 μ long.

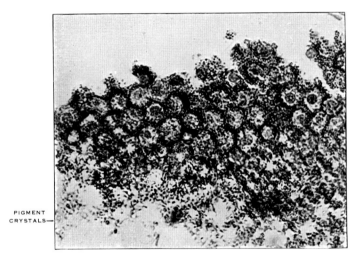

PIGMENT
CRYSTALS—

FIG. 101.—FLAT SECTION OF THE PIGMENT LAYER OF THE RETINA.
    Note that the pigment is much denser at the periphery of each cell, leaving the central nuclear portion almost free, and so appears as a network.   This pattern can at times be made out with the ophthalmoscope (see p. 156).

The rounded granules are found in the base of the cell.   The spindles are found in the processes.   Their elongated form, which makes them different from the pigment of the choroid, immediately stamps any pigment, for instance in pathological processes, as retinal.   At the macula the spindle form predominates, while as we travel towards the periphery the order becomes reversed (Fig. 62). But there are spindles, although very few, both in the pars ciliaris retinæ and the pars iridica retinæ (Fig. 83).

The pigment granules are present in albinos but are colourless. So also during development there are colourless fore-runners. A similar state of affairs is seen in the colourless chromatophores of the white races of mankind at the limbus. In all these the granules can be demonstrated by the dopa reaction or silver stains (see Raehlmann).

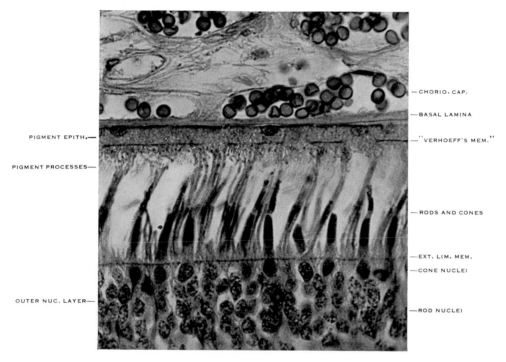

FIG. 102.—VERTICAL SECTION OF THE OUTER PART OF THE RETINA AND INNER PART OF CHOROID. (ZENKER. PHOSPHOTUNG. HÆM.)

Note that to the right of the figure and in the centre where the basal lamina has become artificially detached from the pigment epithelium, its dual nature is clearly seen. Note also " Verhoeff's membrane."

(*Wolff's preparation.*)

Fuscin differs from the melanin of the choroid in its greater resistance to heat and chemicals. It is, however, more easily affected by light which bleaches it in the presence of acid. Under the ultra-microscope the round granules are deep reddish brown ; the spindles, light yellowish brown.

Eichner (1958) considers the pigment granules to be of lipoid nature, and believes that during dark adaptation they pass into the outer segments of the visual cells—thus the pigment actually has a visual function (Fig. 106).

This is not confirmed by electron micrographs (Fig. 103), which show pigment-cell processes with pigment spindles therein ; but these lie between and not within the outer segments.

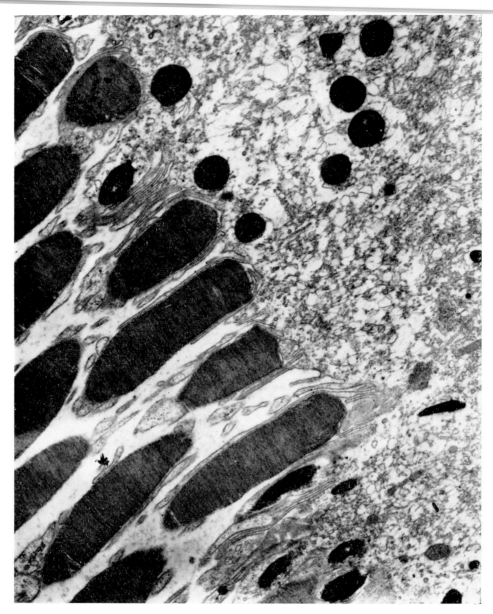

Fig. 103.—Pigment Epithelium and Outer Visual Segments. (Electron Micrograph, Somewhat Oblique, of the Baboon Retina shown in Fig. 98. × 14,000).

Processes of the pigment cells, some containing pigment spindles, project between the outer segments.

(*By courtesy of Dr. C. Pedler, Institute of Ophthalmology, London. Preparation by Mrs. R. Tilly.*)

At the macula the pigment cells are higher (11–14 μ) and narrower (9–11 μ), hence the darker colour of this region.

Near the ora serrata exceptionally large cells, some 60 μ in diameter, occur. They may have several nuclei. Here there are often changes like those which occur in mild choroiditis : partly a disappearance, partly a hyperplasia of the pigment epithelium and a fusion of it with the retina (Salzmann).

At the optic nerve the pigment epithelium does not reach quite as far as the basal lamina of the choroid (Fig. 298). The terminal cells may be somewhat depigmented or may be heaped up. In this case they form the so-called " choroidal " ring at the edge of the disc (Fig. 171).

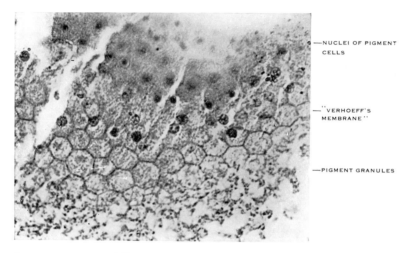

—NUCLEI OF PIGMENT CELLS

—"VERHOEFF'S MEMBRANE"

—PIGMENT GRANULES

FIG. 104.—FLAT (ALMOST TANGENTIAL) SECTION OF THE PIGMENT EPITHELIUM OF THE RETINA TO SHOW " VERHOEFF'S MEMBRANE."

2. **The Visual Cells,** i.e. the rods and cones, constitute the true receptive part of the retina, the remainder being for the transmission of the impulse. Both rods and cones may be called " Neuro-epithelium," designating a specialised form of epithelium capable of transforming physical energy into a nerve impulse, similar to the hair cells in the internal ear or the epithelial cells of taste buds. They transmit the impulse by synapse to the bipolar cells, in the outer molecular zone. The rods and cones are placed in a palisade-like manner on the external limiting membrane, which gives this layer under the low power of the microscope a characteristic finely striated appearance at right angles to the choroid.

Transformation of light energy into the (visual) nerve impulse depends on breakdown of a " visual " pigment contained in the visual cells of the neuro-epithelium. The rods contain *visual purple*, known as *rhodopsin*, which combines vitamin-A with protein. Rhodopsin functions for vision in a dim light and for the registration of movement at the periphery of the visual field.

The cones contain no visual purple. They register acute vision in bright light, and there is good evidence that a pigment takes part in the process. *Iodopsin* is the name given to the visual pigment thought to be present in the cones (in far less concentration than the rhodopsin of the rods).   It is a vitamin-A protein, like rhodopsin, but the protein part is slightly different.   Much ignorance still exists, and current views incline to regarding rhodopsin and iodopsin and other visual pigments as " belonging to one variable family ", as they cannot be distinguished by any single physical or chemical test (Dartnall, H. J. A. and Lythgoe, J. N.—Ciba Symposium on Colour Vision, 1965. *J. & A. Churchill Ltd.*).

Indeed, electron microscopy in its present state of progress suggests that " the concept of the ' rod ' and ' cone ' no longer fits the morphological facts well enough, and is due for replacement ".   In particular the one-to-one synapse between cones and bipolar cells while actual in places appears to be far from universal.   The foveal cones of man may have rod-like form, but stain like cones ; yet they have complex (i.e. multichannel) feet (Pedler, C. 1965, *ibid*.).   Electron microscopy, in current interpretation and understanding, is not yet in a position to be iconoclastic, and the hitherto accepted views based on light microscopy are meanwhile retained in this edition.

Each *rod*, whose length varies from 40 μ to 60 μ, consists of two segments, an outer and an inner.   The outer is cylindrical, highly refractile, and transversely striated, and contains the visual purple.   It is surrounded by a very fine sheath of neurokeratin.   The outer segment stains with osmic acid ; the inner segment takes on nuclear stains.   Apart from this, a longitudinal striation can also be made out.   This, according to Schultze, is due to furrows, which lodge the processes of the pigment epithelium.

The inner segment is slightly thicker than the outer.   In the fresh state its protoplasm is transparent and homogeneous, but soon after death becomes finely granular.

A longitudinal striation seen near the external limiting membrane is due to the fibre baskets of Schultze formed by an extension of this membrane (see below).

Held describes a diplosome near the outer end of the inner member, which sends an *outer thread* through the outer member, and an *inner thread* to the external limiting layer (Fig. 115).

From the inner end of each rod runs a thin varicose *rod fibre* which passes through the external limiting membrane (Figs. 99, 105), swells out into its densely staining nucleus, the *rod granule*, in the outer nuclear layer, and then terminates in a small end knob in the outer molecular layer, where dendrites of the bipolar cells arborise round it.

According to Balbuena, the terminal spherules of the rods are in contact with the cone feet.   In certain regions where the cones are surrounded by a palisade of rods, one sees a bunch of spherules enveloping the cone feet.

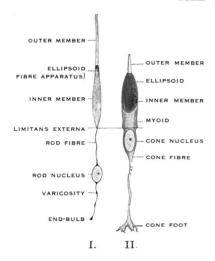

OUTER MEMBER

ELLIPSOID
FIBRE APPARATUS)

INNER MEMBER

LIMITANS EXTERNA

ROD FIBRE

ROD NUCLEUS

VARICOSITY

END-BULB

OUTER MEMBER

ELLIPSOID

INNER MEMBER

MYOID

CONE NUCLEUS

CONE FIBRE

CONE FOOT

I.   II.

FIG. 105.—HUMAN ROD (I) AND CONE (II).
(*After Greeff.*)

Note.—Outer member of cone ought to be longer.

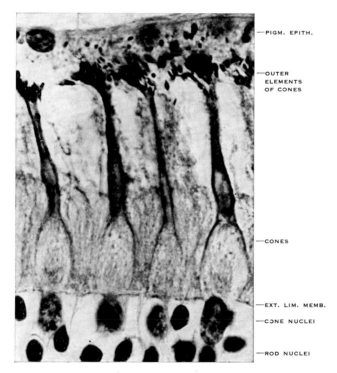

PIGM. EPITH.

OUTER
ELEMENTS
OF CONES

CONES

EXT. LIM. MEMB.

CONE NUCLEI

ROD NUCLEI

FIG. 106.—THE PASSAGE OF RETINAL PIGMENT INTO THE CONES.
The funnel-shaped expansions of the outer elements are receiving pigment spindles.

(PHOTOMICROGRAPH OF "DARK-ADAPTED" HUMAN RETINA.)

(*D. Eichner: Zeitschrift für Zellforschung.*, 1958.)

The Visual Purple is absent in the rods in a zone 3–4 mm. wide at the ora serrata. It is also, of course, missing at the fovea centralis, where there are no rods. The whole of a retina which has just been removed from an eye kept in the dark will therefore appear purplish red except at these places.

The visual purple bleaches rapidly after death.

Each *cone*, whose length varies from 85 μ at the fovea to 40 μ at the periphery, also consists of two segments. Classically the outer segment of the cone is described as conical in shape and much shorter than that of the rod (Fig. 114, A and B), but it has, however, been shown that the outer segment of the cone is much like that of the rod (Fig. 98), only it is very much more fragile. It does, in fact, reach to the pigment epithelium everywhere in the fundus and not only in the macular region. It contains no visual purple. But Eichner (1958) shows that *during dark adaptation* in man the outer segment of the cone is an expanded funnel lying in contact with the surface of a pigment cell and directly absorbing pigment granules (Fig. 106). The lipoid from the granules lies in zones which produce the cross-striations seen in the outer segment. In its passage through the cones this altered pigment takes on a "visual-receptor" function, being presumably elaborated into the visual pigment (iodopsin) of the cones (but see p. 107).

The inner portion of the cone is bulged, and unlike the rod is directly continuous with its nucleus, the cone granule staining differently from the rod granule, and situated just on the inner side of the external limiting membrane (Figs. 96, 102, 122). Striation, etc., is like that of the rods. The shape of the cones varies greatly, depending on which part of the retina they come from (see Macular Cones).

The stout cone fibre runs from the nucleus to end in the *cone foot* provided with lateral processes which arborise with the dendrites of the bipolar cells in the outer molecular layer.

The visual cells with their nuclei and processes are not vascularised but get their nourishment from the chorio-capillaris.

According to Østerberg there are 147,300 cones per sq. mm. at the fovea. At the point where the rods commence, that is at 130 μ from the centre of the fovea, there are 74,800 cones per sq. mm. ; 3 mm. farther 6,000 cones per sq. mm., and 10 mm. from the fovea about 4,000. There is a ring-shaped zone 5-6 mm. from the fovea where the rods are most numerous (160,000 per sq. mm.). (See Livingston, *Trans. O.S.U.K.*, 1943.)

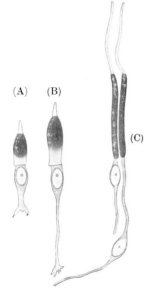

(A)   (B)

(C)

Fig. 114.—Human Cones from different Areas of the Retina.

A = from near the ora serrata. B = from midway between ora and disc. C = from the fovea centralis.

(*After Greeff.*)

Note.—The outer member in A and B ought to be longer.

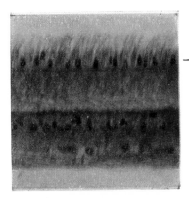 RODS AND
— CONES

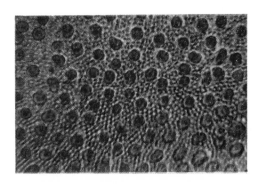

FIG. 107.—DIFFERENTIAL STAIN-
ING OF RODS AND CONES. (ZENKER.
MALLORY.)

Inner ends of cones red ; rods
blue.

FIG. 108.—DIFFERENTIAL STAINING OF RODS
AND CONES. (MALLORY'S TRIPLE STAIN.)

Cones larger and red ; rods smaller and blue.

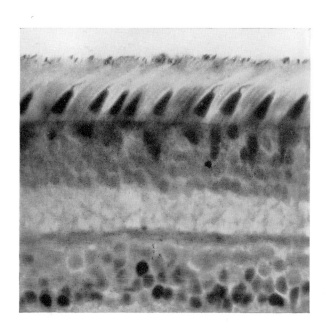

FIG. 109.—DIFFERENTIAL STAINING OF RODS AND CONES OF RHESUS MONKEY. (WEIGERT-PAL.)

Inner segment of the cones stains well.

Fig. 110   Fig. 111 *Trans. Section.*

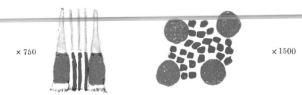

× 750   × 1500

DIFFERENTIAL STAINING OF RODS AND CONES. (ZENKER. MALLORY'S TRIPLE STAIN.)
Cones red; rods blue.

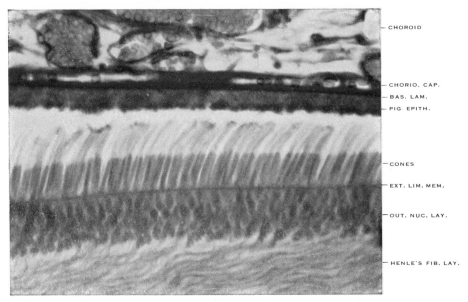

— CHOROID

— CHORIO. CAP.
— BAS. LAM.
— PIG. EPITH.

— CONES

— EXT. LIM. MEM.

— OUT. NUC. LAY.

— HENLE'S FIB. LAY.

FIG. 112.—VERTICAL SECTION OF THE OUTER PART OF THE RETINA AND INNER PART OF CHOROID AT
THE MACULA. (ZENKER. MALLORY'S TRIPLE STAIN.)

Note that the cones here look like rods but stain like cones. The space between the pigment
epithelium and the outer part of the cones is an artefact. (*Photomicrograph.*)

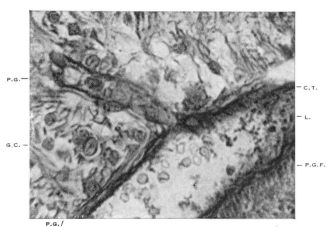

P.G.—

G.C.—

— C.T.

— L.

— P.G.F.

P.G./

FIG. 113.—FLAT SECTION OF THE GANGLION LAYER OF THE RETINA. × 600.
(ZENKER. MALLORY'S TRIPLE STAIN.)

To show the perivascularis gliæ (stained red). P.G. = perivascularis gliæ; P.G.F. = perivascularis gliæ
and feet of glial fibres; G.C. = ganglion cell; C.T. = connective tissue in wall of vessel (stained blue);
L. = lumen of vessel. (*Photomicrograph.*)

[A.E.—113

Actually they are densest directly below the disc, i.e. 170,000 per sq. mm.

From here to the periphery the rods become less dense, but are more plentiful in the upper nasal portion of the retina than in the lower temporal (23,000 to 50,000 per sq. mm.).

The total number of cones is about 7 millions while the rods number about 125 millions.

Differential Staining of the Rods and Cones.—Kolmer, who has done most work on the differential staining of the neuro-epithelium, after stating that he does not believe that there are transition forms between rods and cones, writes :

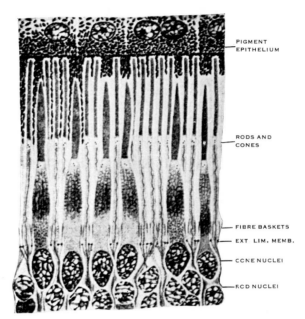

FIG. 115.—VERTICAL SECTION OF RETINA, STAINED MOLYBDIC ACID HÆMATOXYLIN.

(*From the Kurzes Handbuch.*

PIGMENT EPITHELIUM

RODS AND CONES

FIBRE BASKETS

EXT. LIM. MEMB.

CONE NUCLEI

ROD NUCLEI

" By means of certain stains, for instance Unna's Orcein-polychrome methylene blue-tannin stain, I succeeded in the human and many animals in colouring the outer limbs of the cones deep blue, while the rods were entirely uncoloured—which indicates a physico-chemical difference between the two.

" With Mallory's stain and often with Heidenhain's azan a distinct difference is seen in the cone and rod nuclei, for the former stain red with fuchsin, while the latter stain orange.

" The above differences can already be made out in cyclostomes, for instance in Petromyzon, as distinctly as in the human.

" That the cones are made of different material from the rods I was also able to demonstrate in man and the primates in the following way. After fixation in

A.E.—8

chrome-containing fluids and treatment with nascent chlorine, Unna's epithelial stain coloured the inner and outer portions of cones a deep blue (with Wasserblau), while the inner and outer portions of the rods were coloured red (with safranin).

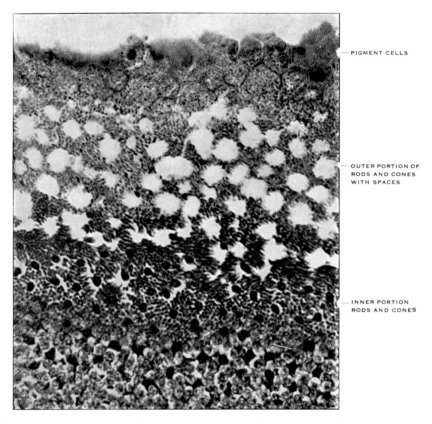

FIG. 116.—FLAT (ALMOST TANGENTIAL) SECTION OF THE OUTER PORTION OF THE RETINA TO SHOW THE SPACES BETWEEN THE OUTER PORTIONS OF THE RODS AND CONES.

(*From the Proc. Roy. Soc. Med.*, 1938, **31**, 1101.)

" Shaffer, indeed, showed as early as 1890 that after fixation by Kulschitsky's fluid and staining in a similar way to Weigert's method for medullated nerve fibres (see Fig. 109), he coloured the cones and cone fibres electively in the human retina.

" Also in many fishes the chemical differences between the rods and cones are striking. Thus in brosmius—a shellfish-like fish—the rods cut easily while the larger cones, due to their extremely large albumen content, become so hard with similar fixation that they, like the lens nucleus, jump out of the section during cutting.

"It seems to me that the above criteria, demonstrated in an extensive range of vertebrates, are quite sufficient to distinguish (with but few exceptions) between rods and cones."

The author (Eugene Wolff) succeeded, in the human, in colouring the inner portions of the cones red with Mallory's triple stain after Zenker fixation, while the corresponding portion of the rod stained blue. This was done both in vertical and in flat sections. This method of staining proved especially interesting in the

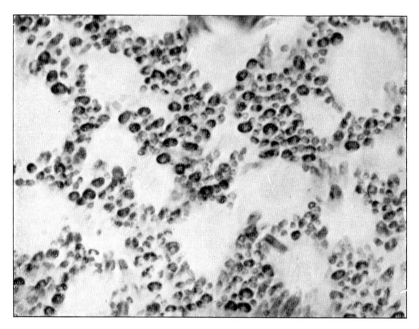

FIG. 117.—As FIG. 116; SHOWING THE SPACES UNDER HIGHER POWER. × 1,500. THE LARGER CIRCLES REPRESENT THE CROSS-SECTIONS OF THE CONES, THE SMALLER ONES THOSE OF THE RODS.

macular region, where the inner limbs of the rod-like cones stained red (Figs. 107, 108, 110, 111).

In another eye where the sections stained with Mallory's triple stain were inadvertently left washing for a long time, the outer elements of the cones stained reddish brown while the corresponding part of the rod stained blue.

Submicroscopic Structure of Visual Cells.—Electron microscopic investigations are still too recent for the significance (and sometimes even the interpretation) of the observed appearances to be clear. Reports are usually descriptive only ; comprehension may come in time. The electron microscopic appearances are strikingly similar in both rods and cones. In each the outer segment contains a pile of lamellæ, or "discs", some 33 per micron (Figs. 118, 119). It may be that a lamella consists of a series of lipid globules enclosed in protein (opsin) envelopes,

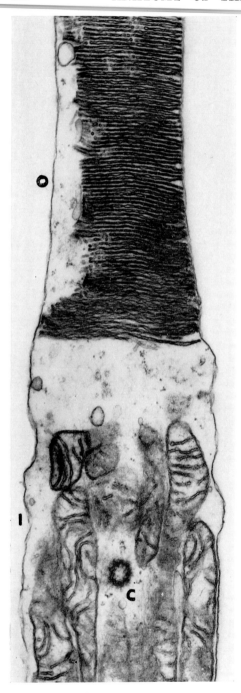

FIG. 118.—JUNCTIONAL ZONE BETWEEN OUTER
AND INNER SEGMENTS OF A ROD (RHESUS MON-
KEY, ELECTRON MICROGRAPH, × 30,000).

The outer segment (O) shows the characteristic discs, the inner segment (I) contains mitochondria. Here there is continuity, within the
plasma membrane, between outer and inner
segments. Such continuity has been observed
also in man. A cilium-like filament joins the
two segments; it is not cut through in the plane
of this section, but its centriole (a pale-centred
dark ring—C) lies centrally between the mitochondria of the inner segment.

*(By courtesy of Dr. C. Pedler, Institute of Ophthalmology,
London. Preparation by Mrs. R. Tilly.)*

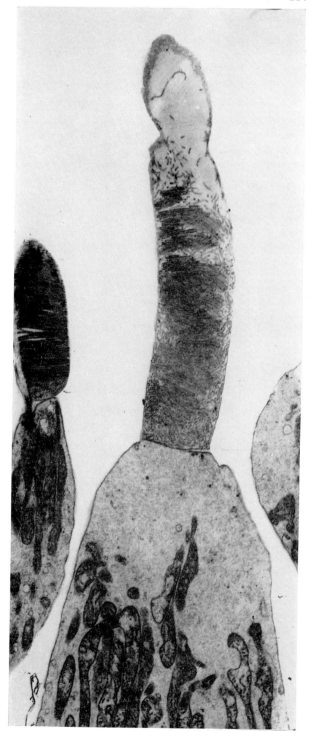

FIG. 119. — JUNCTIONAL ZONE
BETWEEN OUTER AND INNER SEG-
MENTS OF A CONE (RHESUS MON-
KEY, ELECTRON MICROGRAPH, ×
30,000).

The tip of the outer segment
has no discs. The broad inner
segment contains mitochondria.
The cone on the left is cut in
almost tangential section, and this
traverses the fibre joining inner
and outer segments.

(*By courtesy of Dr. C. Pedler, Institute
of Ophthalmology, London. Preparation
by Mrs. R. Tilly.*)

but no certain conclusions are yet possible. Adjacent " discs " of the cone (but not of the rod) appear to be connected at part of their circumference to form a continuum through the outer segment (Sjöstrand, F. S., 1965, *Ciba Symposium on Colour Vision*). Outer and inner segments are connected by a fibre, with filaments similar in appearance to an ordinary cilium of ciliated epithelium. The inner segment consists of a portion near the connecting cilium which is rich in mitochondria, and a basal portion containing a large Golgi complex.

Spaces between the Outer Limbs of the Rods and Cones.—Schäfer in Quain's *Anatomy*, writes :

" The intervals between the rods and cones are only partially filled by the processes of the hexagonal pigment cells ; the remaining part appears to be occupied by a clear substance which, according to Henle and H. Müller, is of a soft elastic consistency during life, and in the fresh condition, but soon liquefies after death ; but according to Schwalbe is normally liquid."

Van der Stricht also found spaces here free from rods and cones in sections stained by silver methods.

My own[1] preparations show that these spaces have a definite shape : hexagonal or polygonal in cross-sections, mirroring as it were the hexagonal pigment cells. This would seem to suggest that the rods and cones diverge towards the periphery of the pigment cells, and indeed if Max Schultze's figure (Fig. 100) be examined with a magnifying glass it will be seen that the rings which represent the cross-section of the apices of the rods and cones are largely to be found at the periphery of the cell (similarly in Fig. 101). It is possible, however, that the spaces, although

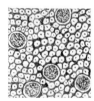

FIG. 120.—FLAT SECTION OF THE EXTERNAL LIMITING MEMBRANE × 1,000, SHOWING LARGE HOLES FOR CONE FIBRES AND SMALL HOLES FOR ROD FIBRES.
(*Wolff's preparation.*)

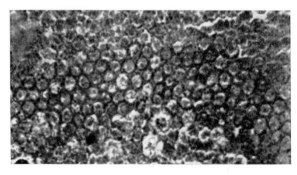

FIG. 121.—FLAT SECTION OF EXTERNAL LIMITING LAYER AT MACULA.

present in all my[1] preparations, may be produced as an artefact by clumping of the rods and cones as a result of fixation. In any case the matter requires further investigation. Electron microscopy on the whole tends to confirm the existence of such spaces.

[1] Eugene Wolff.

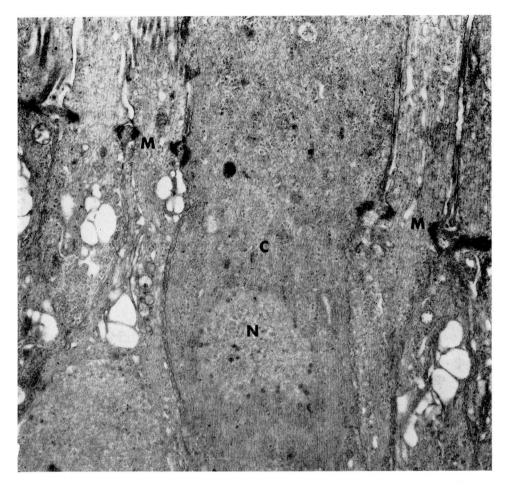

FIG. 122.—THE EXTERNAL LIMITING MEMBRANE (ELECTRON MICROGRAPH OF THE BABOON RETINA SHOWN IN FIG. 98. × 27,000).

In spite of photomicrographic appearances, no actual " membrane " exists. The external limiting membrane (M) is formed by dark tonofibrillar aggregations in the cell bodies of a cone (C) and the adjacent radial fibre processes. The cone nucleus (N) lies near the " membrane ".

(*By courtesy of Dr. C. Pedler, Institute of Ophthalmology, London. Preparation by Mrs. R. Tilly.*)

3. **The External Limiting Membrane.**—The external limiting membrane of the retina has the form of a wire netting. One prefers this analogy to that of a fenestrated membrane, as the holes take up a larger area than the actual membrane itself.

Through the holes in the net pass the processes of the rods and cones. In a section at right angles the membrane appears as a series of dots (Fig. 122) ; if the section is slightly oblique, it may appear as a line. Its true form can only be appreciated in a flat section parallel to the surface. Such a section shows clearly that the diameter of each aperture in the net depends on the structure which passes through it. Thus a rod has a small aperture, while a cone (Fig. 120) has a much larger one.

In the macular region the holes are all more or less of the same size except at the fovea, where the cones are exceptionally fine and the holes correspondingly small. At the fovea, also, the greater length of the cones pushes the external limiting membrane inwards and causes a posterior concavity which is called the fovea externa.

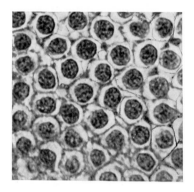

FIG. 123.—FLAT SECTION OF THE OUTER NUCLEAR LAYER IN THE MACULAR REGION, × 1,000, SHOWING THE CONE NUCLEI WITH THEIR NEUROGLIAL SURROUND. NO VESSELS.

(*Wolff's preparation.*)

The external limiting membrane is usually described as being formed by the fibres of Müller. But, according to Seefelder, the external limiting membrane is already present at the formation of the secondary optic vesicle when the fibres of Müller have not yet reached this region. It seems, therefore, that Leboucq is probably correct when he states that both the external limiting membrane and the fibre baskets of Oscar Schultze are the remains of the original intercellular cement of the fœtal retinal cells.

At the edge of the optic nerve the external limiting membrane may bend round and become continuous with the pigment epithelium, that is, with Verhoeff's membrane with which it is homologous, or with the intermediate tissue of Kuhnt. It should be pointed out that embryologically the membrane ought to pass into the glial tissue at the edge of the optic nerve.

Anteriorly at the ora serrata the external limiting membrane ends at the same level as the pigment epithelium by becoming continuous with the cement substance between the pigmented and non-pigmented portions of the ciliary epithelium (Wolfrum).

4. **The Outer Nuclear Layer.**—This consists essentially of the rod and cone granules (nuclei). The rod granule is round, and consists of practically nothing but nucleus with very little protoplasm around it. The cone granule is larger, oval, and stains differently. As the cone fibres are very short, the granules lie as a single layer situated close to the external limiting membrane (Figs. 96, 106).

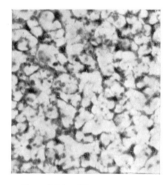

FIG. 124.—FLAT SECTION OF THE OUTER MOLECULAR LAYER × 1,000. (PHOSPHOTUNG. HÆM.)

Avascular and much looser in texture than the inner nuclear layer (compare Fig. 130).

(*Wolff's preparation.*)

Occasionally, most commonly in the macular region, cone nuclei may be found on the outer side of the external limiting membrane (Extruded Nuclei).

The rod and cone fibres continue beyond the granules and end in the outer molecular zone among the dendrites of the bipolar cells. The rod fibre ends in a

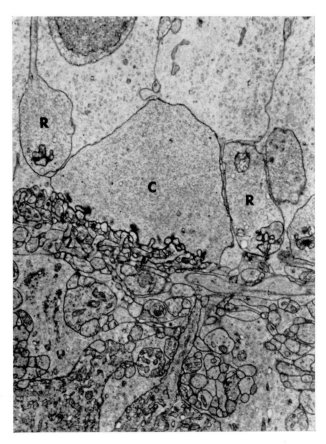

Fig. 125.—The Outer Plexiform Layer (Rhesus Monkey, Electron Micrograph, × 6,000).

Cone (C) and rod (R) pedicles are seen. The outer plexiform layer contains the processes of horizontal cells and many fibres.

(By courtesy of Dr. C. Pedler, Institute of Ophthalmology, London. Preparation by Mrs. R. Tilly.)

small knob, while the cone fibre terminates in a conical swelling with lateral processes.

Generally the granules are about eight deep. Directly to the temporal side of the disc the layer becomes thinner and then increases again, till it is thickest close to the centre of the fovea centralis. At the centre of the fovea it practically disappears (see p. 139, and Figs. 148, 149, and 150).

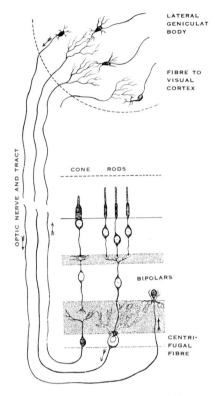

LATERAL
GENICULAT
BODY

FIBRE TO
VISUAL
CORTEX

OPTIC NERVE AND TRACT

CONE   RODS

BIPOLARS

CENTRI-
FUGAL
FIBRE

FIG. 126.—SCHEME TO SHOW THE COURSE
OF THE VISUAL FIBRES FROM THE RODS
AND CONES TO THE LATERAL GENICULATE
BODY.

(Greeff and Cajal modified.)

Note that each cone makes connection
with one bipolar only, but electron
microscopy throws much doubt on this
(FIG. 125).

5. **The Outer Molecular (Plexiform) Layer.**—This consists essentially of the arborisation of the axones of the rod and cone granules with the dendrites of the bipolar cells.

Comprising it also are :
> (a) The processes of the horizontal cells.
> (b) The fibres of Müller.

The outer molecular layer has a reticular structure, the outer part of which is much looser in texture than the inner (Figs. 96, 97, 127).

The denser inner portion is formed for the most part of the horizontal processes of the horizontal cells and the lateral processes of the fibres of Müller.

As we approach the macular region, however, the reticular structure is lost and the layer takes on a fibrous structure (Figs. 112, 149, 150, 155). This is due to the fact that the rod and cone fibres, instead of running vertically, become more and more oblique. Finally, the fibres from the fovea are almost parallel with the surface. Owing to this change in structure the outer molecular layer in the region of the macula has received the name of Henle's fibre layer.

The outer molecular layer, which is thickest at the macula, almost disappears at the fovea.

The outer fibre layer is very liable to take up fluid and become swollen on the slightest provocation, both during life and as the result of post-mortem or fixation changes. This is especially seen in the central area where the swelling of Henle's fibre layer produces the common post-mortem detachment of the macula. This forms a fold, the plica centralis, which runs from the lateral side of the disc to and including the macula.

6. **The Inner Nuclear Layer.**—This consists essentially of the sensory bipolar cells.

Comprising it also are :
> (a) The horizontal cells.
> (b) The amacrine cells.
> (c) The nuclei of the fibres of Müller.
> (d) Capillaries of the central retinal vessels.

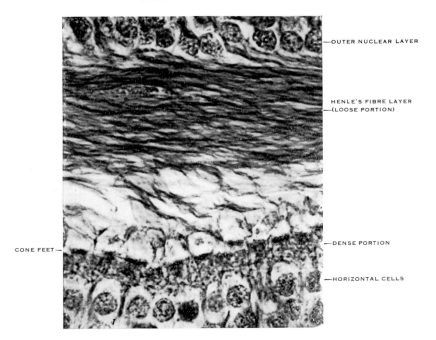

OUTER NUCLEAR LAYER

HENLE'S FIBRE LAYER
(LOOSE PORTION)

CONE FEET

DENSE PORTION

HORIZONTAL CELLS

FIG. 127.—VERTICAL SECTION OF PORTION OF RETINA AT MACULA.

The bipolar cells are neurones of the first order. They have their nuclei in the inner nuclear layer and their dendrites arborise in the outer molecular layer with the rod and cone fibres. Their axones form synapses with the dendrites of the ganglion cells in the inner molecular zone. There are two main types of bipolar cells : the " midget " bipolars which form synapses with footplates of individual cone cells only and the other bipolars which form synapses with both rod spherules and cone feet (see Polyak (1941), The Retina and Pedler, 1965, *Ciba Symposium on Colour Vision*).

The bodies of the bipolar cells resemble the granules of the outer nuclear layer, and consist almost entirely of nucleus with very little surrounding protoplasm. The whole layer, therefore, on ordinary microscopic section resembles the outer nuclear layer but is generally much thinner. As we approach the macula this layer gradually becomes thicker and then thins again towards the fovea, where it practically disappears.

In the batrachians, reptiles, and birds one sees a

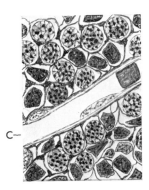

C—

FIG. 128.—FLAT SECTION OF THE INNER NUCLEAR LAYER × 1,000.

The nuclei of the fibres of Müller stain darker and are more angular than the bipolar nuclei. Note the capillary (C) with a deformed blood corpuscle ; and the neuroglial surround to the cells.

(*Wolff's preparation.*)

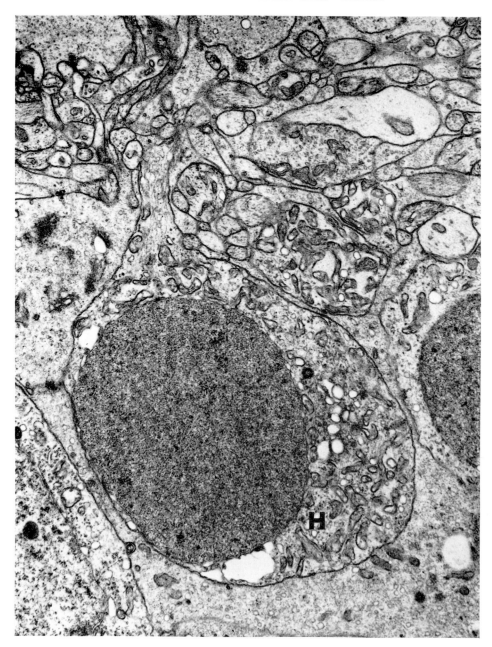

FIG. 129.—A HORIZONTAL CELL (H) (RHESUS MONKEY, ELECTRON MICROGRAPH, × 20,000).
(*By courtesy of Dr. C. Pedler, Institute of Ophthalmology, London. Preparation by Mrs. R. Tilly.*)

non-ramifying fibre coming from the rod-bipolar and passing through the external limiting membrane to end between the inner segments of the rods and cones by an enlargement, known as the Mass of Landolt.

Some time ago Balbuena discovered a new type of bipolar—the synaxique bipolar. The outer end forms a mass directly opposite the cone feet in the external molecular layer. Fortin believes that the bell- or stirrup-like structures (petits appareils) formed by the cone feet and fibres deep to them are little dioptric apparatuses (Figs. 96, 97, 127).

The Horizontal Cells are flat cells whose processes spread out horizontally—that is, parallel to the surface of the retina. They are placed next the outer molecular layer (Figs. 96, 97, 127).

The Amacrine Cells have a pear-shaped body and a single process which passes inwards and ends in the inner molecular layer. Some of them make connection with the centrifugal fibres of the optic nerve. They are placed next the inner molecular layer (Figs. 96, 99).

Both the horizontal and amacrine cells are probably associational in function. They appear to form horizontal connections between adjacent rods and cones ; i.e., they are actual nerve cells (Walls (1942) The Vertebrate Eye). But even this concept is uncertain (*Ciba Symposium on Colour Vision*, 1965, p. 87). It may be that they play a role in colour discrimination (*Ciba Symposium*, p. 192).

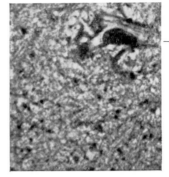

—CAPILLARY WITH NUCLEUS OF ENDOTHEL. CEL

FIG. 130.—FLAT (HORIZONTAL) SECTION OF THE INNER MOLECULAR LAYER × 1,000.

Vascularised and much denser in structure than the outer molecular layer (compare Fig. 124).

(*Wolff's preparation.*)

Electron Microscopy.—This reveals a system of connexions between the visual, horizontal and bipolar cells so complex that it has by no means been unravelled (Figs. 125, 126, 131).

7. **The Inner Molecular (Plexiform) Layer.**—This consists essentially of the arborisation of the axons of the bipolar cells with the dendrites of the ganglion cells. Comprising it also are :

(*a*) The distal processes of the amacrine cells.
(*b*) Fibres of Müller.
(*c*) Branches of the retinal vessels.
(*d*) A few scattered nuclei.

The inner molecular zone forms a reticulum which is divided into several substrata by the horizontally coursing processes of the amacrine cells and the dendrites of the stratified ganglion cells. (This subdivision into layers is better seen in some animals, especially birds, than in man.)

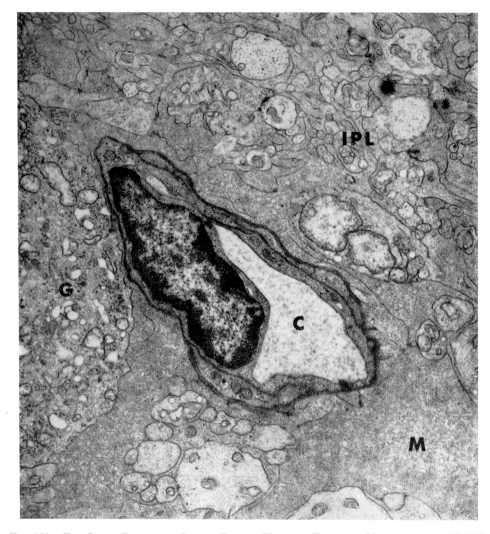

FIG. 131.—THE INNER PLEXIFORM LAYER (RHESUS MONKEY, ELECTRON MICROGRAPH, × 10,000).

The section includes a typical capillary and shows the complexity of the fibres of the inner plexus. IPL—inner plexiform layer. G.—a ganglion cell. C.—a capillary. M—Müller's fibres.

(By courtesy of Dr. C. Pedler, Institute of Ophthalmology, London. Preparation by Mrs. R. Tilly.)

It has practically the same thickness everywhere in the retina, except at the ovea centralis, where it is absent.

The nuclei present in this layer are those of the endothelium of the vessels (Fig. 130) or possibly those of displaced ganglion (Fig. 96) or amacrine cells.

8. **The Ganglion Cell Layer.**—This consists essentially of the ganglion cells

of the retina. In it are also
found :

(a) Fibres of Müller.

(b) Neuroglia or spider cells.

(c) Branches of the retinal
vessels.

The ganglion cells of the retina are multipolar nerve cells,
which resemble those of the
central nervous system. They
have a clear, round, or slightly
oval nucleus with a well-marked
nucleolus. Nissl granules are
well developed (Fig. 133). The

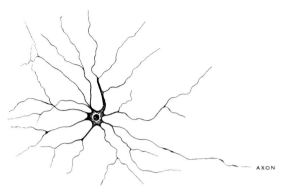

FIG. 132.—A GANGLION CELL OF THE RETINA.

(After Dogiel.)

cells vary greatly in size and shape. Generally large, they may reach up to 30 μ
in diameter, but may be much smaller, especially in the macular region. They
may be round, pyriform, or oval.

From the rounded inner end of the cell the axis cylinder (axon) comes off and

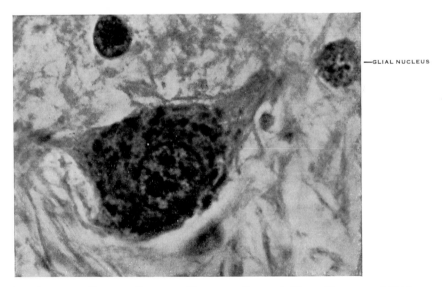

FIG. 133.—GANGLION CELL OF RETINA. (ZENKER. BORELL'S METH. BLUE. × 2,000.)

To show Nissl's granules. Also note nucleus and nucleolus.

(Wolff's preparation.)

passes into the nerve fibre layer. From the opposite extremity (which is usually
embedded in the inner molecular layer) one or more dendrites, which are thicker
than the axis cylinder, come off and ramify in the inner molecular layer. The

processes of the ganglion cells may be *stratified* when they run horizontally in one to three layers, or *diffuse* when they branch like a tree and end anywhere in the inner molecular layer.

The ganglion cells are neurones of the *second order* and correspond to cells in the *nucleus gracilis* and *cuneatus*. Their axons arborise on cells in the lateral geniculate body (Fig. 126), superior colliculus, etc. (p. 355). In the retina generally the ganglion cells form a single row, but on the temporal side of the disc we find two layers. As we approach the macula they increase in depth, so that up to eight layers may be formed at its margin. They decrease again towards the fovea, where they disappear entirely (Figs. 148–150).

Thus, if in any microscopic section we find two or more layers of ganglion cells, we know not only that we are on the temporal side of the disc, but that we are near the macula.

Towards the ora serrata the ganglion cells are sparser and gradually make their way into the nerve fibre layer.

The neuroglia or spider cells have bodies which are smaller than the ganglion cells, and have more densely staining nuclei. They have a large number of fine processes.

Electron Microscopy.—This confirms what is seen in the light microscope (Fig. 146).

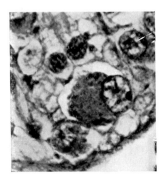

Fig. 134.—Flat Section of the Ganglion Cell Layer of the Retina. (Zenker. Phosphotungstic Acid. Hæm.)

The large ganglion cell has shrunk somewhat and so shows the glial surround very clearly.

9. **The Stratum Opticum or the Nerve Fibre Layer.**—This consists essentially of the axons of the ganglion cells which pass through the lamina cribrosa to form the optic nerve.

But there are also :

    (*a*) Centrifugal fibres.
    (*b*) Fibres of Müller (*q.v.*).
    (*c*) Neuroglial cells.
    (*d*) Retinal vessels.

The nerve fibres are arranged in bundles which run parallel to the surface of the retina. This structure can be made out with ordinary stains, and makes it obviously different from that of the molecular layers. The bundles inosculate with each other, forming a network in whose meshes are the feet of the fibres of Müller (Figs. 135, 136). The fibres all converge towards the optic disc. Those from the nasal side reach it without interruption ; those from the temporal side do not pass through the macula, but have to go round it. The fibres above the horizontal meridian pass above the macula and those below under it.

Thus we find to the lateral side of the macula a sort of raphé from which the nerve fibres arise in a pennate manner (Greeff) (Fig. 137). Those just to the lateral

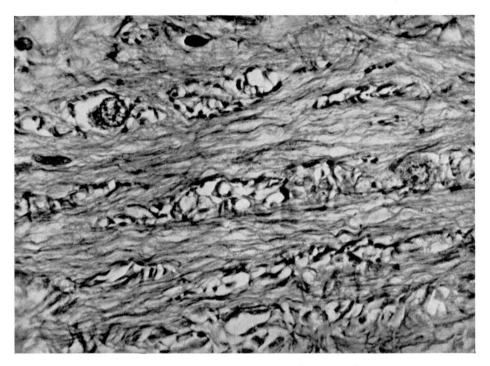

FIG. 135.—FLAT SECTION OF NERVE FIBRE LAYER OF RETINA.

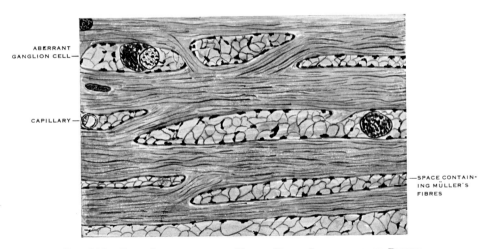

ABERRANT
GANGLION CELL—

CAPILLARY—

—SPACE CONTAIN-
ING MÜLLER'S
FIBRES

FIG. 136.—FLAT SECTION OF THE NERVE FIBRE LAYER OF THE RETINA.

(Wolff's preparation.)

A.E.—9

side of the macula encircle this structure closely, while the more lateral ones pass above and below in ever-increasing arcs.

The fibres from the macula itself pass straight in towards the temporal side of the disc and constitute the important *papillo-macular bundle.*

The nerve fibre layer is thickest around the margins of the optic nerve, 20–30 μ, and here differs in the different quadrants. Thus it is thinnest directly lateral, i.e. in the region of the papillo-macular bundle. Next in thickness are the upper and lateral quadrant and the lower and lateral quadrant, then the most medial part of the edge of the disc, and finally the thickest parts are the upper and

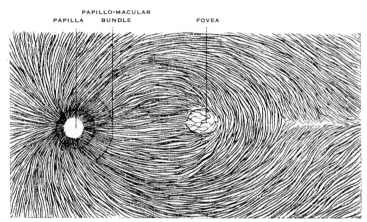

PAPILLO-MACULAR
PAPILLA   BUNDLE   FOVEA

FIG. 137. — THE NERVE FIBRE LAYER OF THE RETINA (SURFACE VIEW OF THE PAPILLO - MACULAR REGION).

(*From Poirier, after Dogiel and Greeff.*)

medial quadrant and the lower and medial quadrant. *The relative thickness most probably determines at which part of the disc papillœdema commences. The swelling is first visible in the thicker parts, that is, at the upper and medial lower and medial quadrants ; next comes the medial edge, then the upper and lower lateral quadrants, while the last part of the disc to show visible swelling will be directly lateral.*[1]

From the disc the nerve fibre layer becomes thinner as we pass towards the periphery, and near the ora serrata is invaded by the sparse ganglion cells—the two layers becoming one. As has been said, it is thinner on the lateral side of the disc than in the other quadrants, and as we pass towards the macula it becomes thinner still. At the bottom of the fovea it seems to disappear entirely, although Dogiel, using methylene blue, showed that even here a fine network of fibres exists.

The nerve fibres are non-medullated (except when the so-called congenital opaque fibres are present) (Fig. 295).

They are mostly very fine, but some may reach 3–5 μ in thickness.

The Centrifugal Fibres are thicker than the centripetal (Ramon y Cajal). They pass through the ganglion cell layer and inner plexiform layer, and end by ramifying in the inner molecular layer around an amacrine cell or among the elements of the inner nuclear layer (Fig. 126).

[1] See Wolff and Davies (1931), *Brit. J. Ophthal.,* **15,** 609.

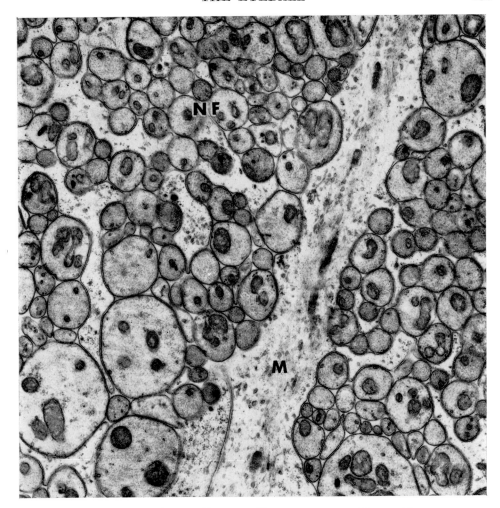

Fig. 138.—The Nerve Fibre Layer (Electron Micrograph of the Baboon Retina shown in
Fig. 98. × 15,000).

N.F.—nerve fibres.   M—Müller's fibres.

(By courtesy of Dr. C. Pedler, Institute of Ophthalmology, London.   Preparation by Mrs. R. Tilly.)

The Neuroglial or spider cells have an oval nucleus with little protoplasm and
numerous fine processes.   The glial fibres form a kind of membrane (limitans
perivascularis of Krückmann) around the vessels (see p. 155 and Figs. 147, 168).

The retinal vessels are found mainly in the nerve fibre layer, but may also lie
in part in the ganglion cell layer (Fig. 169).   They do not as a rule project on
the inner surface of the retina, but rarely may do so very slightly.

10. **The Internal Limiting Membrane.**—Between the retina and the vitreous
is a membrane which forms both the inner limit of the retina and the outer

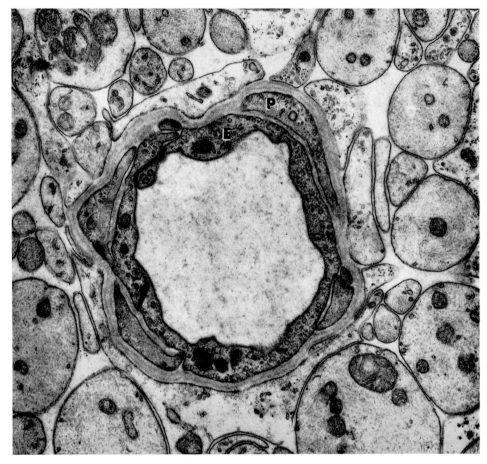

FIG. 139.—A CAPILLARY IN THE NERVE FIBRE LAYER (ELECTRON MICROGRAPH OF THE BABOON
RETINA SHOWN IN FIG. 98. × 20,000).

The capillary endothelium (E) is thin, and pericytes (P) lie outside this.

(*By courtesy of Dr. C. Pedler, Institute of Ophthalmology, London.   Preparation by Mrs. R. Tilly.*)

boundary of the vitreous (Figs. 96, 97, 143, 146).   It has, therefore, been called with
equal justification the internal limiting membrane of the retina and the hyaloid
membrane of the vitreous.   Here the former term will be used.   According to
Redslob (*Traité d'Ophtalmologie*, 1939), the membrane has a double contour.   The
outer, he holds, is formed by the feet of the fibres of Müller, and is thus the true
internal limiting membrane, while the inner is the hyaloid membrane.   It is quite
true that with the denser stains a double contour can often be made out as seen
in Fig. 140.   The inner portion may even separate from the outer and cells may
be seen between the two.   But if we follow this method of description we must
always in illustrations label the membrane with both names (which is complicated)

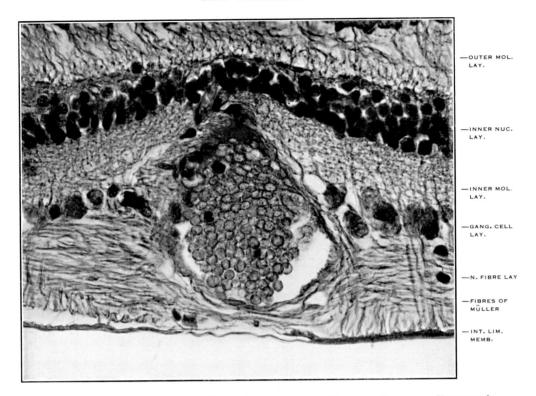

—OUTER MOL. LAY.

—INNER NUC. LAY.

—INNER MOL. LAY.

—GANG. CELL LAY.

—N. FIBRE LAY

—FIBRES OF MÜLLER

—INT. LIM. MEMB.

FIG. 140.—VERTICAL SECTION OF THE INNER PORTION OF THE RETINA. (ZENKER. VERHOEFF'S ELASTIC STAIN.)

Note the thinning of the internal limiting membrane where the vessel lies close to it. No fibres of Müller (well seen to the right of the section) come to it in this region.

(*Trans. O.S.U.K.*, 1937, **57**, 186.)

FIG. 141.—VERTICAL SECTION OF INNER PART OF RETINA.

The internal limiting membrane has become detached as an artefact and so the normal reticulum formed by the foot-pieces of the fibres of Müller on its outer surface has become visible (see Fig. 145).

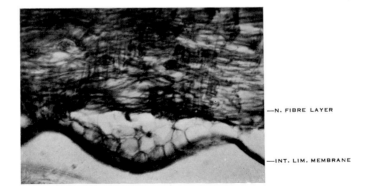

—N. FIBRE LAYER

—INT. LIM. MEMBRANE

and call the membrane, which separates the *outer* part of the disc from the vitreous, the hyaloid, since there are no fibres of Müller here. Also the internal limiting membrane will be absent where a large vessel comes close to the hyaloid (as in Fig. 140).

At the outset it must be emphasised that the membrane stains like collagenous tissue. Thus with Mallory's triple stain it is coloured blue (Fig. 143).

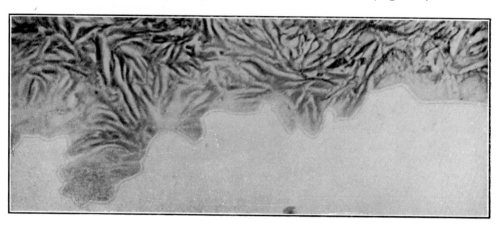

FIG. 142.—FLAT SECTION OF THE INTERNAL LIMITING MEMBRANE.
The inner portion is homogeneous (glass-like); the outer shows the characteristic mosaic.
(*Trans. O.S.U.K.*, 1937.)

In an ordinary section of the retina this membrane appears as a thin line some 1–2 μ thick, perfectly smooth towards the vitreous but having marked irregularities towards the retina. The exact significance of these irregularities has not been decided. They may either be the foot-pieces of the fibres of Müller themselves (Salzmann) or the material which binds these to the membrane proper.

In a flat section of the retina the membrane appears in two parts : (*a*) a homogeneous portion, and (*b*) a curious and rather characteristic mosaic which seems to be due to the irregularities on the retinal aspect. Sometimes on the surface of this mosaic (or lying loose where the membrane has become detached as an artefact, which happens quite frequently, especially in paraffin sections) (Figs. 141, 145, 169), one sees a honeycomb of fibres, forming, no doubt, the material which binds the foot-pieces of the fibres of Müller together (see Van der Stricht).

A very interesting and instructive picture is often seen if one examines a section of the retina where a large vessel comes close to the membrane. Here, opposite the vessel, the membrane is very thin. *It is smooth both on its retinal and vitreous aspects and no fibres of Müller go to it* (Fig. 140).

Further, when it is remembered that the fibres of Müller stain red with Mallory's triple stain, as does neuroglia, it becomes clear that the membrane, which is labelled the internal limiting membrane in all or nearly all modern

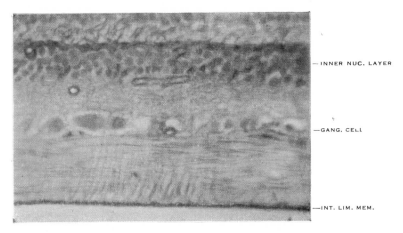

INNER NUC. LAYER

GANG. CELL

INT. LIM. MEM.

Fig. 143.—Vertical Section of Retina. (Zenker. Mallory.)
Note internal limiting membrane stains blue; fibres of Müller stain reddish.

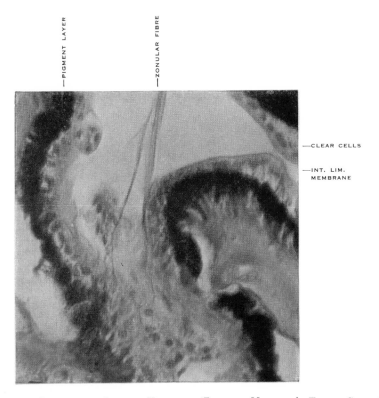

PIGMENT LAYER

ZONULAR FIBRE

CLEAR CELLS

INT. LIM.
MEMBRANE

Fig. 144.—Coronal Section of Ciliary Valley. (Zenker. Mallory's Triple Stain.)
To show the attachment of a zonular fibre to the limitans ciliaris, both of which stain blue.
(*Photomicrograph.*)

textbooks of anatomy, cannot be formed by the apposition of the bases of the fibres of Müller as is usually and classically described (see also Salzmann and Kolmer). The feet of the fibres of Müller are in fact only attached to this membrane.

The internal limiting membrane is a typical glass-like (hyaloid) membrane. It is present at the fovea but is gradually lost at the nerve head where it is continuous with the neuroglia forming the central connective tissue meniscus of Kuhnt (Fig. 298).

THE RETINAL NEUROGLIA

Apart from the actual nervous elements, the retina, like all parts of the central nervous system, contains glial elements which act as its connective and supporting tissues. The glia forms a sheath to each nervous element and thus serves to insulate the various neurones from each other (Figs. 123, 128, 134). Perhaps also it has a trophic function.

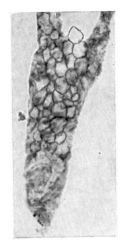

FIG. 145.—TO SHOW THE NETWORK OF (RED STAINING) FIBRES LYING ON A DETACHED (BLUE STAINING) INTERNAL LIMITING MEMBRANE. (FLAT SECTION. ZENKER. MALLORY'S TRIPLE STAIN.)
(*Trans. O.S.U.K.*, 1937.)

The newer methods of staining have taught us that in the retina as well as in the central nervous system there are different types of glial cells.

There are (1) the fibres of Müller, (2) Golgi's spider cells, (3) astrocytes, (4) horizontal bands of glial tissue alone or associated with the smaller vessels, (5) the microglia.

1. **The Supporting Fibres of Müller.**—The fibres of Müller are long, narrow, very complicated structures which pass through the whole thickness of the retina from the internal to the external limiting membranes.

The nucleus is situated at the level of the inner nuclear layer. It can be distinguished from the rounded bipolar nuclei among which it lies by its elongated angular form (Figs. 96, 97), and its staining reactions. Thus with Mallory, phosphotungstic acid hæmatoxylin it stains much darker than the nuclei of the bipolar cells.

The nucleus of Müller's fibre is bipolar in character. It sends a radial process internally and one externally. Both the nucleus and the processes send branches laterally which may be in the form of lamellæ or fibrillæ. The lamellæ occur in the region of the inner and outer nuclear layers and neighbouring lamellæ unite to form a honeycomb in the alveoli of which the cellular elements are contained (Figs. 128, 134). Numerous short branches are also given off to the plexiform layers.

As the inner process passes through the ganglion cell and nerve fibre layers, it

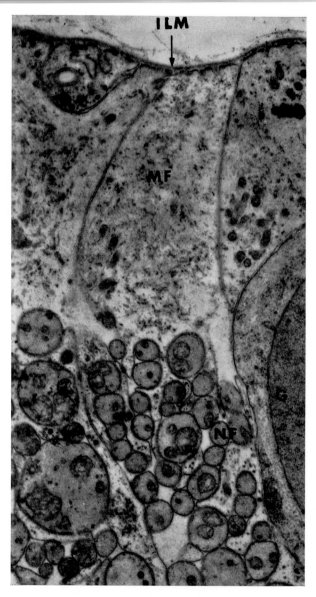

Fig. 146.—The Inner Limiting Membrane (Electron Micrograph of the Baboon Retina shown in Fig. 98. × 12,000).

NF—nerve fibres.   G—ganglion cell.   MF—Müller's fibre.   ILM—inner limiting membrane.

(By courtesy of Dr. C. Pedler, Institute of Ophthalmology, London.   Preparation by Mrs. R. Tilly.)

gives off no lateral branches, or only a few, and thus can be seen here without any special stain (Figs. 96, 140).

At the level of the inner molecular layer the inner process bifurcates or divides into several branches which are attached to the internal limiting membrane by a hollow base or foot. It is usually stated that the bases, or foot-pieces,

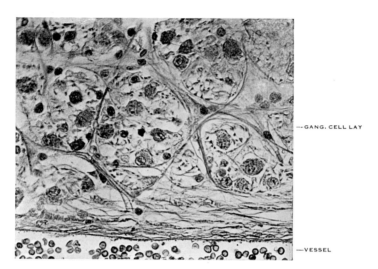

Fig. 147. — Flat Section of the Ganglion Cell Layer of the Retina, to show the Horizontal Bands of Glial Fibres.

The glial feet ending on the vessel wall can be made out but are not very clearly demonstrated.

—GANG. CELL LAY

—VESSEL

of adjoining fibres are united by their edges to form the internal limiting membrane of the retina. This view is denied by both Salzmann and Kolmer (see also p. 135).

Traced externally the outer process reaches the external limiting membrane. Some hold that it forms this membrane and is then continued on as fine fibrillæ which invest the base of the rods and cones and are called the fibre baskets of Oscar Schultze. According to Leboucq, however, this view is not tenable (see p. 120).

Bielschowsky preparations show the diplosome of the fibres of Müller to be directly beneath the limitans externa (Fig. 115).

Near the fovea the fibres of Müller, instead of running at right angles to the layers of the retina, become oblique, following, though not exactly, the slope of the clivus.

Electron Microscopy.—Inomata (1966, *Jap. Jour. Ophth.*, **10** : 1, 26) confirms the "fibre baskets" around the bases of the rods and cones. On the inner (vitreous) side of the retina Müller's fibres "terminate in fan-shaped processes". Inomata postulates that Müller's fibres are comparable to Schwann cells, since they enclose the peripheral processes of the receptor cells in the form of "mesaxons".

2. **The Golgi spider cells** are small glial cells with a round or oval nucleus and

numerous cytoplasmic processes similar to those found in the grey and white matter of the central nervous system. They are most numerous near the disc, in the inner molecular, ganglion cell, and nerve fibre layers. Perivascular glia appear to curl around the capillaries like the tentacles of an octopus.

3. **Astrocytes or star cells** are found here and there in the ganglion cell layer. They are most numerous in the disc and optic nerve.

4. **Horizontal Bands.**—One also often finds well-developed bundles of glial fibres in the nerve fibre and inner molecular layers either alone (Fig. 147) or accompanying the precapillary and capillary vessels.

5. **The Microglia** (del Rio Hortega's *third* [1] glial element).—The cell body is most often triangular but may be round, oval, or rod shaped. It may have one or many processes. Hortega believes the microglia to be derived from mesoderm and not from ectoderm. They constitute wandering cells which are phagocytic and hence act as scavengers, especially to fatty granules, in pathological processes. It has also been suggested that the microglia belongs to the reticulo-endothelial system.

The foregoing is a general description of the retina.

We must now consider the changes that take place in its structure at :

(*a*) The optic disc.

(*b*) The macula lutea and fovea centralis.

(*c*) The ora serrata.

(*a*) At the **Optic Disc** the only layer that is present is the stratum opticum or nerve fibre layer (*q.v.*), and hence if light falls here it will not excite visual impressions and so the disc is known as the blind spot. There are no fibres of Müller here, which has an important bearing on the swelling of the disc in papillœdema. Also at the centre of the physiological cup, the internal limiting membrane gives place to the central connective tissue meniscus of Kuhnt (Fig. 298).

(*b*) **The Macula lutea** is a shallow oval depression about the same size as the disc. Its centre lies 3·5 mm. lateral to the edge of the disc and just *below* its middle.

The side wall of the depression is called the clivus, and slopes gradually towards the fovea centralis.

At the macula lutea, around the fovea, the ganglion cells are much more numerous, being arranged in several layers (five to seven) ; the outer molecular layer is thicker than elsewhere, and forms the outer fibre layer of Henle (p. 122) ; and lastly there is a progressive disappearance of the rods, which are replaced by the cones.

---

[1] Del Rio Hortega divides the neuroglia into three kinds :

1. *The Macroglia or Fibroglia.*—This consists of the fibrillary and protoplasmic astrocytes to which class the fibres of Müller belong.

2. *The Oligodendroglia* is constituted by cells poor in dendrites. They usually occur in association with myelinated fibres but may be found in the ganglion cell layer.

3. *The Microglia.*

At *the Fovea centralis* itself the retina is thinner than elsewhere. This is due to the fact that here there are no supporting fibres of Müller, no ganglion cells, and no nerve fibre layer, though Dogiel, by his methylene-blue stain, showed that even here a fine network of nerve fibres exists.

Also the inner and outer molecular and inner nuclear layers are gradually reduced to thin membranes. The outer nuclear layer, just next the fovea (some hold *at* the fovea), actually increases in thickness, but at the fovea itself is reduced to a single layer (see Figs. 149, 150, and 151).

There are no rods at the fovea, only cones (Fig. 152), and these are much more slender and longer than elsewhere, with the result that they form an elevation which encroaches on the other layers. The " bouquet " of central cones is 200 mm. in diameter (Rochon-Duvigneaud).

It will thus be seen that at the fovea centralis the layers of the retina are spread aside, so that light may fall directly on the true percipient elements, namely the cones.

At the fovea centralis each cone is connected to only one ganglion cell. Its impulse is therefore much purer, and the image received by the brain much sharper than elsewhere in the retina, being as it were insulated from the impulses of neighbouring cells. It is these facts that make the fovea the point of most acute vision. It should be noted, however, that electron microscopists do not agree that such a single cone to ganglion cell connexion exists, except perhaps occasionally. *In the retina generally each ganglion cell is connected with many (up to 100 rods) visual cells.*

The pigment layer is thickened, and so is the chorio-capillaris.

The increased choroidal blood-supply is

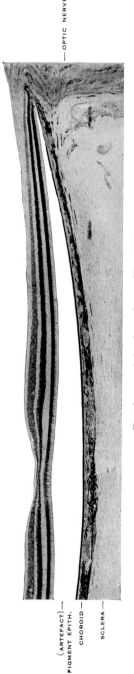

Fig. 148.—Section of the Edge of the Optic Nerve and the Macula.

(*Wolff's preparation.*)

For the remaining legends, see Fig. 149.

Note especially the gradual increase in thickness of the ganglion layer as we pass from the optic nerve.

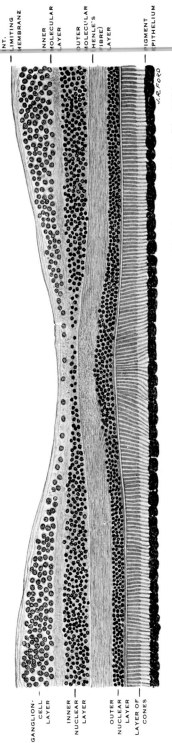

INT. LIMITING MEMBRANE
INNER MOLECULAR LAYER
OUTER MOLECULAR (HENLE'S FIBRE) LAYER
PIGMENT EPITHELIUM

J. R. FORD

GANGLION-CELL LAYER
INNER NUCLEAR LAYER
OUTER NUCLEAR LAYER
LAYER OF CONES

Fig. 149.—Section through the Macula near the Centre of the Fovea. (Based on same slide as Fig. 148)

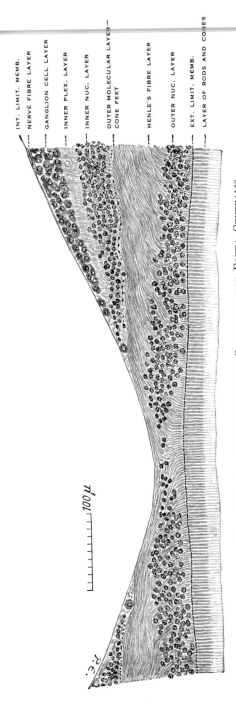

INT. LIMIT. MEMB.
NERVE FIBRE LAYER
GANGLION CELL LAYER
INNER PLEX. LAYER
INNER NUC. LAYER
OUTER MOLECULAR LAYER
CONE FEET
HENLE'S FIBRE LAYER
OUTER NUC. LAYER
EXT. LIMIT. MEMB.
LAYER OF RODS AND CONES

P. C.

100 μ

Fig. 150.—Section through the Centre of the Fovea Centralis.

Note that here the outer nuclear layer is also reduced to a few scattered cells.

(From Eisler, in the Kurzes Handbuch der Ophthalmologie.)

140

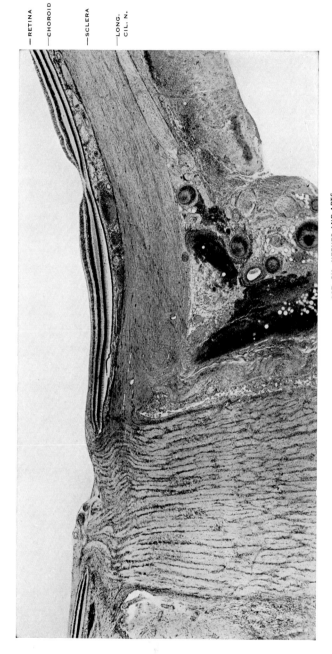

RETINA

CHOROID

SCLERA

LONG. CIL. N.

OST. CIL. NERVES AND ARTS

Fig. 151.—Antero-posterior (horizontal) Section of the Optic Nerve and Macula, passing through the Fovea Centralis. (Zenker. Weigert's Hæm. and Ponceau S.)

Note the increased thickness of the choroid at the macula and especially at the fovea.

(*Wolff's preparation.*)

141

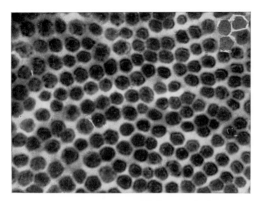

FIG. 152.—THE CONE MOSAIC AT THE MACULA. FLAT SECTION THROUGH THE INNER PORTIONS OF THE MACULAR CONES. × 1,000.

necessary as the macula has no retinal blood-vessels.

The external limiting membrane is sometimes pushed inward, forming a depression which faces the choroid, and has been called the *fovea externa*.

The yellow colour of the macula lutea is best seen in post-mortem eyes in which the retina has already become clouded. But it can be seen in eyes freshly removed from the living. For if one detaches the retina from the choroid and examines it by transmitted light, one sees the yellow colour of the macula with its centre or fovea colourless. Spread on a glass slide with the choroid uppermost the yellow spot can be quite easily examined with the microscope and measured (Rochon-Duvigneaud). It is about 2 mm. in diameter. Its coloration is more intense in brunettes than in blondes

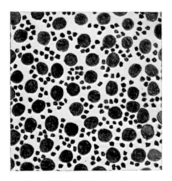

FIG. 153.—FLAT SECTION THROUGH THE INNER LIMBS OF THE RODS AND CONES IN THE MACULAR REGION CLOSE TO THE ROD-FREE AREA. × 1,000. ONLY A FEW RODS TO EACH CONE.

(*Wolff's preparation.*)

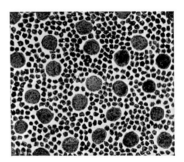

FIG. 154.—FLAT SECTION THROUGH THE INNER LIMBS OF THE RODS (SMALLER) AND CONES (LARGER) NEAR THE MACULA.

Note that the cross-section of the rods is not circular. × 1,000.

and it fades gradually into the surrounding retina. The central clear area is about 0·2 mm. in diameter (Rochon-Duvigneaud). With sufficient magnification it is even possible to see the pattern formed by the bases of the central cones.

With red-free light in ophthalmoscopic examinations the macula is seen as a greenish-yellow area in the pale green of the surrounding retina. The fovea

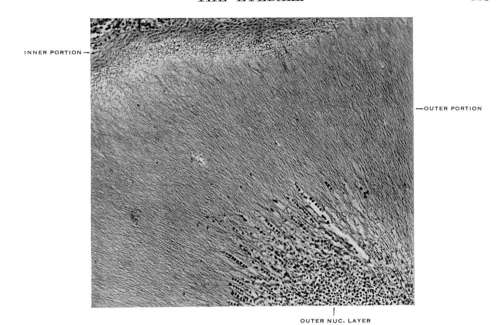

INNER PORTION —

—OUTER PORTION

OUTER NUC. LAYER

FIG. 155.—FLAT SECTION OF HENLE'S FIBRE LAYER AT THE MACULA. (ZENKER. PHOSPHOTUNG. HÆM.)

Note the difference between the inner and outer portions. The outer portion has the structure of fibrous tissue, the inner forms a net. (See also Fig. 156.) Note also the columns of cone nuclei invading the fibre layer.   (*Wolff's preparation.*)

appears yellowish brown. But here we see two membranes superimposed and it is difficult to be sure to which the effect is due.

(*c*) **The Ora Serrata.**—The ora serrata is the dentate fringe which marks the termination of the retina proper. It is some 8·5 mm. from the limbus, about 6 mm. from the equator, and 25 mm. from the optic nerve. Nasally it is 1 mm. nearer the root of the iris than on the temporal side. The teeth of the ora serrata are best marked where the ciliary body is narrowest, i.e. on the nasal side, and particularly in the upper nasal quadrant (Fig. 57). "On the temporal side they often fail completely and the border is often finely and irregularly wavy and angular. The teeth correspond in position to the intervals between the ciliary processes, and all the irregularities of the development in the corona ciliaris are reflected in the ora serrata" (Salzmann). On section the ora serrata appears as a tongue-shaped process which may end

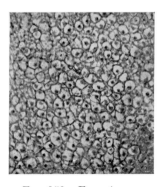

FIG. 156.—FLAT (TANGENTIAL) SECTION THROUGH THE INNER (DENSER) PORTION OF THE OUTER (HENLE'S) FIBRE LAYER AT THE MACULA. × 1,000.
(*Wolff's preparation.*)

in a rounded or right-angled border or may be overhanging. The thickness of the retina here is about 140 μ.

At the ora serrata the retina is firmly adherent to the choroid, which is responsible for the fact that a detachment of the retina ends here.

Here also the vitreous is firmly adherent to the retina. The cells of the

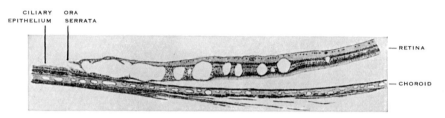

FIG. 157.—THE RETINA AT THE ORA SERRATA, SHOWING CYSTIC DEGENERATION.
(*From Salzmann.*)

pigment epithelium tend to be irregular and the pigmentation varies in intensity.

The numbers of rods diminish and disappear first, but the cones although malformed may continue to the ora. Usually, however, both types cease 1 to 2 mm. from the ora. Yet the retina is blind for about 7 mm. in a normal eye and only 3·5 mm. in an aphakia eye (Maggiore).

The nuclear layers become thinner and eventually fuse. The ganglion cells become sparser, invade the nerve fibre layer, and both end 0·5–1 mm. from the ora serrata. There is a great increase in the neuroglial supporting tissues, thus differing from the central area where there is very little.

The external limiting membrane is continued between the two layers of ciliary epithelium. The internal limiting membrane becomes thinner but is continued over the ciliary epithelium.

According to Maggiore, the ora serrata at three months is placed at the level of the limbus ; but with the development of the ciliary body, it gets pushed farther and farther backwards.

At the ora serrata all the essential elements of the retina cease, so that beyond this point (and indeed slightly posterior to it) it does not give rise to the sensation of vision. The retina is in fact continued forward over the inner aspect of the ciliary body as two layers of cells, an outer cubical and pigmented, an inner columnar and non-pigmented. This portion is called the *pars ciliaris retinæ*.

Similarly, the prolongation of these two layers of cells behind the iris is called the pars iridica retinæ. The most anterior portion of the optic cup forms the fringe of pigment round the margin of the pupil (Fig. 90), which can be seen with the naked eye, especially when the pupil is small.

Peripheral Cystoid Degeneration

(*Iwanoff's Retinal Œdema ; Blessig's Cysts*)

Cystic spaces are not infrequently found in the retina, at or close to the ora serrata. They may be regarded as physiological, and although best marked in

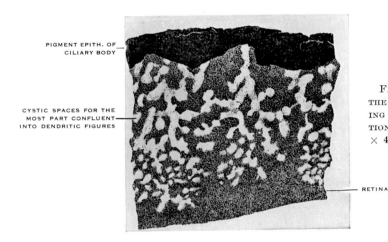

PIGMENT EPITH. OF CILIARY BODY

CYSTIC SPACES FOR THE MOST PART CONFLUENT INTO DENDRITIC FIGURES

RETINA

Fig. 158.—Retina of the Ora Serrata, showing Cystic Degeneration ; Surface View. × 47.

(*From Salzmann.*)

the old, they may be found in quite young people. They usually commence in the outer molecular layer and gradually increase in size till they fill the whole space between the inner and outer limiting membranes. Cystic degeneration is much more marked on the temporal side where the teeth of the ora serrata are small, than on the nasal where they are best developed (Fig. 57).

It has been suggested that the bursting of one of these cysts may induce a detachment of the retina, which so commonly starts at the ora serrata and most often in the lower temporal quadrant.

Their origin is probably associated with the relatively poor blood-supply of the region, and their formation may be regarded as an atrophic phenomenon.

The Blood-supply of the Retina

The retina gets its main blood-supply from the arteria centralis retinæ, but its outer portion, namely, the rods and cones and the outer nuclear layer, is avascular and nourished by the chorio-capillaris, which exists in fact for this purpose. The outer molecular layer, also for the most part avascular, is fed partly from the choroidal, partly from the retinal vessels. (See also cilio-retinal artery and other branches from circle of Zinn, p. 149.)

The double vascular supply of the retina brings it into line with the double supply to the brain, namely, a cortical and a basal system of vessels which do not anastomose. The choroid may be regarded as the forward continuation of the pia-arachnoid.

A.E.—10

The Arteria Centralis Retinæ.—The central artery of the retina is a slender vessel some 0·28 mm. in diameter (Henle), which comes off the ophthalmic close to the optic foramen, usually in company with one or other branch, most commonly the medial ciliary trunk (Quain). It runs a wavy course forward,

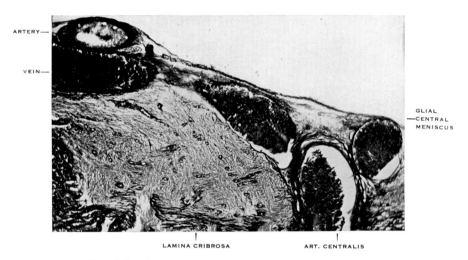

FIG. 159.—ANTERO-POSTERIOR SECTION OF NERVE HEAD.

Note that as the vessels pass into the retina they are covered by only a thin layer of glia.

below the optic nerve, outside but adherent to the dural sheath to some 10–15 mm. behind the eye.   Here, at a point on the under and medial aspect of the nerve, it bends upwards to pierce the dura and arachnoid, from both of which it receives a covering.   There has been much argument as to which aspect the artery pierces.   All are agreed that it is the under side, but some hold with Vossius that it is the under and lateral aspect.   This author says that the fœtal cleft in the optic nerve rotates through 90° during fœtal life.   Leber (in *Graefe-Saemisch*) points out that there is no foundation for this, and agrees with Deyl that it is the under and medial aspect.

Having reached the subarachnoid space clothed by the above membranes, it bends forwards and also to one or other side.   This is probably the reason why one has never been able to get an antero-posterior section which shows the artery passing through the membranes *and* in the nerve.   After a very short course, it again bends upwards at nearly a right angle and passes through or rather invaginates the pia to reach the centre of the nerve.   The entering vessel is thus clothed by the whole thickness of the pia (and at first by some subarachnoid trabeculæ as well), and takes with it the contained (pial) vessels.   It is also surrounded by a sympathetic nerve plexus (Krause) which is called the nerve of Tiedemann.   In this portion of its course the connective tissue carrying the artery (and perhaps also the central vein) can be seen by the naked eye as a radius to the cross-section of the nerve (Figs. 160, 162).

At the centre of the nerve the artery bends forwards, and then, in company with its vein which lies on its temporal side, it passes anteriorly to the lamina cribrosa which it pierces to appear inside the eye. It lies quite superficial in the

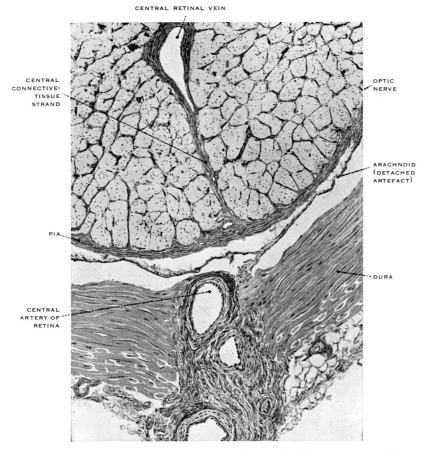

FIG. 160.—CENTRAL ARTERY PASSING THROUGH DURA. THE VEIN IS IN THE NERVE.
(*Wolff's preparation.*)

nerve head, not being covered by nerve fibres but only by that layer of glia (the connective tissue meniscus of Kuhnt), which closes the physiological cup on the side of the vitreous (Figs. 159, 298). It climbs up the *nasal* side of the cup and at about this point divides into two branches (superior and inferior) which, bending at a right angle or nearly so, pass into the retina (Fig. 171).

It will thus be seen that from the point on the under and medial aspect of the

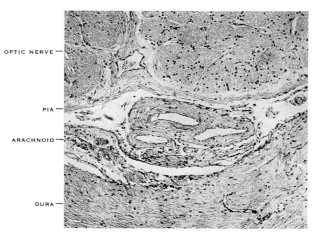

OPTIC NERVE—

PIA—

ARACHNOID—

DURA—

FIG. 161.—THE CENTRAL VESSELS OF THE RETINA ARE IN THE
SUBARACHNOID SPACE.

(*Wolff's preparation. From Wolff and Davies, Brit. J. Ophthal.,* 1931.)

nerve where the artery lies outside the dura to and including its bifurcation, it makes five bends (Fig. 354).

Branches.—(1) Some of the branches referred to as Group A (p. 386).

(2) The central collateral arteries (arteriæ collaterales centralis retinæ) (see p. 387).

(3) Terminal branches.

The superior and inferior branches of the arteria centralis subdivide into nasal and temporal branches, of which the nasal are usually the smaller. This second division usually takes place about the margin of the disc but may occur in the nerve, in which case four branches appear on the disc.

The retinal vessels divide dichotomously, as they proceed towards the ora serrata, where they end in capillaries *which do not anastomose with any other system of vessels.*

From the arteries in the nerve-fibre layer twigs are given off which pass into the ganglion layer, and capillaries from them pass just to the outer side of the inner nuclear layer, but no farther, the retina to the outer side of this point being avascular (Figs. 96, 169).

It will thus be seen that in general the main branches of the retinal arteries have a similar direction to the corresponding nerve fibres. On the nasal side the arteries run roughly radially from the disc. On the temporal side they arch over and under the central area, sending in twigs towards the horizontal meridian.

The macular region is supplied by twigs from the superior and inferior temporal vessels ; but the fovea itself is entirely free of all blood-vessels (Fig. 165).

The small vessels which run radially from the superior and inferior macular vessels form (according to Leber) capillary loops which leave an avascular zone from 0·4 to 0·5 mm. at the fovea. The superior and inferior macular branches supply the perifoveal capillaries almost equally so that a horizontal division exists through the fovea, *which, according to Roenne, accounts for the horizontal division of the fixation area frequently seen in obstruction of an arterial branch.*

To the temporal side of the macula, however, i.e. in the region of the raphé formed by the nerve fibres, the distribution of these arterial twigs is not limited exactly to the horizontal meridian of the retina, but overlaps it both upwards and downwards so that the watershed or vascular division follows a wavy line and corresponds only approximately to the straight nerve fibre raphé (Traquair).

The arteria centralis is an end artery, for if it is blocked blindness results. It does, however, send a few twigs to Zinn or Haller's vascular circle.

Circulus Vasculosus Nervi Optici (circle of Zinn or Haller) is formed by a circular anastomosis between two, four, or more short ciliary arteries which have pierced the sclera for the most part on the medial and lateral sides of the optic nerve. The ring of vessels so formed lies in the sclera close to the nerve (Fig. 354).

From it numerous branches pass forwards to the choroid, inwards to the optic nerve, and backwards to the pial network.

The branches which pass inwards invade the lamina cribrosa and also send branches to the nerve head and neighbouring retina.

These last branches are usually very small and only supply a very small area of retina ; but they may be larger—anything up to a cilio-retinal artery, which is not uncommon.

A cilio-retinal artery can be seen with the ophthalmoscope as a vessel with a hook-shaped origin, running from just within the temporal edge of the disc towards the macula and supplying this area.

There is a capillary anastomosis (but no more than that) between the branches of the circulus arteriosus and those of the arteria centralis in the region of the lamina cribrosa and nerve head (Fig. 163).

A cilio-retinal vein is rare.

The Retinal Veins follow the course of the arteries more or less. A vein may run parallel to the corresponding artery for a short distance (Fig. 171), but they never, or almost never, run next each other (see p. 159). Here and there a vein will cross the artery either superficially or deeply or may be at some distance from it. The diameter of the artery is, as a rule, about two-thirds to three-quarters that of the vein with which it runs, and this applies to the arteria and vena centralis also. The retinal veins do not anastomose, but near the ora serrata their terminal twigs bend round, run circularly parallel to the periphery of the retina, and form an incomplete ring. The most peripheral retinal vessels are capillary arches, but even these do not reach the ora, so that an avascular zone is present here. The arteries end farther back than the veins. The formation of the **vena centralis** from the superior and inferior retinal veins takes place at about the level of the lamina cribrosa (Fig. 171), i.e. somewhat proximal to the division of the artery into its primary branches, which occurs in the retinal portion of the optic nerve.

The vena centralis lies on the temporal side of the artery in the nerve and leaves it somewhat proximally. The artery and vein may cross the subarachnoid space together, but more often they part company at right angles to each other (Fig. 162) in the nerve and reach its periphery at different points. The vein

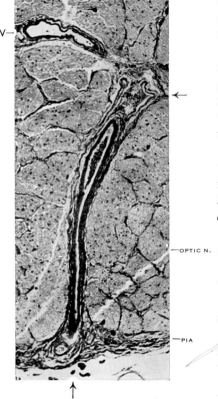

V—

←

—OPTIC N.

—PIA

FIG. 162.—TRANSVERSE SECTION OF
THE OPTIC NERVE.

To show the central artery passing into
the centre of the nerve along a radius of its
cross-section. V = the central retinal
vein which is diverging from the artery to
a different point on the periphery. The
arrows point to the central collateral
vessels.

(*Wolff's preparation.*)

always has a longer course in the subarachnoid space and pierces the dura
farther from the globe than the artery.

It most commonly opens directly
into the cavernous sinus, after having
given a branch to the superior ophthalmic vein, but may drain into the latter
vein entirely. Very rarely it opens into
the inferior ophthalmic veins.

It is the anastomosis with the orbital
veins (as shown by Sesemann) which
negatives *von Graefe's theory that papil-
loedema is produced by pressure on the
cavernous sinus.*

A branch of the vena centralis known
as the **post-central vein** of Kuhnt passes
backwards in the centre of the nerve to
the optic foramen.

The diameter of the central artery is
about 200 μ, that of the vein about 225 μ.

Structure.—In structure the central
retinal artery in the optic nerve resembles
that of a medium-sized vessel (Parsons).[1]

The Intima.—The artery is lined by a
layer of *endothelium* whose nuclei, placed
so that their long axis is that of the
vesels, project into the lumen of the vessel.
Beneath this is a *subendothelial* or intermediate layer, which is not present at birth
but develops with increasing age.

It consists of connective tissue which
stains homogeneously with hæmatoxylin
or van Gieson, but shows circularly
arranged fine elastic fibres with Weigert's elastic stain.

Outside this is the usual (Henle's) elastic fenestrated membrane (membrana
elastic stain.

The Middle Coat or Media consists of circularly arranged unstriped muscle
fibres with rod-like nuclei having their axis at right angles to the length of the
vessel. There is a *very little* white fibrous connective tissue and some elastic fibres.

The Outer Coat or Adventitia.—Directly next the muscle fibres is an indefinite
membrana elastica externa, which fades off into the *adventitia* proper. This consists

[1] See Parsons, J. H., *Pathology of the Eye*, **1–2**, 659.

of connective tissue with many elastic fibres arranged in circular and longitudinal bundles. Externally it passes gradually into the connective tissue sheath.

The Vein has an endothelial lining, a thin subendothelial layer, a media with very few muscle cells but many elastic fibres, and a thin adventitia with fine fibres but little elastic tissue. There is neither membrana elastica interna nor externa.

After division into its branches the walls of the retinal arteries get much thinner, and in the nerve fibre layer the walls, especially the muscularis, are but little developed. The muscle, however, can be followed to the finer branches.

The adventitia is sharply demarcated from the surrounding nerve tissue, which is bounded by a kind of border membrane formed by glia (limitans perivascularis of Krückmann) (Figs. 113, 168).

Between the glia (derived from ectoderm) and the adventitia (derived from mesoderm)

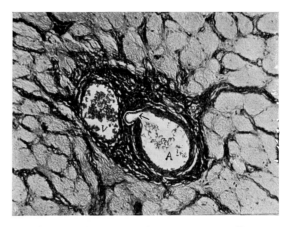

Fig. 163.—Transverse Section of the Central Vessels just behind the Lamina Cribrosa.

To show that the arteria centralis *does* give off a branch (marked by an arrow) in this region, a fact denied by a number of authors. This vessel, followed anteriorly in serial sections, was found to break up into branches which passed into the lamina cribrosa.

(*Wolff's preparation.*)

there is a potential space, which becomes apparent in atrophic conditions of the retina resulting from obliteration of the vessels, and in such conditions as retinitis pigmentosa becomes filled with pigment.

The Retinal Capillaries.[1]—The major branches of retinal artery and vein run peripherally from the disc at a superficial level in the nerve fibre layer. Successive divisions of the vessels remain at this level until the immediate precapillaries are reached ; these fall into two groups : one, the superficial group, gives rise to a capillary net which remains at the same level—the superficial capillary net ; the other or deep group runs usually at a steep angle to a deeper level, where it gives rise to the deep capillary net, lying in the boundary plane between inner nuclear layer and outer molecular layer. The two capillary nets are not, however, independent : anastomotic capillaries run from one to the other ; and the same capillary may run for part of its course in one layer and then change to the other. The markedly lamellar structure of the retina causes these capillary nets to be largely two-dimensional, in contrast to the three-dimensional net found in most other organs, including the brain.

[1] From Michaelson, I. C. and Campbell, A. C. P. (1940) *Trans. Ophthal. Soc. U.K.*, **60,** 71.

This basic two-layered pattern of the vascular architecture is modified in certain parts of the retina—by the addition of other layers and by the reduction to a single layer.

Small arterioles and venules—the arteriæ afferentes and venæ efferentes of His—run from or to the larger arteries and veins. The larger arteries and veins do not, of course, run together ; and in the spaces between them their arterioles and venules run towards each other in a rather regular interdigitating pattern.

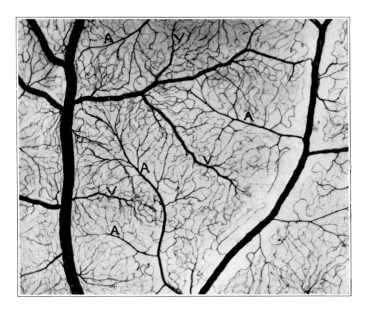

FIG. 164.—FIELD FROM EQUATORIAL ZONE OF RETINA, SHOWING A VEIN ON THE LEFT AND AN ARTERY ON THE RIGHT.

Note the interdigitation of the venæ efferentes (V) with the arteriæ afferentes (A). Note also the capillary-free zone around the artery. × 30.

(*From Michaelson and Campbell, Trans. O.S.U.K.* 1940.)

From these interdigitating arteriæ afferentes and venæ efferentes, precapillaries arise which feed and drain the superficial and deep capillary nets. His, in his classical paper, described the superficial net as arterial and the deep net as venous ; but Michaelson and Campbell cannot support this. Both arterial and venous precapillaries run to both superficial and deep nets, and there is no arterial or venous predominance in one or the other. Venous precapillaries are, of course, more noticeable and striking than arterial precapillaries since, in view of the much slower blood-flow in them, they are of larger calibre ; and hence a fallacious impression may be given that the only precapillaries in the deep net are venous.

The deep capillary net is in general a denser and more complex one than the superficial net. In the equatorial zone of the retina, where the two-layered pattern is most distinct, the difference can be most easily demonstrated. In general, one may say that the capillary pathway between arterial and venous precapillary is a more direct and simple one in the superficial than in the deep net.

In all parts of the retina the capillary nets show regularly varying density in the following way : firstly, as His pointed out, around the arteries of all calibre down to the arterial precapillaries there is a zone *which is quite free from capillaries.* This zone extends on either side of the artery for an average of 50 μ (at the extreme periphery it becomes much wider—about 120 μ). The capillaries do not avoid the neighbourhood of the veins in this way. Secondly, within both superficial and deep capillary nets, the nearer one approaches to the venous precapillaries and their draining venæ efferentes the denser the capillary net becomes ; so that the capillary net shows a regular alternation of dense areas

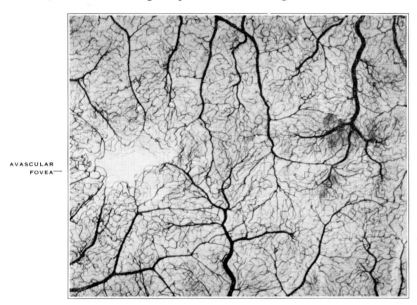

AVASCULAR
FOVEA—

FIG. 165.—THE BLOOD-SUPPLY TO THE LATERAL PORTION OF THE MACULA.
(From Michaelson and Campbell, Trans. O.S.U.K., 1940.)

centred round venæ efferentes and open areas (or areas completely devoid of capillaries) around arteriæ afferentes. This is only to be expected, since the poorer oxygenation of the blood in the venous ends of the capillaries must be compensated for by a denser distribution of capillaries in this region if the tissue is to be uniformly supplied with oxygen.

Modifications of the Basic Two-layered Pattern.—In the posterior, thicker part of the retina, the pattern is considerably modified. The deep layer is un-altered, remaining as a remarkably flat, two-dimensional net. The superficial layer, however, becomes increasingly three-dimensional; fewer capillaries run from arteriole to venule entirely in the nerve fibre layer ; and many capillary loops come to run at the superficial (internal) boundary of the inner nuclear layer. A three-layered pattern therefore appears, of which, however the two superficial layers are much less perfectly two-dimensional than the deep layer. This three-layered pattern is particularly well developed in the macular region.

Furthermore, in and around the disc, where the nerve fibre layer is thick, yet another most superficial capillary net appears, lying in this layer ; precapillaries and capillaries from the superficial layer proper turn superficial to the plane of this layer and break up into an extremely dense net of close-set, radially arranged capillaries. This network is the densest of all those present in the retina. In this central zone, therefore, there are four capillary nets at four different levels : the peripapillary radial net in the superficial part of the nerve fibre layer, the superficial net proper in the deeper part of the nerve fibre layer, the reduplication of the superficial net at the inner boundary of the inner nuclear layer, and the deep net at the outer (deep) boundary of the inner nuclear layer. The extent of the peripapillary radial net is asymmetrical ; it extends on the medial side for 4 mm. from the nerve head and on the lateral side for 7 mm. ; it avoids the macula, however, so that its lateral margin is deeply indented, and in the horizontal plane it only extends 2 mm. lateral to the nerve head.

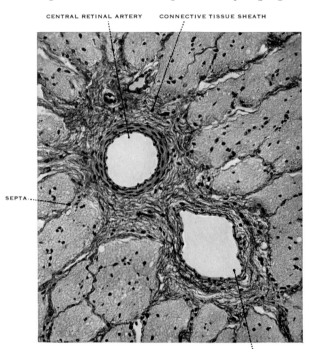

CENTRAL RETINAL ARTERY CONNECTIVE TISSUE SHEATH

SEPTA

CENTRAL RETINAL VEIN

FIG. 166.—THE RETINAL VESSELS IN THE CENTRE OF THE OPTIC NERVE.
(*Wolff's preparation.*)

In the macular region the fovea, as is well known, shows a completely avascular area, varying from 0·4 to 0·5 mm. in diameter. Towards the periphery of the retina the mesh of the capillary nets becomes wider and the peri-arterial space increasingly prominent. Eventually the two-layered pattern becomes intermittent, the deep net being present only around the venæ efferentes. Still farther towards the periphery the deep net disappears entirely, and there is only a single net of wide mesh and wide calibre capillaries. The peripheral margin of the retinal vascular system is formed by wide calibre capillary arches joining the terminations of the arteries and the veins. There are no anastomoses with the vessels of the ciliary body.

The double net extends peripherally for a distance from the nerve head, varying from 11·5 mm. to 14·5 mm., its greatest extent being in the lateral horizontal axis, and its least in the infero-medial quadrant. The extreme margin of the retinal vascular system lies about 1 mm. behind the ciliary body, leaving a narrow peripheral zone of the retina entirely without blood vessels.

Each capillary according to Krückmann has three distinct layers surrounding it.

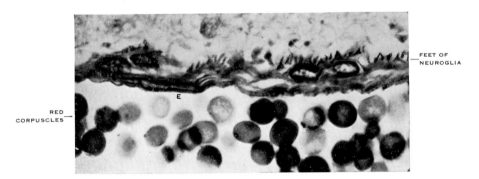

FIG. 167.—LONGITUDINAL SECTION OF PRECAPILLARY VEIN. E = ENDOTHELIAL CELL LINING VESSEL. (MALLORY'S PHOSPHOTUNG. ACID HÆM.)

Note also bilobed endothelial nuclei in lymphatic space in vessel wall.

There is (1) the endothelial lining containing Rouget cells (Schaly 1926). Around this is (2) a membrane continuous with the adventitia of the larger vessels, and lastly (3) comes the limitans perivascularis formed by the glia. Between (1) and (2) is the perivascular lymph space containing loose connective tissue and a few endothelial cells (His) (Figs. 167, 168).

Nerve Supply to the Retinal Arteries.—Although still disputed, Tinel with the silver nitrate method has shown that there is a network of nerve fibres around the central artery and its branches. This has been confirmed by Mawas using methylene blue. The fibres probably come from the sympathetic plexus around the internal carotid artery in the cavernous sinus (see Schiff-Wertheimer (1950) *Trans. Intern. Congress of Ophthal.*, p. 40).

The Lymphatics of the Retina.—There are no true lymphatic vessels. The lymph, however, circulates between the various elements of the retina, and in the perivascular sheaths, and, following the veins, is carried through the lamina cribrosa into the lymphatic spaces of the optic nerve. According to Schieck, the lymphatics of the retina run with the central retinal vessels and open into the subarachnoid space. Levinsohn, on the other hand, believes that they pass out through the dura with these vessels.

The Appearance of the Fundus as seen by the Ophthalmoscope

The fundus, or back of the eye, appears red, owing partly to the blood of the choroid, partly to the pigment epithelium. The colour is lighter in fair people, darker in dark people, depending on the amount of pigment in the pigment epithelium and in the choroid.

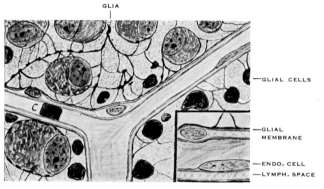

GLIA

GLIAL CELLS

GLIAL MEMBRANE

ENDO. CELL
LYMPH. SPACE

Fig. 168.—Flat (horizontal) Section through the Ganglion Cell Layer of the Retina.

Note the structure of the capillary and the glial fibres. *Inset* semi-schematic enlarged view of section of capillary (Phosphotung. Hæm.) C = deformed red-blood corpuscle in capillary.

(Wolff's preparation.)

If there is much pigment in the pigment epithelium the choroid is hidden altogether, and the fundus appears a uniform brownish red. In extreme cases, as in the dark races, the fundus is almost dark grey.

The fundus has a finely granular appearance, due to the fact that the pigment epithelium varies in thickness and thus is not equally dark all over. A finer mottling is also often seen since the pigment tends to collect at the periphery of each pigment epithelial cell (Figs. 100, 101). "The pigment of the retinal pigment epithelium (when viewed on the flat) tends to collect towards the periphery of the cell, leaving the central nuclear portion relatively free of pigment. It is probable that the darker the fundus the more the central portion is invaded. In not too highly pigmented fundi, therefore, the pigment forms a network, the individual holes of which are constituted by a single living epithelial cell. Now the diameter of a hexagonal cell is about 16 μ ; this multiplied by 15, which is the magnification given by the direct method of ophthalmoscopy, makes 240 μ, i.e. about 0·25 mm.

" If we take into consideration the shrinkage produced by the preparation of a microscopic section, I think we shall not be far wrong if we make this figure 0·3 mm. or 1/75 in., which is well within the visual limits. I have seen this network quite often, and so have my colleagues to whom I have spoken about it. I believe it can be made out best in fair fundi, in the macular region."—Wolff, Eugene (1938), *Proc. R. Soc. Med.,* **31,** 1104.

If the pigment in the pigment epithelium is less marked, and that of the choroid profuse, a tessellated fundus is produced. This consists of dark areas surrounded by red, apparently anastomosing (see p. 93) bands, produced by the choroidal vessels, for the most part the veins. These bands are not sharply defined as they are to a certain extent obscured by the pigment.

The less pigment there is in the pigment epithelium and the choroid the more the sclera shows through and the fairer will be the fundus.

In very fair people, and more so in albinos, in whom there is little or no pigment, the choroidal vessels can be seen distinctly. The vessels are broader and less sharply defined than the retinal vessels which run superficial to them. Moreover, they appear flat and ribbon-like, and show no light reflex. Also, unlike the retinal vessels which branch dendritically and do not anastomose, the choroidal vessels *appear* to form a dense network (see p. 94), except anteriorly, where the *straight* vessels pass towards the ora serrata.

The Optic Disc is pink, owing to the numerous capillaries which it contains (Fig. 298). It must be emphasised, as it is curiously often forgotten, that the white element in its colour is due to the *lamina cribrosa*, and not to the nerve fibres of the " papilla," which are of course non-medullated.

The optic disc under normal conditions lies in the same plane as the retina, and does not therefore form a projection as the name " papilla " would lead one to suppose (Fuchs, Testut, and others. See also Wolff and Davies (1931), *Brit. J. Ophthal.*, **15**, 609).

The optic disc is excavated by a funnel-shaped depression, called the physiological cup, which varies much in form and size. It is most often not in the centre of the disc but displaced slightly to the temporal side. It tends to be absent in high hypermetropia. Its colour is whiter than the rest of the disc, because there are fewer vessels and nerve fibres obscuring the lamina cribrosa. Very often the holes in this membrane for the passage of the nerve fibres can be seen as grey dots. *They become more evident in glaucoma and atrophy of the disc.*

The optic disc is pinker in colour to the medial side of the physiological cup than to the lateral. This is due to the greater thickness of nerve fibres and more capillary vessels. For the same reason the medial edge of the disc tends to be less well-defined than the lateral.

The Retinal Vessels climb up the medial side of the physiological cup. The arteries are easily distinguished from the veins. The arteries are narrower, of a

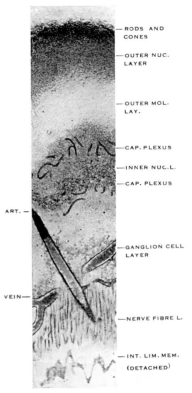

RODS AND CONES
OUTER NUC. LAYER
OUTER MOL. LAY.
CAP. PLEXUS
INNER NUC.L.
CAP. PLEXUS
ART.—
GANGLION CELL LAYER
VEIN—
NERVE FIBRE L.
INT. LIM. MEM. (DETACHED)

FIG. 169.—FLAT (ALMOST TANGENTIAL) SECTION OF THE RETINA TO SHOW ITS VASCULARISATION. (ZENKER. MALLORY'S TRIPLE STAIN.)

Note.—The main vessels lie in the nerve fibre and ganglion cell layers. The capillary plexus in the ganglion cell layer is not visible here, but the plexuses at the inner and outer parts of the inner nuclear layer are well shown.

brighter red colour, and have a well-marked light streak or reflex along their middle.   The light streak along the veins is much less marked.   It is the image of the source of light used in the ophthalmoscopic examination.

When the scleral canal is straight, the end of the arteria centralis is seen in optical section, and the branches appear to come off at 180°.

If the intra-mural portion of the optic nerve is directed laterally as well as forwards (temporally oblique scleral canal) the nasal border of the physiological cup is steep or overhanging.   The arteria centralis is usually invisible, and its first divisions make an angle which is open towards the temporal side.

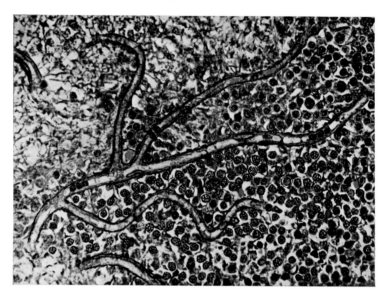

FIG. 170.—FLAT SECTION OF THE CAPILLARY PLEXUS IN THE INNER NUCLEAR LAYER.
(*Wolff's preparation.*)

If the scleral canal runs forwards and medially (nasally oblique canal) the artery can be seen for some distance and the central vessels appear displaced towards the temporal side.

It should be noted carefully that as the disc is on the same plane as the retina, the light streak is not normally lost as the vessels pass over the edge of the disc.   With the slightest amount of swelling of the disc (as in papillœdema) the vessels bend over its edge, and the image of the source of light is thrown beyond the pupil. It thus does not reach the examining eye, and the bent portion of the vessel appears dark.   In this way we get the loss of light reflex so important in the diagnosis of papillœdema.

As the vessels pass out into the retina the nasal vessels run a more or less direct (if wavy) course, while the temporal ones are arcuate.

It will be noted that although an artery is accompanied by the corresponding

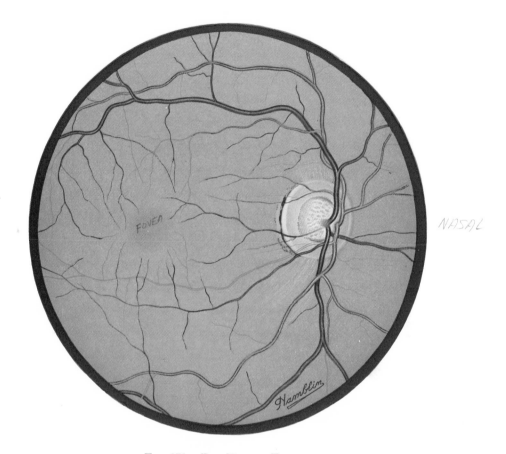

FIG. 171.—THE NORMAL FUNDUS.

(Direct image of the right eye.)

The central vessels climb up the nasal side of the physiological cup. The central artery appears as a single stem which is just visible here and then divides into two branches which appear to separate at an angle of 180°. (Often the stem is invisible where the scleral canal is quite straightforward, or it may be seen for some distance in a very oblique canal ; more rarely it appears as two or more trunks.)

The central vein, on the other hand, appears as two trunks, since its formation (seen hazily) is in the lamina cribrosa. It is lateral to the artery.

As the vessels pass over the edge of the disc they do not lose their light streak.

The macula is seen as an area darker red than the rest of the fundus. Its centre (the fovea), seen as a whitish reflex, lies below the centre of the disc.

At the edge of the disc are a pigmented " choroidal " crescent and a scleral ring.

The normal striation which is often seen above and below the disc and due to the *non-medullated* nerve fibres has come out much too prominently in the figure.

vein, they never or almost never run next to each other for this would cast too much of a shadow on the rods and cones.

Pulsation in the veins is physiological. In the arteries it is pathological, and occurs especially in *glaucoma* (or when the tension of the eye is artificially raised by pressing on it with the finger), in *aortic regurgitation* and anæmia when syncope is imminent.

The *connective tissue* or *scleral ring* is the white ring or part of a ring seen often next the disc. This may be due to the border tissue not covered by the epithelium or to the side-wall of an oblique scleral canal.

The Choroidal Ring is a dark ring (or portion of a ring) outside the scleral ring. It is produced by a heaping up of the retinal pigment epithelium ; hence " choroidal " is a misnomer (Elschnig).

The Macula appears as a small oval area devoid of vessels, of a deeper red than the rest of the fundus, and often slightly stippled with pigment.

The retinal reflexes, which usually change their position with the slightest movement of the eye or ophthalmoscope, are fixed in the macular region.

The oval macular reflex comes from the wall which surrounds the macula. The fovea forms a small concave mirror, and so produces the bright foveal reflex (which at times may be so bright as to deserve the name of bull's-eye lantern reflex).

The region of the clivus is, however, darker than the surrounding retina, because light falling on it from the ophthalmoscope is not reflected back through the pupil ; also the retina here is very thin and the pigment epithelium much denser.

The Anterior and Posterior Chambers

The space in front of the lens and suspensory ligament is divided into two by the iris (Fig. 21).

In front of the iris is the anterior chamber, behind it the posterior chamber.

The Anterior Chamber is bounded in front by the cornea and a small portion of the sclera.

The amount of sclera entering into the formation of the anterior chamber is about 2 mm. above, 1·5 mm. below, and 1 mm. at the sides. Rochon Duvigneaud, measuring from the limbus to the angle, finds 2·25 mm., 2 mm., and 1·25 mm. ; while Lagrange finds (from limbus to a point opposite the attachment of the iris) 1·75 mm., 1·45 mm., and 1 mm. as the corresponding figures.

Behind is the iris, a part of the ciliary body, and that portion of the lens which presents through the pupil.

At the periphery of the anterior chamber is its so-called *angle*, and it is here that we find the sponge-work of the ligamentum pectinatum iridis, with the spaces of Fontana which drain into the sinus venosus scleræ (canal of Schlemm). The anterior chamber is about 3 mm. deep at its centre and is narrowest not at the angle but slightly central to this (Fig. 48).

The Posterior Chamber is somewhat triangular on section, the apex of the triangle being where the edge of the iris rests on the lens. The base is formed by the ciliary processes and the valleys between them, in which are the recesses of Kuhnt.

The posterior wall is formed by the lens and suspensory ligament and the anterior by the iris.

Both anterior and posterior chambers are filled with aqueous humour, which consists essentially of 98·1 per cent. of water, with a trace of sodium chloride and albumen.

THE LENS

The lens of the eye is a transparent bi-convex body of crystalline appearance placed between the iris and the vitreous.

The diameter of the lens is 9–10 mm. ; its thickness, from 4 to 5 mm., varies greatly as the eye is focused for distant or near objects.

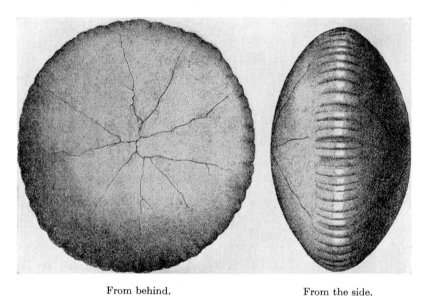

From behind.   From the side.

FIG. 172.—THE LENS.

Note that the equator is not smooth.

(*From Rabl.*)

Like all lenses, that of the eye presents for examination two surfaces, anterior and posterior, and a border where these surfaces meet, known as the equator (æquator lentis).

The anterior surface, less convex than the posterior, is the segment of a sphere whose radius is 9 mm.

It is in relation in front, through the pupil with the anterior chamber of the eye, with the posterior surface of the iris, the pupillary margin of which rests on the anterior surface, with the posterior chamber of the eye, and with the ciliary processes.

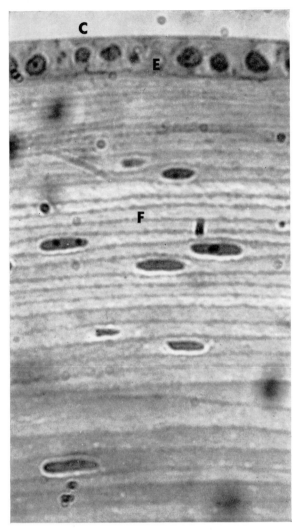

FIG. 173.—THE LENS CAPSULE, EPITHELIUM AND FIBRES (PHOTOMICROGRAPH, × 500).
(*By courtesy of Dr. C. Pedler, Institute of Ophthalmology, London. Preparation by Mrs. R. Tilly.*)

The centre of the anterior surface is known as the anterior *pole,* and is about 3 mm. from the back of the cornea.

The posterior surface, more curved than the anterior, forms the segment of a sphere whose radius is 5·5 mm. It is usually described as lying in a fossa lined by the hyaloid membrane on the front of the vitreous, but it is separated from the vitreous by a slight space filled with " primitive " vitreous (p. 452). This post-lenticular space was described long ago by Berger, and is confirmed by the slit-lamp (see p. 250).

A.E.—11

The Equator of the lens forms a circle lying 0·5 mm. within the ciliary processes. The equator is not smooth, but shows a number of dentations corresponding to the zonular fibres (Fig. 172). These tend to disappear during accommodation, when the zonular fibres are loose.

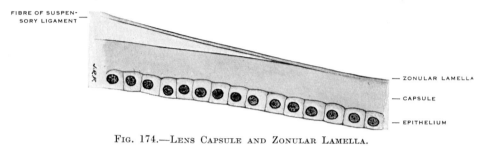

FIBRE OF SUSPENSORY LIGAMENT

ZONULAR LAMELLA

CAPSULE

EPITHELIUM

FIG. 174.—LENS CAPSULE AND ZONULAR LAMELLA.

Structure of the Lens

The lens consists of :

1. Its capsule.
2. The anterior epithelium.
3. The cement substance or amorphous material.
4. The lens fibres.

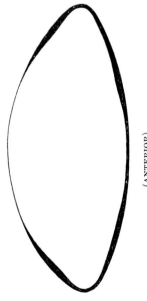

(ANTERIOR)

FIG. 175.—VERY SCHEMATIC ANTERO-POSTERIOR SECTION OF THE LENS CAPSULE TO SHOW RELATIVE THICKNESS OF VARIOUS PORTIONS (FINCHAM).

The Capsule of the lens forms a transparent, homogeneous, highly elastic envelope.

When cut or ruptured its edges roll out and then curl up, so that the outer surface is innermost. It is much thicker in front than behind, and the anterior and posterior portions are thicker towards the periphery (equator), just within the attachment of the suspensory ligament, than at the poles. It is this difference in the thickness of the central and peripheral parts of the anterior capsule which Fincham believes is responsible for the hyperbolic form of the anterior surface of the lens during accommodation.

A lamination of the capsule has been described, and seems to be confirmed by the fact that the zonular or anterior lamina may be separated from the remainder pathologically.

Also with age the capsule gets thicker, and on cross-section a faint longitudinal striation may be seen (Ginsberg).

The Anterior Epithelium (Figs. 173, 174, 176).— This consists of a single layer of cubical cells spread over the front of the lens deep to the capsule. There

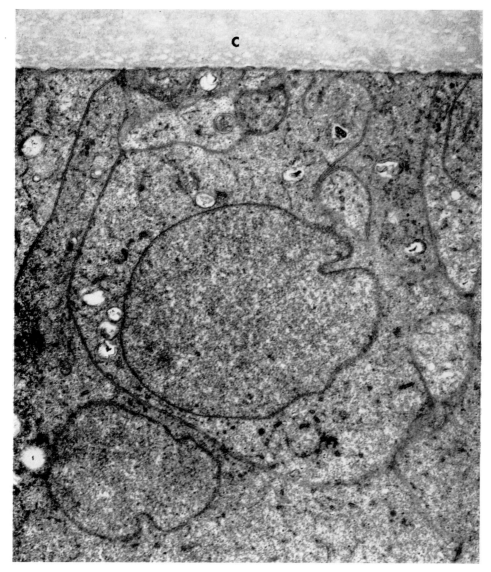

FIG. 176.—THE LENS CAPSULE (C) AND EPITHELIUM (RHESUS MONKEY, ELECTRON MICROGRAPH, × 20,000).

(By courtesy of Dr. C. Pedler, Institute of Ophthalmology, London. Preparation by Mrs. R. Tilly.)

is no corresponding posterior epithelium, since the posterior cells were used up in filling the central cavity of the lens vesicle.

Electron Microscopy of Lens Epithelium.—There is quite considerable inter-digitation between adjacent cells, especially at the equator. A typical epithelial cell is shown in Fig. 176.

If we trace the cells of the anterior epithelium towards the equator we find that they gradually become columnar, and elongating are eventually converted into lens fibres. In Fig. 178 all the stages of development of the lens fibres can be seen.

It will be noted that the base of the cell, i.e. the part in contact with the capsule, becomes the posterior part of the lens fibre, while the opposite end grows into the anterior portion of the lens fibre. The nuclei form a somewhat S-shaped nuclear zone at the equator (see also p. 439).

The Cement Substance or Amorphous Material.— The various elements forming the lens are bound together by an amorphous substance. It is not visible in ordinary sections, and it must be emphasised that anything but a minimal amount of this material must be taken as a post-mortem or pathological change. The cement substance glues the various fibres to each other and is found in the following positions :

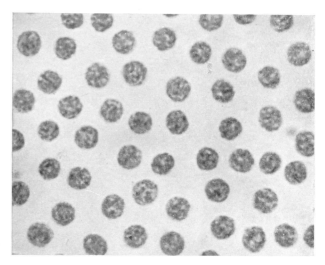

FIG. 177.—PORTION OF ANTERIOR CAPSULE OF LENS VIEWED ON THE FLAT TO SHOW THE EPITHELIUM.

(*a*) Beneath the capsule both in front and behind (Testut).

(*b*) A thin layer just deep to the anterior epithelium (Schwalbe). This probably represents the debris of cells in the embryonic lens vesicle (Fig. 452).

(*c*) The central strand.

The central strand occupies the axis of the lens running from the anterior to the posterior pole. Then jutting out from this axial collection towards the equator we find three shelves of amorphous material which divide the lens into sectors.

Looking at these shelves end-on, in the foetus or infant, we find that they form a Y, the arms of which are separated by angles of 120°. The anterior Y is vertical, the posterior Y inverted, which is the contrary of the classical anatomical description.

These figures are known as the anterior and posterior lens stars or sutures.

In the adult, towards the anterior and posterior surfaces the rays are much more complicated, there being six or more primary and many subsidiary ones, but in front and behind the embryonic nucleus the original Ys persist throughout life (see slit-lamp picture, Fig. 232).

It is into these shelves of amorphous material that the ends of the lens fibres are inserted.

It should be noted that electron microscopy fails to reveal this amorphous material.

The Lens Fibres.—Each lens fibre is a long, prismatic, six-sided band, but the usual description of the lens fibres as bands with parallel sides is incorrect for they always taper from the equator towards the poles (Rochon-Duvigneaud) (see p. 490). Each consists of an albuminoid material enclosed in a pseudo-membrane—pseudo, because it consists of the same material as its contents, only is more dense.

The first lens fibres were formed from the posterior epithelium and ran from the back to the front of the vesicle. But the later ones are derived from the equatorial portion of the anterior epithelium.

Here, as we have seen, we find all stages in the formation of a lens fibre from its cell (Fig. 178).

The newest lens fibres are laid on externally to the older deeper ones, and so the lens acquires a laminated structure. On equatorial section the laminæ are cut transversely, forming the radial lamellæ of Rabl (Fig. 179), while antero-posterior section shows them as long

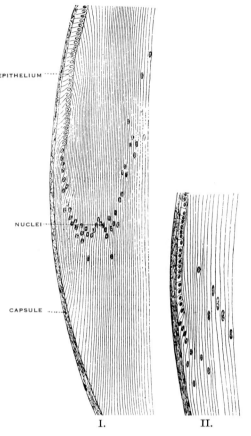

Fig. 178.—Meridional Section of the Equatorial Region of the Lens.

I. New-born.   II. Old man.

(*From Poirier, after Otto Becker.*)

fibres placed one on the other in concentric layers. The fibres belonging to each lamina are of the same length.

The superficial (youngest) fibres, too, are nucleated, their nuclei lying near the equator, and arranged so as to form a letter S in meridional section. Moreover, their sides are quite smooth. The nuclei are at first rounded or slightly oval. As the fibre ages the nucleus becomes longer, often narrower at its middle, and then breaks down into granules.

The deeper, older fibres lose their nuclei, become less succulent as it were, and their edges become serrated, the serrations of one fitting into those of its neighbour. Thus the oldest fibres are irregular in thickness and their contours serrated due to shrinkage. Outside these fibres we see cross-sections of fibres

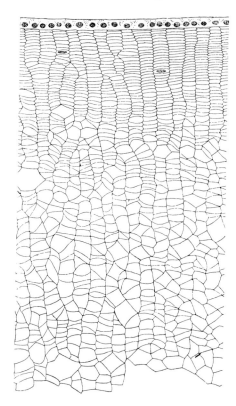

FIG. 179.—PERIPHERAL PORTION OF AN EQUATORIAL SECTION OF THE HUMAN LENS TO SHOW THE RADIAL LAMELLÆ.
(*From Rabl.*)

having four, five, or six sides. They are of irregular thickness, but get thinner towards the periphery. Finally, at the periphery itself is a concentrically striped layer. This appearance must not lead one to think that the whole lens has a concentrically layered structure; for else this appearance ought to be found in equatorial as well as meridional sections. As Rabl has shown (in all vertebrates), only radial lamellæ occur in equatorial sections. Hence here the lens appears built after the manner of an orange rather than like an onion.

The splitting of the lens into concentric lamellæ is due, according to Rabl, to the fact that fibres of the same age have more or less the same physical qualities.

Although the first-formed lens fibres go from pole to pole, of the later ones none do.

In the infantile lens, each starts and finishes on the anterior and posterior Ys respectively in such a way that the nearer the axis of the lens it commences the farther away it ends (Fig. 393).

The fibres formed later, for instance the superficial ones of the adult lens, start and finish on the more complicated stellate figures, conforming, however, to the above rule.

Two of the sides of the hexagonal lens fibres are longer than the remainder, and adhere much less firmly to the neighbouring fibres than do the short sides. It follows that if we treat the infantile lens with alcohol, which dissolves the cement substance, it will first of all divide into three sectors, and then each of these will separate into laminæ like the layers of an onion.

New lens fibres are laid on throughout life, and as the central portion which corresponds to the keratin layer of the skin cannot be shed, the lens keeps on growing. This, however, is not proportional to the number of fibres, for the older ones, as we have seen, shrink. According to Priestley Smith the lens at the 65th year is one-third larger than at 25.

The consistency of the lens varies, the more superficial portion or *cortex* being softer than the central part or *nucleus*. The nucleus increases with age. The lens becomes flatter with age, but its refractive power is retained by an increase in the refractive index of the nucleus.

The sclerosing of the nuclear portion, which starts in earliest youth, continues with increasing speed with age, while new nucleated fibres are laid on around. These in turn lose their nuclei, to be surrounded again by younger nucleated fibres.

As stated before, some new fibres are laid on throughout life, but more slowly with advancing age ; hence there are more nucleated fibres in the young than in the old.

Hence also, the nuclear bow which in young embryos extended right across the lens shows a greater and greater gap with advancing age (Figs. 25, 380).

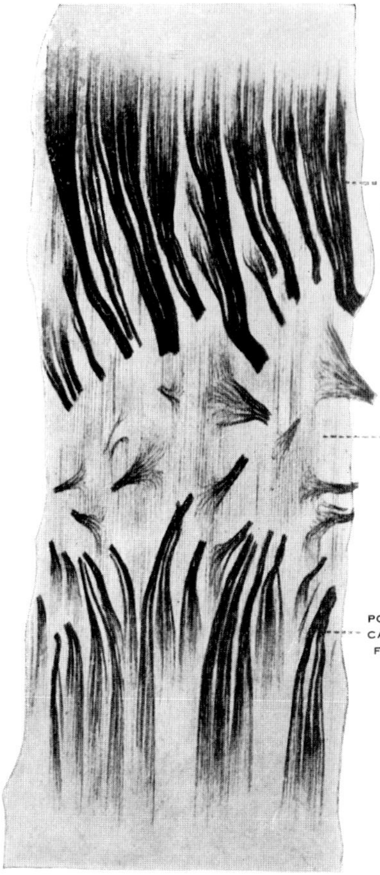

In a well-stained meridional section through the normal adult lens we see at its centre a relatively narrow

ORBICULO-ANTERIOR CAPSULAR FIBRES

EQUATORIAL FIBRES

POSTERIOR CAPSULAR FIBRES

FIG. 180.—EQUATORIAL ZONE OF THE LENS CAPSULE WITH THE INSERTION OF THE ZONULAR FIBRES.
(*From Salzmann.*)

area of axially directed fibres which become more and more convex outwards as we pass laterally.

The colour of the lens, too, changes with age. In the infant and young adult it is usually stated to be quite colourless but, according to Hess, a *very faint* yellow tinge can be made out even here. After about thirty-five years the central portion gets a definite yellow tinge, which becomes darker and more extensive as time goes on. In the old man the lens often has an amber colour.

One other point of practical importance must be mentioned. In old people the lens often appears grey when viewed by indirect illumination. *This appearance may easily be mistaken for a cataract by the uninitiated.*

Electron Microscopy.—Conflicting interpretations exist, and no definite conclusions can yet be drawn (see *Symposium on The Lens*, 1965, *Invest. Ophth.* **4,**

4, 433–451). In general it may be said that cross-sections of young fibres show the hexagonal outline (with two opposite longer sides) already known by light microscopy. The serrated contours of the older lens fibres prove to be a highly tortuous series of mutual interdigitations (Fig. 183).

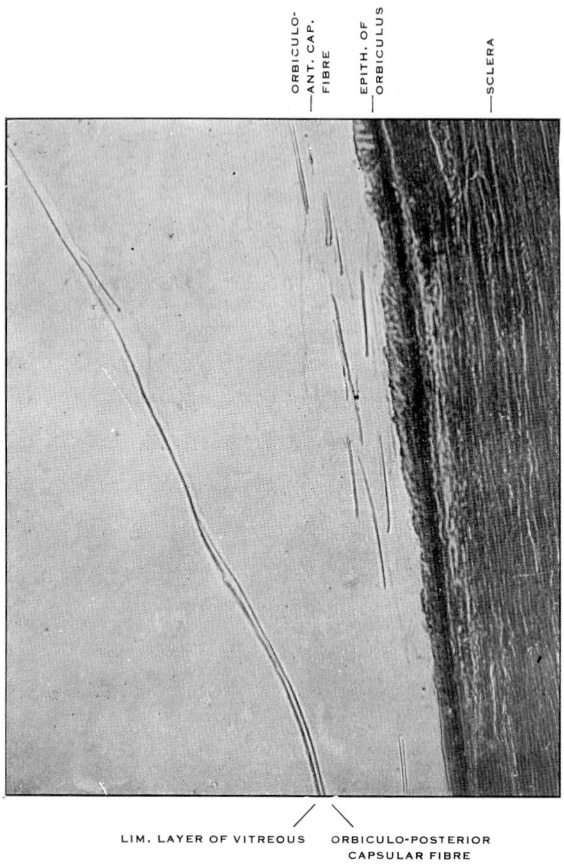

FIG. 181.—ANTERO-POSTERIOR SECTION TO SHOW SOME FIBRES OF THE ZONULE AND THE LIMITING LAYER OF VITREOUS.

THE CILIARY ZONULE (Zonule of Zinn, Suspensory Ligament of the Lens)

The Ciliary Zonule consists essentially of a series of fibres passing from the ciliary body to the lens. It holds the lens in position and enables the ciliary muscle to act on it. The lens and zonule form a diaphragm which divides the eye into a smaller anterior portion which contains aqueous and a larger posterior portion filled with vitreous. As a whole the zonule forms a ring which is roughly triangular on meridional section. The base of the triangle is concave, and occupies the equator and portions of the anterior and posterior surfaces of the lens. The apex is elongated, curved, and follows the posterior border of the ciliary processes and then the orbiculus ciliaris to the ora.

The antero-external side forms part of the posterior boundary of the posterior chamber and then follows the whole of the inner surface of the corona ciliaris. The postero-internal border is in close contact with the anterior limiting layer of the vitreous. The zonular fibres do not fill this triangle uniformly. They are collected mainly into anterior and posterior layers lying along the antero-lateral and postero-medial sides of the triangle. The space between these layers is known as the canal of Petit, but actually it is subdivided into larger and smaller spaces by the crossings of the zonular fibres.

Although the above is now the usual description, Petit himself thought that

Fig. 182.—Lens Fibres in Longitudinal Section (Rhesus Monkey, Electron Micrograph, × 13,500).

(By courtesy of Dr. C. Pedler, Institute of Ophthalmology, London. Preparation by Mrs. R. Tilly.)

the hyaloid membrane split at the ciliary body, the anterior portion forming the suspensory ligament, the posterior continuing over the front of the vitreous, and that he had injected the space between the two. It was Hannover who actually showed that one could inject the space between the anterior and posterior portions of the suspensory ligament.

The zonule consists of fibres which are transparent, straight for the most part, stiff in appearance and inextensible. Viewed along their length they appear roughly rounded or flattened and faintly grooved. The cross-section has

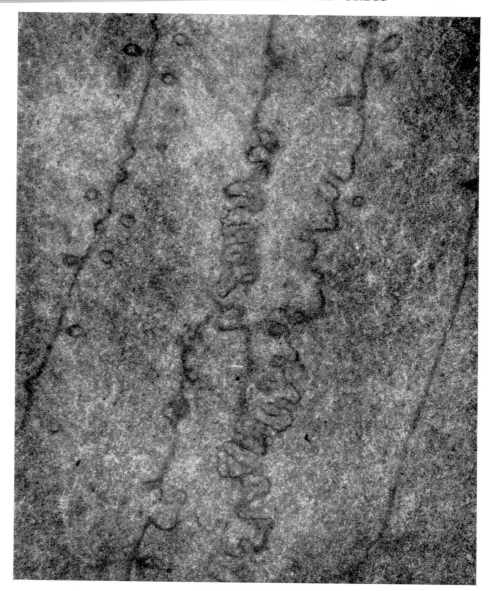

FIG. 183.—LENS FIBRES CUT IN LONGITUDINAL SECTION. (RHESUS MONKEY, SAME AS FIG. 182, ELECTRON MICROGRAPH, × 11,000).

These older fibres show the highly tortuous interdigitations between adjacent surfaces. There is no " amorphous substance " to be seen between the fibres.

(By courtesy of Dr. C. Pedler, Institute of Ophthalmology, London. Preparation by Mrs. R. Tilly.)

an irregular outline corresponding to the grooves and indicating the composite nature of each fibre. Their calibre, which is very constant for each fibre, varies from 2 to 8 μ and may reach 40 μ (Salzmann).

On ordinary histological examination the fibres appear homogeneous, but actually each consists of extremely fine fibrils so closely united that it requires maceration in alcohol, permanganate of potash, etc., to demonstrate this. Only at times can a faint longitudinal striation be made out in the stained section.

Electron microscopy shows that each zonular fibre is a bundle of fine fibrils of uniform size.

Fig. 184.—To show the relation of an Orbiculo-posterior Capsular Fibre (*a*) and the Anterior Limiting Layer of Vitreous (*b*) ; (Ant.-post. Section).

Note fibrillar appearance of latter.

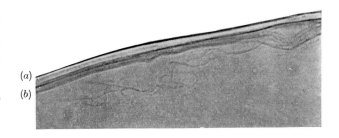

The composite nature of each fibre is again seen at its attachments. To the side of the lens it breaks up in a fan-shaped manner into a series of extremely fine fibrils (Fig. 180), which become continuous with the zonular lamella ; to the side of the ciliary body it may do this too or give off its fibrils like the barbs of a feather but on one side of the fibre only (Salzmann, and Fig. 185).

Among the fibres, or attached to them, one may find white cells which are probably endothelial cells or wandering leucocytes.

In the zonule, Main and Auxiliary Fibres may be distinguished.

The Main Fibres may be classified as follows :

1. Orbiculo[1]-posterior capsular.
2. Orbiculo[1]-anterior capsular.
3. Cilio[1]-posterior capsular.
4. Cilio[1]-equatorial.

1. *The orbiculo-posterior capsular fibres* are the most posterior and also the innermost fibres of the zonule. They take origin from the ora serrata. As regards their thickness they are of the second order. They lie throughout their extent in close contact with the anterior limiting layer of the vitreous, which, exercising a pressure on them, causes their forward convexity. They are inserted together with the vitreous (ligamentum hyaloideo-capsulare of Wieger) to the posterior lens capsule. In meridional sections they may easily be taken for a hyaloid membrane (Figs. 181, 184), but they are hyaline in nature and discontinuous in a section, whereas the limiting layer of the vitreous is fibrillar

[1] Orbiculo = from the orbiculus ciliaris.   Cilio = from the corona ciliaris.

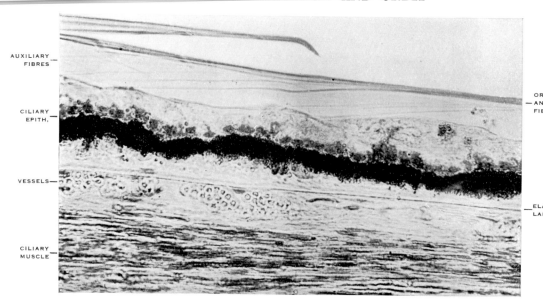

AUXILIARY
FIBRES

CILIARY
EPITH,

VESSELS

CILIARY
MUSCLE

ORBIC
— ANT. C
FIBRE

ELAST
LAMIN

FIG. 185.—MERIDIONAL SECTION OF ORBICULUS CILIARIS WITH ORBICULO-ANTERIOR CAPSULAR AND
AUXILIARY FIBRES.

and continuous. Also, if one looks at oblique meridional (tangential) sections in which the posterior attachments of these fibres are cut it may appear as if they have their origin in the vitreous, which is not the case (Garnier).[1]

2. *The Orbiculo-anterior capsular fibres* are the thickest and strongest of the zonular fibres ; they arise from the orbiculus ciliaris, a great number from a slight ridge known as the posterior zonular border which lies 1·5 mm. in front, and imitates the indentations, of the ora serrata. They are inserted into the anterior capsule of the lens. They receive supporting (auxiliary) fibres along their whole course. They lie in the valleys between the taller ciliary processes at whose sides they form well-marked bundles (Figs. 63, 186). They are attached to the valleys and the sides of the processes by their supporting fibrils. Some cross the heads of the ciliary processes, which they depress like a finger on the string of a harp (Rochon-Duvigneaud).

3. *The Cilio-posterior capsular fibres* are the most numerous zonular fibres. As regards their thickness they are of the third order. They arise from the valleys and less from the sides of the ciliary processes, pass posteriorly, cross the anteriorly directed fibres, and are inserted into the posterior capsule, anterior to the insertion of the orbiculo-posterior capsular fibres. In posterior dislocation of the lens these fibres pull on the ciliary processes.

4. *The Cilio-equatorial fibres* are really only present in youthful eyes. They arise from the ciliary valleys, a few from the orbiculus, and run to the equator of

---

[1] Salzmann, however, says that some zonular fibres do arise in the vitreous.

the lens. Sometimes they occupy the whole interval between the anterior and posterior groups of fibres. With age these fibres largely disappear and only a few sparse bundles eventually remain. Their thickness is much that of the previous group.

The Auxiliary Fibres.—Some of these strengthen the *main* fibres and help to anchor the individual portions of the zonule ; others hold the various portions of the ciliary body together. The auxiliary fibres are for the most part very fine. They run as a rule from without inwards and forwards. But from the posterior part of the corona ciliaris fibres run from without backwards and inwards to the orbiculo-anterior capsular fibres, crossing the auxiliary fibres that run anteriorly.

The zonular fibres here, therefore, have a double attachment which makes for strength; and so always or nearly always the zonular fibres break just beyond this area.

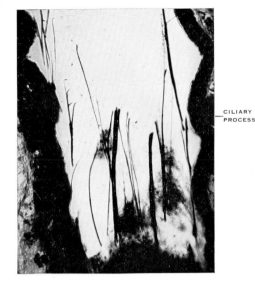

CILIARY
PROCESS

Fig. 186.—Coronal Section of a Ciliary Valley to show Orbiculo-anterior Capsular Fibres.

Over the orbiculus ciliaris the auxiliary fibres run almost parallel with the inner surface of the ciliary body, but more anteriorly they become more and more vertical while the most anterior ones are almost perpendicular to the surface.

The Orbiculo-ciliary fibres run from the orbiculus to the posterior ciliary processes, whose forward movement they tend to prevent.

The Inter-ciliary fibres tend to prevent the separation of two neighbouring processes (Fig. 187).

The great majority of zonular fibres have a meridional or radial direction. Salzmann describes some *circular zonular fibres* which, lying on the anterior limiting membrane of the vitreous, are often hidden in the folds of this layer.

The zonular fibres are firmly attached to the ciliary epithelium and if they are torn away some of the epithelium comes away with them. The exact method of insertion is still much disputed. They appear, however, to run into the internal limiting membrane of the ciliary body (*q.v.*) (Fig. 144). This interpretation is confirmed by electron microscopy.

Czermak showed that in a six and a half months' fœtus the zonular fibres not only came from the inner surface of the ciliary body but from the posterior aspect of the iris as well.

Also Garnier demonstrated that in the new-born child the number of zonular fibres is much larger than in the adult; that fibres pass to the anterior capsule from the most anterior ciliary process and even from the angle of the posterior chamber. In childhood these last disappear, so that in the adult the anterior ciliary process lies free and sends no fibres to the anterior capsule.

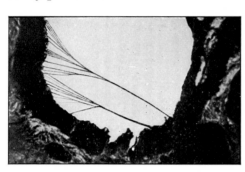

FIG. 187.—CROSS-SECTION OF CILIARY VALLEY TO SHOW INTER-CILIARY FIBRES.

In old age a large number of zonular fibres disappear, but in the process some fibres are much thickened.

Macroscopic Appearances.—The zonular fibres can be seen with the naked eye and better with a (magnifying) loupe. To do this, divide the eye equatorially, remove the vitreous, place the anterior part on a slide, remove the cornea as peripherally as possible, pull out the iris and illuminate the perilental space from below.

Looked at in this way each ciliary process is seen to be flanked on each side by a bundle of zonular fibres. As there are seventy processes, there are one hundred and forty bundles.

These bundles (consisting of orbiculo-anterior capsular fibres) are seen to run to the anterior capsule; they appear, however, to arise from the valleys between the processes. But, as we have seen, they come from farther back; in fact, from the orbiculus ciliaris.

If the preparation be now reversed the zonule can be seen from behind. In the anterior part of the orbiculus the (orbiculo-anterior capsular) fibres give rise to a fine silky meridional striation (better seen in the hardened than in the fresh specimen) which extends into the ciliary valleys leaving the processes free (Salzmann). From the ciliary processes again fibres are seen to run to the posterior capsule. These are the cilio-posterior capsular fibres; for the orbiculo-posterior capsular fibres have been removed with the vitreous. (If the vitreous had not been removed in the preparation the spaces between the zonular fibres would be filled in and therefore they would not be so clearly visible.)

The zonular fibres can also be seen in the living (especially with the help of a slit-lamp) in cases of coloboma of the iris and dislocation of the lens.

THE VITREOUS [1]

The vitreous humour is a perfectly transparent, colourless, gelatinous mass of a consistency somewhat firmer than egg-white, which fills the posterior [2]

[1] For an exceedingly detailed account of the vitreous, see Jokl (1927) *Über Den Bau und die Entwicklung des Glaskörpers, Upsala,* and Busacca and Goldmann (1957) *Biomicroscopie du Corps Vitré et du Fond de l'Œil, Paris.*   [2] Not the posterior chamber.

four-fifths of the globe.   Its shape is that of the cavity in which it lies, that is, of the space behind the diaphragm formed by the lens and suspensory ligament. Thus it has the form of a sphere flattened frontally and indented anteriorly by a saucer-shaped depression known as the fossa patellaris which lodges the lens. At the sides it supports the ciliary body (covered by the zonule) and the retina. Through its central region runs the hyaloid canal, which in the fœtus lodges the hyaloid artery.

The vitreous lies in contact with, but only slightly adherent to, the retina.   It is, however, attached to the optic disc, and more especially to the ciliary epithelium in a zone 1·5 mm. broad immediately adjacent to the ora serrata.   This area is known as the base (Salzmann) or origin (Wolfrum) of the vitreous, for it is here that, as the result of fixation or hardening fluids, or under pathological conditions, the vitreous remains adherent.   Even severe injuries do not tear the living vitreous from this situation, and when it does give way it takes part of the ciliary epithelium with it (Salzmann).   Also, as will be seen later, all vitreous fibrils can be traced back to this region.

From the ora to the lens the vitreous is convex forwards.   This portion is in contact all the way with the postero-internal fibres of the zonule.   It is held away from the orbiculus ciliaris by the zonular fibres.   More anteriorly the ciliary processes although separated by zonular fibres press on and form radial grooves in this portion of the vitreous (Fig. 24).

The vitreous is adherent [1] to the lens in a circle some 9 mm. in diameter, while posteriorly within the circle of adhesion the capillary space of Berger (see p. 250) appears to separate the lens from the vitreous.

The hyaloid canal (canal of Cloquet or Stilling) starts in front of the disc as a funnel-shaped area (area Martegiani), passes through the vitreous as a narrow canal 1–2 mm. wide, and expands again anteriorly in the fossa patellaris of the vitreous.   It is probable that in the adult the canal does not run a direct sagittal course as is usually depicted.   It probably sinks with gravity and moves about with movements of the eye and head.   Its walls are formed of a condensation of the vitreous and not by an actual membrane (Ida C. Mann, Busacca and Goldmann).

MICROSCOPIC STRUCTURE OF THE VITREOUS

It is extremely difficult to get a satisfactory microscopic preparation of the vitreous. This is due to the following facts : it contains a higher percentage of water than any other tissue in the body ; it is very liable to artefacts, and it stains badly with ordinary dyes.

The eye must be fixed as a whole without opening.   One of the best fixatives is the acetone fluid of Szent-Györgi (1914).   The eye should be embedded in celloidin and stained preferably with Held's phospho-molybdic acid hæmatoxylin.

Mallory's triple stain following fixation with Zenker's fluid also gives good results.

Under the microscope the vitreous is seen to consist of a denser limiting layer or rind and a central portion or nucleus.

[1] This adhesion is very weak and does not prevent the lens being removed with its capsule.

The limiting layer is simply a condensation of the vitreous and not a hyaloid membrane, but it does act as a fragile envelope. It is present everywhere, except just in front of the origin of the vitreous (zonular cleft of Salzmann) and at the area Martegiani. It is divided by Salzmann into anterior and posterior limiting layers.

The Posterior limiting layer starts at the origin or base of the vitreous and runs backwards in contact with, but only very slightly adherent to, the internal limiting membrane of the retina. In its course backwards the posterior limiting layer becomes thinner owing to its constituent fibrils gradually peeling off into the vitreous. Around the optic nerve, however, it is firmly attached to the internal limiting membrane, which therefore becomes detached when the vitreous is torn away here.

The Anterior limiting layer starts some 2 mm. from the ora, just anterior to the mass of fibrils passing into the vitreous from its origin or base but continuous with the most anterior of these.

It passes inwards to the posterior aspect of the lens, to which it is attached in the form of a ring some 9 mm. in diameter. This attachment is known as the ligamentum hyaloideo-capsulare of Wieger.

Up to this point the anterior limiting layer is narrow, well defined, and has a constant thickness. Traced inwards from here it becomes thinner through its fibrils peeling off into the vitreous, and almost (but not quite) disappears at the middle of the patellar fossa.

From its start to its attachment to the lens the anterior limiting layer is in contact with and, in fact, adherent to, the most posterior (the orbiculo-posterior capsular) fibres of the zonule. It thus comes about that if the vitreous is removed with forceps the posterior zonular fibres are usually removed with it ; on the other hand, if the vitreous is merely allowed to flow away some vitreous remains attached to the zonular fibres (Garnier).

Busacca and Goldmann (1957) maintain emphatically that the " hyaloid " membrane exists only anteriorly ; from its attachment at the ora serrata it clothes the back of the zonule and of the lens, being adherent to both. They base their views on histological as well as biomicroscopical appearances. Behind this anterior " hyaloid " membrane, and over the posterior convexity of the vitreous, as well as along the hyaloid canal, there is a condensation of vitreous that, while perhaps acting physiologically as a membrane, has no *anatomical* structure, and differs absolutely from the " anterior hyaloid." This surface condensation encloses the definitive vitreous. *Behind* their " hyaloid " membrane the retrolental space consists of the anterior end of the hyaloid canal, expanded into a funnel, containing what they call " hyaloid " vitreous. This is the " primitive " vitreous discussed on p. 452.

The anterior limiting layer is not a hyaloid membrane, for a hyaloid membrane must be transparent, homogeneous, with sharp contours.

But the anterior limiting layer has more the structure of connective tissue and shows a striation due to its constituent fibrillæ parallel with the surface. It is the close relation of the hyaline zonular fibres which is at any rate partly responsible for the error of calling the anterior limiting layer a hyaloid membrane (see Garnier and Figs. 181, 184). But the zonular fibres are not continuous in a section, whereas the anterior limiting layer is.

Although the anterior limiting layer differs from the posterior in not being in close contact with the corresponding internal limiting membrane, being, in fact, separated from it by zonular fibres, it does send fine processes of vitreous between the fibres to the membrane. In the region of the corona ciliaris these vitreous processes (called here the ligamentes cordiformes of Campos) pass between the processes to the ciliary valleys.

The main mass of the vitreous appears under the microscope as a reticulum of extremely fine fibrils, in the meshes of which presumably a fluid was present during life. It would seem that in the adult human eye these fibrils, probably for the most part at any rate, only cross each other without forming any actual connexions.

At more or less regular intervals there occur on the fibrils somewhat spherical thickenings, which stain better than the fibrils themselves.

The swellings have been regarded as granular deposits (artefacts) from the fixative or stain, as optical cross-sections of the fibrils, or as junctional points between the fibrils. As stated above, they are probably actual thickenings of the fibrils.

That the vitreous does consist of a firmer material enclosing in its meshes a more fluid portion is shown by the fact, as H. Virchow demonstrated, that if either the whole or a piece of the vitreous humour be thrown on a filter a small portion always remains on the latter ; although by far the larger portion drains away and may be collected as a clear watery fluid.

The Zonular Cleft lies between the origin or base of the vitreous and the commencement of the anterior limiting layer. It is circular in form in close relation to some of the zonular fibres and marks a place where the vitreous nucleus comes to the surface, i.e. is not covered by a limiting layer.

The Vitreous as seen with the Ultra-microscope.—While the above description is what one finds by ordinary histological methods, the work with the ultra-microscope of Baurmann 1923–26, Comberg 1924, Heesh 1926, Redslob 1927–32, and Duke-Elder 1929, has led them to the following conclusions. Macroscopically the vitreous has the appearance of a colour-less transparent jelly. Microscopically absolutely fresh vitreous has no structure at all. With the ultra-microscope perfectly fresh vitreous is optically empty. Soon, however, fibrillæ of colloidal dimensions, such as are seen in soap gels, appear. When the vitreous has been standing for some time the fibrillæ break up into separate particles.

Thus the appearances seen with various fixatives they suggest are artefacts : the vitreous has no structure in the ordinary sense of the word. The appearance seen with the slit-lamp is due to the fact that the fibrillæ become evident when large numbers of them are arranged in a direction perpendicular to the incident light as obtains near the surface of the vitreous. The optical effect of this arrangement is that of a waved or moiré appearance, suggestive of marcelled hair or watered silk. Where the arrangement of the fibrillæ is haphazard the vitreous appears optically empty. A similar appearance is seen when any gel of like constitution is examined by the slit-lamp in a glass vessel which is gently shaken. This appearance, it must be remembered, is an optical illusion, for the fibrillæ are far too small, being somewhat of the size of molecules, to be seen with the slit-lamp. The vitreous humour consists of 98·5 per cent. of water, with traces of albumen, NaCl, etc.

It has in fact practically the same composition as the aqueous, except that it contains in addition a small amount of residual protein of the collagen-gelatin type (called vitrein by Friedenwald) and hyaluronic acid which is a viscous polysaccharide (see Pirie (1949) *Brit. J. Ophthal.*).

But while many of the properties of the vitreous are those of a gel, there are a number of facts which suggest that this cannot be the whole explanation of its structure. There is the constancy of the microscopic appearances which is against their being artefacts ; there is the firm attachment at the origin or base ; then there is the difference between the central and peripheral portions and the changes with age. Also there are certain pathological considerations which speak for a definite structure of the vitreous ; important among these is the definite arrangement in rows of the blood corpuscles which distinguishes an intra-vitreous from an extra-vitreous hæmorrhage in the region of the ora serrata.

So gross is the optical change on coagulation of a gel, that observation of the *living* vitreous should give the best approximation to reality. Busacca[1] reports that in the anterior half of the vitreous there is a dense luminous substance, morphologically stable, floating in a more fluid dark substance. The luminous substance is heavier, and at rest tends to sink and become arranged vertically in a framework of fine sheets like veils, better seen behind the lens and at the coronal equator. Between the two lies a series of sacs enclosing clear lakes. The sheets are best developed around the hyaloid canal.

Electron Microscopy.—Very thin fibrils and spherical bodies (probably proteins) can be seen. Immediately behind the lens there are very few fibres ; this is the optically empty space. Then is a narrow zone of closely packed fibres (the " hyaloid " membrane). The vitreous appears to be a spongework of delicate fibrils with hyaluronic acid and protein in the interstices.

The Vitreous Corpuscles.—These are rather curious cells found between the vitreous and the internal limiting membrane of the retina and also at the origin or base of the vitreous. The majority show amœboid movement and are probably wandering cells. Some of these cells are round with one or more nuclei, others are branched terminating at times in a varicose tendril-like structure ; some are remarkable for their very large vacuoles which distend the body of the corpuscle pushing the nucleus to one side (see Magitot and Mawas, 1914).

[1] Busacca (1958) : " La Structure Biomicroscopique du Corps Vitré normal," *Annales d'Oculistique*, **191**, 477.

The Lymphatic Drainage of the Eye

The aqueous humour must be regarded as the lymph of the eye, although its composition is not that of lymph in the body generally : it contains less albumen, and does not clot unless pathologically altered.

There are three main theories with regard to the formation of the aqueous :

(a) That it is a *filtrate* from the ciliary vessels.

(b) That it is *secreted* by the ciliary epithelium (see p. 80).

(c) That it is a dialysate through the endothelium of the capillaries of the ciliary body (Duke-Elder).

However formed, the aqueous passes from the ciliary body into the recesses of the posterior chamber and thence anteriorly or posteriorly. Current views are that about 50 microlitres per minute of aqueous are produced. Of this, less than 3 microlitres enter and leave the anterior chamber by flow ; the remaining 47 escape by diffusion and filtration (Adler, 1959, quoting Kinsey and others).

Anterior Drainage.—From the recesses the aqueous flows into the posterior chamber, then through the pupil into the anterior chamber. From here it may pass at the angle through the spaces of Fontana into the sinus venosus sclerae, and thence to the aqueous veins and anterior ciliary veins. Another way open to it is viâ the crypts of Fuchs, where we remember the anterior epithelium and anterior border layer are wanting, directly into the iris. From here the flow is partly into the ciliary veins, partly into the supra-choroidal lymphatic space. From the latter the drainage is viâ the perivascular lymphatics around the venæ vorticosæ through the sclera to Tenon's space.

Posterior Drainage.—From the posterior chamber again the lymph passes backwards through the slit-like spaces of the suspensory ligament into the canal of Petit, around the equator of the lens. From here it passes (perhaps) into the post-lental space of Berger, and then down the hyaloid canal to the perineural lymphatics of the optic nerve.

BIBLIOGRAPHY

Adler, F. H. (1959) : Physiology of the Eye, 3rd edit., *St. Louis, U.S.A.*

Balbuena (1930) : *Bull. Soc. Ophtal., Paris*, 286. Quoted by Redslob in *Traité d'Opht.*, 1939, **1.**

Baurmann (1923) : *v. Graefe's Arch. Ophthal.*, **111,** 352 ; (1924), **114, 276.**

Berger (1882) : *v. Graefe's Arch. Ophthal.*, **28** (2), 28.

——— (1887) : Beiträge zur Anatomie des Auges im normalen und pathologischen Zustande, *Wiesbaden.*

Berliner (1943) : Biomicroscopy of the Eye, *London.*

Bowman (1849) : Lectures on parts concerned in operations on the eye . . . , *London.*

Brücke (1846) : *Arch. Anat. Physiol. wiss. Med.*, 370.

Busacca, Goldmann and Schiff-Wertheimer (1957) : Biomicroscopie du Corps Vitré et du Fond de l'Œil, *Paris.*

CIBA SYMPOSIUM ON COLOUR VISION (1965) : J. & A. Churchill Ltd., *London*.

COMBERG (1922) : *Ber. dtsch. Ophth. Ges.*, **43**, 259.

—— (1924) : *Klin. Mbl. f. Augenheilk.*, **72**, 692.

CORNEA WORLD CONGRESS (1965) : Butterworth, *London*.

DIMMER (1907) : *v. Graefe's Arch. Ophthal.*, **65**, 486.

DOGIEL (1890) : *Anat. Anz.*, **5**, 483.

—— (1891) : *Arch. mikr. Anat.*, **37**, 602.

DUKE-ELDER (1927) : The Nature of the Intra-ocular Fluids, *London*.

—— (1930) : The nature of the vitreous body, *London*.

—— (1932) : Textbook of Ophthalmology, *London*, Vol. 1.

EHLERS, N. (1965) : *Acta. Ophth. (Kobenhavn)*, 81, 60–66.

EICHNER (1958) : " Zur Histologie und Topochemie der Netzhaut des Menschen," *Zeit für Zellforsch*, **48**, 137–186.

ELSCHNIG (1888) : " Optico-ciliares Gefäss," *Arch. Augenheilk.*, **18**, 295.

—— (1897) : " Cilio-retinale Gefässe," *v. Graefe's Arch. Ophthal.*, **44** (1), 144.

—— (1898) : " Über optico-ciliare Gefässe," *Klin. Mbl. Augenheilk.*, **36**, 93.

—— (1900) : *Denkschr. Akad. Wiss.*, *Wien*, **70**.

—— (1902) : "Histologische Artefakte im Sehnerven," *Klin. Mbl. Augenheilk.*, **40** (2), 81.

ELSCHNIG and LAUBER (1907) : *v. Graefe's Arch. Ophthal.*, **65**, 428.

FINCHAM (1925) : *Trans. Ophthal. Soc. U.K.*, **26**, 39 ; (1929), **30**, 101.

—— (1937) : " The Mechanism of Accommodation," *London*.

FORTIN, E. P. (1938) : Rétine Humaine, *B. Aires*, contains list of publications by the author.

FUCHS, E. (1885) : *v. Graefe's Archiv. Ophthal.*, **36** (3), 39.

—— (1917) : Textbook of Ophthalmology, 5th Engl. edit., *Philadelphia*.

FUSZ (1906) : *Virchow's Arch.*, **183**, 465.

GREEFF (1900) : " Mikroskopische Anatomie des Sehnerven und der Netz-Haut," in Graefe-Saemisch. Handbuch d. ges. Augenheilk., 2nd edit., **1**, pt. 2, chap. 5.

GRYNFELTT (1899) : Le Muscle dilatateur de la pupille, *Montpellier*.

HENLE (1866) : Eingeweidelehre. In his Handbuch d. systematischen Anatomie des Menschen, *Braunschweig*, **2**.

HESS (1910) : *Arch. Augenheilk.*, **67**, 341.

HIPPEL (1898) : *v. Graefe's Archiv. Ophthal.*, **45**, 286.

HOLMBERG (1959) : *Arch. of Ophthal.*, **62**, 6, 935–958.

HUECK (1841) : Bewegung der Krystallinse, *Leipzig*.

IWANOFF (1865) : *v. Graefe's Arch. Ophthal.*, **11** (1), 135 ; (1869), **15** (3), 284.

—— (1874) : Handbuch d. ges. Augenheilk, 1st edit., **1**, chap. 3.

KEY and RETZIUS (1875–76) : Studien in der Anatomie des Nervensystems, 2 vols., *Stockholm*.

KRÜCKMANN (1905) : *v. Graefe's Arch. Ophthal.*, **60**, 350 ; 452. (1917) *Z. Augenheilk*, **37**, 1.

KUHNT (1877) : *Zbl. med. Wiss.*, 337.

KUNTZ, A. (1953) : The Autonomic Nervous System, 4th edit., *Philadelphia*.

LAGRANGE (1920) : *Arch. Ophtal.*, *Paris*, **37**, 641.

Leber (1903) : in Graefe-Saemisch, Handbuch der gesamten Augenheilkunde, 2nd edit., **2**, pt. 1, chap. 11.

De Lieto Vollaro (1907) : *Ann. Ottalm.*, **36**, 713.

Maggiore (1917) : *Ann. Ottalm.*, **40**, 317.

——— (1924) : *Ann. Ottalm.*, **52**, 625.

Magitot (1946) : Physiologie Oculaire Clinique, *Paris*.

Mann, Ida C. (1927) : *Trans. Ophthal. Soc. U.K.*, **47**, 172.

Mawas, Jaques (1910) : " Region Ciliare de la Rétine," *Thése de Lyon*.

Mawas and Magitot (1912) : *Arch. Anat. micr.*, **19**.

Meibomius (1666) : De Vasis palpebrarum, *Helmstadi*.

Müller, H. (1855) : *v. Graefe's Archiv, Ophthal.*, **2** (2), 1 ; (1857), **3** (1), 1.

——— (1875) : *Z. wiss. Zool.*, **8**, 1.

——— *Verh. phys.-med. Ges., Würzburg*, **10**, 179.

Nuel : *Arch. Ophtal., Paris*, **12**, 70.

Petit (1723) : *Hist. Acad. Sci. Paris, Mém.*, 38.

Østerberg (1935) : Topography of the Layer of Rods and Cones in the Human Retina, *Acta ophthal., Kbh.*, supp. 6.

Polyak, S. L. (1941) : The Retina, *Chicago* ; (1957) The Vertebrate Visual System, *Chicago, U.S.A.*

Redslob (1927) : *Ann. Oculist., Paris*, **164**, 107 ; 721.

——— (1932) : Le Corps Vitré, *Paris*.

——— (1939) : in *Soc. franç. Ophtal.*, Traité d'Ophtalmologie, *Paris*, **1**, 369.

Rochon Duvigneaud (1903) : *Encyclop. française d'Opht.*, **1**.

——— (1943) : Les Yeux et la Vision des Vertébrés, *Paris*.

Salzmann (1912) : Anatomy and Histology of the Human Eyeball, Transl. by E. V. L. Brown, *Chicago*.

Sattler (1876) : *v. Graefe's Archiv. Ophthal.*, **22** (2), 1.

Schaly (1926) : Thesis, *Gröningen*.

Schwalbe (1887) : Lehrbuch der Anatomie der Sinnesorgane, *Erlangen*.

Structure of the Eye (1961) : Academic Press, *New York*.

Shanthaveerapa and Bourne (1965) *Acta anat.*, **61** 379 (Squamous cells of the choroid seem in all ways identical with those covering the ciliary muscle, the iris, the trabecular meshwork and the arachnoid mater).

Thomson (1912) : Anatomy of the Human Eye, *Oxford*.

Tscherning (1898) : Optique physiologique, *Paris*.

Uribe-Troncoso (1909) : *Ann. Oculist., Paris*, **142**, 237.

——— (1921) : *Amer. J. Ophthal.*, **55**, 321 ; (1925), **8**, 433.

Van der Stricht (1922) : *Arch. d. Biol.*, **32**, 346.

Virchow, H. (1906) : Graefe-Saemisch, Handbuch der gesamten Augenheilkunde, 2nd edit., **1**, pt. 1, chap. 2.

Vogt (1921) : *Klin. Mbl. Augenheilk.*, **66**, 321, 718, 838.

Wolfrum (1907) : *v. Graefe's Arch. Ophthal.*, **65**, 220 ; (1908), **67**, 370.

——— (1908) : *v. Graefe's Arch. Ophthal.*, **67**, 307.

——— (1908) : *v. Graefe's Arch. Ophthal.*, **69**, 145.

——— (1906) : *Ber. dtsch. ophthal. Ges.*, **33**, 341.

CHAPTER III

THE APPENDAGES OF THE EYE

THESE comprise the eyelids, the eyebrows, the conjunctiva, and the lacrimal apparatus.

THE EYELIDS

The eyelids are movable folds which act as curtains protecting the eye from injury or excessive light. They also aid the pupil in regulating the amount of light which reaches the retina. Only when they are shut can the visual cortex really be at rest.

But essentially the lids perform a dual function concerning tears : (1) by blinking, the upper lid acts like a swab to spread a film of tears over the cornea, and this " blinking reflex " is fired off rhythmically by evaporation and consequent dryness of the cornea ; (2) where excessive tears are present, blinking empties the conjunctival sac by its pumping effect on the lacrimal sac (p. 239).

The upper eyelid extends above to the eyebrow, which separates it from the forehead—the lower passes usually without line of demarcation into the skin of the cheek. Often, however, especially in the old, two furrows, the naso-jugal and malar folds, occur just beyond the orbital margin, and limit it below.

At the furrows the skin is tied to the periosteum (on the medial side, at the naso-jugal fold, the band of fascia passes to the interval between the orbicularis oculi and the levator labii superioris). The furrows mark the line of junction between the loose tissues of the lid and the denser tissues of the cheek ; and because the skin

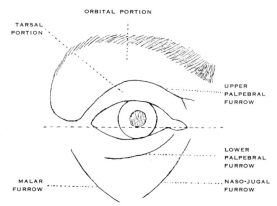

FIG. 188.—THE SURFACE ANATOMY OF THE EYELIDS.
(L. W.)

is tied down tend to limit effusions, and, especially in the old, fat which has escaped from the orbit.

The upper eyelid is much the more movable of the two, being served by a special elevator muscle (levator palpebræ superioris). When the eyes are open and looking straight ahead, it just covers the upper part of the cornea ; when they are closed it covers the whole. The lower lid, on the other hand, is just free of the cornea when the eye is open and rises only slightly when it shuts (see also table on p. 184).

When the eye is open an elliptical space, the palpebral fissure, remains between the lid margins, which meet in the medial and lateral " angles " or canthi of the eye.

The lateral angle is acute. It measures about 60° when the eye is widely open, and about 30–40° normally. The lateral angle is often continuous with a groove which passes laterally and downwards from it, that is a continuation of the line of the margin of the upper eyelid. It is around this groove that the furrows of the " crow's foot " are placed. The lateral canthus is some 5–7 mm. from the orbital margin and about 1 cm. from the fronto-zygomatic suture (Fig. 18).

The medial angle.—The lower boundary is horizontal, while the upper passes downwards and medially—as do, therefore, the corresponding canaliculi. The medial angle is continued medially by the *ridge* produced by the medial palpebral ligament (Fig. 18).

The lateral angle is placed directly against the globe. The medial, more rounded, is separated from it by a little bay—the tear-lake (lacus lacrimalis). In this is a yellowish elevation called the *caruncle,* to the lateral side of which is a reddish semilunar fold, the *plica semilunaris.*

The Caruncle is really a small piece of skin containing large modified sweat glands, and sebaceous glands that open into the follicles of fine hairs (see also p. 221).

The Plica semilunaris represents the third eyelid, membrana nictitans of the lower animals. It often contains plain muscle tissue supplied by the sympathetic (see also p. 222).

At a point in the lids corresponding to the plica semilunaris is a small elevation known as the *papilla lacrimalis,* the centre of which is pierced by a hole, the *punctum lacrimale,* which, as we shall see, serves to carry the tears down into the nose.

The puncta divide the lid margins into *ciliary* and *lacrimal portions.*

Most normal eyes are practically the same size. When we speak therefore of eyes appearing small or large, we usually refer, not to their actual size, but to the amount visible, which depends on the size of the palpebral fissure.

With the eyes open the lateral angle is about 2 mm. above the medial, and thus the axis of the fissure is not horizontal, but slopes from medially upwards and laterally.

An increase in this obliquity is characteristic of the Chinese and Japanese. Moreover, these races have a fold passing from the medial end of the upper lid to the lower, hiding the caruncle—a condition known as epicanthus.

Epicanthus occurs normally in the human fœtus (Keith), but disappears with the development of the bridge of the nose. It is also seen in congenital ptosis (Pockley, 1919). Indeed, it has been regarded as dependent upon the flatness of the nasal bones ; but Duckworth (1904) points out that in the Negroid races, whose nasal bones are even flatter than those of the Mongols, it is usually absent.

When the eyes are open, too, the palpebral fissure, which measures about 30 mm. by 15 mm. (see table below), is seen to be asymmetrical. Its greatest width above the line joining the two angles is on the medial side, while below it is on the lateral side.

When the eyes are shut the lateral angle drops till it lies lower than the medial and the fissure becomes sinuous, concave upwards in its central portion. The roots of the lashes give the shape of the fissure except in the lacrimal portion where it is horizontal. In its lateral part the fissure slopes downwards.

The portions of the eye that are normally visible in the palpebral opening are the cornea, the iris and pupil, a triangle of sclera to the lateral side and a crescent of it to the medial, the caruncle and the plica.

The most exposed portion of the globe is a zone just below the centre of the cornea ; for this remains relatively uncovered even when the eyes are " screwed up." *Hence it is the common site of those congestive or degenerative changes which result from exposure.* At the approach of danger the eyes tend to turn up. Here the exposed portion will be below, and it is thus this region which will be most *affected by injuries due to burns and caustics, and is also the site of ulceration seen sometimes in the coma vigil of typhoid and other severe illnesses.*

The following table shows some of the characteristics of the palpebral opening and its relation with certain parts of the globe (from Winckler).

	Length	Height	Pupil	Cornea	Lacus lac. and Plica	Position of Transverse Axis
Newborn .	18·5–19 mm.	10 mm.	Touches free border of lower eyelid	Upper border at level of free margin of upper eyelid	Not visible	Middle of pupil
Infant .	24–25 mm.	13 mm.	Equidistant from free borders of eyelids	Upper and lower borders covered to same extent	Slightly visible	Below middle of pupil
Adult .	28–30 mm.	14–15 mm.	Near free border of upper eyelid	Lower border at level of free margin of lower eyelid	Visible	Lower border of pupil
Old man .	28 mm.	11–12 mm.	Touches free margin of upper eyelid	Lower border a little distance from free margin of lower eyelid	Very visible	Near lower border of cornea

Here we see that the portion of the globe visible between the eyelids is lower as age increases.

The Free Margin of each lid is about 2 mm. broad, and has an anterior and a posterior border.

From the anterior rounded border jut the eyelashes, which are stiff hairs arranged in two or three rows. The upper lashes are longer and more numerous and curl upwards, while the lower ones turn downwards, so that they do not interlace when the eyes are shut. The lashes are as a rule darker than the hair, and

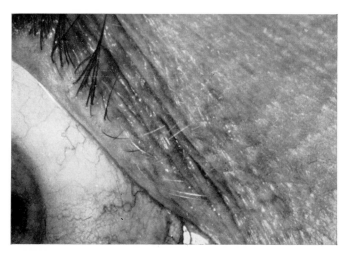

Fig. 189.—Skin of Nasal Portion of the Right Upper Eyelid.
Note almost devoid of hairs.

do not become grey with age, although they may do so after some diseases (e.g. alopœcia areata). It takes about ten weeks for a lash which has been epilated to grow to its full size. The lashes are longest and most curled in childhood.

The Follicles of the Lashes.—Although generally like those of hairs elsewhere, the lashes have no arrector muscles. They pass into the lid obliquely in front of the palpebral muscle (of Riolan) to reach the tarsus. The lashes are very sensitive, being richly supplied with nerves. Young lashes are knob-shaped, and a persistence of this condition is seen in many chronic inflammatory conditions. Each lash remains about five months.

The Posterior Border of the lid margin is sharp and placed against the globe. Just in front of it can be seen the small orifices of the tarsal glands. Between these and the eyelashes is a thin grey line, where the lid can be quite easily split into an anterior and a posterior portion.

The free margins of the lids have the above characteristics in the *ciliary* portion, i.e. up to the puncta. To the medial side of these, i.e. in *the lacrimal portion*, there are as a rule no cilia or tarsal glands. Rarely after the age of ten years lashes are found on the lacrimal portion of the lid margins.   This portion is rounded, hence has no borders.   In its thickness is the lacrimal canaliculus.

The Structure of the Lids.—The lids consist of a series of layers placed one in front of the other like the leaves of a book.

From before backwards we find :

    1. The skin.
    2. A layer of subcutaneous areolar tissue.
    3. A layer of striped muscle (orbicularis oculi).
    4. The submuscular areolar tissue.
    5. The fibrous layer—including the tarsal plates.
    6. A layer of unstriped muscle.
    7. The mucous membrane or conjunctiva.

1. *The Skin* of the eyelids is about the thinnest in the body.   It is less than

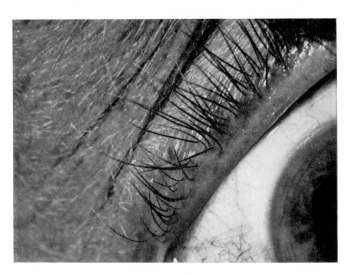

FIG. 190.—SKIN OF LATERAL PORTION OF UPPER EYELID.
Note numerous hairs.

1 mm. in thickness and almost transparent.   Hence it forms folds, and is easily wrinkled.   A well-marked fold is often seen on the lateral side of the upper lid in old people.   It may overhang the lid margin.   The skin also is very elastic so that it recovers rapidly after being distended by fluids, etc.   When the eye is open the upper lid is marked at the upper border of the tarsal plate by a furrow, the mouth of which gets nearer the lid margin the wider the eye is opened.   This furrow is produced by the pull of the tendon of levator palpebræ superioris (p. 238).   The skin of the upper lid is thus furrowed when the eye is open—the skin of the upper lid is wholly in view only when the eye is closed.   The corresponding furrow in the lower lid is ill-marked and often broken up.

Also, as has been mentioned before, furrows exist at times—especially in the old—just beyond the lower orbital margin ; these are emphasised when the lower lids are puffed out with fat escaped from the orbit (see also p. 270). They are due to attachment of the skin to the orbital margin. It is also attached at the medial and lateral canthi to the medial and lateral palpebral ligaments, especially the former.

It should be carefully noted that the nasal portion of the eyelid (Fig. 189) differs quite markedly from that of the temporal side (Fig. 190). It is smoother, shinier, and greasier. Also it has practically no hairs and those that are present are very feeble and have only rudimentary sebaceous glands attached to them. On the other hand, the skin here is well provided with those unicellular sebaceous glands which the author (Eugene Wolff) described as occurring normally in the basal layer of the human epidermis (*Lancet*, 1951, p. 888) (Fig. 191).

Structure.—The epithelium forms a relatively thin layer. The stratum corneum is well developed. The stratum granulosum is present ; the stratum mucosum consists of three or four layers of cells. Then comes the stratum germinativum resting on a basement membrane.

At the lid margin the epithelium becomes modified as we trace it from the anterior to the posterior border. It thickens and contains some 7–10 layers of cells. The dermis is denser and richer in elastic fibres ; it becomes folded to form papillæ which become higher and narrower, and the basement membrane is correspondingly wavy (Winckler).

The muco-cutaneous junction lies at the level of the posterior margin of the openings of the tarsal glands, i.e. at the junction of " dry " and " moist " portions where the marginal strips of tear fluid end in a sharp line (see p. 210).

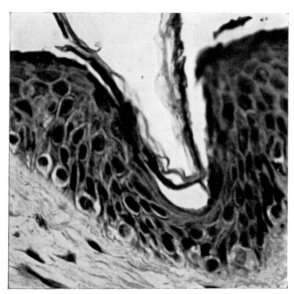

FIG. 191.—SECTION OF SKIN FROM THE NASAL SIDE OF THE EYELID TO SHOW NUMEROUS UNICELLULAR SEBACEOUS GLANDS IN THE BASAL LAYER OF THE EPIDERMIS.

The hairs on the lids, although comparatively large in the fœtus, are more like down in the adult, and have small sebaceous glands connected with them.

The sweat glands, although numerous, are of small size.

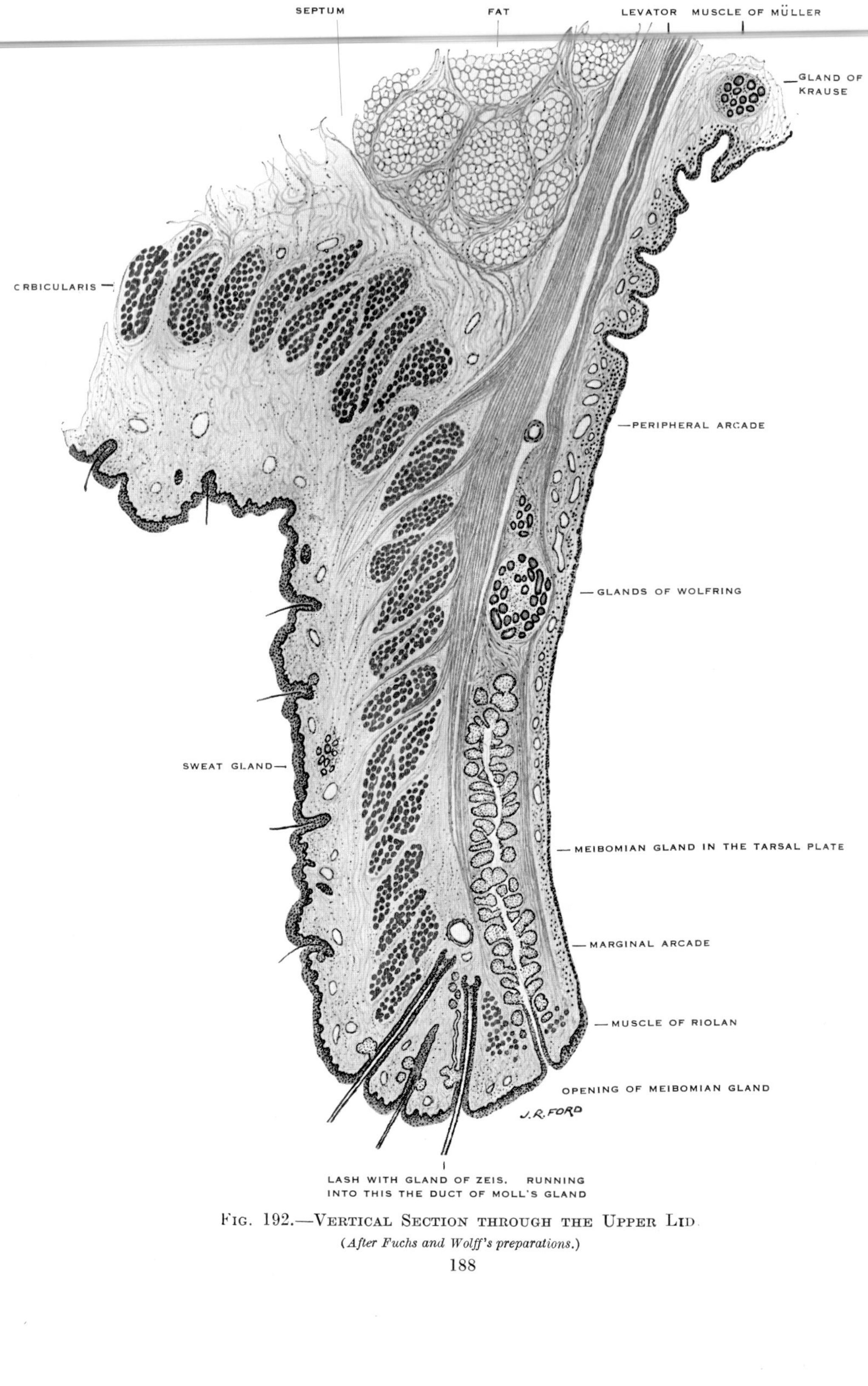

SEPTUM   FAT   LEVATOR   MUSCLE OF MÜLLER

GLAND OF KRAUSE

ORBICULARIS

PERIPHERAL ARCADE

GLANDS OF WOLFRING

SWEAT GLAND

MEIBOMIAN GLAND IN THE TARSAL PLATE

MARGINAL ARCADE

MUSCLE OF RIOLAN

OPENING OF MEIBOMIAN GLAND

J. R. FORD

LASH WITH GLAND OF ZEIS. RUNNING
INTO THIS THE DUCT OF MOLL'S GLAND

FIG. 192.—VERTICAL SECTION THROUGH THE UPPER LID.
(*After Fuchs and Wolff's preparations.*)

Waldeyer described in the skin of the eyelids, in the connective tissue tracts which accompany the vessels, and in the hair follicles, large pigment cells with processes. These cells are found in the skin in most regions of the body but generally are rare, while here they are regularly met with. They are more numerous in brunettes than blondes. The pigment is golden yellow or brown. These chromatophores may wander and so determine the changes more or less marked in the coloration of the eyelids seen in the same individual in different states of health, etc. (Dor).

2. *The Subcutaneous Areolar Layer* consists of loose connective tissue containing no fat ; so the skin can easily be lifted off the underlying muscle and also be distended with œdema or blood. It is absent near the ciliary margin, at the palpebral furrows, and at the medial and lateral angles where the skin is adherent to the palpebral ligaments.

3. *The Layer of Striated Muscle.*—These are the fibres of the orbicularis palpebrarum supplied by the 7th nerve. The muscle fibres are arranged concentrically around the palpebral opening. The fibres are placed obliquely in relation to each other and overlap as do tiles on a roof. The part of this muscle which lies next and occupies nearly the whole thickness of the lid margin is called the ciliary part (muscle of Riolan) (Fig. 192). It is traversed successively by the follicles of the lashes, the glands of Moll, and the excretory ducts of the tarsal glands (Fig. 165) (see also p. 203).

4. *The Submuscular Areolar Tissue* resembles the subcutaneous layer. It lies between the orbicularis and the tarsal plate, and communicates above with the sub-aponeurotic layer (the dangerous area) of the scalp (Trotter, in Choyce's *Surgery*). Hence pus or blood can make its way into the upper lid from the dangerous area (see also p. 207). It is through this plane, which is reached by entering the knife at the grey line, that the lid may, with the greatest ease, be split into anterior and posterior portions. This space is traversed by the fibres of the levator, some of which pass on to the skin through the orbicularis, while others gain attachment to the lower third of the tarsus. The main nerves to the eyelids also lie in this areolar tissue ; *hence, when injecting a local anæsthetic to anæsthetise the lids, it is necessary to inject deep to the orbicularis.*

In the lower lid this tissue lies in a single small space (the preseptal space) in front of the septum orbitale. In the upper lid the space in which the tissue lies is divided by the levator into the pretarsal and preseptal spaces (Charpy and Claremont).

The pretarsal space is small. It contains the peripheral arterial arcade (Figs. 192, 251). It is bounded anteriorly by the levator tendon and the orbicularis ; posteriorly by the tarsal plate and the muscle of Müller. Its upper end corresponds to the place where the muscle of Müller arises from the levator. Its lower limit is formed by the attachment of the fibres of the levator to the front of the tarsal plate. On vertical section the space is fusiform.

The preseptal space is triangular on vertical section. It is bounded in front by the orbicularis, behind by the septum and those tendinous fibres of the levator which pierce the orbicularis. Above is the preseptal cushion of fat.

The preseptal cushion of fat is a well-defined agglomeration of fat different from the subcutaneous fat. It is for the most part in front of the septum and behind the orbicularis. Crescent-shaped, it lies along the orbital margin which it may overlap at times. Its lower, thicker border is parallel to the upper palpebral furrow. The fat is adherent to the orbicularis and the epicranial aponeurosis and this, according to Charpy, separates the preseptal space from the dangerous area of the scalp.

The pre-muscular and retro-muscular spaces communicate between the fibres of the orbicularis, but are separated by the septum and tarsal plates from the orbit. Also infiltrations of the eyelids do not extend on to the cheek and forehead.

5. *The Fibrous Layer.*—The fibrous layer may be regarded as the framework of the lids. It consists of a thickened central portion, the tarsal plates, and a thinner peripheral part known as the palpebral fascia or septum orbitale. Although the term septum orbitale is usually applied to the palpebral fascia only, it is the whole fibrous layer which, when the eyes are shut, forms a septum to the orbital opening.

The Tarsal Plates—one for each of the lids—form the skeleton of the lids, giving them their shape and firmness. They are often called the tarsal cartilages, but consist of dense fibrous and some elastic tissue, found mainly around the acini, in which are embedded the tarsal glands. They contain no cartilage. The lateral ends are 7 mm. from Whitnall's tubercle. The medial ends terminate at the lacrimal puncta, some 9 mm. from the anterior lacrimal crest.

The tarsus is well delimited from the surrounding tissues, but laterally at the ciliary margin its connective tissue is closely united with that round the follicles of the lashes to form a characteristic thickening at the margin of the lid (ciliary mass of Whitnall).

The upper tarsus, which is shaped like the letter **D** placed on its side, is much larger than the lower, being 11 mm. in height at its middle. The corresponding measurement in the lower tarsus, which is somewhat oblong in form, is 5 mm.

Each tarsus, some 29 mm. long and 1 mm. thick, may be described as having an anterior and posterior surface, a free and attached border, and a medial and lateral extremity.

The anterior surface of the tarsus is convex, and is separated from the orbicularis by loose areolar tissue, so that the muscle moves freely on the tarsus.

The posterior surface, which is concave, clothed by and adherent to the conjunctiva, moulds itself on the globe of the eye.

The free border, forming the margin of the lid, is thick, almost horizontal, and co-extensive with the ciliary portion of the lid margin ; *the attached border* is thin, and gradually runs into the septum orbitale, with which it is held by some to be continuous, except where it is pierced by the levator in the upper lid and the prolongation of the inferior rectus in the lower (see below).   The superior border of the upper tarsus gives attachment to the unstriped superior palpebral muscle (Figs. 192, 193, 251), while similarly to the inferior border of the lower tarsus the inferior palpebral muscle is inserted.

The extremities of the tarsal plates are attached to the orbital margin by strong fibrous structures known as the medial and lateral tarsal, or palpebral, ligaments.

The Medial Palpebral Ligament is a somewhat triangular band which is attached to the frontal process of the maxilla from the anterior lacrimal crest to near its suture with the nasal bone (Figs. 18, 225, 274, 275).

The ligament has a lower free border (under which some of the fibres of the orbicularis insinuate themselves), while above it is adherent to and continuous with the periosteum.

At the base of the triangle, that is, at the anterior lacrimal crest, the ligament divides into anterior and posterior portions.   The posterior portion is continuous with the lacrimal fascia, and thus helps to roof over the upper part of the lacrimal sac.

The anterior portion is continued at the medial canthus into two bands, which pass across the lacrimal fossa (but not in contact with the sac), to attach it to the medial extremities of the tarsal plates.   These bands make an angle open laterally with the lacrimal fascia.   They form with the main ligament a letter Y placed on its side.   The two branches, which correspond to the lacrimal portions of the lid margins, and in fact are tubular, contain the lacrimal canaliculi, enclose the caruncle, and delimit the medial canthus.

The anterior surface of the ligament is free and adherent to the skin.   It looks forwards and laterally ; the two branches look forwards and medially and thus make with it an obtuse angle open forwards.

A deep or reflected portion of the medial palpebral ligament is usually described.   This is said to arise from the main ligament as it crosses the sac and is attached behind the sac.   The author (Eugene Wolff) has never been able to demonstrate this posterior portion satisfactorily,[1] *apart* from the lacrimal fascia, and Whitnall (1932) describes it as very thin and of secondary importance, appearing in dissections merely as the fascia clothing the front of the pars lacrimalis muscle.   Only in one full-term fœtus did he find it better developed than the anterior portion.

When the lateral canthus is pulled laterally and upwards the medial palpebral ligament forms a well-marked prominence.   It should be carefully noted that this prominence lies almost entirely on the frontal process of the maxilla.

A finger placed in the lacrimal fossa lies under the medial angle of the eye.

---

[1] Meller also describes the reflected portion of the ligament as being *part of* the deep or lacrimal fascia.

According to Meller the medial canthus corresponds more or less to the anterior lacrimal crest. Also, if a vertical incision is made 2 mm. medial to the medial canthus, *the whole of the dissection to expose the sac is made under the lateral lip of the wound.*

It follows from this, and from what has been said above, that the lower prominent portion of the medial palpebral ligament does not lie in front of the lacrimal sac, at any rate not for more than a millimetre or two, and a probe pressed backwards below its prominence hits the bone and not the sac.

The Lateral Palpebral Ligament is attached to the orbital tubercle on the zygomatic bone 11 mm. below the fronto-zygomatic suture. It is some 7 mm. long and 2·5 mm. broad. It consists of fibrous tissue which is not very dense. Indeed, it is rather a descriptive verbiage than an anatomical reality ; it does not exist in the sense of the strong and well-developed medial palpebral ligament. It is no more than the areolar tissue of the septum orbitale behind the lateral palpebral raphé.

It lies deeper, and does not form a prominence as does the medial palpebral ligament. Its anterior surface is fused with the preciliary fibres of the orbicularis. Superficial also to this ligament are a few lobules of the lacrimal gland and the lateral palpebral raphé formed by the orbicularis and strengthened by the septum orbitale.

The posterior surface is in front of the lateral check ligament, separated, however, from it by a lobule of the lacrimal gland (Fig. 252). Its upper border is united with the expansion of the levator (Fig. 275) ; its lower border with an expansion from the inferior oblique and the inferior rectus (Winckler). It may or may not bifurcate at its medial end to reach the tarsal plates. In the former case the two portions are separated by the lateral termination of the palpebral muscle of Riolan.

THE PALPEBRAL FASCIA OR SEPTUM ORBITALE (Figs. 193, 194, 274)

The palpebral fascia or septum orbitale is attached to the orbital margin at a thickening called the arcus marginale, which is formed where the periorbita is continuous with the periosteum ; centrally it is generally held to be continuous with the tarsal plates, except where it is pierced by the fibres of the levator in the upper lid and the expansion from the inferior rectus in the lower. But the continuity of the septum, with the tarsus between the fibres of the levator, can only be made out with difficulty by dissection under water and is denied by many observers.

A portion of the septum is also carried forwards with the fibres of the levator, and a portion reflected back along its upper surface (Fig. 192).

The palpebral fascia must not be regarded as a fixed and rigid structure. It is a floating membrane, which takes part in all the movements of the lids, and has been regarded (though this is doubtful) as the deep fascia of the palpebral portion of the orbicularis. It consists of two layers, the fibres of which, running in arcades, cross each other more or less at right angles.

The septum is thicker and stronger on the lateral side than on the medial and in the upper lid than in the lower. In the upper lid, in fact, two tendon-like thickenings can be seen starting from the lateral side and gradually becoming lost as we trace them medially.

It is the weak portions of the septum orbitale which determine the site of herniæ

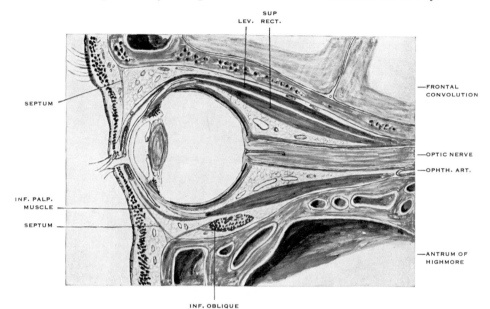

FIG. 193.—VERTICAL ANTERO-POSTERIOR SECTION OF THE ORBIT.
(*After Sattler.*)

of the orbital fat which lies just deep to it. These herniæ are seen frequently, especially in old people.

The attachment of the septum while more or less following the orbital margin does not do so exactly. It does, however, mark the junction of periorbita and periosteum (Fig. 194).

Starting on the lateral side we find the septum attached to the orbital margin in front of the lateral palpebral ligament which goes to Whitnall's tubercle, being separated from it by loose connective tissue containing a lobule of fat. From here the line of attachment runs upwards, crosses the fronto-zygomatic suture, and then follows the posterior lip of the upper orbital margin to the supraorbital notch which it bridges over, converting it into a foramen. Again following the supraorbital margin, the attachment of the septum passes in front of the pulley of the superior oblique and then, leaving the bone, bridges over the upper and medial angle of the orbital opening with its vessels and nerves, to become again

A.E.—13

attached to the bone behind the upper part of the posterior lacrimal crest. It now runs down on the lacrimal bone behind Horner's muscle and thus behind the lacrimal sac and the medial palpebral ligament and in front of the medial check ligament (Fig. 225). The line of attachment crosses the lacrimal sac (or rather the fascia covering it) about its middle, to reach the anterior lacrimal crest at about the level of the lacrimal tubercle. From here it follows the lower orbital margin to the point where the zygomatic portion starts ascending. Here the attachment

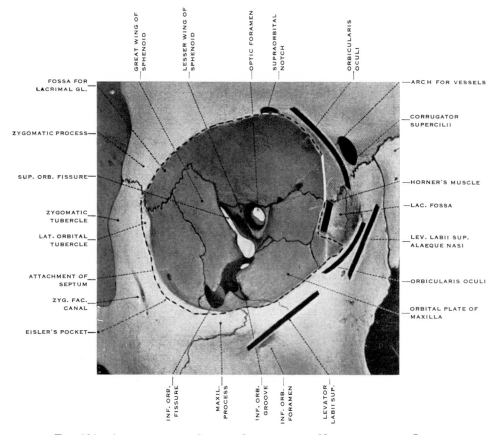

FIG. 194.—ATTACHMENT OF SEPTUM ORBITALE AND MUSCLES AROUND ORBIT.

leaves the margin and lies actually a few millimetres from it on the facial aspect of the zygomatic bone ; so that here the septum forms an osteofibrous pocket, the pre-marginal recess of Eisler, which contains fat. The line of attachment again reaches the lateral orbital margin just below the level of Whitnall's tubercle.

It will be noted that on the lateral side the septum is superficial, lying anterior to the lateral palpebral ligament, while on the medial side it is deep, lying behind Horner's muscle.

Where the two parts of Horner's muscle diverge to reach the upper and lower eyelids the portions of the septum belonging to the upper and lower eyelids meet behind the caruncle and plica. The inferior medial palpebral artery runs here in a plane between the caruncle and Horner's muscle.

Relations.—In the upper eyelid the septum is mainly in contact with orbital fat (continuous with the upper and lateral mass of perimuscular fat). This separates the septum from the lacrimal gland, the levator, and the tendon of the superior oblique. On the medial side the septum is in contact with that portion of the orbital fat which tends to pass out of the orbit between the pulley of the superior oblique and the medial palpebral ligament, pushing the palpebral fascia in front of it (Fig. 255).

In the lower eyelid the septum lies in contact with those portions of the orbital fat which tend to escape through three orifices and also with the expansion of the inferior rectus and inferior oblique (Figs. 193, 251).

In the lower lid there is only one space, bounded behind by the septum orbitale and the tarsal plate, and in front by the orbicularis.

The Septum Orbitale is pierced by the following structures :

(*a*) The lacrimal vessels and nerves.

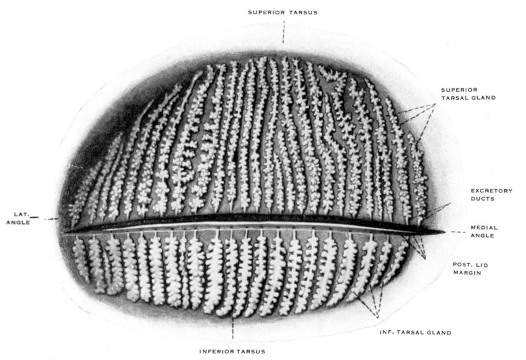

FIG. 195.—THE POSTERIOR SURFACE OF THE TWO EYELIDS WHICH HAVE BEEN MADE TRANSPARENT BY SODA-GLYCERINE TO SHOW THE MEIBOMIAN GLANDS.
(From Sobotta.)

(*b*) The supraorbital vessels and nerves.

(*c*) The supratrochlear nerve and artery.

(*d*) The infratrochlear nerve.

(*e*) The anastomosis between the angular vein and the ophthalmic.

(*f*) The superior and inferior palpebral arteries above and below the medial palpebral ligament.

(*g*) The levator palpebræ superioris in the upper lid and in the lower by a prolongation of the inferior rectus. It must be pointed out that many hold that the lower border of the septum and the upper border of the tarsus are not continuous between the fibres of the levator. The muscle would then pass between these two structures.

6. *The Layer of Unstriped Muscle Fibres*, known as the muscle of Müller, lies just deep to the septum orbitale in both upper and lower lids, and, running for the most part vertically, takes origin among the fibres of the levator in the upper lid and the prolongation of the inferior rectus in the lower. It is inserted into the attached margins of the tarsal plates (Figs. 192, 193, 251).

The inferior palpebral muscle can, according to Fuchs, be seen through the conjunctiva. The muscle of Müller is supplied by the sympathetic, and when in action widens the palpebral fissure. Fibres of unstriped muscle are also found bridging over the inferior orbital fissure and (?) in the capsule of Tenon. The whole system represents the retractor bulbi of some mammalia (see pp. 22, 267).

7. *The Conjunctiva* which lines the lids is called the palpebral conjunctiva. It is firmly adherent to the tarsus (see also p. 207).

THE GLANDS OF THE LIDS

Apart from the glands of the skin, which have already been considered, and those of the conjunctiva, we find the following glands in the lids named after those anatomists who first described them :

1. The Meibomian glands.

2. The glands of Moll.

3. Zeis's glands. (Note spelling—not as Zeiss, the instrument maker.)

1. **The Meibomian Glands** (now called **Tarsal Glands**) are

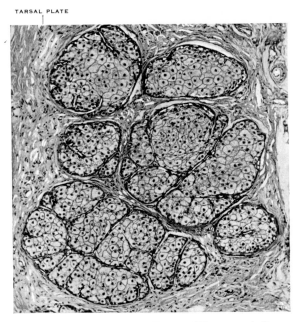

TARSAL PLATE

FIG. 196.—LOBULES OF THE TARSAL (MEIBOMIAN) GLAND.
(*Wolff's preparation.*)

long sebaceous glands which are remarkable in not being connected with hairs ; this, however, is due to the fact that they take the place of a row of lashes (see p. 494). They are situated actually *in* the tarsal plates and run from their attached to their free margins (Fig. 192). The upper ones are therefore the larger. They are arranged vertically parallel with each other, about twenty-five for the upper lid and twenty for the lower. Each consists of a central canal, into the sides of which open numerous rounded appendages which secrete sebum. The small orifices of the canals, whose number is exactly that of the Meibomian glands, can be seen on the margin of the lid just in front of its posterior border (Figs. 192 and 195).

It is here that the sebaceous material is poured *to prevent the overflow of tears, to make for an airtight closure of the lids, to prevent the tears from macerating the skin* (Fuchs) *and after blinking to leave a film* (p. 243) *over the moistened cornea to retard*

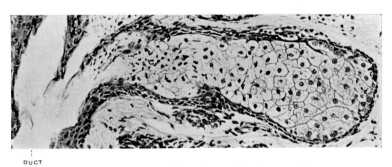

DUCT

FIG. 197.—SECTION OF SACCULE OF MEIBOMIAN GLAND.

Note how nuclei in gland become darker and then break up as we trace them to the duct.

evaporation of the underlying tears. The duct is lined by four layers of cells situated on a basement membrane. The mouth of the duct is lined by six layers of cells, of which the deepest are cylindrical. Keratinisation increases as we approach the lid margin. The acini are usually globular, 10–15 in number and placed irregularly round the central canal till near its orifice and so resemble a chain of onions (Winckler). Each acinus is said to be surrounded by a lymphatic space. The structure of a Meibomian gland is like that of a gland of Zeis (*q.v.*). *The Meibomian glands can be seen easily, showing through the conjunctiva as yellow streaks.*

2. **The Glands of Moll** (now called **Ciliary Glands**) consist of unbranched spiral or sinuous tubules which begin in a simple spiral and not in a glomerulus as do ordinary sweat glands. They may be considered as sweat glands which have become arrested in their development. They are some 1·5 to 2 mm. long and placed obliquely in contact with and parallel to the bulbs of the cilia. They are more numerous in the lower lid, but even here there is not one to every lash.

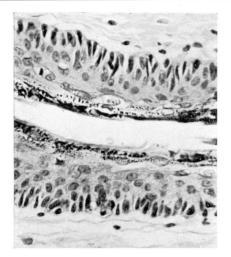

FIG. 198.—LONGITUDINAL SECTION OF PORTION OF MEIBOMIAN DUCT.

Each has a fundus, a body, an ampullary portion, and a neck. The cavity is singularly large (Figs. 199, 200, 223) but gets narrower at the neck. The duct passes through the dermis and epidermis and may terminate separately between two lashes or between the lash and its epithelial covering or into the duct of a gland of Zeis (Fig. 192).

Structure.—The structure of a ciliary gland is much like that of an ordinary sweat gland. The secretory portion is lined by a layer of cylindrical cells which contain secretory granules and fatty granulations ; and between these cells and the basement membrane is placed an ill-defined layer of longitudinal or obliquely placed cells and fibres which are muscular (myo-epithelial) in character.

The duct is lined by one or two layers of cells, the most superficial of which are cylindrical. There are no muscle fibres.

3. **Zeis's Glands** are modified rudimentary **sebaceous glands** which are attached directly to the follicles of the eyelashes (Figs. 192, 199, 202). Each is reduced

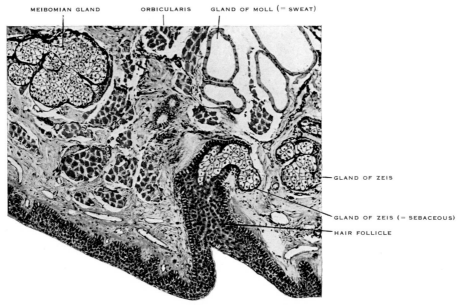

FIG. 199.—SECTION OF THE LID MARGIN TO SHOW THE THREE TYPES OF GLANDS.
(*Wolff's preparation.*)

to a simple cul-de-sac or to two or three lobules only (in general there are 10 to 20 or more). Usually there are two to each cilium. Each gland consists of epithelium placed on a basement membrane. Next to this membrane is a layer of small cubical cells which are actively dividing. The cells resulting from this division enlarge, become polygonal and filled with sebaceous granules. The nuclei, which at first enlarge, become rounded, paler, and usually contain one well-marked nucleolus, diminish in size, stain more densely, become star-shaped, and disappear. The degenerative cells lose their cell walls and are pushed towards the centre of the gland and then towards the secretory duct. The sebum passes out between the lash and its epithelial covering. The purpose of this oily secretion, as elsewhere in the body, is to prevent the hair (eyelash in this case) from becoming dry and brittle.

The Blood-vessels of the Lids

Arteries.—The blood-supply to the lids is derived mainly from the *ophthalmic* and *lacrimal* arteries by their *medial* and *lateral palpebral* branches.

The medial palpebral arteries—superior for the upper lid, inferior for the lower—pierce the septum orbitale above and below the medial palpebral ligament (Fig. 214).

Each anastomoses with the corresponding lateral palpebral artery from the lacrimal to form the *tarsal arches*, whose plane in the lids is in the submuscular areolar tissue (i.e. between the orbicularis and the tarsal plate), close to the lid margin (Figs. 192 and 215).

The Tarsal Arches (*Arcades*) receive anastomosing twigs from the superficial temporal, transverse facial, and infraorbital arteries.

In the upper lid a *second arterial arch* is formed from the superior branch of the medial palpebral. It is called the arcus tarseus superior, and is situated in front of the upper margin of the tarsal plate (Figs. 192 and 215).

From the arches branches pass forward to supply the orbicularis and skin, backward to the conjunctiva and tarsal glands.

The Veins of the lids are larger and more numerous than the arteries. They are arranged in pretarsal and post-tarsal sets, and form a dense plexus (which can be seen in the living) in the region of the upper and lower fornices of the conjunctiva.

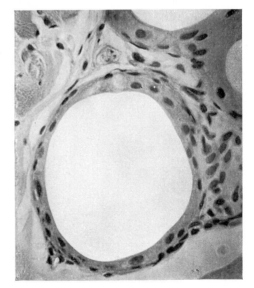

Fig. 200.—Section of Ciliary Gland (of Moll).

Some of them empty into the veins of the forehead and temple, others pass through the orbicularis to reach radicles of the ophthalmic vein.

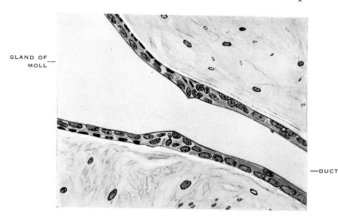

GLAND OF MOLL

—DUCT

FIG. 201.—JUNCTION OF CILIARY (MOLL'S) GLAND AND DUCT.

Note funnel-shaped termination of gland.

Lymphatics.—Like the veins, the lymphatics are arranged in *pre- and post-tarsal plexuses*, connected, however, by cross-channels. According to Fuchs the former have many valves, the latter none.

The *post-tarsal* drain the conjunctiva and tarsal glands ; the *pretarsal* the skin and skin structures.

FIG. 202.—SECTION OF SEBACEOUS GLAND (OF ZEIS).

Note how nuclei in gland become dark and then break up as we trace them to hair follicle.

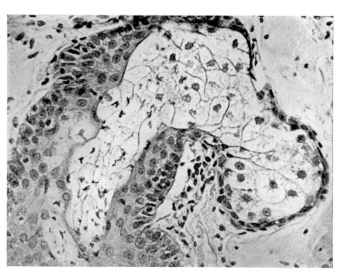

HAIR FOLLICLE

Both groups drain as follows : those for the lateral side run into the pre-auricular and parotid nodes ; those from the medial side into the submandibular lymph glands.

Nerves.—*Motor.*—The orbicularis is supplied by the 7th cranial ; the levator by the upper division of the 3rd, and the plain muscle tissue by the sympathetic.

Sensory.—The upper lid is supplied mainly by the supraorbital. On the medial side the supra- and infratrochlears, and on the lateral side the lacrimal branches of the ophthalmic division of the trigeminal assist. The lower lid gets its supply from the infraorbital, with minimal overlap near the angles by lacrimal and infratrochlear.

The plane of the main branches of the nerves is between the orbicularis and the tarsal plate. From here branches pass forwards to the skin, backwards to the conjunctiva and tarsal glands.

THE PALPEBRAL AND NEIGHBOURING MUSCLES

The Orbicularis Oculi is the sphincter muscle of the eye. It forms an elliptical sheet, which surrounds the palpebral fissure, covers the lids, and spreads out for some distance on to the forehead, temple, and cheek.

It consists of two portions :
(*a*) Palpebral.
(*b*) Orbital.

The Palpebral Portion is the essential part of the muscle. It is confined to the lids, consists of pale muscle fibres, and may itself be divided into pretarsal and preseptal portions. The junction of the two, the thinnest portion of the muscle, lies at the upper- and lower-lid furrows.

It takes origin from the medial palpebral ligament and the neighbouring bone, and passes across the lids in a series of half ellipses, which meet outside the lateral canthus in the lateral palpebral raphé. This consists of inter-digitating muscle fibres strengthened by the septum orbitale (Whitnall).

The Orbital Portion has a curved origin from the medial side of the orbit : from the medial portion of the upper orbital margin medial to the supraorbital notch ; from the maxillary process of the frontal bone ; from the frontal process of the maxilla ; from the medial palpebral ligament, and from the lower orbital margin medial to the infraorbital foramen.

The origin is by actual fleshy fibres or short tendon, and is not continuous.

From this origin the peripheral fibres sweep across the orbital margin in a series of concentric loops, while the more central ones form nearly complete rings.

Relations.—*The Palpebral Portion* of the orbicularis has a layer of areolar tissue containing *no fat* both in front and behind. The anterior, subcutaneous layer, separates it from the skin. The posterior, submuscular areolar layer, which separates it from the tarsal plates and palpebral fascia, contains the main vessels and nerves of the lids and fibres of the levator. This portion of the muscle is only adherent to the skin at the medial and lateral canthi.

The fibres of the levator pass through the palpebral portion to reach the skin (Fig. 192).

The Orbital Portion spreads upwards on to the forehead, where it takes part in the formation of the eyebrow and covers the corrugator supercilii laterally on to the temple, where it covers the anterior part of the temporal fascia, and downwards on to the cheek, where it lies on the zygomatic bone and the origin of the elevator muscles of the upper lip and ala of the nose.

Anteriorly it is separated from the skin, *not* by areolar tissue, but by a layer of *fat*, to which it is adherent, and so acts on the skin, which actually receives only the following fibres, mostly from the periphery of the muscle :

(*a*) *The Musculus superciliaris* (Merkel), or depressor muscle of the head of the eyebrow (Arlt), comprises some of the upper medial peripheral fibres which pass to the skin of the medial portion of the eyebrow.

(*b*) *The Malaris* (of Henle) is constituted by some of the medial and lateral lower peripheral fibres which are attached to the skin of the cheek. Also Merkel has described some fibres which are attached to the skin round the medial canthus, which produce a series of fine lines on the medial part of the lids, especially in those who have small eyes and are subject to frequent blinking (Poirier).

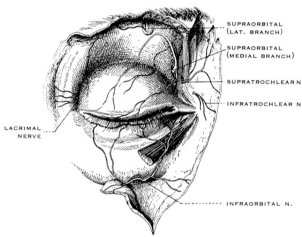

FIG. 203.—NERVES OF THE EYELIDS OF THE RIGHT EYE.
(*From Poirier, after Merkel.*)

Horner's Muscle,[1] or the **Tensor tarsi,** is also called the **pars lacrimalis** of the orbicularis, because it is regarded by some anatomists as forming the deep origin of the pretarsal portion of the muscle.

It consists of a thin layer of fibres which arises behind the lacrimal sac from the upper part of the posterior lacrimal crest (Figs. 224, 225), which often shows a roughening here. The muscle passes laterally and forwards,[2] and divides into two slips, which surround the canaliculi and become continuous with the pretarsal portions of the orbicularis of the upper and lower lids and with the muscle of Riolan. The lacrimal fascia and Horner's muscle prevent ectropion of the

[1] First described by Duverney in 1749. Gerlach also described an anterior lacrimal muscle which arises from the posterior aspect of the medial palpebral ligament and passes laterally and backwards above and below the reflected portion of the ligament (?) to mingle with the orbicularis.

[2] Students often find difficulty in picturing the relations of Horner's muscle. This can be done by closing one's eyes and thinking of one's own lacrimal fossa with Horner's muscle arising behind it. It is not difficult then to picture the muscle passing forwards and outwards lateral to the lacrimal sac and after dividing into two portions reaching the medial ends of the marginal portions of the upper and lower eyelids.

lower lid after excision of the lacrimal sac when the medial palpebral ligament has been divided (see Whitnall).

The Muscle of Riolan is the ciliary portion of the orbicularis, and consists of very fine striped muscle fibres which lie in the dense tissue of the lids near their margin. The ciliary glands (of Moll) separate them from the palpebral portion of the orbicularis (Fig. 192).

A part of the muscle lies superficial to the tarsal (Meibomian) glands and a part (the subtarsal portion) deep to them (Figs. 192, 208).

The muscle of Riolan is continuous medially with Horner's muscle (Fig. 224).

Actions.—The orbicularis is the sphincter muscle of the eyelids. Its two parts have each a dilator muscle in opposition.

The Palpebral Portion is used in closing the eye without effort. Usually it is an involuntary movement, as in blinking, which goes on continuously almost without our being aware of it. People also blink their eyes when they want to see more clearly, often when they are thinking rapidly, to get, as it were, a sharper mental picture of the situation. The eyes are closed reflexly when there is any danger to them, and curiously enough on hearing a loud noise.

The Orbital Portion is used to close the eyes tightly. When this portion of the muscle is in action the skin of the forehead, temple, and cheek is drawn towards the medial side of the orbit, the eyelids being firmly closed. Radiating furrows are formed, especially on the lateral side and below the eye. In the young they are only seen when the muscle is acting ; later they become permanent, and have received the name of " crow's feet." The muscle comes into play in sudden, short-lived conditions, bringing an increased supply of blood to the head and eye, and giving rise to a strong expiratory effort. Thus it is seen in action in crying children, in coughing, in blowing the nose, sneezing, and *excessive* laughing. Charles Bell thought that the eye was shut tightly to lessen the vascular dilatation which accompanies these efforts, and thus act as a protective bandage. *This action of the orbicularis can be greatly curtailed by drawing the lateral canthus laterally or dividing it.*

One portion of the orbicularis may be paralysed without the other. The orbicularis also holds the lower lid in contact with the globe, since in paralysis of the muscle it falls away and epiphora results.

The normal, rhythmical, blinking reflex (palpebral portion of orbicularis) is fired off by dryness of the cornea, and the lids, especially the upper, spread a film of tears over the surface to moisten it. Blinking, moreover, has a further use —to pump away excessive tears (see p. 239). Contraction of the orbital portion of orbicularis depresses the eyebrow—a common defence, this, against excessive light from above. The relaxed palpebral portion meanwhile allows the lids to remain open. Only when both parts contract together are the eyelids " screwed up ".

The two parts of the muscle exercise different effects on the *volume of the conjunctival sac.* The palpebral part, in closing the lids gently, does not diminish the volume of the sac, so that " an eye brimful of tears " is pumped empty by blinking, and no tears spill. " Screwing up the eye " by the orbital fibres compresses the conjunctival sac, and causes an eye brimful of tears to spill down over the cheek. The full contraction of the orbital portion, pressing the thickened lids tight against the globe and orbital outlet, is more strongly protective against external violence than is mere blinking.

The palpebral portion, which closes the lids gently into marginal apposition, is opposed by levator palpebræ superioris. The orbital portion is opposed by frontalis (occipito-frontalis).

Nerve-supply.—The orbicularis is supplied by the *7th cranial nerve*. The upper part of the muscle is supplied by the temporal and upper zygomatic branches of the facial, the lower by the lower zygomatic branches. These branches enter the muscle from the lateral side and on its deep surface.

The former cross the zygoma, as several branches, $\frac{3}{4}$ in. behind the frontal, run a little above the lateral canthus, and then parallel with the supraorbital margin (see Fig. 289).

The lower zygomatic branch (or branches) reaches the lower part of the muscle by crossing the cheek. By the time these nerves actually enter the muscle they have divided into a fair number of branches (Fig. 273).

The Corrugator supercilii (Fig. 199) is a small, darkly coloured muscle situated at the medial side of the eyebrow under cover of the frontalis and orbicularis. *Arising* from the medial end of the superciliary ridge, it passes upwards and laterally, and then through the overlying muscles (Fig. 273), to be *inserted* into the skin of the eyebrow about its middle. It is responsible for the gaping of a vertical wound of the eyebrow.

Action.—The corrugators pull the eyebrows towards the root of the nose, making a projecting roof over the medial angle of the eye and producing characteristic vertical furrows in the middle of the lower part of the forehead and a dimple at its point of insertion.

The muscle is used primarily to protect the eye from the glare of the sun by forming a projecting shelf above it. It is well developed in those farm children who go about in the open without hats. These acquire permanent vertical furrows between the eyebrows quite early in life. In relation to facial expression it is *par excellence* the muscle of " *trouble.*" It is used to express opposition to anything uncomfortable, and is seen in action in the crying child, in sorrow and pain, in frowning, and in retrospect on difficulty. As Froriep points out, it is often used in conjunction with the medial part of the frontalis and procerus, producing a peculiar oblique lie of the eyebrows well seen in the head of the Laocoön.

Nerve-supply.—The 7th cranial, through its superior zygomatic branch.

The Occipito-frontalis consists of the two occipital and two frontal muscles, united together by a large, thin aponeurosis (the galea aponeurotica), which covers and is moulded on the upper part of the cranium.

Each *occipital muscle*, small and of a quadrilateral form, arises from the lateral two-thirds of the highest nuchal line of the occipital bone and from the base of the mastoid process above the insertion of the sterno-mastoid. It is inserted above into the epicranial aponeurosis (galea aponeurotica).

The frontalis, also somewhat quadrilateral in shape, *arises* by a convex upper border from the epicranial aponeurosis midway between the coronal suture and the orbital margin. It is *inserted* into the skin of the eyebrows, mingling with the fibres of the orbicularis and the corrugator. Above, there is a distinct triangular interval between the two frontal muscles. Below, the medial fibres are joined and intermingle with the procerus, but it must be remembered that the latter muscle is running upwards, and is the antagonist of this medial part of frontalis.

Action.—The frontalis raises the eyebrows and draws the scalp forwards, throwing the forehead into a number of transverse wrinkles. These furrows are convex upwards on either side, joined by a piece in the centre, usually convex downwards. The lines are often absent in the triangular interval between the two muscles above. The occipitalis draws the scalp back. By the alternate contraction of the two muscles the scalp may be drawn forwards and backwards, a power possessed, however, by very few. By the raising of the eyebrows the eyes are widely opened, the white tending to show above the cornea.

Occipito-frontalis is thus the opponent of the orbicular portion of orbicularis oculi ; it is especially used in gazing upwards, to *elevate the eyebrows* above the line of vision. Note that levator palpebræ superioris is the true elevator of the upper *lid*, and so opposes the palpebral portion of the orbicularis.

More light thus reaches the eye, and more therefore is reflected from it, making it brighter and animating the gaze. The frontalis is brought into action when vision is rendered difficult, either by the distance of the object or the absence of sufficient light.

From the point of view of facial expression, the frontalis, as Duchenne has so well described it, is the muscle of " attention." It is used in expressing surprise, admiration, fear, and horror, in all of which the element of " attention " is present. If the eyebrows are raised, the lids being half-closed, the appearance of forced attention results.

Surface Form.—The frontalis is the only muscle of facial expression that can be seen on the surface, and this only in certain individuals (usually the thin intellectual type). When visible its upper curved border and the triangular interval can be easily made out, especially when the muscles are in action.

Nerve-supply.—7th cranial.

Procerus muscle.—The two muscles of this name, placed symmetrically on either side of the midline, occupy the bridge of the nose and the interval between the lower portions of the two frontales. The muscles arise from the lower portion of the nasal bones, and run upwards, to be inserted into the skin of the lower part of the forehead on either side of the midline (Fig. 273).

They pull the skin of this region downwards, producing transverse furrows in the lower part of the forehead and root of the nose. It is for this reason that the somewhat wave-like wrinkles of the forehead are convex upwards on either side, due to the frontales, and tend to be convex downwards in the middle.

The procerus is closely associated with the corrugator supercilii. It increases the prominence of the eyebrows as a protection when the eyes are exposed to bright light. From the point of view of facial expression Duchenne calls it the muscle of " aggression " or " menace." Associated with other muscles it expresses painful and similar emotions.

Nerve-supply.—7th cranial.

The frontalis, orbicularis oculi, corrugator supercilii, and procerus have been called by Howe (1907) the *accessory muscles of accommodation*, since they are brought into play when vision is carried out under difficulties. It is possible that the attachment of the frontalis to the occipitalis may explain certain cases of occipital headache due to eye-strain (see also p. 315).

The Eyebrows

Each eyebrow is a transverse elevation clothed with hairs, and situated at the junction of the forehead and upper lid. In structure it resembles the hairy scalp.

It consists of the following layers :

1. Skin.
2. Subcutaneous tissue.
3. Layer of muscles.
4. Submuscular areolar layer.
5. Pericranium.

1. **The Skin** is thick, very mobile, and richly supplied with sebaceous glands. Like that of the scalp, it is closely adherent to the superficial fascia.

The hairs of the eyebrow are hard but silky. Taken as a whole eyebrows are comma-shaped. The *head* of the comma, the hairs composing which run upwards, is placed typically *under* the medial end of the orbital margin. The *body* of the comma lies along the orbital margin, and the hairs composing it run horizontally outwards. The *tail* of the comma usually lies somewhat above the lateral orbital margin, whose prominence can be made out *below* it. Many variations exist. The higher the eyebrow the more curved does it become, the lower its position the more horizontal. Many muscles of facial expression are attached to the mobile skin of the eyebrows, so that they may be raised, lowered, or drawn towards the midline.

Usually the space between the eyebrows is smooth and hairless (hence glabella), but not infrequently they are joined across the midline.

2. **The Subcutaneous Tissue,** like that of the scalp, contains little fat and much fibrous tissue. It is strongly connected to the skin on the one hand, and

to the underlying muscles on the other. Thus, in movements of the eyebrow, the skin, subcutaneous, and muscle layers move on the submuscular areolar layer.

3. **The Layer of Muscles.**—This is constituted by the vertical fibres of the frontalis, the arched horizontal fibres of the orbicularis, and the oblique darker coloured corrugator supercilii.

4. **The Submuscular Areolar Layer.**—This is a continuation of the dangerous area of the scalp, and since the frontalis is *not* attached to the orbital margin, it is further continued into the upper lid in the plane between the septum orbitale and the orbicularis (Trotter).

Charpy, however, holds that a deep portion of the epicranial aponeurosis is attached to the orbital margin, and cuts off the dangerous area from the lids.

The difference between these opposite views is no doubt due to the fact that while clinically blood and pus find their way from the dangerous area into the upper lid, the coarser particles of the injection fluid, as used by Charpy, were held up.

Vessels.

Arteries :
Supraorbital.
Superficial temporal.

Veins :
Medially—to the supraorbital or angular vein.
Laterally—to the superficial temporal veins.

Lymphatics.
Medially they follow the facial vein to the submandibular group.
Laterally they go to the parotid lymphatic glands.

THE CONJUNCTIVA

The conjunctiva is a thin, transparent mucous membrane which derives its name from the fact that it attaches the eyeball to the lids.

It lines the posterior surface of the lids, and is then reflected forwards on to the globe of the eye. Its epithelium becomes continuous anteriorly with the epithelium of the cornea.

It thus forms a (potential) sac, the conjunctival sac, which is open in front at the palpebral fissure, and only closed when the eyes are shut.

Although all parts of the conjunctiva are continuous with each other, it is divided for purposes of description into three portions.

That which belongs to the lids is called the **Palpebral Portion,** that clothing the eyeball is the **Bulbar Portion.** The intermediate part, forming the redoubled fold of the conjunctival sac where the reflection on to the globe takes place, is called the **Fornix.**

1. **The Palpebral Portion** lining the lids may itself be subdivided into *marginal, tarsal,* and *orbital* zones.

The conjunctiva of the margin of the lid is actually a transition zone between skin and conjunctiva proper (see p. 210). The structure of the marginal zone is continued on to the back of the lid for about 2 mm.[1] (Parsons) to a shallow groove known as the subtarsal fold,[2] at which the perforating vessels pass through the tarsus to reach the conjunctiva.

The puncta open on to the marginal portion of the conjunctiva, and through them the conjunctival sac becomes directly continuous with the inferior meatus of the nose viâ the lacrimal passages.

Thus disease from the conjunctival sac may spread to the nose and vice versa.

The Conjunctiva Tarsi is thin, transparent, adherent and very vascular.

The vascularity gives the region its reddish or pinkish colour, and accounts for the fact that it is examined in cases of suspected anæmia.

As the conjunctiva is transparent, the tarsal glands can be seen through it as yellowish streaks.

The conjunctiva tarsi is intimately adherent to the superior tarsus ; in fact, it is almost impossible to separate the two by dissection ; for this reason too it is impossible to cover up gaps in the conjunctiva tarsi, as one can with the bulbar portion, simply by dissecting up neighbouring flaps and drawing them over the bare area. Unlike the upper tarsal conjunctiva, which is closely adherent to the tarsus in almost its whole extent, the lower is only so adherent for half the width of the tarsus.

The Orbital Zone of the conjunctiva of the upper lid lies between the upper border of the tarsal plate and the fornix. It lies loosely on the underlying involuntary muscle of Müller (Fig. 192). Its surface is thrown into horizontal folds. They are folds of movement, and are deepest when the eyes are open and almost disappear when the eyes are shut (Fuchs). The folds appear after birth.

If the area just above the superior tarsal plate be examined with a loupe it will be found marked by a series of shallow grooves, which divide it up into a mosaic of low elevations (Stieda's [3] plateaux and grooves). These elevations are not true papillæ, although they may become so in inflammation. This area may encroach on the conjunctiva tarsi, but never beyond the middle of the tarsus.

2. **The Fornix Conjunctivæ** is a continuous circular cul-de-sac, which is broken only (on the medial side) by the caruncle and the plica semilunaris.

It is divided for purposes of description into superior, inferior, lateral, and medial portions.

The Superior Fornix reaches to the level of the orbital margin some 8–10 mm. from the limbus.

---

[1] Virchow, however, reckons this admarginal zone as only 0·5 mm.

[2] In the fold foreign bodies are very liable to lodge.

[3] See H. Virchow, Graefe-Saemisch, Handbuch der gesamten Augenheilkunde, 2nd edit., **1,** pt. i.

The Inferior Fornix extends to within a few millimetres of the inferior orbital margin, 8 mm. from the limbus.

The Lateral Fornix is placed at a depth of 5 mm. from the surface, i.e. 14 mm. from the limbus, and extends to just behind the equator of the globe.

The fornix conjunctivæ is in contact with and adherent to loose fibrous tissue, which is derived from the fascial expansions of the sheaths of the levator and recti muscles, and which is easily distensible.

In it are found the glands of Krause and the unstriped muscle of Müller. By means of this fibrous tissue the levator and recti can act on the fornix, deepening it when they contract.

Centrally, the fibrous tissue becomes continuous with the tarsus.

In the intertendinous interval, that is, in the diagonal regions of the fornix, the conjunctiva is in contact with the orbital fat, and it is in this region that infiltrations and hæmorrhage, such as arise in fracture of the base of the skull, reach the conjunctiva and may extend to the cornea (Charpy).

The fornix is well supplied with vessels, and a rich venous network can be especially well seen in the inferior fornix, where also the whitish aponeurotic expansion from the inferior rectus and inferior oblique shows through the conjunctiva (Fuchs).

A knife passed through the upper fornix will enter the fibrous tissue between the levator and superior rectus, while through the inferior fornix the knife will hit the interval between the inferior palpebral muscle and the inferior rectus, and if pushed on the aponeurotic expansion from the inferior rectus and inferior oblique (Figs. 193 and 251).

3. **The Bulbar Conjunctiva** is thin, and so transparent that the white sclerotic shows through it, giving rise to the " white of the eye."

It lies loosely on the underlying tissues, so that it can easily be moved apart from them. This movement takes place slightly with all movements of the eye ; it is made evident in the living by pressure on the conjunctiva through the lower lid, and the operator knows how easy it is to pick up a fold of bulbar conjunctiva with forceps.

The bulbar conjunctiva is at first in contact with the tendons of the recti muscles covered by the fascia bulbi (Tenon's capsule).

Thus, in exposing these tendons, for instance in tenotomy, we must divide the conjunctiva, then the capsule of Tenon before they are reached.

In front of the insertion of the recti tendons the bulbar conjunctiva lies on the anterior portion of Tenon's capsule. Up to a point about 3 mm. from the cornea the conjunctiva is separated from the capsule of Tenon by loose areolar tissue, in which we find the subconjunctival vessels, and between it and the sclera is the loose episcleral tissue in the anterior portion of Tenon's space. In this space we find the anterior ciliary arteries, which form the pericorneal plexus, and the tendons of insertion of the recti muscles.

A.E.—14

At about 3 mm. from the cornea, the conjunctiva, Tenon's capsule, and sclera become much more closely united. For this reason, although it is more difficult to raise a fold of conjunctiva close to the cornea, a much firmer hold can be obtained here with forceps than elsewhere.

At the point of union the conjunctiva is sometimes raised by a slight ridge, which becomes very apparent in certain inflammatory conditions, notably spring catarrh. This portion of the conjunctiva is known as the *limbal conjunctiva*. At the limbus in the angle between the epithelium and the sclera, the corium of the conjunctiva, Tenon's capsule, and the episclera are fused into a dense tissue.

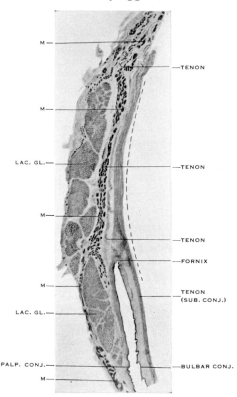

FIG. 204.—MERIDIONAL SECTION UPWARDS AND OUTWARDS THROUGH THE SOFT PARTS SURROUNDING THE EYE.

M = unstriped muscles.

(From Hesser.)

The Structure of the Conjunctiva varies fundamentally in its different portions. On this depends the limitation of certain pathological processes to definite areas (Parsons).

Only in the new-born is the conjunctiva really normal, for owing to its exposed condition slight pathological changes are apt to take place from the earliest age.

The conjunctiva, like all other mucous membranes, consists of two layers—the epithelium and the substantia propria.

The Epithelium.—The greater portion of the free margin of the lid is covered by skin and therefore keratinised.

The muco-cutaneous junction (Figs. 208, 209, 210) lies at the level of the posterior margin of the openings of the tarsal glands, i.e. at the junction of " dry " and " moist " portions where the marginal strips of tear fluid end in a sharp line. Here the eleidin and keratin layers of the skin end quite sharply, giving place to about five layers of non-keratinised squamous epithelium, the most superficial cells of which still retain their nuclei. The deeper portion of the epithelium does not alter at all at the muco-cutaneous junction. Also the first papilla beyond it is just as narrow, consists of the same dense connective tissue and is just as sparingly infiltrated with lymphocytes as the papillæ of the skin (Virchow).

At this point, then, the mucous membrane is much like that of the mouth, i.e. the deepest layer consists of high cylindrical cells as in the epidermis ; this is followed by several layers of polyhedral cells, while the most superficial cells are flattened but still retain their nuclei.   As we travel backwards (Fig. 208) the number of layers of squamous cells is gradually reduced and replaced by columnar and cubical ones.   The total number of layers is also reduced, but the deepest layer remains cylindrical.   In this region also goblet cells, which, however, never reach the muco-cutaneous junction, begin to appear and are particularly numerous just beyond the subtarsal fold.

The epithelium of the tarsal conjunctiva of *the upper eyelid* consists, as classically described, of two layers. The deeper layer is composed of *cubical* cells whose oval nuclei lie with their axes parallel to the surface. The superficial layer consists of tall *cylindrical* cells, whose oval nuclei lie near the base of the cells and have their long axis at right angles to the surface.

As the fornix is approached, there is a tendency for a third layer of polyhedral cells to be inserted between the other two.   So that at the fornix, although generally the structure is like that of the palpebral conjunctiva, we often find three layers instead of two.

The epithelium of the tarsal conjunctiva of *the lower eyelid* differs from the upper in having three or four layers of cells over nearly the whole of its extent; a two-layered arrangement as in the upper is only rarely present ; sometimes five layers may be found.   When four layers are present the basal cells are cubical as in all the tarsal conjunctiva (except the admarginal zone), the next layer is polygonal, superficial to this are elongated wedge-shaped cells, their narrow ends jutting between the cells of the most superficial layer which are cone-shaped.

From the fornix to the limbus the epithelium becomes less and less glandular with a disappearance of the goblet cells, and more like that of the epidermis, but it never becomes keratinised.

More and more polyhedral layers are added between the superficial and deep cells.   The superficial cells become flatter, while the deep cells grow taller.   At the limbus the epithelium is definitely stratified with the formation of papillæ, which give the deep aspect of the epithelium a characteristic wavy outline (Fig. 28).   Here the deepest or basal cells form a single layer of small cylindrical or cubical cells, with a large, darkly staining nucleus and little protoplasm.   It is this fact that produces the *dark line* or seam seen under the low power of the microscope, and characteristic of the limbal conjunctiva (Figs. 25, 28).   Moreover, the basal cells often contain pigment granules.   There are several layers of polygonal cells, and superficially one or two layers of flattened cells with oval nuclei parallel to the surface.   The polygonal cells differ from those of the cornea in having no prickles between them.

Goblet Cells occur in all portions of the conjunctiva, including the plica semilunaris (Fig. 218).   They are large, oval, or round cells which look like fat-cells.   The nucleus is flattened, and is near the base of the cell (Fig. 205).

They are said to be formed from the deepest [1] layer of the conjunctiva, i.e. from the cylindrical cells, and then to pass towards the surface, tending, however, to remain attached to the basement membrane by a pointed process.

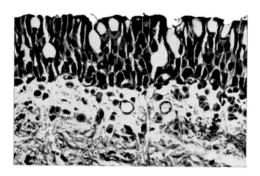

FIG. 205.—SECTION OF THE PALPEBRAL (ORBITAL) CONJUNCTIVA TO SHOW GOBLET CELLS.

At first rounded, they grow larger and more oval as they approach the surface, where they resemble the goblet cells of the large intestine, but differ from these in being destroyed once they have discharged their contents.

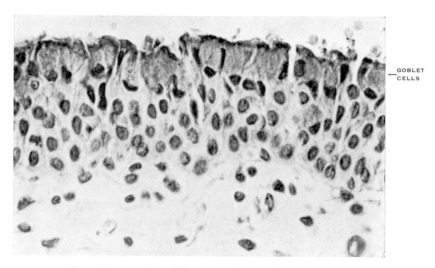

GOBLET
CELLS

FIG. 206.—AS FIG. 205 UNDER HIGHER POWER.

The superficial goblet cells, too, have a stoma, through which the content of the cell, mainly mucin, is discharged.

The goblet cells are true, unicellular mucous glands, moistening and protecting

[1] While this is the usual description, Löhlein, Wolff, and others have never seen goblet cells in the basal layer.

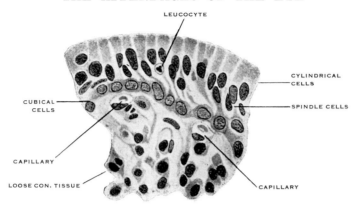

FIG. 207.—EPITHELIUM OF CONJUNCTIVA OF UPPER EYELID AT UPPER END OF TARSUS (VIRCHOW).

the conjunctiva and cornea, so that even extirpation of the lacrimal gland becomes innocuous, whilst on the other hand xerosis of the conjunctiva, involving their destruction, leads to desiccation, in spite of a copious flow of tears (Parsons, Greeff).

Although goblet cells occur normally in the conjunctiva they are greatly increased in inflammatory conditions.

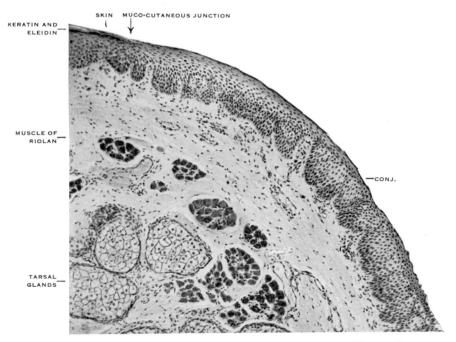

FIG. 208.—VERTICAL SECTION OF POSTERIOR EDGE OF LOWER LID MARGIN (LOW POWER).

Note how the layers of squamous cells diminish in number when traced to the right.

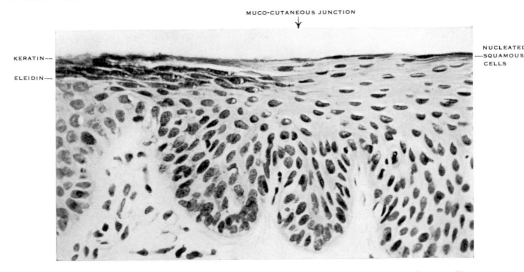

FIG. 209.—VERTICAL SECTION OF THE MUCO-CUTANEOUS JUNCTION OF THE LOWER EYELID.

Note sudden termination of keratin and eleidin layers at arrow. To the right of this nucleated squamous cells.

Kessing (1966) from studies of the whole conjunctiva has mapped out the density of goblet cells. He finds them to be most dense nasally, least dense in the upper temporal fornix, and absent from the bulbar conjunctiva to the nasal and temporal sides of the limbus.

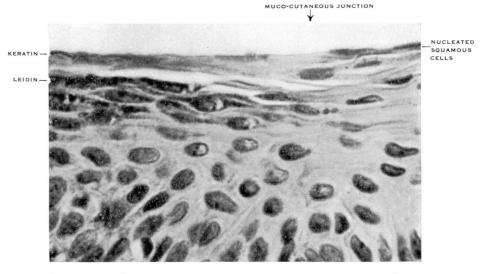

FIG. 210.—AS FIG. 209, BUT ACTUAL JUNCTION UNDER HIGHER POWER (OIL IMMERSION).

Melanophores [1] are present in the conjunctiva of the coloured races. In the white races the cells are present but not usually pigmented. The melanin can, however, always be brought out by the Dopa reaction or silver stains (Fig. 213).

These cells are found at the limbus, at the fornix, in the plica and caruncle, and at the site of perforation of the anterior ciliary vessels.

THE CONJUNCTIVAL GLANDS

The glands of Krause are accessory lacrimal glands having the same structure as the main gland. They are placed deeply in the subconjunctival connective tissue (mainly) of the upper fornix between the tarsus and the inferior lacrimal gland, of which they are offshoots. There are some 42 in the upper and 6 to 8 in the lower fornix (W. Krause). They are thus found largely on the lateral side. Their ducts unite into a rather long duct or sinus which opens into the fornix. Similar glands are found in the caruncle.

The Glands of Wolfring or Ciaccio are also accessory lacrimal glands, but larger than the glands of Krause. There are 2 to 5 in the upper lid situated actually in the upper border of the tarsus about its middle between the extremities of the tarsal glands or just above the tarsus. There are two glands in the inferior edge of the lower tarsus. The excretory duct is large and short and lined by a basal layer of cubical cells and a superficial layer of cylindrical cells like the conjunctiva on which it opens.

Henle's "Glands" occur in the palpebral conjunctiva between the tarsal plates and the fornices. They are probably not true glands, but folds of mucous membrane cut transversely. They resemble Lieberkuhn's crypts in the large intestine, and are lined by epithelium, which is like that of the surrounding conjunctiva.

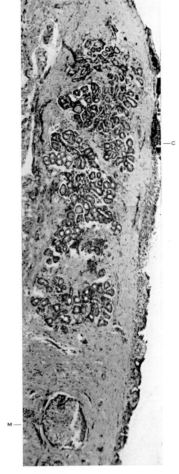

FIG. 211.—GLAND OF WOLFRING OR CIACCIO SITUATED IN UPPER PART OF TARSAL PLATE.

C = conjunctiva;
M = acinus of tarsal gland.

The Glands of Manz are saccular or utricular glands found at the limbus in the pig, calf, and ox. They have also been described in the human, but this is not generally accepted.

[1] These are for the most part actually melanoblasts.

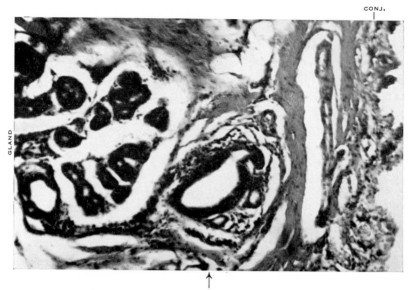

FIG. 212.—GLAND OF CIACCIO OR WOLFRING AND ITS DUCT (ARROW).

The Substantia Propria consists of two portions—a superficial adenoid layer and a deeper fibrous layer. Both end at the limbus ; neither layer passes over the cornea. The adenoid layer is not present at birth, but is formed first in the region of the fornix at 3 to 4 months. It is the formation of this adenoid layer, together with a general increase in the surface area of the conjunctiva, that produces the folds in the upper part of the palpebral conjunctiva at the fifth month (Raehlmann).

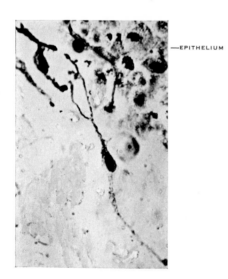

FIG. 213.—FLAT SECTION AT LIMBUS TO SHOW SUBCONJUNCTIVAL MELANOPHORES (STAINED BIELCHOWSKY).

The Adenoid Layer is thin, but most developed in the fornix, being here 50–70 μ in thickness (Villard). It consists of a fine connective tissue reticulum, in the meshes of which the lymphocytes lie. This layer ceases at the subtarsal fold, so that the lymphocytes which are normally present under the conjunctiva in large numbers are not found in the marginal conjunctiva (Fig. 192).

Although nodules of lymphocytes are found in the human conjunctiva, especially towards the angles, they usually fade off at the periphery, and do not form true follicles such as are found especially in the lower fornix of the dog, cat, rabbit, etc. Pathological development of these nodules leads to the formation of undulations on the surface—pseudo papillæ (Parsons).

The Fibrous Layer is generally thicker than the adenoid, but is almost non-existent over the tarsus, with which it is continuous. In it are found the vessels and nerves to the conjunctiva, the unstriped muscle of Müller, and Krause's glands, which are, as it were, encapsuled by it (Villard).

Conjunctival Papillæ.—True papillæ are found only at the limbus (Fig. 28) and at the lid margins.

Those near the limbus are finger-like extrusions of the substantia propria, the interspaces of which are filled with epithelium, whilst the surface of the epithelium remains flat. There are usually only four or five large papillæ (50 μ high) near the cornea, and three or four smaller ones more peripherally (Villard, quoted by Parsons).

The plateaux (and grooves) found at the upper border of the tarsus are not true papillæ, but may become so pathologically. Virchow also described papillæ over the whole of the conjunctiva tarsi, but this is denied by most other observers.

Arteries.—The arterial supply of the conjunctiva comes from three sources.

1. The peripheral arterial arcades.
2. The marginal arterial arcades.
3. The anterior ciliary arteries.

Of these, so far at any rate as the upper lid is concerned, the peripheral arcade supplies by far the greatest area, i.e. almost the whole of the conjunctiva tarsi, the fornix, and the bulbar conjunctiva up to 4 mm. from the cornea.

The Peripheral Arcade in the upper lid is situated at the upper border of the tarsus, between the two portions of the levator (Figs. 192, 193, 215). It gives off the peripheral perforating branches, which pass above the tarsal plate and pierce the muscle of Müller to reach the conjunctiva, under which it sends branches upwards and downwards.

The descending branches supply nearly the whole of the tarsal conjunctiva. They run perpendicularly to the lid margin, and anastomose with the much shorter branches of the marginal artery which have pierced the tarsus at the subtarsal fold.

The zone of anastomosis is but slightly vascular (Langer).

The ascending branches pass upwards to the fornix, then bending round this, descend under the bulbar conjunctiva as the posterior conjunctival arteries (Fig. 215). They pass towards the cornea, at 4 mm. from which they anastomose with the anterior conjunctival arteries, branches of the anterior ciliaries. The posterior conjunctival vessels are mobile, moving with the bulbar conjunctiva.

The peripheral arcade of the lower lid is, when present, placed in front of the inferior palpebral muscle of Müller and then generally behaves as does that of the upper lid. But it is inconstant and may come from other arteries beside the lacrimal, for instance, the transverse facial or superficial temporal.

It is often absent, in which case the conjunctiva of the lower lid, the lower fornix, and inferior portion of the bulbar conjunctiva get their blood-supply from the marginal arcade or from the muscular arteries to the inferior rectus (Fuchs).

The Marginal Arcade sends its perforating branches through the tarsus to reach the deep surface of the conjunctiva at the subtarsal fold.

These branches divide into *marginal* and *tarsal* twigs.

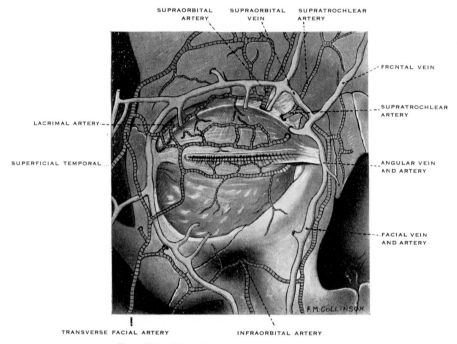

FIG. 214.—THE BLOOD-SUPPLY OF THE EYELIDS.

The marginal arterioles run perpendicularly to the lid margin, forming a very vascular zone ; the tarsal arterioles run perpendicularly to meet the corresponding branches from the peripheral arcade.

The tarsal conjunctiva is well supplied with blood, hence its red colour. The colour diminishes as we pass towards the fornix and the bulbar conjunctiva is colourless except when its vessels are dilated.

The Anterior Ciliary Arteries come from the muscular arteries to the recti (Figs. 87, 215, 216). Each muscular artery gives off two anterior ciliaries, except that to the lateral rectus, which supplies only one.

The anterior ciliary arteries pass forwards on a deeper plane than the posterior conjunctival. They are, however, visible, but appear darker than the superficial vessels. Some 4 mm. from the cornea-scleral junction they bend towards the interior of the eye and pierce the sclera to join the circulus iridis major, which they help to form (Fig. 87). The hole in the sclera is often marked by pigment.

At the bend the anterior ciliaries give off the *anterior conjunctival arteries*, which pass forwards at a deeper level than the posterior conjunctival vessels (Fig. 215). They do not move with the conjunctiva. They pass forwards and, anastomosing with each other, form a series of arcades parallel to the corneal margin

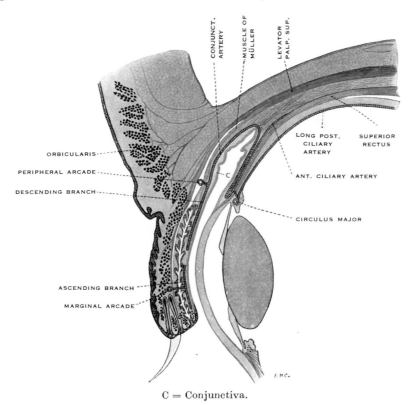

C = Conjunctiva.

FIG. 215.—SECTION OF THE UPPER LID AND ANTERIOR PORTION OF THE EYE TO SHOW THE BLOOD-SUPPLY TO THE CONJUNCTIVA.

which more anteriorly gives place to the pericorneal plexus, while posteriorly they send twigs which anastomose with the posterior conjunctival arteries.

The pericorneal plexus is arranged in two layers : a superficial *conjunctival* and a deep *episcleral* (Figs. 25, 28).

The superficial portion is injected in superficial affections of the cornea, while the deeper portion is hyperæmic in diseases of the iris, ciliary body, or deep portion of the cornea.

It is the dilatation of the deeper portion which gives rise to the characteristic rose-pink band of " ciliary injection." It will be noted that the redness disappears on pressure, but the vessels do not move with the conjunctiva.

In conjunctivitis the bulbar conjunctiva becomes brick-red, due to hyperæmia of the close network of small superficial vessels which, derived from the posterior conjunctival, are normally almost invisible. The redness increases towards the fornices and gets less as we approach the cornea ; it does not fade on pressure. The vessels move with the conjunctiva.

All the above facts are explained by the anatomical arrangements of the vessels.

Thus we see that although joined by anastomoses the area supplied by the palpebral arcades on the one hand and that which gets its blood-supply from the anterior ciliaries on the other hand are more or less sharply differentiated, and in affections of the conjunctiva the vessels of the former area are injected, the redness increasing towards the fornix, while in deep inflammation, that is, of the iris and ciliary body, the network of vessels around the cornea coming from the anterior ciliaries forms a characteristic rose-pink band.

In interstitial keratitis the new vessels that invade the substantia propria of the cornea come from the anterior ciliaries as these are passing through the sclera to reach the iris and ciliary body. They are thus, since the sclera is opaque, only visible up to the limbus.

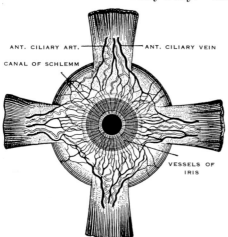

FIG. 216.—ANTERIOR CILIARY ARTERIES AND VEINS.
(*From Poirier after Panas.*)

The Conjunctival Veins accompany but are much more numerous than the corresponding arteries. For the most part, i.e. from the conjunctiva tarsi, from the fornix, and the major portion of the bulbar conjunctiva, they drain into the palpebral veins.

Corresponding to the peripheral arterial arcade of the upper lid, there is an important and well-marked venous plexus, which, placed between the tendons of the levator, sends its blood back to the veins of the levator and superior rectus, which again drain into the ophthalmic (Fuchs).

In the circumcorneal zone supplied by the anterior ciliaries the corresponding veins are less conspicuous than the arteries. They form a network some 5 to 6 mm. wide, which drains into the muscular veins. It becomes apparent in hyperæmia (Merkel).

Lymphatics.—The conjunctival lymphatics are arranged in two plexuses.

A superficial, composed of small vessels, placed just beneath the vascular capillaries ; and a deep, consisting of larger vessels situated in the fibrous layer of the conjunctiva, and receiving the lymph from the superficial plexus.

They drain towards the commissures, where they join the lymphatics of the lids : those from the lateral side go to the parotid nodes, and those from the medial to the submandibular lymph glands.

Nerves.—The nerve-supply of the conjunctiva is derived from the same source as that of the lids generally, but the short ciliaries supply the cornea and circumcorneal zone of the conjunctiva and the lacrimal and infratrochlear supply a much larger area of conjunctiva than of skin.

Nerve Endings.—The nerves may end in :

(a) Free endings

(b) In the end bulbs of Krause, and, according to Crevatin, in

(c) Tufts, or

(d) Ribbons.

(a) *Free Endings.*—The nerves having lost their myelin sheath, form a *sub-epithelial* plexus in the superficial part of the substantia propria. From this fibres pass to form an intra-epithelial plexus around the bases of the epithelial cells and send free nerve fibrils between these cells.

(b) *The End Bulbs of Krause* (Fig. 217) are round bodies from 0·02 mm. to 0·1 mm. in length. Each is surrounded by a connective tissue envelope, continuous with the nerve sheath and lined by endothelial cells. In this is found a twisted mass of fibrils. One or two nerves enter the envelope, lose their myelin sheath, and join the central mass.

These end bulbs are especially abundant in the upper and lateral part of the conjunctiva in the area supplied by the lacrimal nerve (Ciaccio), but are also numerous around the cornea and the marginal portion of the lids.

THE CARUNCLE (Figs. 18 and 218)

The caruncle (diminutive of Latin, *caro*, flesh) is a small fleshy-looking ovoid body some 5 mm. in height and 3 mm. broad, situated in the lacus lacrimalis to the medial side of the plica semilunaris.

It is attached to the plica, and fibres of the medial rectus sheath enter its deep surface. Thus it is most prominent when the eye looks laterally, being pulled on by the plica, and becomes deeply recessed when the eye looks medially *and sometimes following tenotomy of the medial rectus.*

It is really a piece of modified skin, so is covered by modified stratified squamous epithelium, and is supplied with hairs, sebaceous and sweat glands. It differs from the skin in containing glands like those of Krause. In the depths of the caruncle the abundant connective tissue is in contact with the septum orbitale and the medial check ligament. *The epithelium* resembles that of the lid margin, but the superficial layer is not keratinised. Also towards the conjunctiva, goblet cells are found. These may occur singly or in groups, forming a kind of acinus.

The Sebaceous Glands resemble those of Zeis and Meibomius. They produce the characteristic white secretion not infrequently found at the medial canthus.

The Modified Lacrimal Glands are often conspicuous structures. They do not represent the gland of Harder, which is absent in the human. They are placed in the centre of the caruncle, have a typical tubulo-acinous structure, and open by a sinuous duct near the plica semilunaris. Around the lacrimal gland tissue there is usually a thin layer of fat.

The Hairs, some fifteen in number, are fine, colourless, and directed towards the nose.

Blood-supply.—The superior medial palpebral artery. The branches, to reach the caruncle, have to pass through dense connective tissue. This keeps them patent when cut and results in free bleeding, as does a similar arrangement in the scalp.

Lymphatics.—These drain into the submandibular lymph glands.

Nerve-supply.—The infratrochlear nerve.

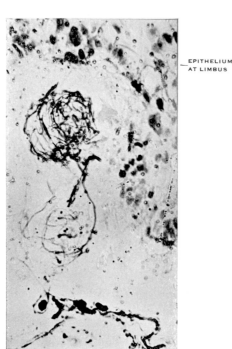

EPITHELIUM AT LIMBUS

FIG. 217.—FLAT SECTION AT LIMBUS TO SHOW END BULB OF KRAUSE (STAINED BIELCHOWSKY).

THE PLICA SEMILUNARIS

The plica semilunaris is a narrow crescentic fold of conjunctiva placed vertically with its concavity facing laterally and lying lateral to and partly under cover of the caruncle. Its lower horn reaches to the middle of the lower fornix, while the upper does not pass up so far. The lateral border is free and separated from the bulbar conjunctiva by a small cul-de-sac some 2 mm. deep, present when the eye looks medially, but almost disappearing when the eye looks laterally. The pink colour of the plica is due to its vascularity (Fig. 218) and contrasts with the white of the sclera. In structure it is like that of the rest of the bulbar conjunctiva, but the epithelium instead of six layers consists of eight to ten, and the deepest layer, instead of being cubical, is cylindrical, and it contains a lobule of fat and some unstriped muscle supplied by the sympathetic. Goblet cells are particularly numerous (Fig. 218).

The goblet cells may be superficial or grouped and then open on the surface by a narrow duct (intra-epithelial gland of Tourneux) (Fig. 219). Melanophores called cells of Langerhans are always present. They may be non-pigmented in fair people but can always be demonstrated by the Dopa reaction and in other ways.

The connective tissue stroma of the plica is loose and contains numerous

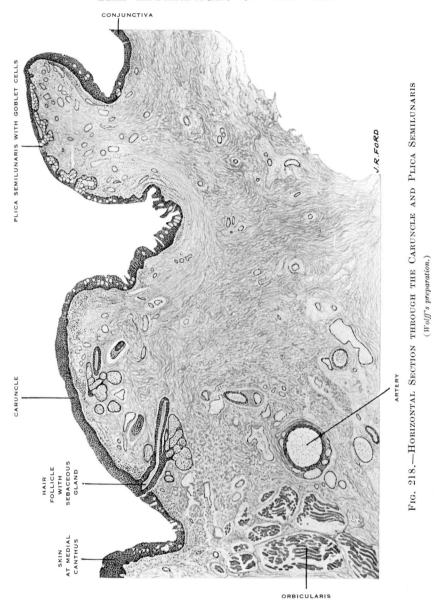

CONJUNCTIVA

PLICA SEMILUNARIS WITH GOBLET CELLS

PLICA SEMILUNARIS

J.R.FORD

CARUNCLE

ARTERY

HAIR FOLLICLE WITH SEBACEOUS GLAND

SKIN AT MEDIAL CANTHUS

ORBICULARIS

Fig. 218.—Horizontal Section through the Caruncle and Plica Semilunaris

(*Wolff's preparation.*)

vessels and sometimes a nodule of fibro-cartilage. At the base of the plica there is a lobule of fat and sometimes some unstriped muscle fibres.

Similar structures are found in the caruncle and come from the medial rectus and more especially from the medial capsulo-palpebral muscle of Hesser.

The plica may represent the 3rd eyelid or nictitating membrane of the lower animals. Lindsay Johnson (quoted by Treacher Collins, *Trans. Ophthal. Soc.*

U.K., 1921, **41**) saw a boy who had an obvious nictitating membrane which reached almost up to the cornea and was capable of slight movement. But developmental abnormalities really prove nothing, and perhaps there is no evolutionary mystery at all. Forty years ago Stibbe (1928) showed that the plica is not homologous with the nictitating membrane. He suggested that the plica acts as a " flap valve " to enable excessive tears to float a foreign body forwards towards the medial canthus.

A still simpler view of the plica semilunaris is that it is an inevitable formation. The conjunctival area here must be generous enough to allow full lateral movement of the eyeball. Thus there is slack to be taken up when the eye looks forwards or medially; hence the fold. No such arrangement exists laterally, for here the fornix is very deep. The absence of a deep medial fornix is a functional necessity to enable the puncta to dip into *superficial* strips of tear fluid (p. 237).

THE LACRIMAL APPARATUS

The lacrimal apparatus is constituted as follows :

The lacrimal gland situated above and to the lateral side of the globe of the eye secretes the tears and pours them through a series of ducts into the conjunctival sac at the upper fornix. The lacrimal gland and its tears are only present in those animals which live in air. In fishes, for instance, there is no lacrimal gland, the water in which they live acting in place of tears.

The tears moisten the front of the eye, lubricate it, prevent friction between globe and lids, and also desiccation of the corneal epithelium (see p. 238).

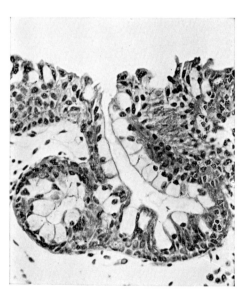

FIG. 219.—SECTION OF PORTION OF PLICA SEMI-LUNARIS TO SHOW GLAND OF TOURNEUX.

Some of the tears evaporate, but the rest make their way medially to the puncta situated in the margin of the lids. From here they are conducted by the (lacrimal) canaliculi to the lacrimal sac, and then pass into the naso-lacrimal duct, which opens into the inferior meatus of the nose.

Under normal conditions almost no tears pass down the naso-lacrimal duct ; just enough tears are produced to replace evaporation from the cornea and exposed conjunctiva. Thus removal of the lacrimal sac, with consequent obliteration of the drainage channels, is little embarrassment to the average individual.

The Lacrimal Gland

The Lacrimal Gland consists of two portions (Figs. 275, 280, and 281) :

(i) A large orbital or superior portion ;

and (ii) A small palpebral or inferior portion ;

which are, however, continuous behind. *The Orbital Portion* is lodged in its fossa on the anterior and lateral part of the roof of the orbit. It is shaped like an almond, and hence we have for examination a superior and inferior surface, an anterior and posterior border, and a medial and a lateral extremity.

The Superior Surface is convex, and lies in the fossa on the frontal bone, with which it is connected by weak trabeculæ.

The Inferior Surface, slightly concave, lies successively on the levator palpebræ, the lateral expansion of its tendon, and the lateral rectus (Figs. 277 and 280).

The Anterior Border is sharp and in contact with the septum orbitale.

Hence, to reach this portion of the lacrimal gland from the front, one has to divide skin, orbicularis, and septum orbitale.

The Posterior Border, more rounded, is in contact with the orbital fat in the same coronal plane as the posterior pole of the eye.

The Medial Extremity rests on the levator—the *lateral* on the lateral rectus.

The Palpebral Portion, also flattened from above down, is about one-third the size of the orbital portion, and placed so that the anterior border lies just above the lateral part of the upper fornix. It can be seen in this situation through the conjunctiva when the upper lid is everted.

It lies for the most part on the fornix and palpebral conjunctiva, but partly also on the superior palpebral muscle.

It is separated from the superior portion by the expansion of the

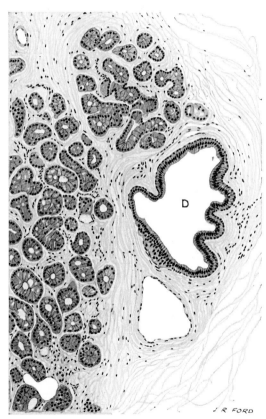

FIG. 220.—SECTION OF THE LACRIMAL GLAND.

D = *one* of the ducts.

(*Wolff's preparation.*)

levator, but behind this its posterior border is continuous with the rest of the gland (Fig. 280).

The Glands of Krause (Fig. 192) are accessory lacrimal glands occurring under the conjunctiva from the fornix to the convex border of the tarsus. They may be regarded as a continuation downwards of the palpebral portion of the lacrimal gland.

Fine Ducts pass from both portions of the lacrimal gland to open by ten to twelve small orifices just in front of the lateral part of the superior fornix. One or two also open into the lateral part of the lower fornix.

Structure.—The lacrimal gland is a tubulo-racemose gland with short branched gland tubules resembling the parotid in structure (Fig. 220). It consists of masses of lobules, each being about the size of a pin's head. It is not very sharply differentiated from the surrounding adipose tissue, and fat is also found between the lobules.

The acini consist of two layers of cells placed on a thin hyaline basement membrane and surrounding a central canal. The cells of the basal layer are myoepithelial in character and are flat and contractile ; the other cells are cylindrical, and form the true secreting cells. At rest these contain granules. After secreting for some time the cells become shorter and the granules disappear. The secretion of the acini passes into very small interlobular ducts, opening into slightly larger ducts which are, however, still intermediary. These finally open into the definitive excretory duct.

The smaller ducts have much the same structure as the acini, but in the large ducts outside the basement membrane is a fibrous coat.

The inter-acinous and inter-lobular connective tissue is hardly present in the young but increases with age. In it are found plasma cells and lymphocytes which may be aggregated into follicles.

The ducts from the orbital portion traverse or are in contact with the palpebral portion. *It thus comes about that removal of the palpebral portion practically does away with the secretion of the whole gland.*

So-called ligaments have been described in connection with the lacrimal gland ; none, however, deserve the name.

(*a*) *Superior* to the lacrimal fossa (= suspensory ligament).

(*b*) *Inferior*—inferior pole to zygomatic bone.

(*c*) *Posterior*—where the lacrimal nerve and vessels enter, to the periorbita.

(*d*) *Internal*—accompanying the ducts.

Vessels.—The lacrimal artery, which enters it on its posterior border, and sometimes a branch of the transverse facial. The corresponding vein joins the ophthalmic.

Lymphatics to the conjunctival lymphatics, and thence to the preauricular glands.

Nerves.—Lacrimal, great (superficial) petrosal, and sympathetic.

The Fibres of the Great (Superficial) Petrosal, the nerve of tear secretion, arise in the cells of the superior salivatory nucleus.

They pass out in the nervus intermedius to the geniculate ganglion (but make no cell station here), from which the great (superficial) petrosal arises.

This runs in a groove on the front of the petrous temporal (Fig. 272), then under the trigeminal ganglion to join the deep petrosal (from the sympathetic

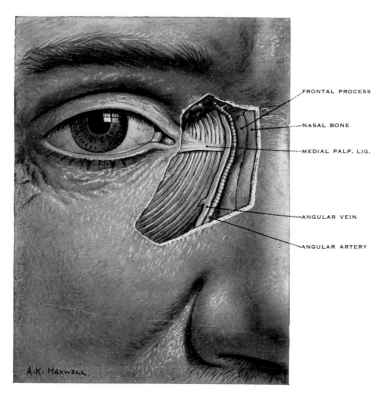

FRONTAL PROCESS

NASAL BONE

MEDIAL PALP. LIG.

ANGULAR VEIN

ANGULAR ARTERY

Fig. 221.—Dissection to show Lacrimal Apparatus. Relation of Angular Vein and Artery to Medial Palpebral Ligament.
(*Wolff's dissection.*)

plexus round the internal carotid artery) to form the (Vidian) nerve of the pterygoid canal in the foramen lacerum (Fig. 287).

The Nerve of the Pterygoid Canal (Vidian Nerve), thus composed of parasympathetic (secretomotor) and sympathetic (vasomotor) fibres, joins the pterygopalatine (spheno-palatine, Meckel's) ganglion. Only the parasympathetic fibres relay in the ganglion. The postganglionic secretomotor fibres pass to the zygomatic nerve and reach the lacrimal gland via the connecting branch with the lacrimal nerve.

The Sympathetic Fibres come from the superior cervical ganglion viâ

    (*a*) Sympathetic nerves on the lacrimal artery.

    (*b*) Deep petrosal.

    (*c*) Sympathetic fibres in the lacrimal nerve.

The Sensory Fibres are carried by the lacrimal nerve ; their cell bodies are in the trigeminal ganglion.

The Puncta

Each punctum lacrimale is a small, round, or transversely oval aperture situated on a slight elevation, *the papilla lacrimalis*, at the medial end of the lid margin at the junction of its ciliary and lacrimal portions.   It is in a line with

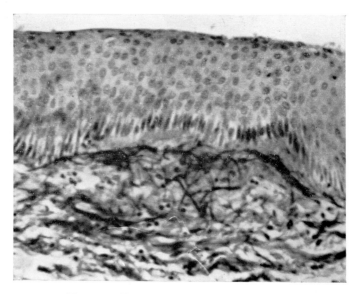

Fig. 222.—Portion of Wall of Canaliculus.
Note elastic fibres deep to epithelium.

the openings of the ducts of the tarsal glands, the nearest of which is only 0·5 to 1 mm. away.

The region of the punctum is relatively avascular, and so is paler than the surrounding area.   This pallor is emphasised on drawing the lower lid laterally, *a fact of great value in finding a stenosed punctum.*

The upper punctum is slightly farther to the nasal side (being 6 mm. from the medial canthus) than the lower, which is 6·5 mm. from this point.   Thus, when the eye is shut the puncta are not in contact, but the upper lies to the medial side of the lower.

The upper punctum looks downwards and backwards, and the lower upwards and backwards. *For this reason a normal punctum is only visible if the lid is everted.*

Each punctum, when the eye is opened or shut, glides in the groove between the plica semilunaris[1] and the globe ; and is kept patent by a ring of very dense fibrous tissue, continuous with the tarsus which surrounds it. Around this again

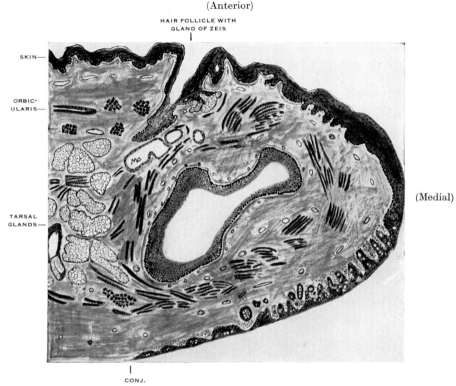

(Anterior)

HAIR FOLLICLE WITH
GLAND OF ZEIS

SKIN—

ORBIC-
ULARIS—

(Medial)

TARSAL
GLANDS—

CONJ.

Fig. 223.—Horizontal Section of the Medial Portion of the Lower Eyelid, showing the Lacrimal Canaliculus at the Junction of the Vertical and Horizontal Portions, surrounded by Fibres of the Orbicularis.

MO = gland of Moll. Note goblet cells in conjunctiva.
(*Wolff's preparation.*)

are fibres of the orbicularis which press the punctum in towards the lacus lacrimalis. Their atrophy in old age makes the papilla lacrimalis more prominent.

The Canaliculi

Each canaliculus consists of a vertical and a horizontal portion. *It is, therefore, of great importance in passing a probe to remember that the canaliculus runs at first vertically.*

[1] i.e. when the eye is looking straight ahead. When the eye looks laterally it glides in the groove between the plica and the caruncle.

The vertical portion is about 2 mm. long and then bends medially almost at a right angle to become continuous with the horizontal portion. At the junction of the two is a dilatation or *ampulla*.

Both horizontal portions slope towards the medial canthus ; thus the upper runs downwards as well as medially, while the lower has a slight inclination upwards. Some 8 mm. long, the upper being slightly the shorter, they lie in the lid margin.

The canaliculi pierce the lacrimal fascia (i.e. the periorbita covering the lacrimal sac) separately as a rule, then unite to enter a small diverticulum of the sac called the sinus of Maier (Fig. 226).

The point of entry lies just behind the middle of the lateral surface of the sac about 2½ mm. from its apex.

Structure.—The canaliculi are lined by stratified squamous epithelium (Figs. 222, 223) placed on a corium rich in elastic tissue. The walls are thus so thin and

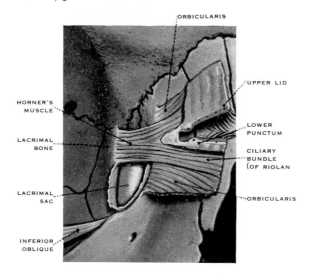

FIG. 224.—THE RELATIONS OF THE LACRIMAL SAC AND HORNER'S MUSCLE. THE LIDS HAVE BEEN TURNED OVER ON TO THE NOSE.

(*Wolff's dissection.*)

elastic that the canaliculus can be dilated three times its normal diameter, which is 0·5 mm. For the same reason, in pulling the lids laterally and in passing a probe the angle between vertical and horizontal portions can be easily straightened. Also being so close to the edge of the lid and covered by translucent tissue, a coloured fluid injected into the canaliculus can be seen.

Like the punctum the canaliculus is surrounded by fibres of the orbicularis (Fig. 223), which on contraction tend to invert the lower lid and draw the punctum inwards.

The medial third of the canaliculi is covered in front by the two bands which connect the medial palpebral ligament to the tarsi, while behind this portion is the lacrimal (Horner's) muscle (Fig. 224).

THE LACRIMAL SAC

The membranous lacrimal sac is placed in the lacrimal fossa (formed by the lacrimal bone and the frontal process of the maxilla) which lies in the anterior part of the medial wall of the orbit (see also p. 4).

The sac is closed above and open below, where it is continuous with the naso-lacrimal duct, a constriction marking the junction between the two.

Looked at *from the side* the sac and fossa are seen to slope backwards 15–25°, the line being given by joining the medial canthus to the 1st upper molar of the same side.

From the front the sac slopes gently laterally, the duct slightly less so. The two thus make an obtuse angle open inwards (Fig. 226).

The sac is enclosed by a portion of the periorbita which, splitting at the pos-

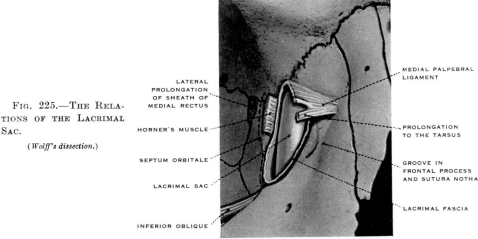

FIG. 225.—THE RELATIONS OF THE LACRIMAL SAC.

(*Wolff's dissection.*)

terior lacrimal crest, encloses the sac to meet again at the anterior lacrimal crest, and thus forms what is called the *lacrimal fascia* (Figs. 224, 225, 226).

The lacrimal fascia is separated from the sac by areolar tissue containing a fine plexus of veins continuous with that around the duct, except at the fundus, where it is closely adherent, and, sometimes, on its medial aspect.

Relations.—*Medially* the sac is in relation above with the anterior ethmoidal air-cells (Fig. 3) (which may also at times lie behind and even in front of the sac), below with the middle meatus of the nose. Between bone and sac, however, we always find periorbita.

Laterally are the skin, fibres of the orbicularis, and the lacrimal fascia.

For the relation of the medial palpebral ligament to the sac see p. 191.

The inferior oblique arises from the floor of the orbit just lateral to the lacrimal fossa, a few fibres often taking origin from the lacrimal fascia.

The angular vein is the great bugbear in the approach to the lacrimal sac. Lying under the skin it crosses the medial palpebral ligament 8 mm. from the medial canthus.   Not infrequently a tributary of the angular vein, which can also be seen in the living, crosses the ligament between the medial canthus and parent vein.   *It is therefore not safe to make the incision for the removal of the sac more than 2 to 3 mm. medial to the medial canthus.*

The lower margin of the medial palpebral ligament is free, but it is continued upwards and laterally as a sheet which blends with the lacrimal fascia covering the fundus of the sac (Fig. 225) (see p. 191).

As Fisher points out, this attachment to the sac may explain how relatively

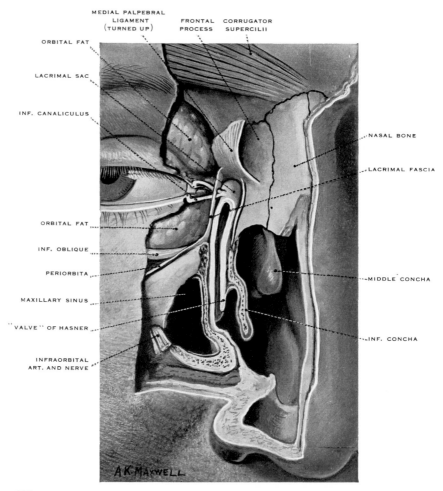

FIG. 226.—DISSECTION TO SHOW THE RELATIONS OF THE LACRIMAL SAC AND THE NASO-LACRIMAL DUCT FROM IN FRONT.
(*Wolff's preparation.*)

slight blows on the eye (as in boxing) may cause swelling of the lids on blowing the nose. A sudden strain is put on the ligament, which pulls on and tears the sac.

The portion of the sac below the level of the ligament is covered by only a few fibres of the orbicularis, which offer little resistance to distension and swellings of the sac. *It is, therefore, in the area below the ligament that abscesses and fistulæ will open.*

Behind the sac are the lacrimal fascia and Horner's muscle which takes origin from the upper half of the posterior lacrimal crest, runs behind the sac and covers the posterior aspect of the medial third of the canaliculi. Behind this again is the septum orbitale, and then comes the check ligament of the medial rectus (Fig. 198).

The Sinus of Maier is a slight diverticulum from the upper part of the sac behind the middle of the lateral surface into which the canaliculi open either together or separately.

THE NASO-LACRIMAL DUCT

The naso-lacrimal duct, the continuation downwards of the lacrimal sac extending from the so-called neck to the inferior meatus of the nose, is only $\frac{5}{8}$ in. in length. It lies in a canal formed mainly by a groove on the maxilla (Figs. 3 and 6) and completed by the lacrimal bone and the lacrimal process of the inferior concha (turbinate). It passes backwards, laterally and downwards, its direction being given in lateral view by a line from the medial angle of the eye to the 1st upper molar of the same side.

The position and shape of the inferior orifice vary greatly. In some cases, where it corresponds to the opening of the bony canal at the highest part of the meatus it tends to be round ; in others it runs as a *membranous* tube for some distance under the mucous membrane, and is then found at different points down the lateral wall of the meatus, becoming more slit-like as it descends. It may be very difficult to find.

The naso-lacrimal duct lies lateral to the middle meatus (Fig. 226), and laterally makes a ridge in the forepart of the maxillary antrum (Fig. 19), *a relation which explains why epiphora is such a frequent symptom of growths of this sinus.*

The Valves.—Numerous so-called valves have been described in the naso-lacrimal duct. They are simply folds of mucous membrane which have no valvular function, since fluids can be blown up the duct to come out at the puncta. The most constant of these folds is the " valve " of Hasner (plica lacrimalis) at the lower end, which represents the remains of the fœtal septum (see also Figs. 226, 227). When well-developed (and it usually is) the plica functions adequately in preventing a sudden blast of air (blowing the nose into a handkerchief) from entering the lacrimal sac.

Structure.—The lacrimal sac and duct are lined by two layers of epithelium, the superficial of which is columnar, the deeper flattened. The bases of the columnar cells pass through the deeper layer to reach the basement membrane. The superficial layer is never ciliated, but in it goblet cells may be found (Rochon-Duvigneaud). Mucous glands have also been described. In the subepithelial layer are lymphocytes, which may be aggregated into follicles (? pathological). The actual membranous wall of the sac consists of fibro-elastic tissue, the elastic portion being continuous with that around the canaliculi. The naso-lacrimal duct is curious in having a rich plexus of vessels around it, forming an erectile tissue resembling in structure that on the inferior concha (turbinate bone). *Engorgement of these vessels is in itself sufficient to obstruct the duct* (Fuchs).

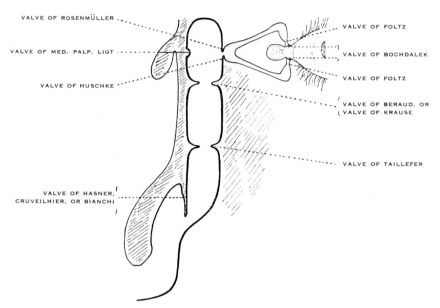

FIG. 227.—SCHEME OF THE SO-CALLED VALVES OF THE NASO-LACRIMAL CANAL.
(From Poirier after Aubaret.)

Whilst at its upper part the naso-lacrimal duct can easily be separated from the bone, below it is closely adherent, forming a muco-periosteum, and *thus disease may pass easily from bone to duct or vice versa.*

Vessels.—The *arterial* supply comes from the superior and inferior palpebral branches of the ophthalmic (Fig. 275); from the angular artery; from the infra-orbital artery, and from the nasal branch of the spheno-palatine.

The Veins above drain into the angular and infraorbital veins, while below they run into the nasal veins.

The Lymphatics pass to the submandibular, and deep cervical glands.

The Nerves.—The nerve-supply of sac and duct comes from the infratrochlear and anterior superior alveolar.

There is probably a reflex relation between the nerve-supply of the lacrimal gland and sac, for extirpation of the latter greatly diminishes the tear flow.

THE DISTRIBUTION OF THE LACRIMAL FLUID

At the posterior margin of both upper and lower eyelids there is a collection or S strip of tear fluid.

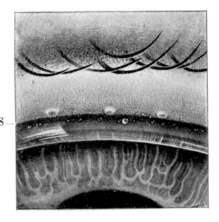

With the naked eye and without the previous instillation of fluorescin these strips of fluid can be made out only with difficulty; but since each acts as a mirror it reflects light strongly so that the brilliant linear reflex that it produces can be seen at some distance. Usually this applies only to the lower strip, since the upper lid margin is normally in shadow.

FIG. 228.—THE SUPERIOR MARGINAL STRIP (S).

Note the oil droplets in it. Also some air bubbles.

The strips of fluid can be made out better with a loupe and, of course, best of all with the slit-lamp.

With the slit-lamp the strip-like collection of fluid is seen to be between the

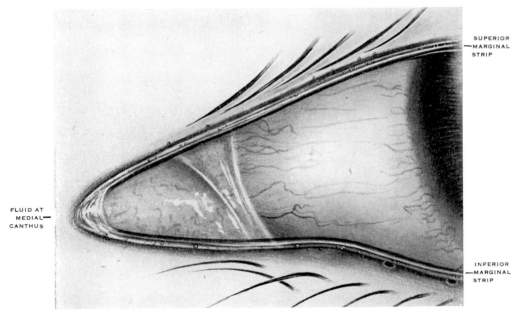

FIG. 229.—WITH THE EYE LOOKING LATERALLY THE MARGINAL STRIPS ARE CONTINUED MEDIALLY BETWEEN THE LID MARGIN ON ONE HAND AND THE PLICA AND CARUNCLE ON THE OTHER. THEY JOIN AT THE MEDIAL CANTHUS.

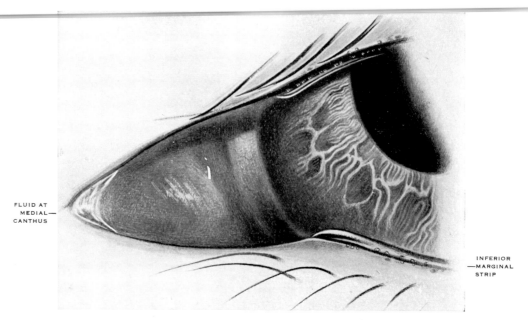

FLUID AT
MEDIAL—
CANTHUS

INFERIOR
—MARGINAL
STRIP

FIG. 230.—WITH THE EYE LOOKING MEDIALLY A CAVITY APPEARS DEEP TO EACH LACRIMAL PORTION
OF THE LID MARGIN AND THE MARGINAL STRIPS STOP SHORT.
(*Trans. O.S.U.K.*, 1946, **66,** 291.)

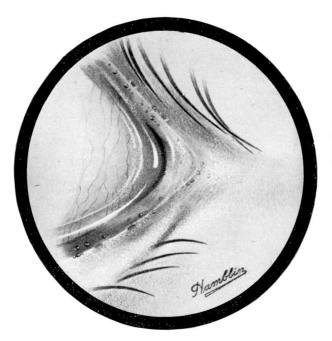

FIG. 231.—THE COLLECTION
OF TEAR FLUID AT THE LATERAL
CANTHUS. IT IS CONTINUOUS
WITH THE FLUID IN THE LATERAL
CUL-DE-SAC.

(*Trans. O.S.U.K.*, 1946.)

236

posterior lid margin of both eyelids and the exposed portion of the globe. That of the lower lid (the inferior marginal strip) runs up on the cornea for a millimetre or so, due to surface tension, and hence the tear fluid appears always, that is normally, to be brimming over. It is prevented from actually overflowing, however, by the secretion of the tarsal glands. The anterior limit is at the posterior margin of the openings of the tarsal glands. When the lower lid is drawn away from the eye the tear fluid sinks down into the lower fornix, but immediately returns when the lid is allowed to return to its normal position. In the adult this collection of fluid, where it is in contact with the conjunctiva, contains some folds of this mucous membrane.

The collection of fluid at the posterior margin of the upper lid (the superior marginal strip) runs down on to the cornea for a millimetre or so and ends in a *sharp line*. One would emphasise the fact that one has never failed to find evidence of oil, that is of the secretion of the tarsal glands, in these strips of fluid. This may take the form of oil drops or of a film of oil which may at times be seen spreading over the cornea as a typical coloured oil film. The amount of Meibomian secretion on the strips of fluid may be increased, sometimes to a startling extent, by the forceful closure of the eyelids.

When the upper eyelid is lifted away from the globe, the tear fluid runs up towards the upper fornix.

On tracing the strips of fluid at the posterior margin of the eyelids laterally, a veritable tear lake is seen at the lateral canthus. This reservoir contains more obvious fluid than the lacus lacrimalis itself, and is of great importance as it is one of the ways by which lacrimal fluid from the upper lid may reach the lower conjunctival cul-de-sac and the strip of fluid at the lower lid margin. Here, too, the fluid on the side of the skin ends in a sharp line.

The strips of fluid at the lid margins are continued medially between the lacrimal portions of the lid margins on the one hand and the plica and caruncle on the other.[1] At least this is true when the eye looks laterally and usually straight ahead. When the eye looks medially a large space appears deep to the lacrimal portion of the lid margins, which now stand right away from the plica and (the lateral part of) the caruncle.[2]

The actual capacity of the lacus lacrimalis is thus greatly increased, but it still contains only a little fluid. This is a thin film covering the plica semilunaris and the slight amount of fluid in the grooves on either side of it and in the little groove to the medial side of the caruncle. One would draw special attention to the fact that it is much more accurate to say that the puncta dip into the strips of fluid at the posterior lid margin than into the lacus lacrimalis. For if it were necessary for them to dip into the tear lake, as universally stated, they could not function in the adducted position of the eye when the puncta are in

[1] Whose oily sebaceous secretion has taken on the function of the Meibomian glands.
[2] The amount of recession of the caruncle varies in different people.

contact with the cornea, and any person with an internal strabismus would of necessity have a watery eye, which obviously is not the case.

The Conduction of the Lacrimal Fluid

From what has gone before, it becomes clear how one would suggest the tears reach the puncta.

Secreted by the lacrimal gland they pass for the most part into the lateral part of the upper fornix, whence they descend to the strip of fluid at the upper lid margin. They reach the upper punctum along this strip or directly under the upper eyelid. The tear fluid reaches the lower lid mainly at the collection of fluid at the lateral canthus and through the lateral conjunctival cul-de-sac. It also communicates at the slight amount of fluid to the medial and lateral side of the caruncle.

Some may also pass from the strip of fluid at the posterior margin of the upper lid to that of the lower at the moment of closure of the lids, and then some ducts of the lacrimal gland actually open into the lower cul-de-sac.

Now the tear fluid is limited by the sebaceous secretion at the muco-cutaneous junctions. It will therefore inevitably fill the reservoirs above described. Among these is the inferior marginal strip into which the lower punctum dips. It is in this manner that Wolff suggested the lacrimal secretion reaches its efferent passages.

It will be noted that it has not been necessary to invoke the massage action of the orbicularis, due to its more mobile lateral portion being drawn towards its fixed origin on the medial side, nor to a *flow* of tears over the exposed portion of the globe.

It is usually stated that the tears flow over the exposed portion of the globe to reach the lower punctum. But this process has never been observed and many explanations have been offered why it has not been seen.

One would say that the reason why no one has seen the tear fluid flow across the eye under normal conditions is that it does not occur. Further, that it is actually prevented from doing so. The main mechanism which stops the tear fluid from flowing down over the cornea is, one would suggest, the oily surface layer of the precorneal film (see p. 243). This is aided by the fact that the upper cul-de-sac acts as a narrow tube, which is closed above.

It seems that if the tears did flow across the eye they could only do so in rivulets, as seen in an exaggerated form in crying, when the above mechanism breaks down with results disastrous for the refraction of the eye.

A thin film of tears is actually *spread* over the cornea by blinking, the upper lid acting in this manner like a swab.

Now we must consider how the tears :
        (*a*) Get into the lacrimal sac.
        (*b*) Are discharged into the nose.

The tears get into the canaliculi partly through capillarity, partly through the canaliculi becoming shorter and wider during contraction of the orbicularis (Halben).

The orbicularis is attached to the medial palpebral ligament, and this is attached to the sac. Hence, when the orbicularis contracts, the ligament is pulled upon and the lacrimal sac is *dilated* and so sucks in the tears.

Similarly, Horner's muscle is attached to the fascia covering the posterior part of the sac, and when it contracts will also dilate the sac. We must, however, add here that some hold that Horner's muscle has the opposite action, namely, that it compresses the sac to *expel* the tears.

The tears are expelled from the sac by its own elasticity. Hence, in those pathological cases in which the lacrimal sac has lost its elasticity (atony of the sac), the downward conduction of tears is arrested, although the naso-lacrimal duct is quite patent (Fuchs).

The tears pass into the naso-lacrimal duct rather than into the canaliculi, because the former has a wider calibre, and moreover the downward direction is helped by gravity and by any of the " flap-valves " of mucous membrane that may be present (p. 233).

The pumping action of the orbicularis is well seen in the blinking movements that remove excess tears. The one-way flow through the canaliculi and duct causes the lacrimal sac to act like a rubber enema syringe, sucking in fluid at one end (the puncta) and squirting it out at the other end (the inferior meatus).

BIBLIOGRAPHY

Aubaret, E. (1908): *Arch. d'Ophtal., Paris*, **28**, 211. (Abstr. in *Ophthalmoscope*, 1908, **6**, 900.)

Ciaccio, G. (1874): *Moleschott's Untersuch. zur Naturlehre des Menschen u. d. Thieren.* **11**, 420

—— (1873): *Mem. Accad. Sci. Ist. Bologna*, 3.s., **4**, 460.

Contino, A. (1907): *v. Graefe's Arch. Ophthal.*, **66**, 505.

—— (1909): *v. Graefe's Arch. Ophthal.*, **71**, 1.

Crevatin, F. (1903): *Anat. Anz.*, **23**, 151.

Dubreuil (1907): Les glandes lacrymales des mammifères et de l'homme, *Thèse Méd., Lyon.*

Duckworth, W. (1904): Morphology and Anthropology, *Cambridge.*

Duverney (1749): L'Art de disséquer méthodiquement les muscles, etc., *Paris.*

Eisler, P. (1930): in Schieck and Brückner, Kurzes Handbuch der Ophthalmologie, **1**, 1.

Fisher, J. H. (1904): Ophthalmological Anatomy, *London.*

Fuchs, E. (1878): *v. Graefe's Arch. Ophthal.*, **24** (3), 1.

—— (1917), Textbook of Ophthalmology (Duane's Translation), *London and Philadelphia.*

GREEN, LEEDHAM (1894) : "Über die Bedeutung der Becherzellen der Conjunctiva," v. Graefe's Arch. Ophthal., **40** (1), 1.

HENLE (1853) : Handbuch der topographischen Anatomie, *Wien.*

HORNER, W. (1824) : "Description of a Small Muscle at the Internal Commissure of the Eyelids," *Philadelphia J. med. and phys. Sci.*, **8,** 70.

JAYLE, G. E. (1939) : "Appareil Lacrymal," in Traité d'Ophtalmologie, *Paris*, **1,** 331.

KEITH, A. (1913) : Human Embryology and Morphology, *London.*

KESSING, S. V. (1966) : *Acta. Ophth. (Kobenhavn)*, **44,** 439.

KRAUSE, C. (1842) : Handbuch der menschlichen Anatomie, *Hanover*, **2.**

—— (1879) : Handbuch der menschlichen Anatomie, 3rd edit. by W. Krause, **2,** 29.

KRAUSE, W. (1854) : *Z. rationelle Med.*, **4,** 337.

—— (1867) : *Jour. Anat. and Physiol.*, **1,** 346.

MANZ. W. (1859) : *Z. rationelle Med.*, 3.s., **5,** 122.

MERKEL, F. (1887) : *Anat. Anz.*, **2, 17.**

—— (1885) : Handbuch der topographischen Anatomie, 2nd ed., *Braunschweig.*

MERKEL and KALLIUS (1901) : "Makroskopische Anatomie des Auges," in : Graefe-Saemisch, Handbuch der gesamten Augenheilkunde, 2nd edit., **1,** chap. 1 (and new ed., 1904, 1, **1,** 1).

MOLL, J. (1857) : *v. Graefe's Arch. Ophthal.*, **3** (2), 258.

MÜLLER, H. (1858) : *Z. wiss. Zool.*, **9,** 541.

—— (1859) : *Verhandl. der phys.-med. Ges.*, *Würzburg*, **19,** 244.

PARSONS, J. HERBERT (1902) : "The Nerve Supply of the Lacrimal Gland," *R. Lond. ophthal. Hosp. Rep.*, **15,** 81.

—— (1904–05) : The Pathology of the Eye, Vols. 1–2, *London.*

POCKLEY, F. (1919) : *Med. J. Aust.*, **1,** 509.

POIRIER (1911) : Traité d'Anatomie Humaine, 3rd edit., **5**; fasc. 2 (" Les organes du sens ").

STIBBE, E. P. (1928) : *J. Anat., Lond.*, **62,** 159.

VILLARD, H. (1896) : *N. Montpellier méd.*, **5,** 651, 672, 693.

VIRCHOW, H. (1902) : *Abhandl. d. Kgl. Preuss. Akad. d. Wiss.*

WHITNALL, S. E. (1932) : Anatomy of the Human Orbit, 2nd ed., *Oxford.*

WOLFRING, E. (1872) : *Zbl. med. Wiss.*, **10,** 852.

ZEIS (1835) : *Z. Ophthal.*, **4,** 231.

CHAPTER IV

NORMAL APPEARANCES AS SEEN WITH THE SLIT-LAMP AND CORNEAL MICROSCOPE

THE CONJUNCTIVA

The Bulbar Conjunctiva shows itself as a transparent membrane in which the most striking feature is the vessels.

These form a superficial bright-red anastomosing system which is easily distinguished from the more deeply placed reddish-blue episcleral vessels. The superficial vessels move with the conjunctiva, which occurs normally with each blinking movement of the lids. Usually it is impossible to distinguish arteries and veins.

Visible streaming of the blood in the vessels can easily be made out. Usually the blood-current has a somewhat granular appearance. But in the smallest vessels, especially at the loops, the blood-column is not infrequently broken up, and one sees clumps of red cells or even individual cells moving in a somewhat staccato manner.

At the limbus the conjunctiva joins the transparent cornea without a sharp line of demarcation.

The Palpebral Conjunctiva—seen by everting the lids—is smooth and transparent, and the corium presents a rich vascular network, in which one can distinguish a fine subepithelial plexus and larger vessels running at right angles to the lid margin, which are derived from the tarsal arches.

THE CORNEA

When the slit-lamp beam passes through the cornea it forms a characteristic prism, or more correctly a parallelopiped.

In this we recognise four surfaces :

The anterior, corresponding to the epithelium ; *the posterior*, corresponding to the endothelium ; and the *lateral surfaces*, which form the areas where illuminated and non-illuminated portions of the cornea meet.

With a certain incidence the light may be reflected from the anterior and posterior surfaces of the cornea with mirror-like brightness, and give rise to what are called the anterior and posterior *zones of specular reflection*.

The Anterior Surface appears smooth, translucent, and on it can be seen tears, mucus, and oil belonging to the precorneal film (but see p. 245).

The Stroma appears somewhat milky, and has a faintly reticular structure, which Koeppe thinks is due to lymphatics, a view which cannot be upheld.

The Posterior Endothelium can be seen quite clearly (in the posterior zone of specular reflection).

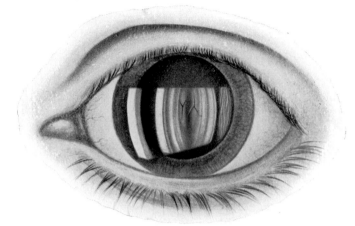

FIG. 232.—OPTICAL SECTION OF THE EYE AS PRODUCED BY A MODERATE BEAM OF THE SLIT-LAMP.

The various portions are represented as being in focus simultaneously. To the left is the optical section of the cornea ; then comes a dark interval representing the aqueous ; next is the optical section of the lens with its bands of discontinuity and Y sutures ; behind this the retro-lental space is represented dark, while the vitreous is most posterior.

The cells appear slightly yellow in colour. They are mostly hexagonal, some-times pentagonal, rarely square, and form a mosaic. Sometimes their nuclei may be visible. (Fig. 235.)

Near the limbus dark areas are seen in the mosaic. These are probably due to the (Hassall-Henle) warts on Descemet's membrane. (Fig. 233.)

Bowman's and Descemet's membranes are normally not seen, but become visible when pathologically altered.

The Line of Türck is a vertical line seen in children from 7 to 16 years old, and due to a deposit of leucocytes at the back of the cornea.

The Limbus appears as a transitional zone and has a dentate border. Its limits are not so well defined with the slit-lamp as with the naked eye.

Here we find vascular loops placed between the brilliant tongue-shaped prolongations of the sclera.

The blood-vessels which come from the conjunctiva and sclera have their connecting loops at the limits of the transparent area.

Veins and arteries are distinguished with difficulty. The colour does not help much. Usually one can decide by the direction of the

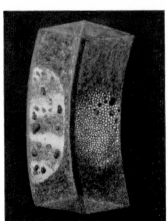

FIG. 233.—THE CORNEAL PRISM (PARALLELOPIPED).

The light is coming from the left. In the anterior zone of specular reflection are tears and mucus ; in the posterior zone one sees the endothelium and Hassall-Henle bodies (seen as black spots).

(*Modified from* Vogt.)

blood-current. But even this may be misleading. For the current in a certain vessel may be at times towards the cornea, at others away from it.

Sometimes a *palisade appearance*, which is due to whitish tracts derived from the sclera, is seen at the limbus, more frequently at its upper and lower parts.

The Corneal Nerves are easily seen. They are most numerous in the middle and anterior layers of the cornea. They appear as about thirty whitish filaments, which are better marked near the limbus where they still have their myelin sheath. The myelin always disappears before the first division of the nerve, which is usually dichotomous. The nerves never appear to inosculate. Not infrequently they present small nodosities, usually at a bifurcation, which Koeppe holds are congenital neuro-fibromata.

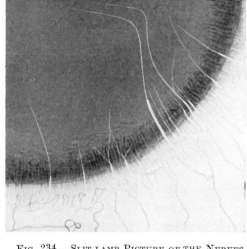

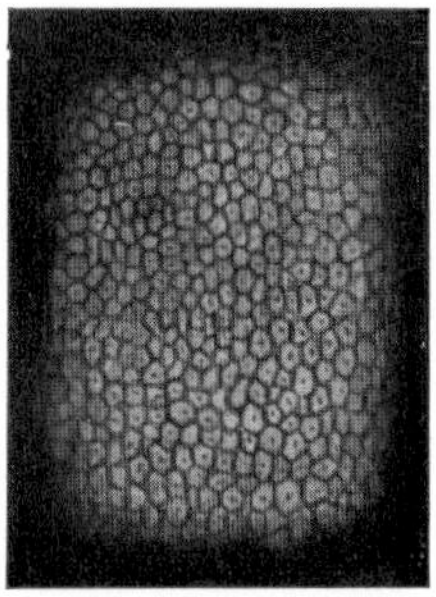

FIG. 234.—SLIT-LAMP PICTURE OF THE NERVES ENTERING THE CORNEA TO SHOW THE CHANGE FROM MEDULLATED TO NON-MEDULLATED PORTIONS.

FIG. 235. — THE ENDOTHELIUM AT THE BACK OF THE CORNEA.

(After Vogt.)

THE PRECORNEAL FILM (WOLFF'S VIEWS)

It is generally emphasised that the precorneal film does not consist of lacrimal fluid alone, but contains also the secretion of the tarsal and conjunctival glands.

One would go further and say that although there is probably some slight admixture, each of these three main constituents must be thought of separately; that is, that the oily tarsal secretion, the watery tear fluid and the mucoid secretion of the conjunctival glands have each their special position and function.

As the upper lid moves down in the act of blinking, the marginal strip of tear fluid, with the oil on its surface, is pushed down over the front of the cornea.

Above the lid margins is the perfectly smooth (see Cuenod and Nataf) surface of the tarsal conjunctiva, and jutting out from the mouths of the goblet cells are plugs of mucus (Fig. 206). Thus the tarsal conjunctiva, impregnated as it were, with the mucoid conjunctival secretion, forms an ideal polishing cloth for the cornea.

As the lid descends, the tarsal conjunctiva passes down in close contact with the corneal epithelium, probably displacing as it does so the watery tear fluid, and then passes up again. In this action the conjunctival secretion is, as it were, rubbed into the corneal epithelium, and forms the deepest layer of the precorneal film. As the lid passes up also, the strip of tear fluid will pass up too, and will form a layer superficial to the mucoid layer. The oily layer remains superficial, floating on the watery tear fluid.

It is as if a master artist, with a single down-and-up stroke of his brush, had laid on to the surface of the cornea three perfectly smooth and even coats of paint (Wolff owed this simile to his daughter).

As the lid passes up also, the small particles of the tear film are drawn up by the upper lid as a surface tension phenomenon, and come to rest when the movement of the lid stops.

The relation of the oily, sebaceous secretion to the tear fluid may be fairly accurately represented by placing on a glass microscope slide some water, and on this a minute drop of oil, and then drawing another slide backwards and forwards on these. The drop of oil spreads out into a characteristic colour film floating on the water. It will be seen that the movement of the slide can draw on this film for some distance.

A similar series of events takes place as, in the act of blinking, the lower lid passes up and then down. But these movements are, of course, not so extensive nor so important as those of the upper.

We see then that the precorneal film consists of three parts :

(1) The mucoid layer is deepest. One would suggest that it is this layer which Fischer says remains when closure of the eyelids has been artificially prevented until the cornea has dried. The precorneal film evaporates to a layer 0·05 mm. in thickness, which remains constant in spite of further evaporation. Fischer points out that this layer has a composition different from that of the freely moving tears and more like that of the corneal epithelium itself.

(2) The watery lacrimal fluid forms the middle layer. It wets the eye and washes away foreign particles from the front of the eye. It contains most of the bacteriocidal lyzozyme and protein which is organ and animal specific (Ridley).

(3) The oily film is the most superficial. It greatly slows the evaporation of the watery layer deep to it which, owing to its great thinness would, one thinks, otherwise disappear immediately the eye was opened.

One would suggest that it is the main mechanism which tends to prevent the tear fluid from flowing down across the cornea.

Also the oily surface layer appears to be the fly-paper to which foreign particles adhere. They can thus, as described above, be drawn out of the way by the movement of the upper eyelid without affecting the layers deep to it, and still less the epithelium of the cornea itself.

It is clear that we may say with Treacher Collins and Rollet that the glands of the eyelids are essentially the glands proper to the cornea, which in the interests of vision have been moved out of the way.

CURRENT VIEWS ON THE PRECORNEAL FILM

Wolff's prescience is exemplified in the foregoing account, left *verbatim* from his own writings. Niels Ehlers (1965) has produced a well substantiated modification of Wolff's views, based on biomicroscopical and histochemical observations, and supported by thoughtful theoretical considerations. The precorneal film is compressible and elastic. It has clinging properties that preserve its stability, and spreading properties that ensure clear vision immediately after blinking. The film is framed by the watery tears along the lid margins. If the margins are everted (as by an operating speculum) the precorneal film spreads, thins out, and evaporates more quickly than normal. Ehlers cannot substantiate the separate layer of mucus that Wolff postulated deepest into the film, on the surface of the corneal epithelium. The aqueous film is about 10 μ thick and may perhaps contain the mucus dissolved within it. The aqueous film is sandwiched between a lipid surface layer of cholesterol ester and a deep layer of phospholipids which enter also the surface layer of living corneal epithelium. These enclosing lipid layers meet at the limbus ; they delay evaporation of the imprisoned water. The two sandwiching lipid layers are derived from the tarsal (Meibomian) glands, and are spread into the precorneal film by the blinking lid margins.

Mishima (1965) is likewise doubtful about the presence of the mucous layer. He concludes that evaporation of the precorneal film produces a hypertonicity that makes water flow from the aqueous through the cornea.

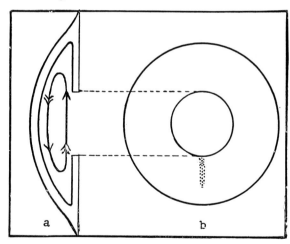

FIG. 236. — DIAGRAM SHOWING THE THERMIC CIRCULATION OF THE AQUEOUS HUMOUR.

On the left (a), sagittal section of the anterior chamber ; on the right (b), frontal view. In b is seen the line formed by microscopic deposits on the posterior surface of the cornea.

(*From Koby.*)

THE ANTERIOR CHAMBER

The anterior chamber is almost, but not quite, optically empty. With the ordinary, broad slit-lamp beam, it appears quite black, but with a very bright, narrow pencil of light, especially if oscillating, a faint relucence along the path of light can be made out (the aqueous flare) (Graves).

This is due to the fact that the normal aqueous contains very small particles which are not big enough to be resolved by the magnification used. When larger particles are present they are lit up like dust particles in a beam of sunlight passing across a darkened room.

Convection Currents.—The cornea is cooled by the air. The aqueous, therefore, behind the cornea is cooler than the aqueous in front of the iris. Convection currents are thus set up, the aqueous sinking behind the cornea and rising in front of the iris. Particles in the aqueous will follow these convection currents, which are no doubt responsible for the line of Türck (see Fig. 236).

THE IRIS

Embryologically and for descriptive purposes we may divide the iris into three layers : two anterior, which are mesodermal in origin, and a posterior, the retinal portion which is ectodermal (Fig. 237).

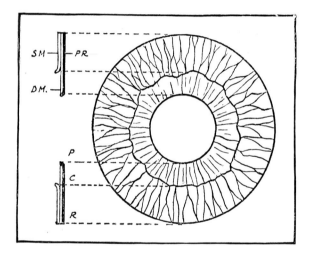

FIG. 237.—DIAGRAM SHOWING THE STRUCTURE OF THE IRIS.

The retinal layer appears at the edge of the pupil, where it forms the pigment border. The mesodermal layer is separable into a deep layer running from the root of the iris to the pupil and a superficial, the axial limit of which forms the collarette. SM = superficial mesodermal layer. DM = deep mesodermal layer. PR = posterior retinal layer. The crypts of the iris situated in the ciliary portion may be considered as openings distributed in the superficial mesodermal layer (anterior). P = pigment border. C = collarette. R =

(From Koby.)

The structure of the iris is seen to differ widely in normal people, and this is essentially dependent on the amount of stroma pigment.

The superficial layers of the blue iris which contains very little stroma pigment appear as a delicate diaphanous tissue, the fibres and trabeculæ of which look like transparent wool (Koby). The dark iris presents a more compact structure on which the vessels are not visible except at the crypts. The surface is smooth, and resembles tinder.

Usually clumps of melanophores producing yellow or brown patches can be seen ; but the structure of individual pigment cells cannot be made out with the slit-lamp in the human.

The superficial mesodermal layer is shorter than the deep, and extends from the ciliary border to the *collarette* (circulus minor), which forms a dentate fringe, separated from the underlying middle layer of the iris to a varying degree.

It is this superficial layer which gives the ciliary portion of the iris its colour. In it one finds the iris crypts, and looking through these and the underlying deep mesodermal layer one can, in slightly pigmented irides, see the dark posterior ectodermal layer. This latter becomes more and more difficult to see as the amount of stroma pigment increases.

The crypts are bounded by the trabeculæ of the collarette, which are the remains of obliterated vessels that passed to the pupillary membrane during embryonic life (Lauber and Vogt).

The Deep Mesodermal Layer extends from the ciliary border to the pupillary edge.

In slightly pigmented irides it has a radial fibrillary appearance, and is transparent, so that the deeply pigmented ectodermal layer is visible through it.

The Collarette (circulus minor) consists of a series of trabeculæ forming a rough

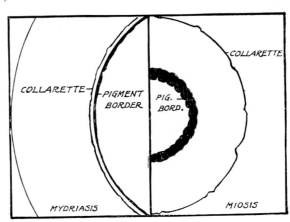

FIG. 238.—DIAGRAM SHOWING THE RELATIONS OF THE PIGMENT BORDER AND COLLARETTE AND THE VARIATIONS IN THICKNESS OF THE FORMER ACCORDING TO THE WIDTH OF THE PUPIL.

To the left, pupil dilated ; to the right, pupil contracted.

(From Koby.)

and broken circle, and varies greatly in form. To it are often attached remains of the pupillary membrane (Fig. 271).

The anterior mesodermal layer is but loosely attached to the deeper one, and glides freely over it. It does not participate to any marked extent in the movements of the rest of the iris. It thus comes about that, as the pupil dilates, the pupillary edge approaches nearer and nearer to the collarette—so, when the pupil is widely dilated, remains of the pupillary membrane may appear to arise from the edge of the pupil when they are actually attached to the collarette.

There are other changes as the pupil dilates.

The pigment ring showing at the pupillary border is thinned and may disappear.

There is a much more decided step between the collarette, whose angles have straightened out, and the pupillary margin ; the crypts become oblique clefts. The vessels are more tortuous, the contraction furrows and the peripheral furrows are deeper, and the border zone disappears.

The vessels of the iris can be made out in non- or very slightly pigmented irides. The radial vessels can be seen passing to the collarette and then following one of its trabeculæ.

They do *not* form a complete circle. Hence *circulus* iridis minor is not strictly correct.

The Sphincter Iridis can be seen if the iris contains little or a moderate amount of pigment.

The Ectodermal Layer, as pointed out above, can be seen through the crypts in slightly pigmented irides. Its edge is seen at the pupillary border as a fringe of pigment with a crenated margin. This is much better marked when the pupil is small, especially above. The slightest pupillary reaction is made manifest with the slit-lamp.

The dilatator pupillæ and the nerves of the iris are invisible.

THE LENS

When the beam of the slit-lamp passes through the lens it is obvious that the portion lit up (the optical section) is not homogeneous. It is divided into a number of bands, some of which are brighter than others. These bands are called by Vogt the zones of discontinuity (Fig. 232). In adults ten bands can usually be made out.

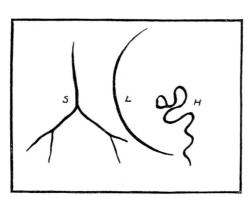

FIG. 239.—DIAGRAM SHOWING THE RELATION OF THE POSTERIOR λ OF THE FŒTAL NUCLEUS (S), OF THE ARCUATE LINE (L), OF THE INSERTION OF THE REMAINS OF THE HYALOID ARTERY (H) IN A RIGHT EYE.

The artery is found on the nasal side, separated from the posterior pole of the lens by the arcuate line, the concavity of which is turned towards the artery.

(From Koby.)

Of these, the anterior and posterior bands (of the lens), corresponding to the anterior and posterior surfaces of the lens, are the brightest.

The Fœtal Nucleus, which represents the condition at birth, appears as two plano-convex lenses with a central dark interval, which is the most homogeneous portion of the lens and the part which has the least optical density.

In front and behind the fœtal nucleus are the *anterior and posterior Y-shaped sutures.*

The anterior Y is upright, the posterior is inverted (λ), contrary to the usual anatomical description.

The farther we go from the fœtal nucleus, the more complicated do the sutures become.

Around the fœtal nucleus are the *anterior* and *posterior peripheral bands* of the fœtal nucleus. More peripheral still are *the anterior and posterior bands of the adult nucleus*, while beneath the anterior and posterior bands of the lens are the *subcapsular bands* or anterior and posterior bands of disjunction (Vogt).

The Anterior Surface of the lens does not appear homogeneous, but is somewhat irregular, and gives an appearance resembling shagreen (anterior lens shagreen).

At the *Posterior Surface* of the lens, as well as the anterior, there is a zone where the light is reflected vividly (*zones of specular reflection*).

In the posterior zone of specular reflection is seen the *Posterior Lens Shagreen*. It has a slightly yellower tint than the anterior. A marked polychromatic lustre in this posterior region is diagnostic of a complicated cataract.

A corkscrew-like remainder of the *Hyaloid Artery*, which moves with the movements of the eye, is often seen fixed by a whitish dot to the posterior aspect of the lens, just below and medial to its centre and in the concavity of the arcuate line (Fig. 239).

The Arcuate Line is a whitish crescent situated below and medial to the posterior pole of the lens. It is found by tracing the nasal branch of posterior λ till it bifurcates.

The Suspensory Ligament of the lens cannot be seen in the normal eye. When the lens is congenitally dislocated or absent, it may be made out as consisting of cobweb-like strands which are attached in front and behind the equator.

THE REMAINS OF THE PUPILLARY MEMBRANE

1. The commonest form consists of a series of brown dots on the anterior capsule of the lens, usually near the centre, which, when seen with the slit-lamp, have a stellate appearance. These are finer than the remains of posterior synechia, which also when present in any quantity tend to be disposed in a circle.

2 Fine filaments arising from the collarette and branching in the anterior chamber are attached to the front of

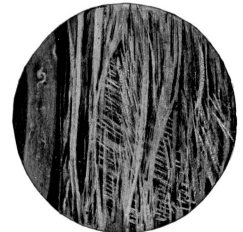

Fig. 240.—THE NORMAL VITREOUS BODY OF A SUBJECT OF TWENTY YEARS, THE LIGHT COMING FROM THE LEFT.

On the left is seen the posterior band of the lens where the zone of specular reflection has been avoided. On its right the vertical bundles of the vitreous, and a second system of bundles chiefly horizontal and finer. Magnification about × 30. Figure slightly schematic.

(From Koby.)

the lens, where they may end in white tufts or pass across the anterior chamber and be attached to another part of the collarette.

3. Thick cord-like remains which are usually associated with anterior polar cataract.

THE VITREOUS

Only the anterior third of the vitreous can be seen with the slit-lamp as ordinarily used.

Directly behind the posterior band of the lens is the " post-lenticular space." This, with the ordinary broad beam of the slit-lamp, appears optically empty, i.e. quite black (Fig. 232). The less the illumination, the deeper does the space appear. On the other hand, with higher intensities of illumination, faint fibrils can be seen crossing this space.

Comberg believes that the space is capillary only. No hyaloid membrane can be made out with the slit-lamp.

The anterior part of the vitreous appears as wavy milky folds of gossamer-like texture separated by intervals which are optically empty—the whole oscillating with the movements of the eye (p. 152). The folds appear to consist of criss-crossing fibrils. Small nodosities may be seen at the intersection of two fibrillæ.

In old age a powdery appearance in the vitreous is quite common.

BIBLIOGRAPHY

The most complete and classical work on Slit-lamp Microscopy is Vogt's beautiful *Atlas of Slit Lamp Microscopy* : Part I (1930) Cornea and Anterior Chamber, *Berlin* ; Part II (1931) Lens and Zonule, *Berlin* ; Part III (1942) Iris, Vitreous and Conjunctiva, *Stuttgart*, or (1941), in English, *Zurich*.

In English there are Berliner's Biomicroscopy of the Eye, 1943 and 1949, *New York*, Goulden and Harris's translation of Koby's Microscopie de l'Œil Vivant (Slit-lamp microscopy of the living eye) (in which there is an extensive bibliography), and Harrison Butler's An Illustrated Guide to the Slit-lamp, 1927 ; also Graves in Recent Advances in Microscopy (Churchill).

Other Standard works by :

Meesman, 1927, *Berlin*.

Lemoine and Valois, 1931, *Paris*.

Koeppe, 1920 and 1922, *Berlin*.

Gallemaerts, 1926, *Paris*.

Busacca, Goldmann and Schiff-Wertheimer (1957) : *Biomicroscopie du Corps Vitré et du Fond de l'Œil, Paris*.

EHLERS, Niels (1965) : *Acta. Ophthalmologica (Kobenhavn)*, Supplementum 81, 9–118.

MISHIMA, S. (1965) : *Arch. Ophth. (Chicago)*, 73, 233.

CHAPTER V

THE EXTRINSIC MUSCLES OF THE EYE

THE *extrinsic* muscles of the eye are so called to distinguish them from the muscles inside the globe, the dilatator and sphincter pupillæ and the ciliary muscle, which are unstriped and named *intrinsic*.

The extrinsic muscles of the eye are six in number the superior, inferior, medial and lateral recti, and the superior and inferior obliques. In the

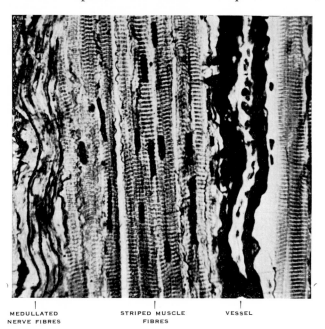

FIG. 241.—STRUCTURE OF HUMAN RECTUS MUSCLE. (STAINED BIELCHOWSKY.)

MEDULLATED NERVE FIBRES   STRIPED MUSCLE FIBRES   VESSEL

case of the superior and lateral recti the fleshy portions end in a V, while in the inferior and medial they end in a dentate line.

The insertions into the sclera are made by glistening tendons whose fibres run almost entirely parallel to the long axis of the muscle. These fibres consist of fibrous tissue supported by thick elastic fibres. Apart from their size they resemble the scleral fibres, being made of the same tissue. But whereas the tendon fibres are practically all longitudinal, the scleral fibres run in many directions (Figs. 40, 64). This results in the tendon having a glistening silky appearance while the sclera is dull white (Salzmann).

The tendon fibres enter the superficial layers of the sclera, and soon become

251

indistinguishable from it (Fig. 64). Only the cessation of the thick elastic fibres marks the place where one begins and the other ends.

Not infrequently one finds fibres which leave the main tendon close to its insertion to be attached farther back. These recurrent fibres may be missed in doing a tenotomy (Motais).

Structure of the Extrinsic Muscles.—These muscles, as are those derived from the branchial arches, are more highly differentiated than any other muscles of the body.

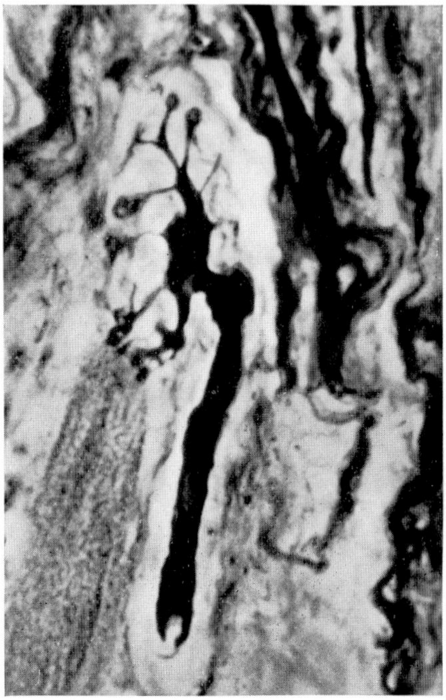

FIG. 243.—MOTOR NERVE ENDING IN HUMAN RECTUS MUSCLE. (STAINED BIELCHOWSKY.)

Instead of being grouped together in bundles separated by dense connective tissue, the fine fibres are but loosely united and hence easily separated by dissection.

In the intervals between the fibres are a great number of nerve fibres (Figs. 241, 242). It must be remembered that each eye muscle receives a nerve which is relatively, compared with the size of the muscle it supplies, much bigger than any in the body.

Each muscle fibre has a diameter of 15·9–22·7 μ, this being less than other striated muscles. Each fibre is surrounded by a sarcolemma which contains a granular sarcoplasm in which myofibrils may be seen. This gives the cross-section of the fibril a punctiform appearance. Directly under the sarcolemma are one or more well-staining nuclei.

The connective tissue around the fibres constitutes the endomysium and contains a large quantity of elastic tissue arranged longitudinally. Similar septa, but surrounding a number of muscle fibres, are called the internal perimysium. This contains larger elastic fibres, the vessels and nerves, and some connective tissue cells. The internal perimysium is continuous with the external perimysium, or epimysium, which surrounds the muscle.

The muscles of the eye are peculiar in the number of nerve and elastic fibres which they contain. Schifferdecker believes that the elastic tissue helps the muscle in action, and regulates the give of its antagonist. This contributes to the making of the delicacy and smoothness of ocular movements. Apart from these mechanical reasons, however, the rich nerve supply (Fig. 242) is surely the main factor. Each motor neurone supplies relatively few muscle fibres.

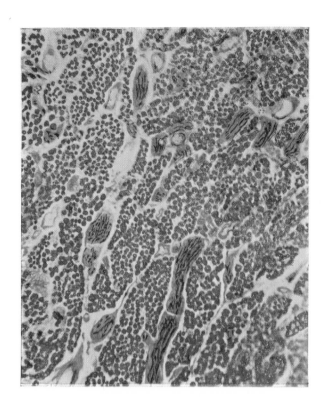

Fig. 242.—Transverse Section of Fibres of a Human Rectus Muscle. (Masson's Stain.)
Note the rich nerve supply.

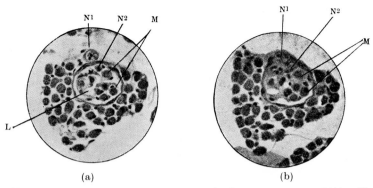

(a)   (b)

FIG. 244.—Reproduction of Farquhar Buzzard's Illustration of 1908. The original
description is as follows :

" Photographs of the Same Spindle at Levels a Short Distance from One Another in an Ocular Muscle.

N[1] is an extra-fusal nerve bundle which in (b) is being incorporated within the spindle sheath.
N[2] Intra-fusal nerve fibres.
M Intra-fusal muscle fibres.
L Lymphatic space.
Note the equality in size between the intra- and extra-fusal muscle fibres, and the thick sheath, with spindle-shaped nuclei."

(*By courtesy of the Honorary Editors of the Proceedings of the Royal Society of Medicine.*)

The Sheaths of the Muscles.—From the origin for two centimetres the sheath
is practically non-existent, being very thin and transparent so that the macroscopic structure of the muscle is easily visible.
From the level of the back of the globe it
becomes thicker, opaque and disposed in two
layers, the outer or orbital layer with circular
fibres and the inner with longitudinal fibres.
The inner is continuous with the internal
perimysium.

PROPRIOCEPTIVE NERVE ENDINGS

Farquhar Buzzard,[1] in 1908, described
and figured muscle spindles in the eye
muscles of man ; he knew they were proprioceptive in function.   For its historical
interest, one of his illustrations is reproduced
here (Fig. 244).   Yet for many years this was
overlooked and the spindles were not seen.
For instance Woollard (1930, *J. Anat.*) described fine nonmedullated fibres to the ocular

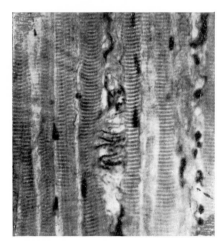

FIG. 245.—Spiral Nerve Ending in
Human Rectus Muscle. (Stained Bielchowsky.)

muscles, seen in stained sections, and he wondered if they were sensory—but he
failed to see or mention muscle spindles.   Daniel (1946), Cooper and Daniel (1949)
and Cooper (1951) again described muscle spindles.   They are, however, only found

[1] *Proc. R. Soc. Med., Neurol. sect.*, **1**, 83.

in certain regions.   Forty-seven have been counted in one inferior rectus muscle. The muscle spindle found in the eye muscles of man is a smaller and more delicate end organ than the comparable structure in the other somatic muscles.   Like its larger counterpart, it consists of a group of fine cross-striated muscle fibres with a rich nerve supply enclosed in a torpedo-shaped capsule of fibrous tissue. The capsule is thin, consisting of two or at the most three laminæ of fibrous tissue with characteristic flattened nuclei, and continuous from end to end of the spindle. The muscle fibres within the capsule, the intrafusal fibres, are usually of smaller diameter than the ordinary extrafusal fibres, generally 7 to 20 μ.   They may

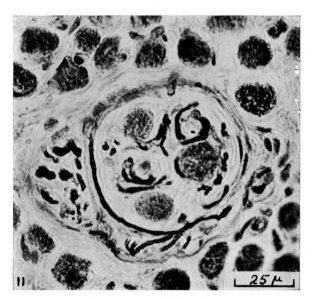

Fig. 246.—Transverse Section of a Muscle Spindle in a Human Medial Rectus Oculi Muscle.

A well-defined capsule is seen with a nerve trunk incorporated in its wall (on the left).   Within the capsule there are three intrafusal muscle fibres, capillaries and intricate arrangement of nerve fibres. One nerve fibre partly encircles the spindle, either just inside or within the walls of the capsule.   (Paraffin section, Holmes' "silver on the slide" method.)

(From Cooper and Daniel (1949 Brain 72, 1.)

end at the termination of the capsule but most often pass out to become continuous with an extrafusal fibre.   The nucleus of the intrafusal muscle fibre is often central instead of being peripheral, as in the extrafusal type (Cooper and Daniel).   Cooper, working with goats (J. Physiol. (1951), **113,** 463) recorded afferent impulses in the 3rd nerve.   The muscles are exquisitely sensitive, the inferior oblique registering at the order of 1 degree of rotation of the eyeball.

The Actions of the Eye Muscles

Movements of the eyeball take place round the centre of movement which corresponds approximately to the centre of the eye.   The eyeball as a whole, therefore, is not displaced.

The movements may be resolved into those taking place round the three *primary axes* which pass through the centre of the movement, and are at right angles to each other.   These are :

(1) The *vertical* axis, round which the centre of the cornea moves laterally (abduction) or medially (adduction).

(2) The *transverse* axis runs from right to left. Round it the centre of the cornea moves either up (elevation) or down (depression).

(3) The *sagittal* or antero-posterior axis corresponds to the line of vision. Round it the movement of wheel-rotation takes place and is called medial (intorsion) or lateral (extorsion) as twelve o'clock on the cornea moves nasally or temporally. It will thus be seen that in naming the movements of the eye about the transverse and vertical axes the centre of the cornea (or the pupil) is taken as the moving point, and will indicate in which direction the eye is made

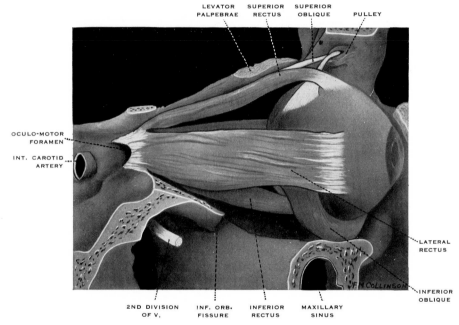

FIG. 247.—DISSECTION TO SHOW THE OCULAR MUSCLES FROM THE LATERAL ASPECT.
Note especially oculo-motor foramen.
(From a specimen in the Anatomy Museum of University College.,

to look ; while *wheel-rotation* about the antero-posterior axis is named from the direction of movement of the upper part of the vertical meridian or, what comes to the same thing, twelve o'clock on the cornea.

This is a necessary convention, for it is obvious that the posterior pole of the eye will go up when the anterior goes down and the lower part of the vertical meridian (or six o'clock on the cornea) will move laterally when the upper moves medially.

Each muscle, except the medial and lateral recti, has a *main* and a *subsidiary* action.

The main action will be greatest when the eye is looking in a certain direction, while in this position the subsidiary actions will be least and vice versa.

Thus the main action of the superior rectus will be elevation, and is greatest when the eye is turned out, while the subsidiary actions adduction and wheel-rotation medially are increased as the eye looks medially.

Synergic Action.—Often in carrying out a certain movement two muscles work together. Thus, in looking directly upwards the superior rectus will act with the inferior oblique, and in looking directly downwards the inferior rectus acts with the superior oblique.

The Four Recti Muscles

The four recti muscles arise from a short funnel-shaped tendinous ring (anulus tendineus communis of Zinn). This is oval on cross-section, and encloses the optic foramen and a part of the medial end of the superior orbital (sphenoidal) fissure, its attachment to the anterior margin of which is marked by the *spina recti lateralis*.

The inner surface of the anulus is thickened in its upper and lower parts by two strong bands or *common tendons*.

The Lower Tendon (of Zinn) is attached to the inferior root of the lesser wing of the sphenoid between the optic foramen and the superior orbital fissure. This attachment may be marked by a tubercle (the infraoptic tubercle) (Fig. 1), a roughness, or a small depression. The lower tendon gives origin to part of the medial and lateral recti and the whole of the inferior.

The Upper Tendon (of Lockwood) arises from the body of the sphenoid, and gives origin to part of the medial and lateral recti and the whole of the superior.

Owing to the slope of the orbital roof the origins of the superior and medial recti are on a plane anterior to the others. *Also these muscles are much more closely attached to the dural sheath of the optic nerve* (Fig. 15). It is this attachment of the superior and medial recti to the nerve sheath which is responsible for the characteristic pain which accompanies extreme movements of the globe in retro-bulbar neuritis.

With regard to their *length*, which is somewhere about 40 mm., the superior is the longest, then the medial, then the lateral. The inferior is the shortest.

The recti muscles run forwards close to the walls of the orbit, and are inserted into the sclera beyond the coronal equator by tendons of different widths and at different distances from the cornea.

These will be discussed with each muscle, and will be found tabulated below :

	Distance from Cornea	Length of Tendon	Width of Tendon
	mm.	mm.	mm
Superior rectus . . .	7·7	5·8	10·8
Inferior rectus . . .	6·5	5·5	9·8
Medial rectus . . .	5·5	3·7	10·3
Lateral rectus . . .	6·9	8·8	9·2

THE SUPERIOR RECTUS

The superior rectus arises from the upper part of the anulus of Zinn above and to the lateral side of the optic foramen and from the sheath of the optic nerve.

This origin lies in the angle formed by the splitting of the dura which lines the optic canal to form the orbital periosteum (periorbita) on the one hand, and the dural covering of the nerve on the other.

It is below that of the levator, and is continuous on the medial side with the medial rectus and on the lateral with the lateral rectus.

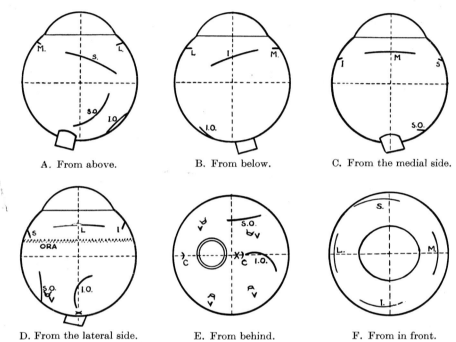

A. From above.   B. From below.   C. From the medial side.

D. From the lateral side.   E. From behind.   F. From in front.

FIG. 248.—To show the Insertions of the Eye Muscles. (Right Eye.)

X = position of the macula.   C = long ciliaries.   V = venæ vorticosæ.   S.O. = superior oblique. I.O. = inferior oblique.   M = medial rectus.   L = lateral rectus.   I = inferior rectus.   S = superior rectus.

Note position of optic nerve.   Its centre is just *above* the horizontal meridian.

The muscle passes forwards and laterally beneath the levator, making an angle of 25° with the visual line, pierces Tenon's capsule, and is inserted into the sclera 7·7 mm. from the cornea by a tendon 5·8 mm. long.

The line of insertion is oblique, 10·8 mm. long, and curved so as to be slightly convex forwards.

Relations.—*Above* the superior rectus is the levator and the frontal nerve, which separate it from the roof of the orbit (Figs. 15, 276, 277).

Below is the optic nerve, but separated by orbital fat, the ophthalmic artery

A.E.—17

and the naso-ciliary nerve (Fig. 277). Farther forwards the reflected tendon of the superior oblique passes between it and the globe to reach its insertion (Fig. 247).

Laterally, in the angle between the superior and lateral recti, are found the lacrimal artery and nerve.

Medially, in the angle between the superior rectus on the one hand and the medial rectus and superior oblique on the other, are found the ophthalmic artery and naso-ciliary nerve (Figs. 277, 278).

Nerve.—The superior rectus is supplied by the superior division of the oculomotor (3rd cranial), which enters the under-surface of the muscle at the junction of the middle and posterior thirds (Fig. 281).

Blood-supply.—This is from the lateral muscular branch of the opthalmic artery.

Actions.—The superior rectus makes the eye look upwards or medially or wheel-rotates it medially (intorts). It also helps the levator to lift the upper lid (see p. 264).

The Main Action is the elevation, which increases as the eye is turned out, and becomes nil when the eye is turned in.

The superior rectus is, in fact, the only elevator in the abducted position of the eye, for the inferior oblique does not elevate the eye in this position. It thus comes about that in a palsy of the right superior rectus, if the patient is asked to look upwards and to the right, he cannot elevate his right eye beyond the middle of the palpebral fissure.

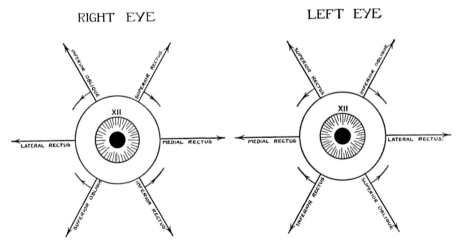

RIGHT EYE   LEFT EYE

Fig. 249.—Diagram to show the possible Actions of the Extrinsic Muscles of the Eyes.

The straight arrows show the direction in which the eye is made to look, i.e. towards which the centre of the cornea is moved. The small curved arrows indicate the direction of wheel-rotation, i.e. about an antero-posterior axis. Thus the medial and lateral recti make the eye look medially and laterally respectively, while the superior oblique makes the eye look downwards or laterally or causes wheel-rotation medially (taking XII o'clock as the moving-point).

Note that the diagram only gives the possible actions from the position of rest; thus the superior oblique cannot depress the eye in the abducted position.

The subsidiary actions are the adduction and intorsion, which increase as the eye is turned in.

THE INFERIOR RECTUS

The inferior rectus is the shortest of the recti muscles. It arises below the optic foramen, from the middle slip of the lower common tendon.

It passes forwards and somewhat laterally along the floor of the orbit, making an angle of 25° with the visual line, and is inserted into the sclera 6·5 mm. from the cornea by a tendon 5·5 mm. in length.

The line of insertion is 9·8 mm. long, markedly convex forwards, always somewhat oblique, so that the nasal end lies nearer the cornea.

The inferior rectus is also attached to the lower lid by means of the fascial expansion of its sheath (see Fig. 280).

Relations.— *Above* are the inferior division of the 3rd nerve, the optic nerve separated by orbital fat, and the globe of the eye (Fig. 280).

Lateral.—The nerve to the inferior oblique runs in front of the lateral border of the inferior rectus or between it and the lateral rectus.

Below is the floor of the orbit, roofing the maxillary sinus. The muscle is in contact with the orbital process of the palatine bone, but more anteriorly it is separated by orbital fat from the orbital plate of the maxilla.

The infraorbital vessels and nerve in their canal also lie below the inferior rectus.

The inferior oblique crosses below the inferior rectus, the sheaths of the two muscles being united here.

Nerve.—The inferior rectus is supplied by the inferior division of the 3rd nerve, which enters it on its upper aspect at about the junction of the middle and osterior thirds (Figs. 279, 281).

Its **Blood-supply** comes from the medial muscular branch of the ophthalmic.

Actions.—The inferior rectus makes the eye look downwards or medially or wheel-rotates it laterally (extorsion). By means of its fascial expansion it also depresses the lower lid.

The Main Action is the depression which increases as the eye is turned out and becomes nil when the eye is turned in. The inferior rectus is the only depressor in the abducted position of the eye.

The Subsidiary Actions are the adduction and extorsion, which increase as the eye is turned in.

THE MEDIAL RECTUS

The medial rectus is the largest of the ocular muscles and much stronger than the lateral. It has a wide origin to the medial side of and below the optic foramen from both parts of the common tendon, and from the sheath of the optic nerve.

It passes forwards along the medial wall of the orbit, and is inserted into the sclera 5·5 mm. from the cornea by a tendon 3·7 mm. in length. The line of insertion is 10·3 mm. long, is straight and symmetrical to the horizontal meridian (as a rule).

Relations.— *Above* is the superior oblique, and between the two muscles are the ophthalmic artery and its anterior and posterior ethmoidal branches and the posterior ethmoidal, anterior ethmoidal and infratrochlear nerves (Figs. 277, 278).

Below is the floor of the orbit.

Medially is some peripheral orbital fat, then the orbital plate of the ethmoid, which bounds the ethmoidal air-cells.

Laterally is the central orbital fat.

Nerve.—The inferior division of the 3rd, which enters it on its lateral surface at about the junction of its middle and posterior thirds.

The **Blood-supply** comes from the medial muscular branch of the ophthalmic artery.

Action.—The medial rectus is a pure adductor. Both muscles act together in convergence.

THE LATERAL RECTUS

The lateral or external rectus arises from both the lower and upper parts of the common tendon from those portions which bridge the superior orbital (sphenoidal) fissure.

This origin is continuous, and is strengthened by its attachment to the spina recti lateralis (of Merkel) on the greater wing of the sphenoid.

The origin thus takes the form of the letter U (or V), placed so that the opening looks towards the optic foramen, the limbs of the U being referred to as the *upper* and *lower heads* of the muscle (Figs. 247, 261).

The lateral rectus passes forward along the lateral wall of the orbit, at first separated only by a small and variable amount of peripheral fat. More anteriorly, however, it passes inwards towards the globe, pierces Tenon's capsule, and is inserted into the sclera 6·9 mm. from the cornea by a tendon 8·8 mm. long.

The line of insertion is 9·2 mm. in length, is vertical or slightly convex forwards, and usually symmetrical.

The lateral rectus can in the living often be seen through the conjunctiva and Tenon's capsule (see also paragraph on the expansions of its sheath, p. 266).

Relations.—(a) *At the Apex of the Orbit.*—Between the origin of the lateral rectus and that portion of the lesser wing which separates the optic nerve from the medial portion of the superior orbital (sphenoidal) fissure is a small though very important interval.

The structures which go through it are described as passing between the two heads of the lateral rectus, within the cone of muscles or anulus of Zinn, or the interval is called the *oculomotor* foramen (Fig. 247).

These structures from above downwards are the *upper division* of the 3*rd nerve*, the *naso-ciliary*, and a branch from the *sympathetic*, then the *lower division* of the 3*rd*, then the 6*th*, and then sometimes the *ophthalmic vein* or veins.

The 6th nerve is actually passing from being below the lower division of the 3rd to lie lateral and in between the two divisions (Fig. 261).

Above the cone of muscles, i.e. above the upper head of the lateral rectus, are the *fourth*, *frontal* and *lacrimal nerves*, the *recurrent lacrimal artery*, and the *superior ophthalmic vein*. According to Hovelacque (1927) these structures do not pass through the outer narrow part of the superior orbital fissure, as is classically represented, since this is closed by dense fibrous tissue (Figs. 259, 260), and with this the author is in entire agreement. (See also the lacrimal nerve, p. 299.) Below the cone of muscles nothing passes as a rule, sometimes the inferior ophthalmic vein.

(*b*) *Farther Forwards.*— *Above* the lateral rectus are the lacrimal artery and nerve. The lacrimal gland lies anteriorly. The lacrimal nerve runs along the upper border for almost its whole length, the artery only for the anterior two-thirds (Fig. 277).

Below is the floor of the orbit, and anteriorly the tendon of the inferior oblique passes below, then medial to the lateral rectus to gain its insertion (Fig. 247).

Medial, near the apex of the orbit between the lateral rectus and optic nerve, are the 6th nerve, the ciliary ganglion and ophthalmic artery. Between the muscle and the inferior rectus is the nerve to the inferior oblique (Figs. 278, 280).

Laterally, it lies directly against periorbita in its posterior part (Figs. 15, 16), while more anteriorly a slight amount of perimuscular fat intervenes ; farther forward still the lacrimal gland lies between it and the bone.

Nerve.—The 6th nerve (abducens) enters it on its medial aspect, just behind its middle.

The **Blood-supply** comes from the lacrimal artery, and from the lateral muscular branch of the ophthalmic artery.

Actions.—The lateral rectus is a pure abductor—that is, makes the eye look directly laterally in the horizontal plane.

THE SUPERIOR OBLIQUE

The superior oblique is the longest and thinnest eye muscle. It arises above and medial to the optic foramen by a narrow tendon which partially overlaps the origin of the levator.

The fusiform muscle belly, more rounded than that of the other extrinsic muscles, passes forwards between the roof and medial wall of the orbit to the pulley or trochlea of the superior oblique (Figs. 277, 278, 279).

The trochlea consists of a U-shaped piece of fibro-cartilage, which is closed above by fibrous tissue, and is attached to the fovea or spina trochlearis on the under-aspect of the frontal bone a few millimetres behind the orbital margin.

Through the pulley the tendon is enclosed in a synovial sheath, beyond which a strong fibrous sheath accompanies the tendon to the eyeball.

The muscle, about 1 cm. behind the trochlea, gives place to a rounded tendon, which passes through the pulley, then bends downwards, backwards, and laterally at an angle of about 55° (the trochlear angle), pierces Tenon's capsule, passes under the superior rectus, and, spreading out in a fan-shaped manner, is attached obliquely in the postero-superior quadrant almost or entirely lateral to the mid-vertical plane. The line of insertion is about 10·7 mm. long, and is convex backwards and laterally. Its anterior end lies about on the same meridian as the temporal end of the superior rectus (Salzmann) (see Figs. 247, 248, A).

Actions.—The superior oblique makes the eye look downwards or laterally or (wheel-) rotates it inwards (i.e. makes twelve o'clock on the cornea move towards the nose).

The Main Action is the depression, and this increases as the eye is turned in. The superior oblique is the only muscle which can depress in the adducted position. Its action is practically nil when the eye is abducted.

The abduction and intorsion are the *subsidiary actions*, and increase as the eye turns out.

The superior oblique acts with the inferior rectus to make the eye look directly down. The abductor component of the action of the oblique muscles is due to their being inserted behind the equator of the globe.

Nerve.—The superior oblique is supplied by the 4th or trochlear nerve which, having divided into three or four branches, enters the muscle on the upper-surface near its lateral border ; the most anterior branch at the junction of the posterior and middle thirds, the most posterior about 8 mm. from its origin (Fig. 277).

The **Blood-supply** comes from the superior muscular branch of the ophthalmic artery.

THE INFERIOR OBLIQUE

The inferior oblique is the only extrinsic muscle to take origin from the front of the orbit ; it is also remarkable in having the shortest tendon of insertion (Figs. 275, 280).

It arises by a rounded tendon from a small depression (sometimes a roughness) on the orbital plate of the maxilla a little behind the lower orbital margin and just lateral to the orifice of the naso-lacrimal duct. Some of its fibres may, in fact, arise from the fascia covering the lacrimal sac.

It passes laterally and backwards, making an angle of 50° with the visual line (that is parallel with the reflected tendon of the superior oblique) between the inferior rectus and the floor of the orbit, then under the lateral rectus to be inserted by a very short tendon[1] (Fig. 85) (often none at all) to the back and lateral

---

[1] As Salzmann points out, one often finds actual muscle fibres inserted into the sclera. The shortness of the tendon of the inferior oblique may be used to determine to which side an excised globe belongs. Having found it, we know which is the upper and which is the lower aspect of the globe : the attached tendons of the obliques will point away from the side to which it belongs.

portion of the globe, for the most part below the horizontal meridian. The line of insertion is oblique, 9·4 mm. long, and is convex upwards.

Its posterior or nasal end is about 5 mm. from the optic nerve, *and thus lies practically over the macula* (only 2·2 mm. from it (Poirier)) (Fig. 248, E). The anterior, temporal end lies in about the same meridian as the lower end of the insertion of the lateral rectus.

Relations.—Near its origin the lower surface of the muscle is in contact with the periosteum of the floor of the orbit, but further laterally it is separated from this by fat. Just before the insertion of the muscle, this surface which now faces laterally is covered by the lateral rectus and the capsule of Tenon.

The upper aspect is in contact with fat, then the inferior rectus, then finally spreading out and becoming concave it moulds itself on the globe.

Nerve.—The inferior oblique is supplied by the inferior division of the oculo-motor, which crosses above the posterior border about its middle to enter the muscle on its *upper*-surface.

The **Blood-supply** comes from the infraorbital artery and the medial muscular branch of the ophthalmic.

Actions.—The inferior oblique makes the eye look upwards or laterally or wheel-rotates it laterally (extorts).

The Main Action is the elevation which increases as the eye is turned in and is nil in abduction. The inferior oblique is the only elevator in the adducted position.

The Subsidiary Actions are the abduction and extorsion, which increase as the eye is abducted.

The inferior oblique acts with the superior rectus to make the eye look directly upwards.

THE LEVATOR PALPEBRÆ SUPERIORIS

The levator palpebræ superioris arises from the under-surface of the lesser wing of the sphenoid above and in front of the optic foramen by a short tendon which is blended with the underlying origin of the superior rectus.

The flat ribbon-like muscle belly passes forwards below the roof of the orbit and on the superior rectus to about 1 cm. behind the septum orbitale (that is more or less at the upper fornix or a few millimetres in front of the equator of the globe), where it ends in a membranous expansion or *aponeurosis*. This spreads out in a fan-shaped manner, so as to occupy the whole breadth of the orbit and thus gives the whole muscle the form of an isosceles triangle. The fleshy part of the muscle is horizontal, the tendinous part is nearly vertical, moulding itself on the globe of the eye, as indeed does the whole of the upper eyelid. The change of direction takes place round the reflected tendon of the superior oblique.

Attachments.—(*a*) The main insertion of the levator is to the *skin* of the upper lid at and below the upper palpebral sulcus. It reaches this by passing through the fibres of the orbicularis (Fig. 192).

(*b*) *To the Tarsal Plate.*—Some of the fibres of the aponeurosis are attached to the front [1] and lower part of the tarsal plate, but the main attachment of the levator here is viâ the unstriped *superior palpebral muscle.* This is continuous with the fleshy part of the levator, and is attached to the upper border of the tarsus (Figs. 192, 193).

(*c*) The attachment of the levator to the superior fornix of the *conjunctiva* is actually viâ the fascial sheath of the muscle (see later).

(*d*) The two extremities of the aponeurosis are called its "*horns.*" The *lateral horn* passes between the orbital and palpebral portions of the lacrimal gland (Fig. 280), which is as it were folded round it, and plays a part in supporting the gland against the orbital roof The lateral horn is attached to the orbital tubercle and to the upper aspect of the lateral palpebral ligament (Fig. 275).

The *medial horn* is much weaker than the lateral. It is attached somewhat below the fronto-lacrimal suture and to the medial palpebral ligament.

The Sheath of the levator has several points of interest. It is attached below to that of the superior rectus (*q.v.*), and it is the tissue between the two muscles which gains attachment to the upper conjunctival fornix (Fig. 215). On the upper aspect of the junction of aponeurosis and muscle the sheath is thickened to form a band (Whitnall), the medial end of which passes up to the pulley of the superior oblique and to the neighbouring bone and sends a slip to bridge over the supraorbital notch. The lateral end of the band passes above the aponeurosis, and is in part joined to it. Part of it passes into the lacrimal gland and part reaches the lateral orbital wall. Whitnall considers these the true check ligaments of the levator.

Relations.— *Above* the levator and between it and the roof of the orbit are the 4th and frontal nerves and the supraorbital vessels. The 4th nerve crosses the muscle close to its origin from lateral to medial to reach the superior oblique (Figs. 15, 277).

The supraorbital artery is above the muscle in its anterior half only.

The frontal nerve crosses the muscle obliquely from the lateral to the medial side.

Below the levator is the medial part of the superior rectus (which, being the larger muscle, has its lateral edge exposed) and the globe of the eye (Fig. 277).

In front of the tendon at its commencement is the retro-septal roll of fat which is continuous with the upper and medial orbital lobe of fat. Below this the front of the tendon of the levator is in contact with the septum. Behind is the pre-tarsal space, containing the peripheral palpebral arcade (Fig. 192), and the palpe-bral portion of the lacrimal gland. The pretarsal space placed behind the tarsal insertion of the tendon is prolonged laterally behind the lateral horn of the levator and contains here the palpebral portion of the lacrimal gland.

Nerves.—(*a*) The *Superior Division of the 3rd*, which reaches the muscle either

---

[1] The fibres of the levator form a definite layer here, *which it is important to realise, especially in exposing the tarsal plate from in front.*

by piercing the medial edge of the superior rectus (and thus forming another bond between the two muscles) or by winding round its medial border.

(b) *Sympathetic Fibres* to the unstriped superior palpebral muscle.

Blood-supply.—This is from the lateral muscular branch of the ophthalmic artery.

Action.—The levator raises the upper eyelid, thus uncovering the cornea and a portion of the sclera, and deepens the superior palpebral fold. Its antagonist is the palpebral portion of the orbicularis.

THE FASCIA BULBI

The fascia bulbi (capsule of Tenon) is a thin, fibrous membrane which envelops the globe from the margin of the cornea to the optic nerve.

Its inner surface is well defined and in close contact with the sclera, to which it is connected by fine trabeculæ.

These opposing surfaces were held by Schwalbe to be lined by endothelium, the capsule of Tenon thus forming an articular socket, in which the eyeball moves freely in all directions. The joint cavity, too, was thought by Schwalbe to be a lymph space continuous behind with the lymph space surrounding the external coat of the optic nerve (supravaginal lymph space). But the capsule of Tenon is attached to the globe in front, to the ocular muscles, and to the sclera by the above-mentioned trabeculæ. It is probable, therefore, that while slight movements take place between the globe and the capsule, in more extensive movements the globe and the capsule move together in the surrounding fat.

The posterior surface of the fascia bulbi is in contact with the orbital fat, from which it is separated with difficulty.

Anteriorly the fascia bulbi becomes thinner, and merges gradually into the subconjunctival connective tissue. It is separated from the conjunctiva by loose connective tissue, and in operations for exposing the ocular muscles can be demonstrated separately from this membrane.

Posteriorly around the optic nerve, where it is pierced by the ciliary vessels and nerves, it becomes very thin, and can be traced only with difficulty to the dural sheath of the optic nerve, with which it is held to be continuous. Schwalbe, however, describes it as being continuous with a membrane which surrounds this sheath to form the supravaginal lymph space—a view which is now held to be very doubtful.

The lower part of the fascia bulbi is thickened to form a sling or hammock, on which the globe rests, and which has received the name of the *suspensory ligament of Lockwood*. That it is effective in supporting the eye is shown by the fact that the globe does not sink down after removal of the maxilla.

The fascia bulbi is pierced posteriorly by the optic nerve (Fig. 250), and around this by the ciliary nerves and arteries ; just behind the equator by the venæ vorticosæ, and anteriorly by the six extrinsic muscles of the eye.

Where the fascia bulbi is pierced by the tendons of the extrinsic muscles it sends round each *a tubular reflection* backwards, which clothes it like the fingers of a glove. The reflections differ in the different muscles. In the case of the recti they gradually become continuous with the perimysium, but send important slips or expansions to surrounding structures.

The lateral expansion of the lateral rectus is attached to the orbital tubercle on the zygomatic bone, while that of the medial rectus passes to the lacrimal bone.

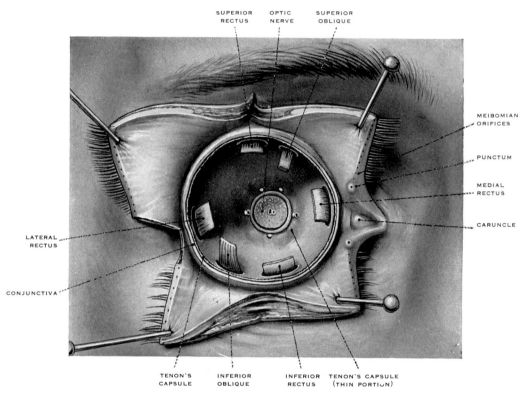

FIG. 250.—DISSECTION TO SHOW THE FASCIA BULBI (TENON'S CAPSULE).
The (right) eye has been removed.
(*Wolff's preparation.*)

These expansions are strong and to some extent limit the action of the muscles. They have therefore received the name of *check ligaments*.

The expansion of the superior rectus is attached to the levator palpebræ by a definite band, in which a bursa may be found (Motais). This band is important physiologically. It ensures the synergic action of the two muscles. Thus, when the superior rectus makes the eye look upwards the upper lid is raised as well.

The expansion from the inferior rectus (Fig. 280) passes from the under-surface of this muscle above the inferior oblique, then deep to the conjunctival cul-de-sac and the palpebral conjunctiva, from which it is separated by the unstriped inferior palpebral muscle (which, according to Fuchs, can be seen through the conjunctiva), and then is inserted between the tarsal plate and the orbicularis. By this means the inferior rectus can act on the lower lid as the levator acts on the upper. The lower lid is, in fact, lowered 2 mm. and pulled down by its action and the lashes tend to be everted. This movement is, however, aided by the lid being in contact with the globe.

The reflection of the superior oblique passes up to its pulley, that of the inferior oblique to the lateral part of the floor of the orbit.

From the anterior end of the expansions of all the muscles, fibrous bands pass, to be attached to the conjunctival cul-de-sac. When the muscles act the conjunctiva is pulled back also, and thus is prevented from folding and strangulation, much in fact as the musculus articularis genu pulls the synovial membrane of the knee-joint out of the way in contraction of the quadriceps and prevents it being nipped by the patella.

The Unstriped Muscles of the Orbit

The capsulo-palpebral muscle of Hesser, forms the peribulbar portion of the unstriped muscles of the orbit. It forms an almost complete ring round the eye, but is missing on the lateral side. It consists of superior, inferior, and medial palpebral portions. Apart from the muscle of Müller there is no definite origin or insertion to the various portions. Also the fibres of any particular portion may run in various directions. *The Superior Palpebral Portion* consists centrally of the superior palpebral muscle of Müller. This arises from the inferior or bulbar aspect of the levator palpebræ just behind the fornix. Some 15 to 20 millimetres wide at its origin, it widens a little towards its insertion to the upper edge of the tarsal plate after an almost vertical course of 10 millimetres (Figs. 192, 251).

It forms a well-defined muscular layer which can be easily dissected, thus differing from other portions of the capsulo-palpebral muscle. It lies in connective tissue and fat between the tendon of the levator in front and the palpebral portion of the fascia bulbi and the palpebral conjunctiva behind. It limits the pretarsal space (see p. 189).

The Supero-lateral Portion of the unstriped musculature extends from the lateral edge of the muscle of Müller to the orbital margin, becoming thinner and less defined. As it does so it divides into two layers which surround the palpebral portion of the lacrimal gland (Fig. 204).

The Supero-medial Portion passes to the medial part of the upper border of the tarsal plate. Its fibres are feeble and placed in the fascia bulbi.

The Inferior Palpebral Portion consists centrally of the inferior palpebral muscle of Müller which passes from the ocular surface of the inferior rectus to the lower border of the tarsal plate. For the most part the inferior portion consists of fibres which are dispersed in that portion of the fascia bulbi which separates the inferior rectus from the inferior oblique. Anteriorly the fibres lie between the palpebral conjunctiva and the inferior portion of the septum orbitale in the palpebral extension of the capsule. The inferior portion of the muscle is more or less feeble, especially in its lateral part.

The Medial Portion of the capsulo-palpebral muscle is the feeblest. The fibres lie scattered in the fascia bulbi and do not reach the eyelids. They stop about a millimetre from the medial fornix (Fig. 252).

PRACTICAL CONSIDERATIONS

From a practical point of view there are four spaces inside the orbit.

(1) Firstly, and most important, is that bounded in great part by the rigid orbital walls, but, anteriorly, by the eye and septum orbitale, including the tarsal plates and tarsal ligaments.

(2) Since the periorbita is for the most part easily detachable there is a potential space between it and the bone.

(3) Inside this is the space bounded by the cone of muscles, the intermuscular membrane and the capsule of Tenon.

The intermuscular membrane (Fig. 253) is described by Poirier as follows : " The sheaths of the four recti muscles are joined to each other by an aponeurotic membrane, which becomes thinner as we trace it backwards and anteriorly is continuous with the capsule of Tenon. It is strongest between the superior and lateral recti muscles. In thin and feeble subjects it may be ill-marked, and hence is neither mentioned nor figured by many authors. At the posterior pole of the eye it separates the fat of the orbit into two layers, one central the other peripheral, and controls to a certain extent the progress of infiltrations."

From the above it follows that the muscle cone forms a separate space. Hence an exploration of the orbit outside it can have but little effect on a lesion situated within it. This is illustrated by a case described by Harrison Butler. The orbit was explored several times in a patient with proptosis and rigors and no pus was found. Later, on removal of the eye, the pus was found inside the muscle cone.

(4) The fourth space to be considered is Tenon's capsule, and Harrison Butler and others have recorded cases where a conjunctival incision has been effective in evacuating pus from this space.

The methods, then, that might be employed to relieve tension in the orbit are :

(*a*) An incision into the orbit outside the muscle cone.

(*b*) An incision into the orbit with splitting of the lid in a vertical direction and division of one or both tarsal ligaments. This was the method used by George Lawson and Tweedy.

(*c*) The division of one or other ocular muscle. This not only allows the eye to move farther forwards and so diminishes the pressure behind it, but also opens up the muscle cone and Tenon's capsule, and gives a good view of the back of the eye and anterior part of the optic nerve.

(*d*) Opening Tenon's capsule by a conjunctival incision.

(*e*) Temporary resection of part of the orbital wall as in Krönlein's operation.

THE ORBITAL FAT

The orbital fat compactly fills all the space not occupied by the other structures. Indeed, in formalin-hardened specimens it forms so firm a mass that ex-

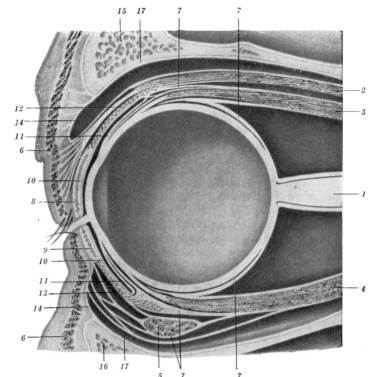

FIG. 251.—SCHEM-
ATIC SAGITTAL SECTION
OF THE EYE AND ITS
SURROUNDINGS.

1. optic nerve.
2. levator.
3. superior rectus.
4. inferior rectus.
5. inferior oblique.
6. orbicularis.
7. fascia bulbi.
8. superior tarsus.
9. inferior tarsus.
10. palpebral conjunc-
    tiva.
11. bulbar conjunc-
    tiva.
12. superior capsulo-
    palpebral muscle.
13. idem, inferior por-
    tion.
14. septum orbitale.
15. frontal bone.
16. maxilla.
17. periorbita.

(From Eisler, after Hesser.)

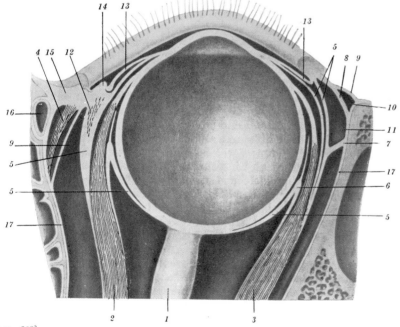

FIG. 252.—SCHEM-
ATIC HORIZONTAL SEC-
TION OF THE EYE AND
ITS SURROUNDINGS.

1. optic nerve.
2. medial rectus.
3. lateral rectus.
4. Horner's muscle.
5. fascia bulbi.
6. fascia bulbi.
7. lateral check liga-
   ment.
8. aponeurosis of
   levator.
9. septum orbitale.
10. superior recess.
11. recess for lacrimal
    gland.
12. medial capsulo-
    palpebral muscle.
13. bulbar conjunc-
    tiva.
14. caruncle.
15. medial palpebral
    ligament.
16. lacrimal sac.
17. periorbita.

(From Eisler, after Hesser.)

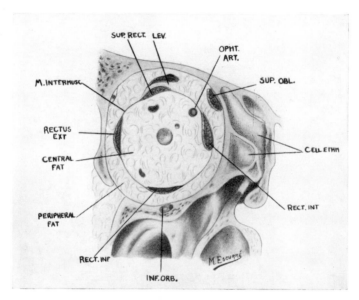

FIG. 253.—THE INTERMUSCULAR MEMBRANE.

Right side, posterior segment. The intermuscular membrane joins the recti muscles and divides the orbital fat into central and peripheral portions. There is a recess containing fat under the levator.

(*From Poirier.*)

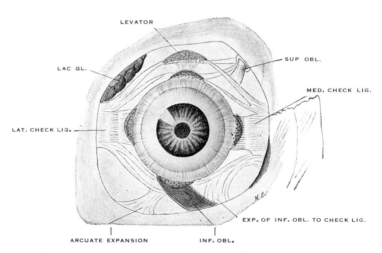

FIG. 254.—ORBITAL EXPANSIONS OF THE MUSCLES OF THE EYE.

Slightly schematised. The recti sectioned with their sheaths surround the globe and are united by the capsule of Tenon, orbital extensions of levator and superior rectus. Expansion of superior rectus to levator. Arcuate expansion of inferior oblique to floor of orbit. Check ligament from medial and lateral recti, strengthened above and below by superior and inferior expansions.

(*From Poirier.*)

cellent sections of the orbital contents can be cut with a razor by hand (Whitnall).

The orbital fat extends from the optic nerve to the orbital wall and from the apex of the orbit to the septum orbitale. Sometimes the fat pushes the septum in front of it, but never passes through it into the eyelids. The fat varies in its different portions in consistency and in the amount of connective tissue it contains.

The fat consists of lobules of different sizes enclosed in a capsule which is better marked laterally, where it forms a kind of sac for the fat (Charpy). From the capsule septa passes inwards and demarcate the lobules. The inter-lobular septa are soft, vascular, and easily distended with œdema fluid. Birch-Hirschfeld having produced an artificial œdema thought that the clefts so formed were lymphatic channels. Although this idea is not generally accepted, these septa provide the route along which orbital phlegmon spreads, and hæmorrhage from a fracture of the base of the skull passes into the depths of the orbit.

The fat is divided by the intermuscular membrane into a *Central* or *intramuscular portion* and a *Peripheral* or *extramuscular portion* (Fig. 253). Posteriorly where there is no intermuscular membrane the two portions run into each other.

The Central Fat around the optic nerve is loose, no doubt to allow for movements of the optic nerve and the ciliary vessels and nerves in excursions of the globe. It is finely lobulated and the septa which surround the lobules are very thin ; which make it easy to separate them from each other. In general the lobules are fusiform with the long axis parallel to the optic nerve. At the back of the globe the septa are inserted into Tenon's capsule so that if an attempt be made to separate the fat from the capsule, dentate processes remain attached to the latter. There is thus no space between the fat and the capsule, so that movement of the globe takes place only slightly in the capsule—for in excursions of any extent the fat moves also. Indeed, the capsule of Tenon may in part be regarded as the thickened limiting membrane of the fat.

At the surface of the optic nerve the central fat has a limiting membrane which separates it from the dural covering of the nerve. Between this membrane and the dura is a space traversed by septa which is the supravaginal space of Schwalbe. It is most probably produced by the movements of the fat and optic nerve (Charpy).

The Peripheral Fat is placed between the periorbita and the recti muscles. It is thickest in the region of the insertion of the muscles. It is limited anteriorly by the septum. This fat is covered by a thin transparent membrane which is united to the periorbita by feeble processes easily torn. In spite of its thinness, as long as it is not ruptured, blood passes between it and the periorbita to reach the deep portions of the eyelids, but not the conjunctiva. But if it is ruptured a subconjunctival ecchymosis is produced. Posteriorly the fat covers the recti muscles near their origin. The peripheral fat is situated in the intermuscular spaces and is in the form of four lobes (Winckler). The posterior portion of each lobe passes deeply to become continuous with the central fat, with which indeed it is united by numerous connective tissue septa. Anteriorly its deep surface is in contact with the intermuscular membrane and Tenon's capsule. Superficially each lobe spreads out to cover partially the two muscles between which it lies. The connective tissue membranes which surround the lobes are in contact with the sheaths of the muscles and their prolongations, with the periorbita, and with the septum orbitale.

The Supero-lateral Lobe is placed between the superior and lateral recti. It just covers the edge of the superior rectus and is separated from the superomedial lobe by the frontal nerve. It covers the lateral rectus, especially anteriorly, while the lacrimal gland separates it from the septum.

The Infero-lateral Lobe is placed between the lateral and inferior recti. Its lower border lies along the nerve to the inferior oblique. The lobe increases

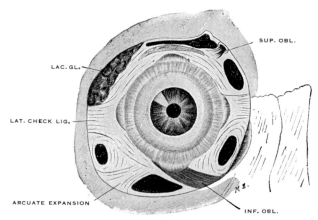

FIG. 255.—THE HERNIAL ORIFICES AT THE BASE OF THE ORBIT.

The eyelids and the septum orbitale have been removed, together with the fat which had herniated through the orifices.

(From Poirier.)

in thickness anteriorly and comes into contact with the inferior oblique muscle. It sends a prolongation to the septum on either side of the arcuate expansion of the inferior oblique.

The Infero-medial Lobe is placed between the inferior and medial recti. It also enlarges anteriorly and sends a prolongation to the septum on either side of the inferior oblique muscle. The remainder of the lobe is placed behind the expansion of the medial rectus to the posterior aspect of the septum, that is, it is posterior to Horner's muscle and the lacrimal sac.

The Supero-medial Lobe lies between the superior rectus and levator laterally, and the medial rectus medially. It is partially separated from the periorbita by the superior oblique. Anteriorly this lobe has two prolongations. One passes under the pulley of the superior oblique and then through the supero-medial aperture for hernia of the orbital fat and so reaches the septum. The other passes above the pulley through the superior aperture. Then it forms a retro-septal roll which lies along the anterior margin of the check ligament of the levator and the lacrimal gland.

THE APERTURES AT THE BASE OF THE ORBIT THROUGH WHICH ORBITAL FAT MAY HERNIATE (Orifices adipeux of Charpy)

If in a dissection of the eyelids the septum orbitale is carefully removed, one sees that the base of the orbit is partially closed by the globe surrounded by its muscles and the fibro-elastic expansions which these send to the walls of the orbit just behind its margins. These expansions and the two oblique muscles bound a series of orifices, five in number, between the orbital margin and the globe (Fig. 255). Through these orifices fat may herniate from the orbit to come into contact with the septum.

The Superior Aperture is in the form of a comma placed on its side. It lies between the roof of the orbit and the upper surface of the levator. The head of the comma, which is medial, is near the pulley and reflected tendon of the superior oblique ; the tail reaches the lacrimal gland. Through this aperture fat from the supero-medial lobe may herniate and form the retro-septal roll.

The Supero-medial Aperture forms an oval with its long axis vertical. It is placed between the reflected tendon of the superior oblique and the medial check ligament. Through it passes that process of the supero-medial lobe which is responsible for the common lobulated prominence in old people, which replaces the normal concavity of the region. Through this aperture pass the infra-trochlear nerve, the dorsal nasal artery, and the angular vein.

The Infero-medial Aperture is also oval. It lies between the medial check ligament, the origin of the inferior oblique, and the lacrimal sac. It is through this aperture that in those animals which have a third eyelid a mass of fat in relation to it passes (Charpy).

The Inferior Aperture is triangular and lies between the inferior oblique, its arcuate expansion, and the floor of the orbit.

The Infero-lateral Aperture is small and lies between the arcuate expansion of the inferior oblique and the lateral check ligament.

In general these apertures form a communication between the cavity of the orbit and the deep portions of the eyelids. It is through them that blood and pus pass out of the orbit from the space between the periorbita and the peripheral fat. They reach the septum but are stopped by it (Charpy).

BIBLIOGRAPHY

BIRCH-HIRSCHFLD (1909) : " Die Krankheiten der Orbita," Graefe-Saemisch, Hand-
    buch der gesamten Augenheilkunde, 2nd edit., **9**, Abt. 1, Teil 1, Kap. 13, 261.
BUTLER, T. H. (1923): *Trans. Ophthal. Soc. U.K.*, **43**.

HESSER, C. (1913): *Anat. Hefte*, **49,** 1.

HOWE, L. (1907) : The Muscles of the Eye, *New York*.

LAWSON, G. (1895) : *Trans. Ophthal. Soc. U.K.*

LOCKWOOD, C. (1886) : *J. Anat. Physiol.*, **20,** 1.

MOTAIS, E. (1887) : L'Appareil moteur de l'Œil, *Paris*.

POIRIER (1911) : Traité d'Anatomie Humaine 3rd edit., **5 ;** fasc. 2. (" Les organes du sens ").

SCHIEFFERDECKER, P. (1905) : Abst. in *Z. Augenheilk.*, **14,** 186.

SCHWARZ (1925) : *Z. f. Anat., Entw Gesch.*, **75,** 361.

TENON (1806) : Mémoires et observations sur l'anatomie, *Paris*.

WHITNALL, S. E. (1932) : Anatomy of the Human Orbit, 2nd ed., *Oxford*.

WOLTER, J. R. (1955) : *A.M.A. Arch. Ophthal.*, **53,** 201.

WOOLLARD, H. (1931) : *J. Anat., Lond.*, **65,** 215.

CHAPTER VI

THE NERVES

THE OCULO-MOTOR OR 3RD CRANIAL NERVE

Superficial Origin.—The oculo-motor nerve arises by a series of 10 to 15 rootlets, for the most part from the sulcus oculo-motorius, which lies on the medial side of the basis pedunculi. A small lateral portion, however, actually takes origin from

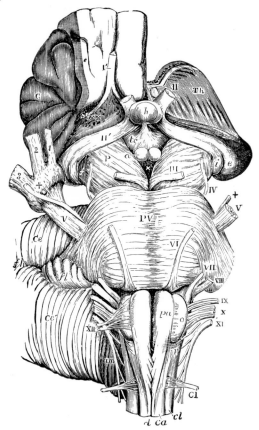

FIG. 256.—VENTRAL ASPECT OF THE BRAIN-STEM, SHOWING THE ATTACHMENTS OF THE CRANIAL NERVES.

The following references apply to the roots of the nerves. I′ = right olfactory tract, divided near its middle. II = left optic nerve springing from the chiasma, which is concealed by the pituitary body. II′ = right optic tract ; the left tract is seen passing back into *i* and *e*, the medial and lateral roots. III = left oculo-motor nerve. IV = trochlear. V,V = sensory roots of the trigeminal nerves. +, + = motor roots, the + of the right side is placed on the trigeminal ganglion. 1 = ophthalmic, 2 = maxillary, and 3 = mandibular divisions. VI = left abducent nerve. VII = facial. VIII = eighth. IX = glosso-pharyngeal. X = vagus. XI = accessory. XII = right hypoglossal nerve ; at *o*, on the left side, the rootlets are seen cut short. C1 = suboccipital or first cervical nerve.

(*After Allen Thomson in Quain's " Anatomy."*)

the neighbouring ventral surface of the peduncle. As pointed out by Zander, the two portions almost meet posteriorly, but separate anteriorly and so practically form a letter **V**.

The posterior part of this origin comes close to the upper border of the pons, near the termination of the basilar artery (Figs. 352, 353).

Between the two nerves is the posterior perforated substance.

The posterior cerebral artery runs along the medial side of the origin of the 3rd nerve, then curls round above the upper rootlets (Figs. 352, 353). It often sends twigs between the rootlets of the nerve. The superior cerebellar artery runs below the origin at the upper border of the pons (Figs. 258, 353).

Course and Relations.—(a) *In the Posterior Cranial Fossa.*—Surrounded by pia and bathed in cerebro-spinal fluid, the 3rd nerve passes downwards and

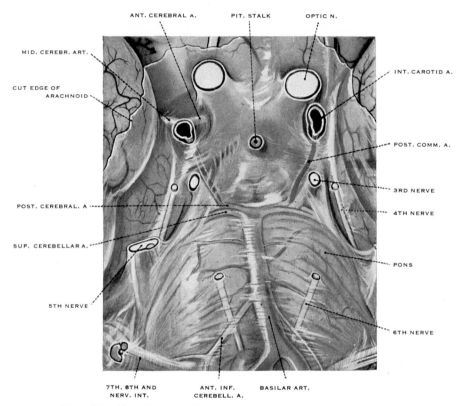

FIG. 257.—THE CISTERNA INTERPEDUNCULARIS AND CISTERNA PONTIS.

A portion of the base of the brain with the arachnoid *in situ* showing the relation of this membrane to the cranial nerves (II to VIII) and to the circle of Willis.

forwards in the cisterna interpeduncularis [1] (Fig. 257), between the posterior cerebral and superior cerebellar arteries (Figs. 258, 259).

At first somewhat flattened in form it twists on itself, so that the inferior fibres become superior, and, leaving the arteries, soon becomes a rounded cord.

It runs above and medial to the free margin of the tentorium cerebelli and

[1] The cisterna interpeduncularis is the large subarachnoid space which is formed by the bridging across of the temporal lobes by arachnoid. It contains the cerebral peduncles, the interpeduncular space, and the circle of Willis (Fig. 257).

4th nerve, and below and lateral to the posterior communicating artery (Fig. 258). It crosses the under-aspect of the optic tract from medial to lateral (Figs. 260, 316). Also above and lateral is the uncus (Fig. 319).

For about 1 cm., i.e. from a point just behind the posterior clinoid

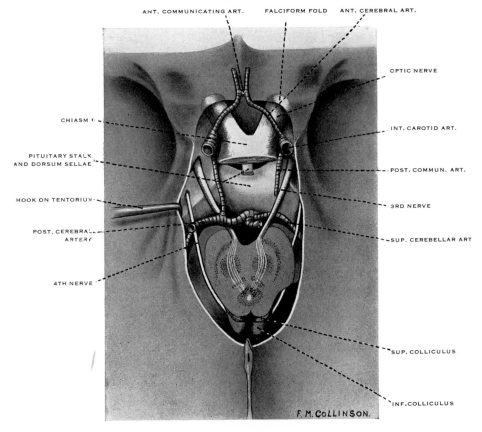

ANT. COMMUNICATING ART.   FALCIFORM FOLD   ANT. CEREBRAL ART.

OPTIC NERVE

CHIASM

INT. CAROTID ART.

PITUITARY STALK AND DORSUM SELLAE

POST. COMMUN. ART.

HOOK ON TENTORIUM

3RD NERVE

POST. CEREBRAL ARTERY

SUP. CEREBELLAR ART

4TH NERVE

SUP. COLLICULUS

INF. COLLICULUS

F. M. COLLINSON.

FIG. 258.—DISSECTION TO SHOW THE COURSE OF THE 3RD AND 4TH NERVES AND THE RELATION OF THE CIRCLE OF WILLIS TO THE PITUITARY FOSSA.

The mid-brain is divided in the aperture of the tentorium, and the cerebrum removed. On the right side the posterior cerebral and posterior communicating arteries are cut short in order to expose the origin of the 3rd nerve. On the left side the tentorium and cerebral peduncle are slightly separated so as to show the 4th nerve more fully.

(After T. W. P. Lawrence in Quain's " Anatomy.")

process to the point where the nerve pierces the dura, it is in contact with arachnoid.

(b) *In the Middle Cranial Fossa.*—The 3rd nerve passes just lateral to the posterior clinoid process and above the attached margin of the tentorium cerebelli. It now lies lateral to the pituitary fossa *above* the cavernous sinus ; then, piercing the dura about midway between the anterior and posterior clinoid processes close to the prolongation forwards of the free margin of the tentorium cerebelli, it passes through the roof and so comes to lie in the lateral wall of the sinus (Figs. 259, 270, 272).

Here it has the 4th nerve and the first and second divisions of the 5th nerve

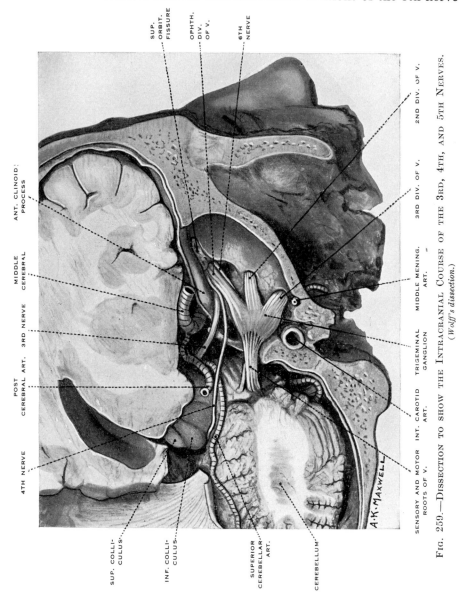

FIG. 259.—DISSECTION TO SHOW THE INTRACRANIAL COURSE OF THE 3RD, 4TH, AND 5TH NERVES. (*Wolff's dissection.*)

below and lateral in that order from above downwards and the 6th nerve, and internal carotid artery actually in the sinus lying below and medial to it (Fig. 366).

While in the lateral wall of the sinus the 3rd nerve receives communications from the first division of the 5th and the sympathetic round the carotid artery.

The 3rd nerve now enters the superior orbital (sphenoidal) fissure, but just before it does so it divides into a small superior and a larger inferior division, and about at this point the 4th nerve crosses the 3rd to lie above and then medial to it. The position of this crossing is variable. Testut holds that at the level of the optic foramen the 4th and 5th nerves are still below and lateral to the 3rd (Fig. 259).

At the anterior part of the cavernous sinus, too, the ophthalmic division of the 5th crosses the 3rd from below upwards, and just about this point divides into its three branches (Figs. 259, 282).

(c) *In the Superior Orbital (Sphenoidal) Fissure.*—The two divisions of the 3rd nerve pass through the fissure within the anulus of Zinn, i.e. between the two heads of the lateral rectus (Fig. 261). They have the naso-ciliary nerve medial and between them, and the 6th nerve at first below, then lateral. The fourth, frontal and lacrimal nerves pass through the *wide* portion of the fissure above the anulus.

(d) *In the Orbit.*—*The superior division* inclines medially above the optic nerve and just behind the naso-ciliary to supply the superior rectus on its under-surface at the junction of the middle and posterior thirds (Figs. 278, 280, 281), and the levator palpebræ superioris. The branch to the latter muscle either pierces or curls round the medial border of the superior rectus.

The inferior division, much larger than the superior, immediately divides into three. These are the branches to the medial rectus, the inferior rectus, and the inferior oblique.

The branch to the medial rectus passes under the optic nerve to enter the muscle on its *lateral* or ocular aspect near the junction of its middle and posterior thirds (Fig. 281).

The branch to the inferior rectus pierces the muscle on its upper aspect near the junction of middle and posterior thirds.

The long branch to the inferior oblique runs along the floor of the orbit on the lateral border of the inferior rectus or between this muscle and the lateral rectus. It crosses above the posterior border of the inferior oblique about its middle, and breaks up into two or three branches which enter the *upper* surface of the muscle.

It is this nerve that gives the short stout branch to the ciliary ganglion, for relay to the sphincter pupillæ and the ciliary muscle (Fig. 279).

Communications and Varieties.—(a) A branch of communication from the 6th to the 3rd in the lateral wall of the cavernous sinus has been described, but must be very rare.

(b) The superior division fairly often has a communicating branch from the naso-ciliary.

(*c*) Volkmann describes a twig from the 3rd to the superior oblique.

(*d*) Generali describes a case where a branch from the 3rd replaced the 6th which was absent.

(*e*) Henle in one case saw the branch to the inferior oblique pierce the inferior rectus, and the same branch was seen by Arnold to pass through the lower part of the ciliary ganglion (Quain).

(*f*) There may be no short branch to the ciliary ganglion, which then sits directly on the nerve to the inferior oblique (Testut).

SUMMARY OF THE OCULO-MOTOR NERVE (Fig. 283)

The superior branch supplies :

> Superior rectus.
> Levator palpebræ superioris.

The inferior branch supplies :

> Medial rectus.
> Inferior rectus.
> Inferior oblique.
> Motor root of the ciliary ganglion.

As a whole, the 3rd nerve supplies all the extrinsic muscles of the eye except the lateral rectus and superior oblique, and also innervates the sphincter pupillæ and the ciliary muscle.

NUCLEUS AND CONNECTIONS (see also p. 509)

The nuclei of the 3rd, 4th, and 6th nerves, with the exception of that portion of the 3rd which supplies the intrinsic muscles, belong to the somatic efferent nuclear column (Fig. 266) and are composed of rather large polygonal cells like those of the anterior horns of the spinal cord.

Each 3rd nerve nucleus forms a small column of multipolar nerve cells some 10 mm. long which lies in the floor of the aqueduct (of Sylvius) beneath the superior colliculus. Its superior extremity reaches to the floor of the third ventricle, while it ends below on a level with the lower border of the superior colliculus.

The dorso-medial aspect of each nucleus is in contact with the grey matter of the aqueduct, its ventro-lateral with the medial longitudinal bundle (Fig. 263). Inferiorly the third nucleus is continuous with that of the fourth.

Localisation within the Nuclei.—Punctate lesions within these small nuclei are very rare ; thus the interest is more academic than clinical.

In fact, exact localization within the *human* pair of nuclei remains highly speculative. Evidence from animal experiments and human ophthalmoplegias is fragmentary and very conflicting. The formerly accepted scheme of Brouwer and others (Fig. 264) has been shown by Warwick to be very different in the monkey. The formerly accepted scheme is reprinted here for its historical interest and

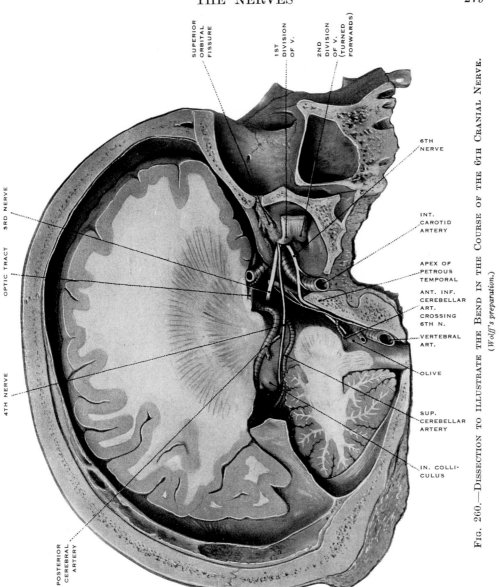

SUPERIOR ORBITAL FISSURE

1ST DIVISION OF V.

2ND DIVISION OF V. (TURNED FORWARDS)

6TH NERVE

INT. CAROTID ARTERY

APEX OF PETROUS TEMPORAL

ANT. INF. CEREBELLAR ART. CROSSING 6TH N.

VERTEBRAL ART.

OLIVE

SUP. CEREBELLAR ARTERY

IN. COLLI-CULUS

3RD NERVE

OPTIC TRACT

4TH NERVE

POSTERIOR CEREBRAL ARTERY

FIG. 260.—DISSECTION TO ILLUSTRATE THE BEND IN THE COURSE OF THE 6TH CRANIAL NERVE.

(*Wolff's preparation.*)

because it is not yet fully refuted *in man*, but this account is followed (*v. inf.*) by that of the monkey nucleus as explored by Warwick (*Ann. R.C.S.* 1956, **19** : 36–52).

Localisation within the Nuclei.—Former Ideas of the Two Nuclei.—The two third nuclei, taken as a whole, consist of five parts : two *main lateral* nuclei ; an unpaired central *nucleus of Perlia* which unites the main nuclei and the paired small-celled *nucleus of Edinger-Westphal* situated anteriorly (Fig. 264).

The Main Lateral Nuclei contain the centres for the motor nerves to the eye muscles. Each muscle[1] is governed by a well-defined group of cells. These from cranial to caudal are *probably* levator palpebræ, superior rectus, inferior oblique, inferior rectus. The centre for the medial rectus (medial movement) is next to the median nucleus of Perlia.

The Central Nucleus of Perlia [2] probably has to do with convergence. Thus convergence and medial movement, whose centres lie close together, although often affected together, are not necessarily so.

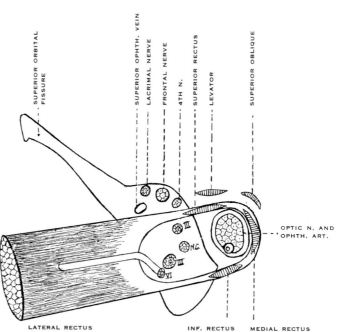

FIG. 261.—DIAGRAM OF THE STRUCTURES PASSING THROUGH THE SUPERIOR ORBITAL FISSURE AND OPTIC FORAMEN (L.W.).

Note that nothing goes through the narrow portion of the fissure.

III = upper and lower divisions of the 3rd nerve. N.C. = Naso-ciliary. VI = 6th nerve.

(labels) SUPERIOR ORBITAL FISSURE — SUPERIOR OPHTH. VEIN — LACRIMAL NERVE — FRONTAL NERVE — 4TH N. — SUPERIOR RECTUS — LEVATOR — SUPERIOR OBLIQUE — OPTIC N, AND OPHTH. ART.

LATERAL RECTUS   INF. RECTUS   MEDIAL RECTUS

The Nucleus of [3] *Edinger-Westphal* [4] probably subserves the pupillary musculature. It is paired and interposed anteriorly between the two lateral nuclei. It is composed of small pyriform cells of the preganglionic autonomic type.

The fibres from the cranial part of the third nucleus are direct, i.e. go to the muscles of the same side ; of those from the caudal part some are held to be direct and some crossed.

Third Nucleus of the Monkey.—Warwick shows that in the monkey a dorso-ventral rather than a cranio-caudal organization exists (Fig. 265). Man has a

---

[1] Le Gros Clark, however, believes that movements rather than muscles are represented in the nucleus (*J. Anat.*, **60**, 1926).

[2] Perlia (1889), *v. Graefe's Arch. Ophthal.*, **35** (4), 287.

[3] Edinger (1885), (*a*) *Arch. ges. Psychol.*, **16**, 858 ; (*b*) *Untersuchungen über d. vgl. Anat. des Gehirns* ; (*c*) (1911), *Vorlesung*.

[4] Westphal (1889), *Centralbl. f. Nervenheil*.

wider midbrain than the monkey and this widens the human nucleus ; it is likely (but not certain) that the general configuration is the same in both.

Pitts (1965 ; *Am. Jour. Optometry* : **42** : 7, 379) summarises the existing literature, from 1846 to 1964, into the following conclusions :

1. The pair of nuclei consist of an artero-median nucleus, two Edinger-Westphal nuclei, two lateral nuclei and a central caudal nucleus. Each lateral nucleus may be subdivided into dorsal, intermediate and ventral columns.

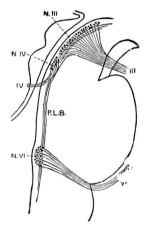

FIG. 262.—PLAN OF THE ORIGINS OF THE 3RD, 4TH, AND 6TH NERVES.

The nerves and their nuclei are projected into the outline of a median section of the mid-brain and pons. III = 3rd nerve. N.III = its nucleus. IV = 4th nerve. N.IV = its nucleus. P.L.B. = medial longitudinal bundle. VI = 6th nerve. N.VI = its nucleus.

(*From Quain's " Anatomy.*")

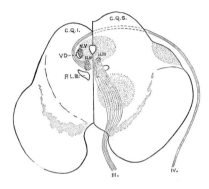

FIG. 263.—PLAN OF THE ORIGINS OF THE 3RD AND 4TH NERVES.

The mid-brain is supposed to be divided at different levels on the two sides, the section on the right side of the figure passing through the superior, and on the left side through the inferior, colliculus. III = 3rd nerve. N.III = its nucleus. IV = 4th nerve. N.IV = its nucleus. V.D. = mesencephalic root of the 5th nerve. N.V. = its nucleus. C.Q.S. = superior, and C.Q.I. = inferior, colliculus. P.L.B. = medial longitudinal bundle.

(*From Thane in Quain's " Anatomy.*")

2. Levator palpebræ superioris is supplied bilaterally from the central caudal nucleus. The superior rectus is suppled from the opposite lateral nucleus (intermediate column). The remaining muscles are supplied ipsilaterally as indicated in Fig. 265.

3. The antero-median and Edinger-Westphal nuclei are parasympathetic and supply the sphincter pupillæ and ciliary muscles, but it is still uncertain whether each muscle is supplied by one or both of these nuclei.

Course of the Fibres.—Whatever may be the truth about the organization of the nucleus the oculo-motor fibres pass in bundles with a lateral convexity through the medial longitudinal bundle, the tegmentum, the red nucleus, and the medial margin of subtantia nigra, to emerge from the sulcus oculo-motorius on the medial aspect of the basis pedunculi (Figs. 258 and 263). The bundles corresponding to the various muscles remain separate in the midbrain and for a little distance beyond the superficial origin of the nerve. Hence they may be affected separately.

Connections.—The third nucleus receives fibres from the superior colliculi viâ the tectobulbar tract, the occipital cortex, the frontal cortex of the opposite side, viâ the pyramidal tract, and the cerebellum viâ the superior peduncle. It sends fibres viâ the medial longitudinal bundle to the 4th, 6th, and 8th nerves of the same and opposite sides, and some which join the 7th, and are said eventually to supply the orbicularis oculi and frontalis. Hence these muscles escape in a supranuclear lesion of the facial. This is very doubtful.

Structure of the 3rd Nerve.—Like the 6th and 4th, the 3rd nerve is very large compared with the muscles it supplies. It contains about 24,000 fibres. Most of them are large, but some destined for the ciliary ganglion are small. Most of the fibres are motor, but some are sensory. Of the latter, some are derived from the 5th nerve, but others are proprioceptive, and can be demonstrated in the orbit, i.e. distal to the point where the branch of the trigeminal joins the 3rd (Sherrington and Tozer, 1910 and see p. 253).

The non-medullated fibres in the nerve were regarded by Boeke (1915, 1921) as sympathetic, but Woollard (but see p. 253) and others hold that they are proprioceptive in function and pass up to the mesencephalic nucleus of the trigeminal nerve.

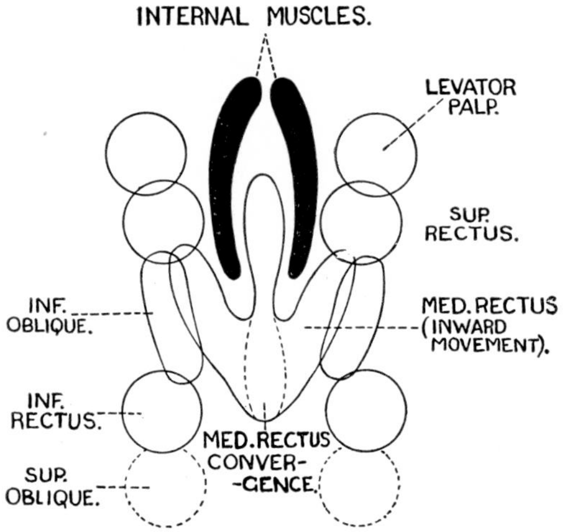

FIG. 264.—SCHEME OF THE 3RD NERVE NUCLEUS.

The portion that supplies the internal muscles is the nucleus of Edinger-Westphal. The median nucleus (of convergence) is the nucleus of Perlia.

(*After Brouwer and Zeeman.*)

Cross-sectional Anatomy.—The rootlets of origin of the 3rd nerve soon join to form a single cord which is surrounded by a thin perineurium and well-marked pial sheath (Fig. 267). On section a few fine interfunicular septa and also a number of small blood-vessels are seen.

Along its course the nerve is intersected by numerous thick irregular septa from the pia, which, however, bear no relation to the future branching. In the cavernous sinus the superior division may at times be seen forming a cap to the nerve; but there is no regular method by which the inferior division separates into its branches (Sunderland and Hughes).

Fuchs placed the pupillary fibres in the centre of the nerve, drawing attention to the fact that the intrinsic eye muscles often escaped involvement in a fracture of the base of the skull.

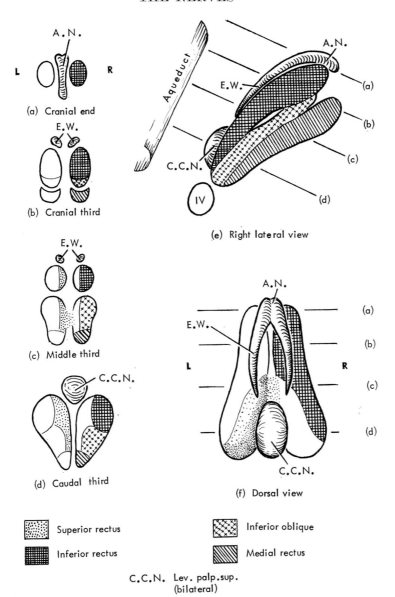

(a) Cranial end

(b) Cranial third

(c) Middle third

(d) Caudal third

(e) Right lateral view

(f) Dorsal view

Superior rectus

Inferior rectus

Inferior oblique

Medial rectus

C.C.N. Lev. palp.sup.
(bilateral)

Fig. 265.—The Oculo-Motor Nucleus of the Monkey (Modified, in conjunction with Professor R. Warwick, from his Original Diagrams in J. Comp. Neur., **98**, 480).

On the left, diagrams of sections of the nucleus at the levels indicated (a–d) on the right lateral and dorsal views. **A.N.**—antero-median nucleus. **E.W.**—Edinger-Westphal nucleus. **C.C.N.**—central caudal nucleus. The extrinsic muscles of the *right* orbit are innervated from the areas shown in the diagrams. The areas for superior rectus show some overlap in the middle third of the oculo-motor nucleus (? nucleus of Perlia).

Sunderland and Hughes (1946, *Brain*, **69,** 301), however, hold that the pupillo-constrictor fibres, which vary in diameter from 3 to 5 μ, are concentrated over the superior arc of the nerve from the cavernous sinus to the mid-brain, and may, therefore, be affected alone in pressure from above.

It should, however, be pointed out that fine medullated fibres are scattered through the cross-section of the nerve and that they also occur in the trochlear and abducens.

THE BLOOD-SUPPLY OF THE 3RD, 4TH, AND 6TH CRANIAL NERVES

All nerves are supplied with blood vessels, which are essential for their normal functioning.

The arteries supplying a nerve are derived from adjacent vessels which most often are of small size and only of moderate regularity of position. On reaching the nerve the nutrient artery breaks up into ascending and descending branches which anastomose in the epineurium with similar branches from other nutrient arteries. From such epineural vessels branches penetrate into the perineurium, where further anastomoses occur, and finally small vessels penetrate into the fasciculi and form there a rich longitudinally disposed capillary network which runs up and down the nerve in unbroken continuity. This intra-fascicular network is reinforced along its length by contributions from the various nutrient vessels which reach the epineurium, *but no part of the intra-fascicular plexus may be regarded as being dominated by any one nutrient artery.*

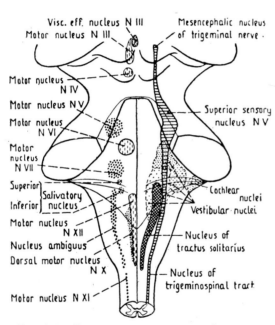

FIG. 266.—DIAGRAM INDICATING THE COLUMNAR ARRANGEMENT OF THE CRANIAL NERVE NUCLEI.

The nuclei belonging to the same categories are indicated by identical symbols.

(From Brodal after Herrick.)

Sympathetic nerve fibres, presumably vasomotor in function, accompany the arteries which supply the vessels (Durward in Cunningham's Anatomy).

The blood-supply to the oculo-motor (Fig. 267), trochlear, and abducens is built on the same principle as described above.[1] It is obvious (although not often men-

[1] But in the place of the epineurium is the pia.

tioned as a likely cause of ocular palsy) that deprivation of blood-supply to the nerves by spasm, thrombosis, or embolism may produce a palsy of the muscles supplied.

PRACTICAL CONSIDERATIONS

1. **Paralysis** of the 3rd nerve results in the following :

(a) Ptosis from paralysis of the levator.

(b) The eye looks laterally, due to overaction of the lateral rectus and superior oblique. Since the eye is in abduction, the depression due to the superior oblique is nil or minimal. There is inability to look upwards, downwards, or medially beyond the midline.

(c) There is wheel-rotation medially on asking the patient to follow the examining finger downwards and laterally (overaction of the superior oblique).

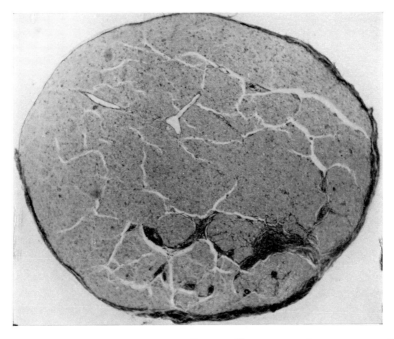

FIG. 267.—TRANSVERSE SECTION OF THE 3RD CRANIAL NERVE ABOUT ¾ INCH FROM ITS ORIGIN.

(d) The pupil is semi-dilated, from unopposed action of the sympathetic, and does not react to light or accommodation.

(e) Sometimes slight proptosis.

2. *The Syndrome of Weber* consists of a 3rd nerve palsy on the side of the lesion with a facial paralysis and hemiplegia of the opposite side. The facial palsy is of the upper motor neurone type, the upper part of the face being

spared. The syndrome is due to a mid-brain lesion, and involves the seventh fibres and those of the trunk and limbs before their crossing.

The Syndrome of Benedikt is like that of Weber, but the hemiplegia is associated with tremors. These may be due to involvement of the red nucleus.

3. It is of interest to note that the 3rd and 4th nerves are more commonly affected by pituitary enlargements than that weakling of the cranial nerves, namely the 6th, which is here protected by the internal carotid artery. A glance at Fig. 260 will explain this.

4. The 3rd nerve may be pressed on by hardening or an aneurism of any of the nearby arteries ; namely, the posterior cerebral, superior cerebellar, basilar, posterior communicating, and internal carotid.

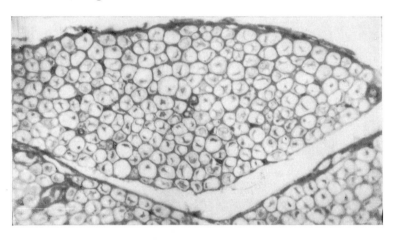

FIG. 268.—PORTION OF TRANSVERSE SECTION OF THE 3RD NERVE UNDER HIGHER POWER.

THE 4TH CRANIAL OR TROCHLEAR NERVE

The trochlear is the most slender of the cranial nerves and yet has the longest intracranial course (75 mm.).

Superficial Origin (Fig. 269).—After having crossed[1] from the opposite side in the superior medullary velum, which forms part of the roof of the 4th ventricle, the trochlear nerve leaves the upper part of this membrane by two or three rootlets medial to the superior cerebellar peduncle and just below the inferior colliculus. Its attachment to the velum is very delicate, and the smallest pull will often detach it from its origin.

It is the only motor nerve, cranial or spinal, which arises from the dorsal aspect of the central nervous system.

Relations.—(*a*) *In the Posterior Cranial Fossa.*—Surrounded by pia and bathed in cerebro-spinal fluid the nerve passes at first laterally behind the superior cerebellar peduncle. In this part of its course it is crossed from below upwards by

---

[1] So that the right nucleus supplies the left superior oblique and vice versa. See also p. 510.

the branch of the superior cerebellar artery to the inferior colliculus. It now runs forwards at the upper border of the pons between and parallel to the posterior cerebral and superior cerebellar arteries (Figs. 259 and 260). It appears on the ventral aspect of the brain, between the temporal lobe and the pons (Fig. 257). At first medial and below the free margin of the tentorium cerebelli, the 4th

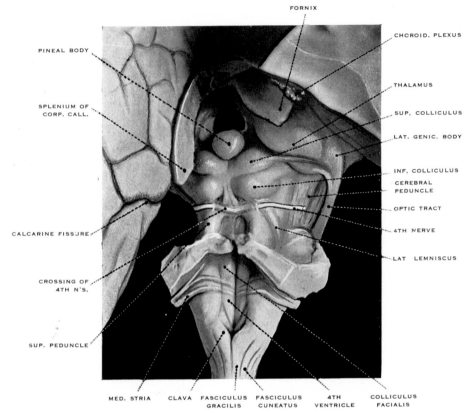

FORNIX

PINEAL BODY

CHOROID. PLEXUS

THALAMUS

SPLENIUM OF
CORP. CALL.

SUP. COLLICULUS

LAT. GENIC. BODY

INF. COLLICULUS

CEREBRAL
PEDUNCLE

OPTIC TRACT

CALCARINE FISSURE

4TH NERVE

LAT LEMNISCUS

CROSSING OF
4TH N'S.

SUP. PEDUNCLE

MED. STRIA   CLAVA   FASCICULUS   FASCICULUS   4TH   COLLICULUS
                     GRACILIS   CUNEATUS   VENTRICLE   FACIALIS

FIG. 269.—DISSECTION TO SHOW THE ORIGIN OF THE 4TH NERVE.
(*Wolff's preparation.*)

nerve soon comes to lie beneath and to be hidden by this membrane (Figs. 258, 316).

The 5th nerve, which takes origin from the lateral aspect of the pons just above its middle, passes forwards below and lateral to the 4th (Fig. 259).

The 3rd nerve is above and medial, but since its direction is downwards and forwards, and that of the 4th almost directly forwards, they approach each other as they proceed anteriorly, and as we shall see, eventually cross (Figs. 258, 259, 260).

Just before entering the middle cranial fossa by passing lateral to the dorsum sellæ and while still under cover of the free margin of the tentorium cerebelli the 4th nerve acquires a very short covering of arachnoid which it loses again where it pierces the dura.

(b) *In the Middle Cranial Fossa.*—The trochlear nerve pierces the dura in the lateral angle between the free and attached margins of the tentorium cerebelli, and then lies in the lateral wall of the cavernous sinus above and medial to the trigeminal ganglion and lateral to the pituitary fossa (Figs. 259, 260, 272).

Here the 3rd nerve is at first above and medial, but just before it enters the superior orbital (sphenoidal) fissure, the 4th nerve crosses it so as to be at first lateral, then above, then medial.

The first and second divisions of the 5th are below and lateral and, in the sinus itself, the 6th nerve and internal carotid artery are below and medial.

(c) *In the Superior Orbital (Sphenoidal) Fissure.*—The 4th nerve enters the orbit through the *wide* portion of the superior orbital (sphenoidal) fissure close to its upper border above the cone of muscles with the frontal and lacrimal nerves which are lateral to it and the ophthalmic vein which is below it (Figs. 261 and 272).

The 3rd, naso-ciliary and the 6th nerves and sometimes the ophthalmic vein pass through the fissure within the anulus of Zinn.

(d) *In the Orbit*, the 4th nerve leaves the frontal nerve, which is at first close to it, at an acute angle, and passes medially and forwards beneath the periorbita (periosteum) (Fig. 276) and above the levator and superior rectus (Fig. 277). It divides up in a fan-shaped manner into three or four branches which supply the *superior oblique* on its upper surface near the lateral border, the most anterior branch entering the muscle at the junction of the posterior and middle thirds, and the most posterior some 8 millimetres beyond its origin.

Nucleus and Connections

The 4th nerve nucleus lies in the dorsal part of the cerebral peduncle, deep to the upper part of the inferior colliculus, ventro-lateral to the aqueduct (of Sylvius) and dorsal to the medial longitudinal bundle with which it is in direct contact (Figs. 262, 263).

Like the 3rd nerve nucleus, which is continuous with it above, it represents the upward continuation of the base of the anterior horn of the spinal cord.

It consists of multipolar nerve cells some 40 to 50 μ in diameter.

From the nucleus the fourth fibres run first laterally to reach the medial surface of the mesencephalic root of the 5th nerve, then downwards parallel to the aqueduct, then at the lower border of the inferior colliculus they pass medially to decussate completely (or almost so) in the superior medullary velum. The 4th nerve thus crosses to the opposite side, and each superior oblique is supplied from the opposite fourth nucleus. The fibres emerge at the medial border of the superior cerebellar peduncle.

The connections are similar to those of the 3rd nerve.

Communications and Varieties.

1. While in the lateral wall of the cavernous sinus the 4th nerve is connected with the sympathetic on the carotid artery, and is joined by a filament probably containing proprioceptive fibres from the ophthalmic division of v.

2. In one case the 4th nerve pierced the levator on its way to the superior oblique (Thane).

3. The nerve has been observed in several cases sending a branch torward to the orbicularis oculi, or to join the supratrochlear, the infratrochlear, or the naso-ciliary nerve (Thane).

4. A communication with the frontal nerve is recorded by Berte (Thane).

Structure.—The 4th nerve consists of about 3,400 fibres, mostly of large size. (Björkman and Wohlfart). It also shows close to its origin the vestiges of a degenerated ganglion (Gaskell). See also structure of the 3rd nerve.

Practical Considerations

Paralysis of the 4th nerve produces palsy of the superior oblique. This results in :

(*a*) The greatest limitation of movement is seen when, in the adducted position, the patient is asked to look downwards. This is because the superior oblique is only depressor in the adducted position.

(*b*) The face is turned downwards and towards the sound side.

(*c*) Diplopia occurs on looking downwards, and is homonymous.

The false image is below, and its upper end is tilted towards the true image, i.e. in the direction of action of the paralysed muscle.

The Abducens or 6th Cranial Nerve

Superficial Origin.—The 6th cranial nerve emerges between the lower border of the pons and the lateral part of the pyramid by seven or eight rootlets, some of which may actually pierce the pons. Unlike the rootlets of the oculo-motor and trochlear nerves, which very soon join up to form a common trunk, those of the abducens join up at varying distances from their origin and some may remain separate (Fig. 243) till the nerve pierces the dura.

Course.—It passes upwards, forwards, and slightly laterally in the posterior cranial fossa to pierce the dura over the basiocciput ; then runs upwards under this membrane on the back of the petrous temporal near its apex, then forwards through the cavernous sinus. Finally it passes into the orbit through the superior orbital fissure within the anulus of Zinn to supply the lateral rectus muscle.

Relations.—(*a*) *At its Origin.*—The two 6th nerves are about 1 cm. apart at their superficial origin, and between them lies the basilar artery at its formation from the two vertebrals. Sometimes an asymmetrical vertebral artery may curve upwards and lie under the nerve. The origin of the 7th nerve to the lateral side of the olive is lateral (Figs. 256, 352, 353).

(*b*) *In the Posterior Cranial Fossa.*—The nerve, at first flat and fasciculated,

A.E.—19

soon becomes rounded and firmer. Covered by pia it passes upwards, forwards, and slightly laterally in the cisterna pontis of the subarachnoid space (Fig. 257) between the pons and the occipital bone (Fig. 260). After a course of 15 mm. it pierces the dura at the back of the basilar portion of the occipital bone about 2 cm.[1] below and slightly to the lateral side of the posterior clinoid process, and

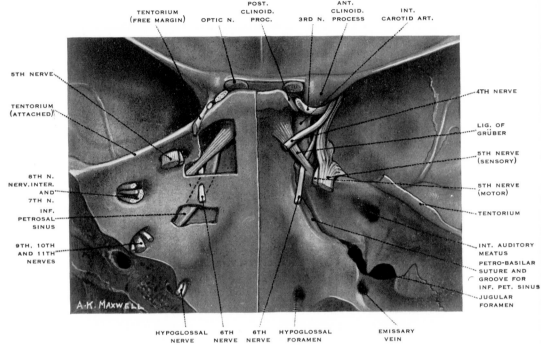

FIG. 270.—DISSECTION TO SHOW RELATIONS OF 6TH NERVE TO THE PETROUS TEMPORAL, INFERIOR PETROSAL SINUS, ETC.

On the right side the dura has been removed to show the bony relations.

(*Wolff's dissection.*)

just to the medial side of or posterior to the inferior petrosal sinus which lies in the petro-basilar suture (Fig. 270).

It is plastered to the pons by the arachnoid (Fig. 257), but does not receive a complete covering of this membrane till a few millimetres from the dural opening.

Just beyond its origin it is crossed by the anterior inferior cerebellar artery (Figs. 260, 271). Usually, i.e. in over four-fifths[2] of the cases, the artery is ventral, but it may be dorsal or pass between the rootlets of the nerve. The 3rd, 4th, and 5th nerves are above, but are gradually approaching the 6th as they pass forwards towards the middle cranial fossa.

[1] The spheno-basilar suture is about 1·5 cm. from the top of the dorsum sellæ (H. A. Harris). Hence the 6th nerve pierces the dura opposite the *occipital* bone.

[2] Stopford, J. S. B., (1915–16) *J. Anat. Physiol.*, **50,** and 1916–17, **51.**

Under the dura the 6th nerve crosses the inferior petrosal sinus from medial to lateral and runs almost vertically up the back of the petrous temporal near its apex. It is placed and held here in a groove [1] (which may be quite well marked, though not infrequently difficult to find). Having arrived at the sharp upper border of the bone, it bends [2] forwards practically at a right angle under the petrosphenoidal ligament of Grüber, and under the superior petrosal sinus to enter the cavernous sinus (Figs. 260, 270). The abducens nerve and the inferior petrosal sinus enter the sinus together by an opening which is known as Dorello's canal (Fig. 270). Very commonly the 6th nerve pierces the inferior petrosal sinus, inside which it then runs to enter the cavernous sinus.

(c) *In the Cavernous Sinus.*—In the cavernous sinus the 6th nerve runs almost horizontally forwards. In the posterior part of the sinus the nerve winds round the lateral aspect of the ascending portion of the internal carotid artery, thus making a *second* bend,[3] this time, however, with a lateral convexity (Fig. 270).

—ARACHNOID

SUB. ARACH. TRAB.

—ARTERY

—ABDUCENS

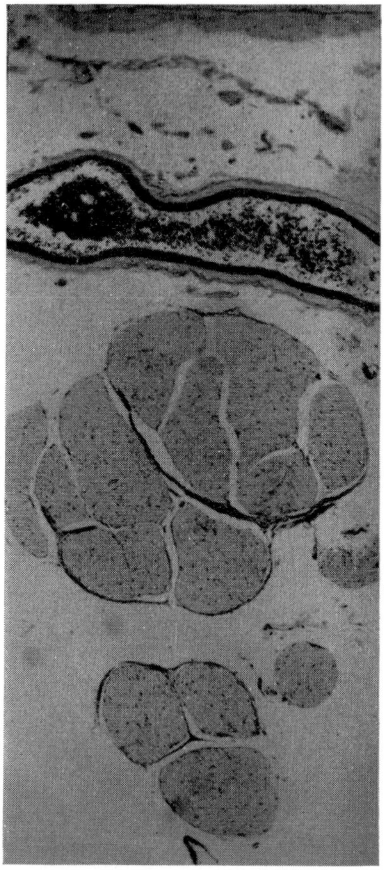

FIG. 271.—RELATION OF 6TH NERVE TO ARACHNOID AND ANTERIOR-INFERIOR CEREBELLAR ARTERY.

Note 6th nerve has not united to form one trunk.

Farther forwards the abducens lies below and lateral to the horizontal portion of the artery (Figs. 260, 366).

The carotid is here surrounded by a sympathetic plexus, which sends branches of communication to the 6th nerve (Fig. 260).

In the lateral wall of the sinus from above down are the third, fourth, and first and second divisions of the 5th nerves (Fig. 366).

Usually the 6th nerve lies actually in the sinus surrounded by a separate

[1] Hovelacque, *Nerfs Craniens, Paris,* 108.

[2] See Wolff (1928) *Brit. J. Ophthal.,* **12,** 22.

[3] This second bend varies greatly. It may be very slight, the ascending portion of the internal carotid just pushing the nerve slightly laterally, or it may (as Wolff saw in one case) approach the right angle.

sheath, but it may be adherent to the lateral wall or attached to it by a septum of fibrous dura mater.

Outside the lateral wall of the sinus is the trigeminal ganglion (Figs. 270, 272).

(d) *In the Superior Orbital Fissure.*—The 6th nerve is placed here within the anulus of Zinn, at first below the two divisions of the 3rd nerve, then lateral and in between the two. The naso-ciliary is medial (Fig. 261).

(e) *In the Orbit.*—The nerve divides into three or four filaments which enter the ocular surface of the lateral rectus muscle just behind its middle.

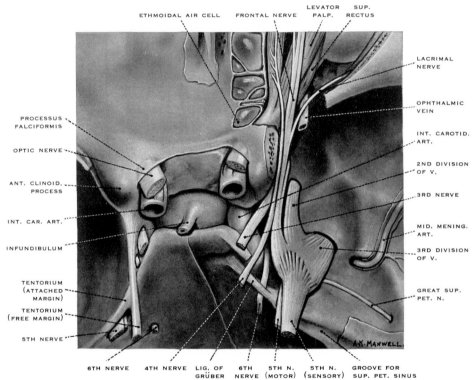

FIG. 272.—DISSECTION TO SHOW NERVES PASSING FROM MIDDLE CRANIAL FOSSA INTO ORBIT.
(*Wolff's preparation.*)

Communications.

From (a) *The Sympathetic* in the cavernous sinus. (b) *From the Ophthalmic* just before entering the orbit.

Variations.

(a) The 6th nerve may arise in two parts, which may remain separate to the superior orbital fissure.

(b) The nerve or part of it may pass above the petro-clinoid ligament of Grüber.

(c) It may give a branch to the ciliary ganglion (Pourfour du Petit).

(d) The nasociliary nerve may be a branch of the 6th (Krause).

(e) The 6th nerve may be absent (Generali), its work being done by the 3rd.

Nucleus and Central Connections

The nucleus of the 6th nerve is a small spherical mass consisting of large multipolar cells lying close to the mid-line in the tegmental portion of the pons under cover of the *colliculus facialis*. This is an elevation in the floor of the fourth ventricle, which is produced by the bend of the fibres of the 7th nerve (Figs. 269 and 290). The nucleus of the abducens is separated from the median plane by the medial longitudinal bundle, which is thus ventro-medial (while it is ventro-lateral to the nucleus of the oculomotor and ventral to that of the trochlear).

The fibres pass forwards through the whole length of the pons, first medial to the corpus trapezoideum, then lateral to the pyramid, some fibres passing through the latter (Figs. 262, 290).

Connections.—Some axons go from the nucleus of the 6th (or as is much more probable from an intercalated neurone in the medial longitudinal bundle) into the medial longitudinal bundle to the 3rd nerve nucleus of the opposite side ; they are concerned with conjugate movements of the eyes, one lateral rectus working with the medial rectus of the opposite side. The following[1] is the probable course of the supranuclear fibres for conjugate movement of the globes. Arising from the cortical centres in the frontal lobe the fibres pass in the anterior limb of the internal capsule, and occupy a medial position in the cerebral peduncle. They cannot be traced farther than the upper part of the pons, but the probability is that they find their way through the tegmentum to the nucleus of the 6th cranial nerve. The 6th nucleus is connected with the other motor nuclei of the brain stem through the medial longitudinal bundle.

The abducens nucleus is also connected to the corpus trapezoideum, bringing it into relation with hearing, to the vestibular nucleus, which makes a communication with the vestibular apparatus; with the visual pathway viâ the superior colliculus and tectobulbar tract.

Structure.—The nerve contains some 6 to 7 thousand fibres as it leaves the brain stem (Björkman and Wohlfart, 1936).

Some Practical Considerations

1. Division of the 6th nerve results in paralysis of the lateral rectus muscle. There is internal strabismus. The eye *can* move to the middle of the palpebral fissure, but no farther. The diplopia is homonymous, and is worse on looking towards the affected side.

2. Fractures of the base of the skull are very liable to involve the 6th nerve owing to its contact with the basi-occiput and the apex of the petrous temporal bone.

3. Paralysis of the 6th nerve alone has no localising value. The abducens is, in fact, the weakling of the cranial nerves, and may be affected in almost any

[1] Head, *Trans. Ophthal. Soc. U.K.*, **18**, 395.

type of cerebral lesion, whether near *or at a distance* from the nerve. Many theories have been evoked to account for this :

(*a*) Collier [1] thought that it was due to the shifting *backwards* of the brain stem. Those nerves whose direction was most nearly fronto-caudal would be involved before the others.

Thus the 6th would be the first, then the 3rd, and lastly the 7th and 8th.

But if this were true the frailer 4th nerve, with its longer antero-posterior course, ought to be first affected. It is suggested that it is protected by the free margin of the tentorium cerebelli, in which it lies for a part of its course, an explanation that will hardly hold for an antero-posterior pull.

(*b*) Cushing [2] showed that the anterior inferior cerebellar artery when it ran ventral to the 6th nerve [3] (a relation present in 86 per cent. on the right side and 81 per cent. on the left) might, as a result of increased intracranial pressure, press on and groove the nerve and the underlying pons, and thus produce a lateral rectus palsy.

(*c*) The author [4] suggested that the important factor was the bend over the sharp apex of the petrous temporal. If we consider a tumour in any position in the cranium there will come a time when, owing to the increase of intracranial pressure, the brain will be forced to its largest outlet—the foramen magnum— and foraminal herniation ensue. As a result of this the medulla and pons will tend to move *downwards*. Now the 6th nerve is fixed to the pons and more or less held in the cavernous sinus. It will therefore be pressed against the sharp upper border of the petrous temporal, with resulting interruption of conduction and palsy of the lateral rectus. Blows on the vault of the skull, quite apart from those which are complicated by basal fractures involving the apex of the petrous temporal, will also tend to force the hind brain downwards, with resulting tension in the 6th nerve. A similar condition of movement towards the foramen magnum will follow compression of the skull in difficult labour with or without forceps, and probably explains the 6th nerve birth palsy.

4. *Gradenigo's Syndrome.*—A palsy of the 6th nerve and severe unilateral headache in suppurative middle-ear disease. The 6th nerve and the trigeminal are involved at the apex of the petrous temporal by direct spread of infection, usually through a pneumatic condition of the bone.

5. An abducens and facial palsy existing together suggest a lesion of the floor of the 4th ventricle—where the fibres of the seventh cross the nucleus of the 6th.

The Syndrome of Millard-Gübler consists of a facial and sixth palsy of the same side as the lesion with a hemiplegia of the opposite side. The facial palsy is of the lower motor neurone type, i.e. involves the whole nerve. The syndrome is due to a bulbo-pontine lesion.

[1] Collier, J., (1904) *Brain*, **27**, 490. [2] Cushing, Harvey, (1910–11) *Brain*, **32**.
[3] Stopford, see p. 384. [4] E. Wolff (1928) *Brit. J. Ophthal.*, **12**, 22.

6. According to Gray, division of the 6th nerve results at times in ptosis and small pupil owing to the sympathetic fibres it contains.

7. Conjugate [1] deviation of the eyes may be due to an *irritative* lesion of the supranuclear fibres, or a *paralytic* lesion of the sixth nucleus [2] or its connection

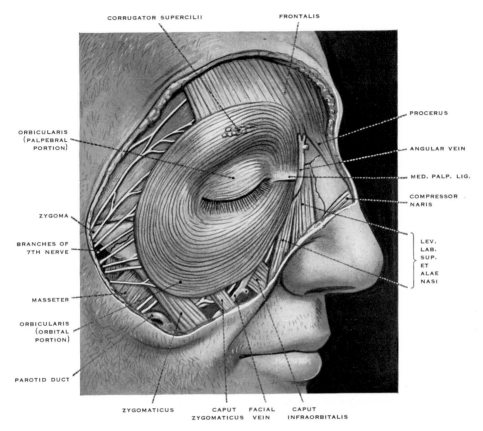

FIG. 273.—DISSECTION OF ORBIT FROM IN FRONT.
Stage 1. Orbicularis oculi.
(*Wolff's dissection.*)

with the 3rd nerve of the opposite side.   In the former case the eyes are forcibly turned to one or other side from tonic spasm of the associated muscles, in the latter the patient is unable to turn the eyes to one or other side owing to paralysis of the associated mechanisms.

Thus in a cortical hæmorrhage the eyes look towards the side of the lesion in

[1] See Head, in Albutt's *System of Medicine*, **6,** 782.

[2] As stated on p. 293, it is much more probable that the fibres which go to the opposite third nucleus arise not in the sixth nucleus but in an intercalated neurone situated in the medial longitudinal bundle above it.

the brain. In a pontine hæmorrhage involving the nucleus of the 6th the patient cannot look towards the side of the lesion, and often has an associated palsy of the facial nerve of the lower motor neurone type on the same side.

THE 5TH CRANIAL OR TRIGEMINAL NERVE

The trigeminal, the largest of the cranial nerves, resembles a typical spinal nerve : it has two roots, sensory and motor, and further, on the sensory root, there is a large ganglion.

Superficial Origin.—The two portions of the 5th nerve arise close together, somewhat above the middle of the lateral surface of the pons. The sensory portion is much larger than the motor, which is placed above and medial to its companion (Figs. 256 and 259).

Course and Relations.—The two portions of the trigeminal pass almost directly forwards, with only a very slight inclination upwards in the posterior cranial fossa towards a notch at the upper border of the petrous temporal, which they reach after a course of about 1 cm. They are surrounded by separate sheaths of pia but enclosed in a common covering of arachnoid which accompanies them to the ganglion. Princeteau has shown that the arachnoid is reflected on to the two roots; but is at first some distance from them, a complete sheath only being formed a few millimetres behind the apex of the petrous temporal. Its relation to the nerve is in fact that of the canvas of a bell-tent to its centre pole (Fig. 257).

The 7th, 8th and nervus intermedius are *below* and diverging towards the internal acoustic (auditory) meatus. *Above* is the cerebellum, the free margin of the tentorium cerebelli, with the 4th nerve close under it.

The 6th nerve, which is at its origin some distance (about $1\frac{1}{2}$ cm.) below and medial to the 5th, gradually approaches it, and comes to lie quite close to its medial side at the apex of the petrous temporal (Fig. 270).

The 5th nerve pierces[1] the dura under the attached margin of the tentorium cerebelli which contains the superior petrosal sinus, and having spread out in a plexiform manner, joins the posterior concave border of the trigeminal (Gasserian) ganglion (Figs. 270, 272).

The Trigeminal (Gasserian) Ganglion is the sensory ganglion of the 5th nerve, corresponding and having a similar structure to the posterior root ganglion of the spinal nerves. It is also liable to the same affections.[2] It is somewhat crescentic or, better, bean-shaped in appearance, the hilum being directed backwards. The ganglion is some 4 cm. medial to a point just above the articular tubercle at the root of the zygoma. It lies in a bony fossa on the front

---

[1] It thus passes through a sort of foramen formed partly by the notch in the sharp upper border of the petrous temporal and partly by the attached margin of the tentorium, which bridges over it Fig. 270).

[2] Notably ganglionitis, producing shingles or herpes.

of the apex of the petrous temporal, and below this covers that part of the foramen lacerum which overlies the internal carotid artery and greater petrosal nerve.

It is enclosed in a sheath of dura mater prolonged from that of the posterior cranial fossa, which loosely invests the two roots and extends forwards to fuse with the anterior half of the ganglion. This sheath of dura is the cavum trigeminale

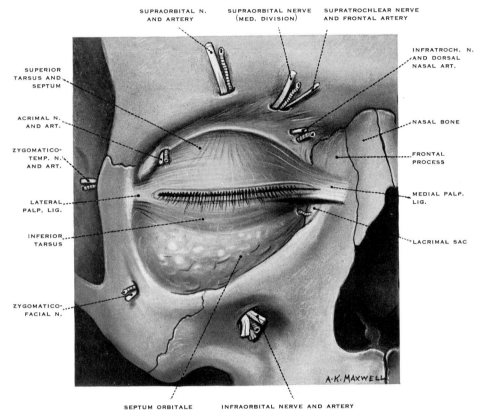

FIG. 274.—DISSECTION OF ORBIT FROM IN FRONT.

Stage 2. Orbicularis removed to show septum orbitale.

(*Wolff's dissection.*)

(Meckel's cave). The dura is lined with arachnoid, so the sensory and motor roots and the posterior half of the ganglion are bathed in cerebrospinal fluid. The sheath of dura (i.e. the cave) lies between the fibrous and endosteal layers of the dura mater of the middle cranial fossa.

To its *lateral side* the ganglion has the foramen spinosum, transmitting the middle meningeal artery, which is, therefore, *an obstruction in approaching it by the temporal route.* To its *medial side* is the cavernous sinus, the internal carotid artery, and the 3rd, 4th, and 6th nerves (Figs. 259 and 260). To the medial side of these again is the pituitary body.

Above the ganglion is the uncus and temporo-sphenoidal lobe, *deep* to it are the greater and lesser (superficial) petrosal nerves, the *motor root of the 5th* and, as has been said before, the internal carotid artery.

After extradural approach to the ganglion across the middle fossa there sometimes results a *facial* paralysis. This is due to pulling on the greater (superficial) petrosal nerve, producing trauma at the geniculate ganglion. Resultant œdema of the ganglion, or interference with the blood supply, blocks the facial nerve. The palsy is transient, and recovery complete.

The Motor Portion of the 5th nerve has no connection with the ganglion, but lies on its deep surface, crossing from the medial to the lateral side to join the third division of the trigeminal.

The posterior border of the ganglion is concave, and receives the expanded sensory root. From its anterior convex border the three divisions of the 5th nerve are given off, namely :

The first or ophthalmic ;

The second or maxillary ; and

The third or mandibular.

Apart from these branches the ganglion receives communications from the sympathetic round the internal carotid artery and from its posterior part a few filaments pass to the dura.

Small *accessory ganglia* may be found along the concave border of the trigeminal ganglion corresponding to the accessory ganglia found on the posterior root between the posterior root ganglion and the spinal cord.

THE OPHTHALMIC NERVE

The Ophthalmic Nerve, the smallest of the three divisions of the trigeminal, comes off the medial and upper part of the convex anterior border of the trigeminal ganglion.

It runs forwards in the lateral wall of the cavernous sinus enclosed in a separate sheath of dura. Hence it is necessary to incise the dura of the lateral wall of the sinus and *then* the proper sheath of the nerve before it is exposed (Hovelacque). The 3rd and 4th nerves are above it, the internal carotid artery and 6th nerve medial, and the maxillary nerve below and lateral.

After a course of about 1 in. (2·5 cm.) it divides, just behind the superior orbital (sphenoidal) fissure into three branches, *lacrimal, frontal,* and *nasociliary,* which pass through the fissure to enter the orbit.

Communications.—*In the cavernous sinus* it is joined by branches of communication from the 3rd, 4th, and 6th nerves (probably proprioceptive) and from the sympathetic round the internal carotid artery. It also sends a *recurrent* branch (the nervus tentorii of Arnold) to the supratentorial dura mater (Figs. 282, 316). This nerve comes off near the origin of the ophthalmic and passes backwards to cross the 4th. It is usually closely adherent to this nerve, and not infrequently passes through it (hence it has been described as a branch of the trochlear) to reach the tentorium.

The Lacrimal Nerve, the smallest of the three terminal branches of the ophthalmic, arises in the anterior part of the middle cranial fossa.

It passes through the *wide* portion of the superior orbital (sphenoidal) fissure above the anulus of Zinn to the lateral side of the frontal and 4th nerves and above and medial to the ophthalmic vein. In the orbit the nerve runs laterally

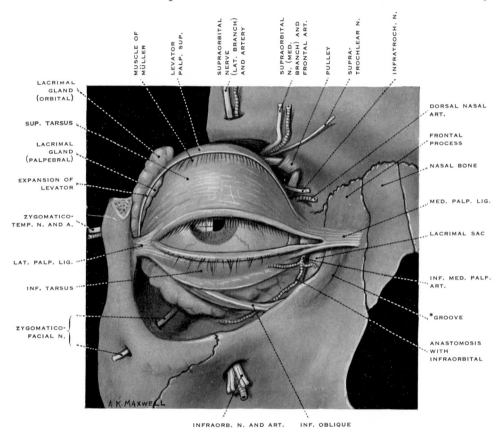

The groove on the frontal process of the maxilla (not the sutura notha) is marked to draw attention to its presence as it is liable to be mistaken for the lacrimal fossa in exposing the lacrimal sac.

FIG. 275.—DISSECTION OF ORBIT FROM IN FRONT.
Stage 3. Septum removed.
(*Wolff's dissection.*)

parallel to and close in front of the narrow portion of the superior orbital fissure, then forwards [1] along or just lateral to the upper border of the lateral rectus muscle to reach the lacrimal gland. In the last portion of its course, i.e. for the distal two-thirds of its relation with the lateral rectus, it is accompanied by the lacrimal artery (Fig. 277).

[1] The course of the lacrimal nerve is well described by the expression " en baïonnette," that is following the shape of the old-fashioned bayonet ⌐ (Hovelacque and Reinhold). (Fig. 282.)

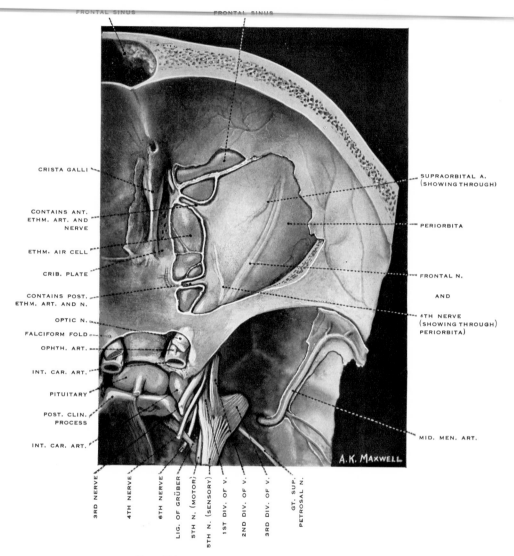

FRONTAL SINUS   FRONTAL SINUS

CRISTA GALLI

CONTAINS ANT.
ETHM. ART. AND
NERVE

ETHM. AIR CELL

CRIB. PLATE

CONTAINS POST.
ETHM. ART. AND N.

OPTIC N.

FALCIFORM FOLD

OPHTH. ART.

INT. CAR. ART.

PITUITARY

POST. CLIN.
PROCESS

INT. CAR. ART.

SUPRAORBITAL A.
(SHOWING THROUGH)

PERIORBITA

FRONTAL N.

AND

4TH NERVE
(SHOWING THROUGH)
PERIORBITA)

MID. MEN. ART.

A. K. MAXWELL

3RD NERVE
4TH NERVE
6TH NERVE
LIG. OF GRÜBER
5TH N. (MOTOR)
5TH N. (SENSORY)
1ST DIV. OF V.
2ND DIV. OF V.
3RD DIV. OF V.
GT. SUP.
PETROSAL N.

Fig. 276.—Dissection of Orbit from Above.
Stage 1.   To show the periorbita, the roof has been removed.
(*Wolff's dissection.*)

Just before reaching the gland the nerve receives an anastomotic twig from the zygomatic nerve (Fig. 281) ; then, having passed through the gland to which it sends branches, it supplies the conjunctiva and the skin of the lateral part of the upper lid, which it reaches by piercing the septum orbitale.

The Frontal Nerve, the largest of the three branches of the ophthalmic, arises in the

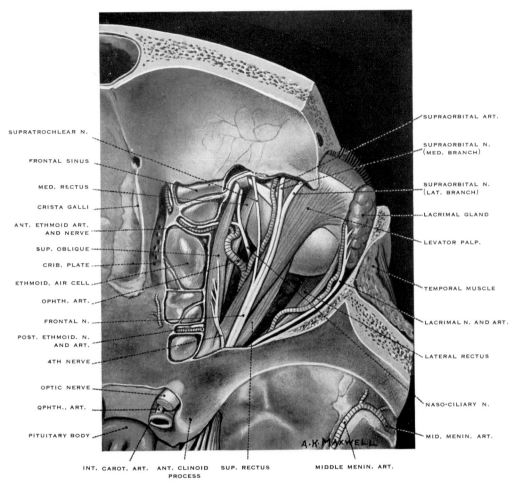

SUPRATROCHLEAR N.

FRONTAL SINUS

MED. RECTUS

CRISTA GALLI

ANT. ETHMOID ART.
AND NERVE

SUP. OBLIQUE

CRIB. PLATE

ETHMOID, AIR CELL

OPHTH. ART.

FRONTAL N.

POST. ETHMOID. N.
AND ART.

4TH NERVE

OPTIC NERVE

QPHTH., ART.

PITUITARY BODY

INT. CAROT. ART. ANT. CLINOID SUP. RECTUS
PROCESS

MIDDLE MENIN. ART.

SUPRAORBITAL ART.

SUPRAORBITAL N.
(MED. BRANCH)

SUPRAORBITAL N.
(LAT. BRANCH)

LACRIMAL GLAND

LEVATOR PALP.

TEMPORAL MUSCLE

LACRIMAL N. AND ART.

LATERAL RECTUS

NASO-CILIARY N.

MID. MENIN. ART.

A.K MAXWELL

FIG. 277.—DISSECTION OF ORBIT FROM ABOVE.

Stage 2.   Periorbita removed.

(*Wolff's dissection.*)

cavernous sinus just behind the superior orbital fissure through which it enters the orbit.

In the fissure it is placed above the anulus of Zinn between the lacrimal and the trochlear.

It runs almost directly forwards under the periosteum (periorbita) and on the levator palpebræ superioris.

Towards the front of the orbit it divides into *supratrochlear* and *supraorbital branches*.   In the specimen drawn in Fig. 277 the division is unusually far back.

The Supratrochlear Nerve (Fig. 277), much smaller than the supraorbital,

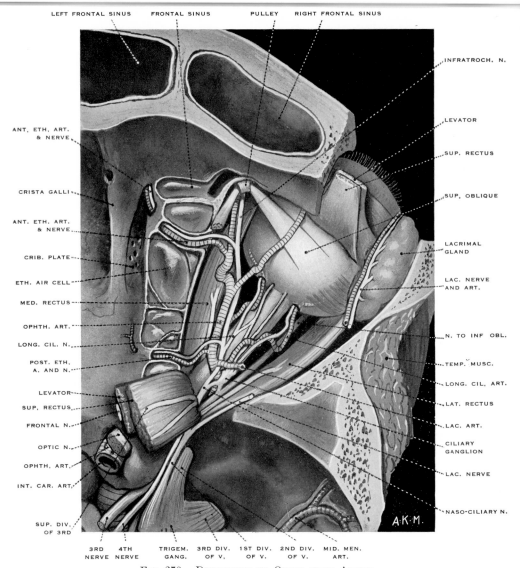

LEFT FRONTAL SINUS   FRONTAL SINUS   PULLEY   RIGHT FRONTAL SINUS

INFRATROCH. N.

LEVATOR

ANT. ETH. ART.
& NERVE

SUP. RECTUS

SUP. OBLIQUE

CRISTA GALLI

ANT. ETH. ART.
& NERVE

LACRIMAL
GLAND

CRIB. PLATE

LAC. NERVE
AND ART.

ETH. AIR CELL

MED. RECTUS

N. TO INF OBL.

OPHTH. ART.

LONG. CIL. N.

TEMP. MUSC.

POST. ETH.
A. AND N.

LONG. CIL. ART.

LEVATOR

LAT. RECTUS

SUP. RECTUS

LAC. ART.

FRONTAL N.

OPTIC N.

CILIARY
GANGLION

OPHTH. ART.

LAC. NERVE

INT. CAR. ART.

NASO-CILIARY N.

A·K·M·

SUP. DIV.
OF 3RD

3RD   4TH   TRIGEM.   3RD DIV. 1ST DIV. 2ND DIV. MID. MEN.
NERVE   NERVE   GANG.   OF V.   OF V.   OF V.   ART.

FIG. 278.—DISSECTION OF ORBIT FROM ABOVE.

Stage 3.   Levator and superior rectus reflected.

(*Wolff's dissection.*)

runs forwards to pass above the pulley of the superior oblique near which it sends a twig of communication to the *infratrochlear* branch of the naso-ciliary.

In company with the supratrochlear artery, and under cover of the orbicularis and the corrugator supercilii, the supratrochlear curls up over the orbital margin about ½ in. (1·25 cm.) from the mid-line. It sends branches of supply to the skin of the forehead and to the upper lid and conjunctiva.

The Supraorbital Nerve, much the larger of the terminal branches of the frontal, continues the direction of the parent nerve. It lies on the levator with the supraorbital artery medial, and leaves the orbit in company with this vessel by the supraorbital notch or foramen (Figs. 274, 275).

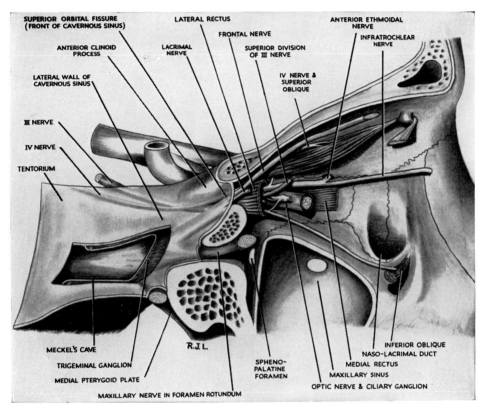

SUPERIOR ORBITAL FISSURE
(FRONT OF CAVERNOUS SINUS)
LATERAL RECTUS
ANTERIOR ETHMOIDAL NERVE
FRONTAL NERVE
INFRATROCHLEAR NERVE
ANTERIOR CLINOID PROCESS
LACRIMAL NERVE
SUPERIOR DIVISION OF III NERVE
LATERAL WALL OF CAVERNOUS SINUS
IV NERVE & SUPERIOR OBLIQUE
III NERVE
IV NERVE
TENTORIUM
MECKEL'S CAVE
R.J.L.
INFERIOR OBLIQUE
NASO-LACRIMAL DUCT
TRIGEMINAL GANGLION
SPHENO-PALATINE FORAMEN
MEDIAL RECTUS
MEDIAL PTERYGOID PLATE
MAXILLARY SINUS
OPTIC NERVE & CILIARY GANGLION
MAXILLARY NERVE IN FORAMEN ROTUNDUM

FIG. 279.—A LONGITUDINAL SECTION THROUGH THE RIGHT ORBIT AND MIDDLE CRANIAL FOSSA VIEWED FROM THE LATERAL SIDE. (From Last's "Anatomy, Regional and Applied," by permission).

(*J. & A. Churchill Ltd.*)

Occasionally the nerve divides within the orbit into medial and lateral branches (Fig. 277). The lateral branch then occupies the supraorbital notch, and the medial passes out of the orbit about midway between the pulley of the superior oblique and the supraorbital notch. Usually it has a notch (frontal notch of Henle) or rarely a foramen of its own.

The supraorbital nerve breaks up into branches which inosculate with each other and supply the forehead and scalp to the vertex or even farther back, the upper eyelid, and the conjunctiva. Those to the *scalp* run up on the bone (sometimes grooving it) under the orbicularis and frontalis, which they pierce at intervals. Those to the upper lid pass through the orbicularis. The nerve also sends a twig to the diploë and frontal sinus viâ a small aperture in the floor of the supraorbital notch.

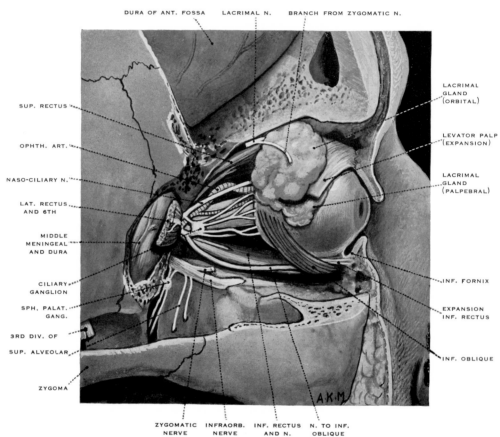

FIG. 280.—DISSECTION OF THE RIGHT ORBIT FROM THE LATERAL SIDE.
(*Wolff's preparation.*)

The Naso-ciliary Nerve arises from the medial and lower part of the ophthalmic, being as a rule the first of the three terminal branches to be given off. Intermediate in size between the lacrimal and frontal, it lies at first in the lateral wall of the *cavernous sinus*. It passes through the *superior orbital (sphenoidal) fissure* within the anulus of Zinn, between the two divisions of the 3rd nerve close to the *sympathetic root* of the ciliary ganglion, which is below and medial.

In the *orbit* it inclines medially, with the ophthalmic artery above the optic nerve, in front of the superior division of the 3rd nerve (Fig. 278), and below the superior rectus muscle. Near the anterior ethmoidal foramen it divides into its two terminal branches, the anterior ethmoidal and infratrochlear.

Branches.—(*a*) *The Long or Sensory Root of the Ciliary Ganglion* is given off in or just in front of the superior orbital (sphenoidal) fissure. It is a slender nerve about $\frac{1}{4}$ in. to $\frac{1}{2}$ in. (·6–1·25 cm.) long, which passes along the lateral side

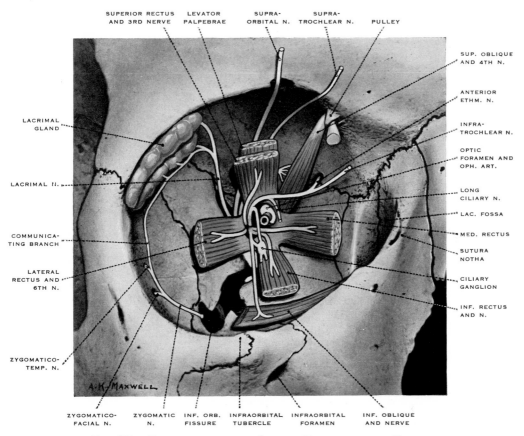

SUPERIOR RECTUS AND 3RD NERVE — LEVATOR PALPEBRAE — SUPRA-ORBITAL N. — SUPRA-TROCHLEAR N. — PULLEY

SUP. OBLIQUE AND 4TH N.

ANTERIOR ETHM. N.

LACRIMAL GLAND

INFRA-TROCHLEAR N.

OPTIC FORAMEN AND OPH. ART.

LACRIMAL N.

LONG CILIARY N.

LAC. FOSSA

COMMUNICA-TING BRANCH

MED. RECTUS

SUTURA NOTHA

LATERAL RECTUS AND 6TH N.

CILIARY GANGLION

INF. RECTUS AND N.

ZYGOMATICO-TEMP. N.

A.K. MAXWELL

ZYGOMATICO-FACIAL N. — ZYGOMATIC N. — INF. ORB. FISSURE — INFRAORBITAL TUBERCLE — INFRAORBITAL FORAMEN — INF. OBLIQUE AND NERVE

FIG. 281.—DISSECTION TO SHOW ORBITAL NERVES FROM IN FRONT.
(*Based on Wolff's dissections.*)

of the optic nerve to reach the upper and posterior part of the ganglion (Figs. 278, 280)

(*b*) *The Long Ciliary Nerves*, two in number, come off as the naso-ciliary crosses the optic nerve, to the medial side of which they come to lie. They run with the short ciliaries, pierce the sclera (Fig. 85), and passing between this and the choroid (Fig. 42), supply *sensory* fibres to the *iris, cornea*, and *ciliary muscle* and *dilatator* fibres to the *pupil* (see p. 91).

(*c*) *The Posterior Ethmoidal Nerve* passes between the superior oblique and

A.E.—20

medial rectus and enters the posterior ethmoidal foramen with its accompanying artery, and supplies the sphenoidal sinus and posterior ethmoidal air-cells.

(d) *The Infratrochlear Nerve* (Figs. 275, 278) is given off as a terminal branch of the naso-ciliary. It runs forward near the lower border of the superior oblique and passes below the pulley of this muscle, near which it gets a communication from the supratrochlear to appear on the face.

It breaks up into its branches, which supply the skin and conjunctiva round the medial angle of the eye, the root of the nose, the lacrimal sac and canaliculi, and the caruncle. It inosculates with the supraorbital and infraorbital nerves.

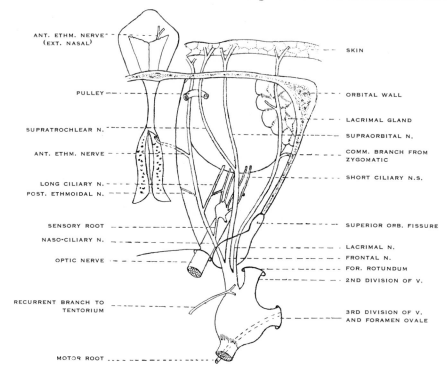

Fig. 282.—Diagram of the First Division of the 5th Nerve (L.W.).

(e) *The Anterior Ethmoidal Nerve* passes between the superior oblique and medial rectus to leave the orbit with the anterior ethmoidal artery by the anterior ethmoidal canal, which lies between the frontal and ethmoid bones. Here it supplies the middle and anterior ethmoidal air-cells and the infundibulum of the frontal sinus. It enters the *anterior cranial fossa* at the side of the cribriform plate of the ethmoid. Inclining medially it passes between the two layers of dura mater to the *nasal slit*, alongside the crista galli. In this part of its course it lies partly under or entirely in front of the olfactory bulb (Fig. 287) but separated from it by dura.

Traversing the nasal slit the nerve reaches the roof of the nose, where it gives *lateral nasal* branches to the upper and anterior quadrant of the lateral wall, and *medial nasal* branches to the anterior part of the septum. The nerve next lies in a groove (Figs. 12 and 287) on the posterior surface of the nasal bone, which it notches to appear on the face as the *external nasal nerve*. This supplies the skin over the cartilaginous part of the nose, down to the tip.

Varieties.—Absence of the infratrochlear nerve has been noted (Testut), its place being taken by the supratrochlear. Branches have been seen passing from the anterior ethmoidal to the levator (Fäsebeck) ; to the 3rd and 6th nerves (Switzer) ; to the mucous membrane of the frontal sinus, as the nerve lies in the anterior ethmoidal canal (Meckel and Langenbeck).

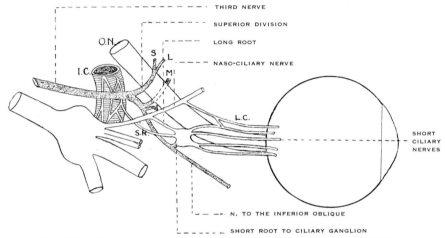

FIG. 283.—SCHEME OF THE 3RD NERVE AND CILIARY GANGLION (L.W.).

O.N. = optic nerve.   I.C. = internal carotid artery.   S = nerve to superior rectus.   L = nerve to levator.   M = nerve to medial rectus.   I = nerve to inferior rectus.   L.C. = long ciliary nerve. S.R. = sympathetic root.

(*After Cuneo.*)

The Naso-ciliary Nerve, *either directly through the long ciliaries or indirectly through the short ciliaries, is the sensory nerve to the whole eyeball.*

Thus there is good anatomical ground for the statement that if the naso-ciliary branch of the ophthalmic (division of the trigeminal) is involved in Herpes ophthalmicus the eye is usually affected as well.

THE CILIARY GANGLION

The ciliary ganglion is most easily found by first isolating the nerve to the inferior oblique. This can be done by exposing the inferior oblique from in front ; then it is quite easy to see the nerve as it crosses the middle of the posterior border. By pulling gently on the nerve it can readily be identified behind the globe and so leads one to the ciliary ganglion.

The Ciliary Ganglion is a small reddish-grey somewhat quadrilateral body about the size of a pin's head (2 mm. in antero-posterior and 1 mm. in vertical diameter), situated at the posterior part of the orbit about 1 cm. from the optic foramen between the optic nerve and the lateral rectus muscle. It is in close contact with the nerve, but separated from the muscle by some loose fat. Usually also it is close to the ophthalmic artery (Figs. 278, 279).

CAPSULE

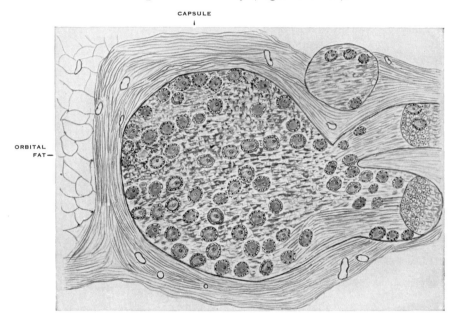

ORBITAL FAT —

FIG. 284.—SECTION OF THE CILIARY GANGLION (MALLORY'S PHOSPHOTUNG. HÆM.)
SLIGHTLY SCHEMATISED.

Note that the ganglion cells are also found in the branches of the ganglion.
(*Wolff's preparation.*)

It receives posteriorly three roots (Fig. 283) :
(1) The long or sensory root ;
(2) The short or motor root ;
(3) The sympathetic root.

(1) *The Long or Sensory Root* comes from the naso-ciliary, and is given off just after that nerve has entered the orbit. It is a slender nerve about 6 to 12 mm. long, which passes along the lateral side of the optic nerve to reach the upper and posterior part of the ganglion. It contains sensory fibres from the *cornea, iris,* and *ciliary body,* and possibly (from the sympathetic fibres which often join it) dilator fibres to the pupil.

(2) *The Short or Motor Root* comes from the nerve to the inferior oblique a few millimetres beyond the point where the nerve arises from the inferior division of the oculo-motor, much thicker than the sensory root, only about 1 to 2 mm. long, and passes upwards and forwards to enter the postero-inferior angle of the ganglion.

It carries the fibres of supply to the sphincter pupillæ and the ciliary muscle. These synapse in the ganglion.

(3) *The Sympathetic Root* comes from the plexus around the internal carotid artery. It passes through the superior orbital fissure within the anulus of Zinn, infero-medial to the naso-ciliary. It lies below and close to the long root, with which it may be blended, and enters the posterior border of the ganglion between the other roots. It carries constrictor fibres to the blood-vessels of the eye, and possibly dilator fibres to the pupil.

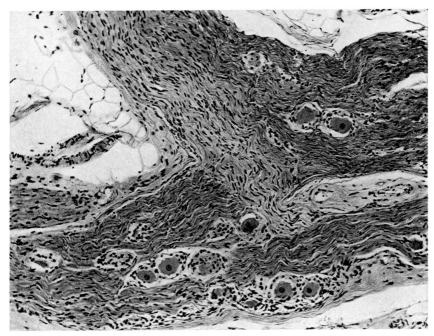

FIG. 285.—SHOWING GANGLION CELLS IN THE SHORT CILIARY NERVES.
(*Wolff's preparation.*)

BRANCHES OF THE GANGLION

Only the parasympathetic fibres relay in the ganglion. Their cell bodies are in the Edinger-Westphal nucleus and they reach the ciliary ganglion through its motor root. Both the sensory fibres (cell bodies in trigeminal ganglion) and the sympathetic fibres (cell bodies in the superior cervical ganglion) pass directly through the ganglion without relay and take part, with the postganglionic parasympathetic fibres, in the formation of the short ciliary nerves (Fig. 364).

The Short Ciliary Nerves, six to ten in number, are delicate filaments which come off in two groups from the antero-superior and antero-inferior angles of the ganglion respectively. They run a wavy course, with the short ciliary arteries, above and below the optic nerve, the lower group being the larger. As they pass forwards they inosculate with each other and with the long ciliaries, and having given branches to the optic nerve and ophthalmic artery pierce the sclera around the optic nerve. They run anteriorly between the choroid and sclera, grooving the latter to reach the ciliary muscle on the surface of which they form a plexus which supplies the iris, ciliary body, and cornea.

The ciliary ganglion which contains multipolar [1] nerve cells forms a cell

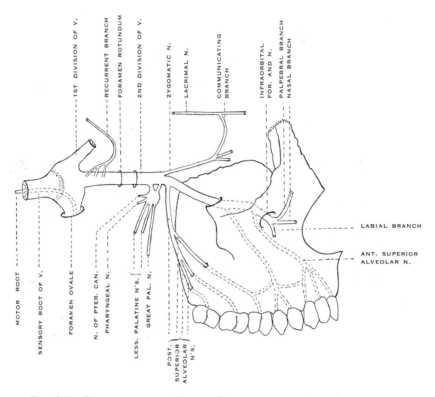

FIG. 286.—DIAGRAM OF THE SECOND DIVISION OF THE 5TH NERVE (L.W.).

station for the relay of the parasympathetic fibres of the 3rd nerve. Yet the short ciliary nerves are medullated (Fig. 361). Thus, as Gaskell pointed out, they are the only medullated post-ganglionic fibres in the body (see also p. 397).

Varieties.—The short root may be absent, the ganglion then sitting on the nerve to the inferior oblique. Additional roots have been described from the trochlear (Krause and Telgman), from the 6th nerve in a case where the oculo-motor was absent (Pourfour du Petit). and from the lacrimal (Quain). There may be multiple sympathetic roots. The *sensory root* may come from the ophthalmic or the supraorbital (Switzer).

[1] Ganglion cells are also often found along the short ciliary nerves (Figs. 284 and 285).

With regard to the accessory ganglia Nathan and Turner (1942) write as follows : " Axenfeld showed in 1907 that just proximal to the sclera or in the scleral canals, ganglion cells were frequently found on the ciliary nerves ; he found up to thirty of them, and named them *episcleral ciliary ganglia*. They not only supply the choroid, but also supply a mass of fibres to the ciliary muscle ; like the other short ciliary nerves, they are myelinated, their terminal divisions losing their myelin sheaths when they come to lie as small bundles of fibrillæ in the stroma of the ciliary body, as originally described by Agababow (1892). More recent work by Givner (1939) shows that these episcleral ganglia are not only common, but are probably a normal structure ; he found them in ten consecutive eyes which he examined ; his paper contains excellent photomicrographs of these nerves and ganglia.

"Here is a possible alternative pathway, which avoids the ciliary ganglion. It is possible that the fibres which take this path are those concerned with the accommodation-convergence synkinetic contraction and not with the light reflex ; but no positive evidence on this point has yet been obtained.

"It may be added that this mode of innervation is typical of the parasympathetic pattern, as seen, for example, in the submandibular gland. Langley (1885) has shown that the parasympathetic fibres supplying the gland arise from the ganglion cells lying within the hilum of the gland and not only from the submandibular ganglion. In the same way it is possible that the parasympathetic pupillo-constrictor fibres relay not only in the ganglion cells of the ciliary ganglion, but also in the more peripherally situated episcleral ciliary ganglia."

THE MAXILLARY NERVE

The Maxillary Nerve, or second division of the 5th nerve, is intermediate in size between the ophthalmic and the mandibular, and comes off the middle of the convex anterior border of the trigeminal ganglion. It runs forwards in the lower angle of the cavernous sinus in a groove (Figs. 259 and 366) on the greater wing of the sphenoid, which leads it to the foramen rotundum.

It passes through this foramen (which is usually a canal) into the pterygo-palatine fossa. It now turns laterally behind the orbital process of the palatine bone and at the inferior orbital fissure divides into its two terminal branches, the infraorbital and zygomatic nerves.

Relations.—(*a*) *In the Cranial Cavity.*—It lies in the lower angle of the cavernous sinus, surrounded by a cuff of dura mater. *Above* it, is the ophthalmic division of the 5th nerve, while *laterally* is the temporal lobe of the brain.

When the sphenoidal sinus is large it may send a prolongation into the great wing of the sphenoid between the foramen ovale and rotundum, *which may account for the nerve being involved in sinus disease* (Hovelacque).

(*b*) *In the Pterygo-palatine Fossa.*—Here the nerve is close to the termination of the maxillary artery and a plexus of veins. It is also close to the ethmoidal air-cells in the orbital process of the palatine bone, *and may be involved in ethmoidal disease here* (Ramadier).

Branches.—(*a*) In the cranial cavity a recurrent branch, the so-called *middle meningeal nerve,* supplies the dura mater of the anterior half of the middle cranial fossa.

(b) In the pterygo-palatine fossa two short branches are attached to the pterygo-palatine (spheno-palatine) ganglion, forming its sensory root (p. 313). These are called the **pterygo-palatine nerves.**

The **posterior superior alveolar** (dental) **nerves,** usually three in number, branch away just before the maxillary nerve divides in the inferior orbital fissure. They sweep down in a curve that carries them laterally through the pterygo-maxillary fissure.   One branch is purely *gingival* and supplies the buccal gum of the three upper molar teeth.   The other two enter foramina in the posterior wall of the maxilla and run in bony canals to supply the three molar teeth, their periodontal membranes (not the gum) and the nearby mucous membrane of the maxillary sinus.

(c) The **infraorbital nerve** runs forwards from the inferior orbital fissure on the orbital plate of the maxilla.   It indents the bone, first into a groove, then into a canal through which it runs with the infraorbital artery to emerge on the face through the infraorbital foramen.

The *middle superior alveolar* (dental) *nerve* is given off in the infraorbital groove and runs down in the lateral wall of the maxilla to supply the two bicuspid teeth and the adjoining sinus mucosa.   It is commonly absent, in which case the anterior superior alveolar takes its place.

The *anterior superior alveolar* (dental) *nerve* arises in the infraorbital canal. Passing first *laterally* in the bone, it curves down and medially below the infra-orbital foramen to supply the canine and both incisors, the mucosa of the sinus, and the anterior inferior quadrant of the lateral wall and nearby floor of the nose.

On the face the infraorbital nerve emerges between levator labii superioris and levator anguli oris.   It breaks up into a leash of branches, some of which join twigs of the facial nerve.   These branches radiate from the overlying cheek downwards, medially and upwards.   The *labial branches* supply the skin of the upper lip and the mucous membrane of the vestibule (including the labial gum) from the mid-line to the second bicuspid tooth.   The *nasal branches* supply the lateral side of the lower part of the nose.   The *palpebral branches* run up to supply the skin and conjunctiva of the lower lid.

(d) The **zygomatic nerve** inclines laterally from the inferior orbital fissure, and soon divides into zygomatico-temporal and zygomatico-facial branches.

The Zygomatico-temporal Branch runs upwards in a groove on the *lateral wall* of the orbit, *gives a communicating twig to the lacrimal nerve,* which carries secretory fibres to the lacrimal gland, and then enters a canal in the zygomatic bone, which leads it to the temporal fossa.   It now ascends, pierces the temporal fascia behind the zygomatic tubercle, and having joined with branches of the facial, supplies the skin over the anterior part of the temporal region up to the lateral orbital margin.

The Zygomatico-facial Branch likewise enters a canal in the zygomatic bone, which leads it to the face where, having joined with branches of the facial and pierced the orbicularis, it supplies the skin over the zygomatic bone.

Varieties.—The whole zygomatic nerve may enter one canal and then divide in the bone itself. The lacrimal communication may replace the zygomatico-temporal branch and a twig from the infraorbital take the place of the zygomatico-facial branch.

The Zygomatico-facial Branch may come out on the face as two or more branches.

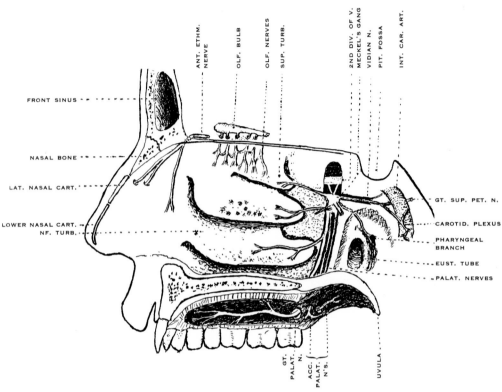

FIG. 287.—NERVES OF THE LATERAL WALL OF THE NOSE.
(*From Wolff's " Shorter Anatomy."*)

THE PTERYGO-PALATINE (SPHENO-PALATINE) GANGLION

The pterygo-palatine or Meckel's ganglion is situated in the upper part of the pterygo-palatine fossa, just lateral to the spheno-palatine foramen and suspended from the maxillary nerve by its pterygo-palatine branches (Figs. 280, 286, 287).

ROOTS

Sensory.—Pterygo-palatine nerves. They pass through the ganglion without relay ; their cell bodies are in the trigeminal ganglion.

Sympathetic and Motor.—From the nerve of the pterygoid canal. This nerve is formed in the foramen lacerum by the union of the great (superficial) petrosal, from the geniculate ganglion of the facial, with the deep petrosal of the sympathetic plexus around the internal carotid artery (Fig. 287). It passes through the pterygoid canal in the sphenoid bone, which commences just above the pterygoid tubercle and ends in the pterygo-palatine fossa, where it joins the ganglion. The deep petrosal nerve (sympathetic) comes from cell bodies in the superior cervical ganglion by way of the carotid plexus. Its fibres are post-ganglionic, and pass without relay directly through the ganglion into the branches of distribution. They are vasco-constrictor.

The great (superficial) petrosal carries fibres which after synapse supply the lacrimal gland, which they reach viâ the branches of the pterygo-palatine ganglion to the zygomatic nerve and its branch to the lacrimal. They supply secreto-motor fibres to the glands in the mucous membrane supplied by the pterygo-palatine ganglion, namely, nose, naso-pharynx, paranasal sinuses and palate. These parasympathetic fibres alone relay in the ganglion ; their cell bodies are in the superior salivatory nucleus of the pons, and the fibres leave the brain stem in the nervus intermedius (Fig. 364).

The result of stimulation of this pathway is not only lacrimation, but secretion from a wide area of nasal and palatal mucosa—hence the name " ganglion of hay fever " commonly given to this ganglion. To treat intractable hay fever the ganglion is sometimes permanently blocked by alcohol or other injection.

BRANCHES OF THE GANGLION

These are five in number—two for the nose, two for the palate, and one for the naso-pharynx. *Each of these carries fibres from all three roots of the ganglion* : sensory, parasympathetic (secreto-motor), and sympathetic (vaso-motor). *Orbital branches*, conventionally described, are rather branches of the maxillary nerve itself ; they supply periosteum at the apex of the floor of the orbit.

1. **The Naso-palatine Nerve** (long spheno-palatine nerve) enters the nose by the spheno-palatine foramen, crosses the roof, then descends in a groove on the vomer, giving branches to the mucous membrane all along its course. It passes through the incisive canal to supply the muco-periosteum behind the two incisor teeth.

2. **The Posterior Superior Nasal Nerves** (short spheno-palatine nerves) enter the nose through the spheno-palatine foramen, and turn forwards to supply the postero-superior quadrant of the lateral wall of the nose.

3. **The Greater Palatine Nerve** descends in the slot (greater palatine canal) between the maxilla and vertical plate of the palatine bone. Here it gives off multiple twigs that pierce each bone, to supply the mucosa of the maxillary sinus and that of the postero-inferior quadrant of the lateral wall of the nose.

The greater palatine nerve, emerging through the greater palatine foramen, runs forward to supply the muco-periosteum of all the hard palate up to the incisive canal.

4. **The Lesser Palatine Nerves,** often branches from the greater palatine, pass through the lesser palatine canals and, behind the crest of the palatine bone, pass back to supply the mucous membrane on both surfaces of the soft palate.

5. **The Pharyngeal Branch** passes back through the palatino-vaginal canal to supply the mucosa of the naso-pharynx.

THE MANDIBULAR NERVE

The mandibular or third division of the 5th nerve is made up of two roots.

The Sensory Portion comes from the trigeminal ganglion, the motor part is the motor root of the trigeminal, the whole of which goes with this division.

The two roots pass through the *foramen ovale,* and almost immediately unite into one trunk, which has the tensor palati and Eustachian tube medial and the lateral pterygoid and middle meningeal artery lateral.

The Foramen Ovale lies to the lateral side of the base of the lateral pterygoid plate. *With the mouth open, so as to get the coronoid process out of the way, pass a needle just below the zygoma and* 1 *in.* (2·5 *cm.*) *in front of the temporo-mandibular joint directly inwards. It strikes the lateral pterygoid plate. Now direct it a little backwards and upwards, and it enters the foramen* 1¾ *in.* (4·5 *cm.*) *from the surface. If pushed too far it enters the Eustachian tube.*

NUCLEUS AND CENTRAL CONNECTIONS OF THE 5TH NERVE

The Sensory Nucleus of the 5th nerve lies in all three parts of the brain stem. The mesencephalic part is slender. The pontine and medullary parts together are shaped like a tadpole (Fig. 288). The head, forming the main sensory nucleus (nucleus sensibilis *a* of Winkler) lies in the lateral dorsal part of the pons beneath the superior cerebellar peduncle. The tail forms the nucleus of the spinal tract (nucleus sensibilis *b* + nucl. gelatinosus of Winkler), and becomes continuous with the substantia gelatinosa of Rolando at the level of the 2nd cervical segment (Fig. 266).

The fibres of the sensory root which come from the trigeminal ganglion, on entering the pons, divide into ascending and descending branches, as does any ordinary spinal nerve. The ascending fibres mostly end in the upper expanded part or main sensory nucleus.

The descending fibres form the *tractus spinalis* of the trigeminal nerve, and enter the nucleus of the spinal tract at various levels.

The main sensory nucleus (nucleus sensibilis *a* of Winkler) most probably has to do with fine discriminative touch. The tail receives heat, cold, pain, and crude touch fibres ; those from the ophthalmic division go to the *lowest* part, those from the maxillary division are next, while those from the mandibular division are uppermost. This arrangement, as pointed out by Paton, explains *how in syringo-myelia involving the upper part of the cord, the forehead and eye may be affected and the buccal area escape.* Also the fact that the great occipital nerve comes from the 2nd cervical segment, where the ophthalmic portion of the nucleus ends, *may explain the frequency of occipital headaches in eye disease.*

The mesencephalic nucleus lies in the grey matter lateral to the aqueduct of the midbrain. It is thought to consist of the cell bodies of the *first sensory neurone* for proprioceptive impulses from the muscles of the face and orbit (the pontine

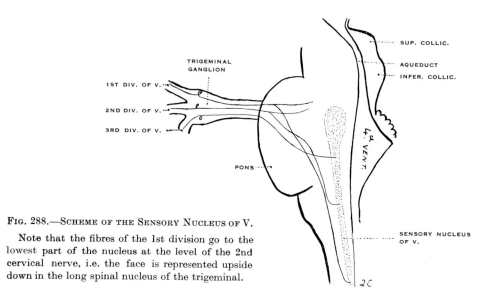

FIG. 288.—SCHEME OF THE SENSORY NUCLEUS OF V.

Note that the fibres of the 1st division go to the lowest part of the nucleus at the level of the 2nd cervical nerve, i.e. the face is represented upside down in the long spinal nucleus of the trigeminal.

and spinal nuclei contain the cell bodies of the *second* sensory neurone, the cell bodies of their first neurone being in the trigeminal ganglion).

The fibres from the sensory nucleus pass for the most part viâ the medial lemniscus to the thalamus of the opposite side, while the heat, cold, and pain fibres pass up in the trigeminal and spinal lemniscus.

The Motor Nucleus lies in the lateral tegmental portion of the pons medial to and nearer the floor of the 4th ventricle than the sensory nucleus. It is in line with the *nucleus ambiguus* and the nucleus of the facial (Fig. 266).

Connections.—The 5th nerve has taken on the sensory function of almost all the nerves of the head. Its connections are therefore very extensive.

Function.—The 5th nerve carries protopathic and epicritic sensation from the areas which it supplies ; probably also proprioceptive impulses from the eye muscles and trophic fibres. Division of the 1st division of the 5th nerve tends to produce neuroparalytic keratitis ; the mechanism of its production is not entirely explained : the trophic fibres no doubt, at any rate, play some part in this. Some hold that it is due to injury to the great (superficial) petrosal nerve which lies beneath the trigeminal ganglion (Fig. 272).

THE 7TH CRANIAL OR FACIAL NERVE

The facial nerve emerges from the brain at the lower border of the pons in the recess between the olive and the inferior cerebellar peduncle (Fig. 352). It is here some distance lateral to the 6th, but medial to the nervus intermedius and the 8th. From its superficial origin it runs laterally and forwards in the posterior

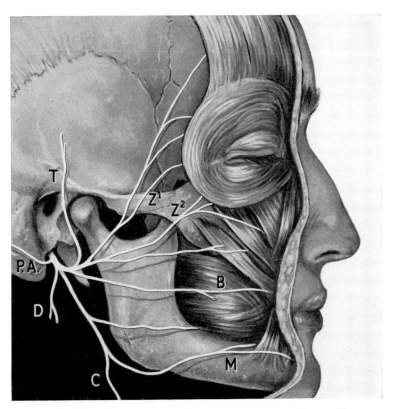

FIG. 289.—THE EXTRACRANIAL DISTRIBUTION OF THE FACIAL NERVE.

P.A.=posterior auricular. D.=branch to posterior belly of digastric and stylohyoid. T.=temporal branch. Z¹.=upper zygomatic branches. Z².=lower zygomatic branches. B.=buccal branch. M.=mandibular branch. C.=cervical branch.

cranial fossa to the internal acoustic (auditory) meatus. In this part of the course it lies in a groove on the upper surface of the 8th, with the nervus intermedius between them (Fig. 353). Accompanied by the labyrinthine artery these structures enter the meatus, at the bottom of which is the lamina cribrosa, divided into four parts by a horizontal and a less-marked vertical partition. The 7th nerve, with the nervus intermedius, passes through the antero-superior quadrant, and enters the facial canal. It, now, for a short distance (4 mm.) continues laterally more or less in the direction of the internal auditory meatus, then bends backwards over the vestibule to reach the middle ear. The geniculate ganglion is placed on this bend of the facial nerve, and here the nervus intermedius fuses with it. In the middle ear it lies in a bony canal, placed between the roof and medial wall, and running above the promontory and fenestra vestibuli (ovalis). The bone may be wanting in parts, and hence the nerve may more easily be affected in inflammation of the tympanum. The fibres affected earliest are those supplying the orbicularis (according to Asherson the winking reflex goes first), which suggests that in the cross-sectional anatomy of the nerve these fibres are most superficial.

At the junction of the medial and posterior walls the 7th nerve makes a second bend, downwards this time, and escapes from the skull through the stylo-mastoid

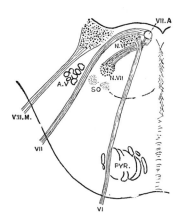

FIG. 290.—PLAN OF THE ORIGINS OF THE 6TH AND 7TH CRANIAL NERVES.

The outline represents a transverse section of the lower part of the pons, on to which the course of the facial nerve is projected. VI = 6th nerve. N.VI = its nucleus. VII = facial nerve. VII.A = the ascending portion of its root, supposed to be seen in optical section. N.VII = its nucleus. S.O. = trapezoid body. A.V. = ascending or pontine root of 5th nerve. VIII.M. = medial root of 8th nerve.

(*After Schwalbe, from Quain's " Anatomy."*)

foramen. The descending portion of this second bend forms a ridge on the medial wall of the aditus, and has above it the bulge formed by the lateral semicircular canal. Having escaped from the skull, the facial nerve gives off two branches (Fig. 289) and then divides into a larger upper and a smaller lower division (temporo-zygomatic and cervico-facial). These run forwards in the parotid, lying here superficial to the retromandibular (posterior facial) vein and the external carotid artery, and divide in the substance of the gland. Classically the temporo-zygomatic is described as dividing into its branches at the neck of the mandible. Actually only the upper branches reach the neck, the lower ones crossing the ramus of the mandible a little above its middle (Fig. 289). It is of practical importance to note that in the infant, who has no mastoid process, the 7th nerve at its exit from the skull lies more on the lateral than the under aspect of the skull, and if the usual incision behind the ear be made to expose the mastoid antrum it will almost certainly be injured.

BRANCHES

In the temporal bone :
  (a) Great (superficial) petrosal.
  (b) Tympanic branches.
  (c) Nerve to the stapedius.
  (d) Chorda tympani.
At its exit from the stylo-mastoid foramen :
  Posterior auricular.
  Digastric.
  Stylo-hyoid.
On the face :
  Temporal.
  Zygomatic.
  Buccal.
  Mandibular.
  Cervical.

The great (superficial) petrosal and chorda tympani contain fibres from only the nervus intermedius, and are not really 7th cranial nerve fibres at all. The tympanic branches are partly 7th (sensory) and partly nervus intermedius (secretomotor), while the nerve to stapedius is true 7th. All the extracranial branches are true 7th, the companion nervus intermedius fibres having been all given off in the intrapetrous course of the nerve.

The Great (Superficial) Petrosal comes off the geniculate ganglion. It passes through a canal, then runs in a groove on the anterior surface of the petrous temporal (Fig. 272) under the trigeminal ganglion to the foramen lacerum. Here it unites with the deep petrosal, from the sympathetic plexus on the internal carotid artery, to form the nerve of the pterygoid canal, which joins the pterygo-palatine ganglion viâ the pterygoid canal (Fig. 287). The great (superficial) petrosal contains taste fibres to the mucous membrane of the soft palate, and also secretory fibres to the palatal, nasal and lacrimal glands (see also p. 227). It has been described as the " nerve of hay fever."

The Tympanic Branches join the plexus on the promontory. Together with the tympanic branch of the 9th nerve they are : (a) secreto-motor viâ the lesser petrosal nerve and otic ganglion relay to the parotid gland, and (b) sensory to the mucosa of the middle ear. These sensory twigs commonly encroach on the external surface of the tympanic membrane and even on the skin of the external auditory meatus and pinna. Thus is explained the presence here of vesicles in some cases of facial herpes.

The Temporal Branch runs upwards (Fig. 289). It supplies auricularis anterior and superior, and gives a few twigs to frontalis.

The Zygomatic Branches are in two groups. The upper of these (Fig. 289, Z¹) run subcutaneously across the zygomatic arch to supply frontalis and the muscles of the upper eyelid (orbicularis oculi, corrugator supercilii, procerus) (Fig. 273). Interruption of these nerves makes closure of the eye impossible, and corneal desiccation and ulceration result. The lower zygomatic branches (Fig. 289, Z²) cross the zygomatic bone to supply the orbicularis fibres of the lower lid and the upper fibres of the elevators of the upper lip.

The Buccal Branch runs forwards below the parotid duct to supply buccinator and the muscles of the upper lip as far as the midline.

The Mandibular Branch commonly runs down in the neck and crosses the lower border of the mandible on the facial artery at the anterior border of masseter. Here it is vulnerable to trauma or surgical incisions. It supplies all the muscles of the lower lip.

The Cervical Branch runs down to supply platysma.

Nucleus and Connections.—The facial nerve is usually regarded as consisting of a motor portion, the facial proper, and a sensory portion, the nervus intermedius. But the nervus intermedius contains secretory fibres as well.

The sensory portion of the nervus intermedius rises in the geniculate ganglion, which consists of unipolar cells, whose axones divide in a **T**-shaped manner. The central processes form part of the nervus intermedius, the peripheral processes, the taste fibres of the chorda tympani, and great (superficial) petrosal.

The central fibres pass through or dorsal to the spinal root of the 5th, to reach the upper part of the tractus solitarius. The motor (somatic) nucleus of the 7th consists of large cells homologous with the nucleus ambiguus, the upward continuation of the anterior horn of the spinal cord. The nucleus of the 7th is situated near its point of exit, but the fibres do not pass straight out. They run first backwards and medially through the pons to the floor of the 4th ventricle, where they cross and run upwards medially to the 6th nerve nucleus, forming the colliculus facialis in the floor of the ventricle. The fibres now turn laterally, cross the 6th nucleus again, pass forwards between their own nucleus and the spinal root of the 5th nerve, to emerge between the olive and the inferior cerebellar peduncle (Figs. 290, 352).

Communications.—(*a*) From the 3rd probably to supply the orbicularis oculi, the frontalis and the corrugator, for in supranuclear lesions of the 7th these are not involved. (*b*) From the 12th to the orbicularis oris (probably). (*c*) From the cortex of the opposite side, viâ the pyramidal tract. The crossing takes place in the pons, *hence unilateral lesions here produce palsy of the face on the same side and on the opposite side of the rest of the body. Note that in the precentral gyrus the face area comes next the hand, but in the internal capsule the shoulder and face fibres are together.*

THE NERVUS INTERMEDIUS

This nerve, unnoticed and unnumbered by earlier anatomists, is really a cranial nerve in its own right. Applied to it, the term "sensory root of the facial nerve" is a misnomer. True it carries a few sensory fibres from the middle ear and external meatus, but almost all its sensory fibres carry *taste* from the mouth and these have, of course, nothing to do with the facial nerve. Moreover, it carries also preganglionic secreto-motor (i.e. parasympathetic) fibres to the lacrimal gland and to the glands of the nose, sinuses, palate and mouth.

Origin.—It leaves the brain-stem between pons and inferior cerebellar peduncle (nearer the 8th than the 7th—Fig. 353) and runs with the 7th into the internal acoustic meatus. It joins the 7th at the geniculate ganglion.

Distribution.—The fibres, a mixture of taste and secreto-motor, leave the 7th nerve in the great (superficial) petrosal nerve (p. 319) and the chorda tympani. The chorda tympani provides the anterior two-thirds of the tongue with taste, and the salivary glands of the floor of the mouth with their secreto-motor fibres.

Nucleus.—This is the *superior salivatory nucleus* for the secreto-motor fibres. It lies lateral to the nucleus of the 7th nerve, beneath the floor of the pontine part of the fourth ventricle. The taste fibres (their cell bodies in the geniculate ganglion) run to the pontine part of the *nucleus of the tractus solitarius.*

THE 8TH CRANIAL NERVE

The 8th cranial nerve consists of two portions, a cochlear division which carries auditory impulses, and a vestibular part, which has to do with equilibrium and sense of position.

It is attached to the brain just below the lower border of the pons lateral to the 7th. The nervus intermedius runs between these, and often curiously enough nearer the 8th. The 8th nerve runs laterally and forwards to the internal acoustic (auditory) meatus, its two portions forming a groove in which the 7th rests, the nervus intermedius lying between them.

Accompanied by the labyrinthine branch of the basilar artery, these structures enter the meatus, at the bottom of which the 8th nerve divides into branches which pass through the lamina cribrosa.

The cochlear portion passes through the lower and anterior quadrant to reach the cochlea. The branches of the vestibular division pass through the two posterior quadrants. Through the supero-posterior quadrant go the nerves to the utricle, superior and lateral semicircular canals. Through the infero-posterior quadrant pass the nerves to the sacculus and posterior semicircular canal.

Nuclei and Central Connections.—The ganglion of the cochlear division, or ganglion spirale, lies in the modiolus of the cochlea. Its peripheral fibres come from the organ of Corti.

The ganglion of the vestibular division, or ganglion of Scarpa, is in the internal auditory meatus. Its peripheral fibres come from the vestibular apparatus. The two nerves are united in the internal auditory meatus, and so run back to enter the brain below the pons lateral to the 7th nerve. The cochlear portion now goes to two nuclei, one dorsal and one ventral to the inferior cerebellar peduncle. From the dorsal nucleus fibres pass through the peduncle to join the lateral lemniscus of the opposite side.

The fibres from the ventral nucleus also join the lateral lemniscus, which makes connection with the inferior colliculus for relay of acoustic reflexes. For conscious hearing the lateral lemniscus relays in the medial geniculate bodies, whence fibres traverse the posterior limb of the internal capsule to reach the anterior transverse gyrus of the temporal lobe.

The vestibular fibres end in (a) the principal dorsal nucleus of the vestibular nerve, which lies in the so-called area acousticæ of the 4th ventricle ; (b) Deiters' and Bechterew's nuclei in the side wall of the 4th ventricle, and (c) the cerebellum.

Both the cochlear and vestibular divisions of the 8th nerve make connection with the medial longitudinal bundle, and thus with the ocular nuclei.

A.E.—21

CHAPTER VII

THE VISUAL PATHWAY

THE visual pathway from the retina (p. 103) may be divided into six parts :

    (1) The optic nerve.
    (2) The optic chiasma.
    (3) The optic tract.
    (4) The lateral geniculate body.
    (5) The optic radiation.
    (6) The sensory cortex.

THE 2ND CRANIAL OR OPTIC NERVE

The Optic Nerve, ensheathed in pia, runs as a flattened band from the antero-lateral angle of the somewhat quadrilateral chiasma forwards and laterally and slightly downwards to the optic foramen (Fig. 258). Actually the cross-section behind the optic foramen is pear-shaped, with the rounded end medial. At its entry into the optic canal it receives a covering of arachnoid (Fig. 257).

Becoming more oval, and acquiring a dural covering, it traverses the optic canal and enters the orbit. As a rounded cord it now runs forwards and slightly laterally and downwards in a somewhat sinuous manner[1] (to allow for ocular movements), and is attached to the back of the eyeball, so that the centre of its cross-section is just *above* and 3 mm. medial to the posterior pole (Fig. 248, E).

Its total length is 5 cm., the intracranial portion being about 1 cm., the intracanalicular 6 mm., the intraorbital 3 cm., and the intraocular 0·7 mm.

Although we speak of the optic *nerve*, it is very important to realise that it is really no nerve at all, but essentially a *fibre tract* joining two portions of the brain.

Relations.—(*a*) *In the Cranial Cavity.*—The nerve lies at first above the diaphragma sellæ, which covers the pituitary body, then on the anterior portion of the cavernous sinus.

Between the two nerves in front of the chiasma is a triangular space in which a variable portion of the pituitary body covered by the diaphragma lies (see p. 343).

Above the nerve is the *anterior perforated substance*, the *medial root of the*

---

[1] Usually two curves can be recognised : a posterior with a lateral convexity, and an anterior with its convexity downwards.

olfactory tract, and the *anterior cerebral artery,* which crosses it from lateral to medial (Figs. 258, 318, 353).

The Internal Carotid Artery is at first below, then lateral.

The Ophthalmic Artery usually comes off the internal carotid under the middle of the optic nerve (Fig. 278), but since its course here is antero-posterior, and that of the nerve laterally as well as forwards, it may appear at the medial border of the nerve before it eventually passes laterally. At any rate, in this first portion of its course it is nearer the medial border than the lateral (Fig. 291). The nearer the origin of the artery is to the optic foramen, the nearer the *medial* side of the nerve is it placed.

(b) In the Optic Canal.—The pia forms a sheath closely adherent to the nerve. The dura constitutes the periosteal lining to the canal and at its orbital

OPTIC NERVE COVERED BY FALCIFORM EDGE

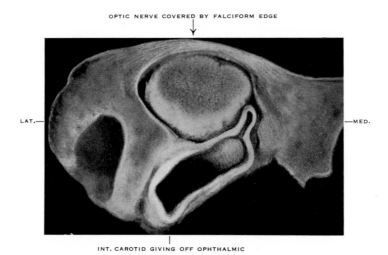

LAT.—   —MED.

INT. CAROTID GIVING OFF OPHTHALMIC

Fig. 291.—Transverse Section of Portion of Sphenoid Bone with Optic Canal at Level of Falciform Edge.

Note ophthalmic artery is medial here.

end splits to become continuous on the one hand with the periorbita and on the other with the dura of the optic nerve.

According to Hovelacque, who quotes Pfister, a small sleeve of arachnoid penetrates the cranial end of the canal for 1 to 2 mm., but for the rest this membrane is absent in the canal. Manschot and Hampe, however, have demonstrated the arachnoid in the canal, and in my own[1] preparations, coloured with Masson's trichome and Mallory's triple stain, the arachnoid although compressed can be seen throughout the canal.

The relations of the sheaths of the optic nerve in the optic canal differ some-

[1] Eugene Wolff.

what in different individuals (Pfister). There is, however, as Schwalbe first pointed out, a well-marked communication between the subarachnoid space inside the skull and that around the optic nerve in the orbit.

The dura is anchored to the bone and to the pia. This forms a point of fixation of the nerve which might otherwise be pushed backwards and forwards in and out of the cranium and thus be liable to injury (Schwalbe).

But this adhesion varies in its position and in its density. Schwalbe held that it was above, so that only in the lower part did the cranial subarachnoid space communicate with that in the orbit.

But Pfister has shown that the adhesion may be anywhere in the circumference of the nerve and indeed most often in the region of the ophthalmic

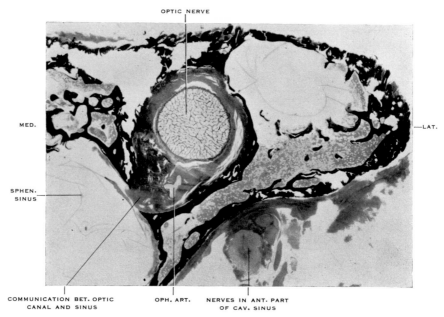

FIG. 292.—Transverse Section of Portion of Sphenoid Bone with Optic Canal (Bone Decalcified).

Note dense connective tissue around artery.

artery (Fig. 292). There are also here and there weaker trabeculæ which cross from the dura to pia.

The ophthalmic artery is crossing below the nerve in the dural sheath to the lateral side. It leaves the dura at or near the anterior end of the canal. It will be seen that the internal carotid artery is anchored to the dural sheath by its ophthalmic branch (Fig. 293) ; and it is also indirectly attached to the optic nerve by the adherence of the sheaths and by branches to the nerve from the ophthalmic artery.

Medially the optic nerve is near the sphenoidal air sinus (Fig. 292) or a posterior ethmoidal air-cell, from which it may be separated by a thin plate of bone only. *This provides the anatomical explanation of the nerve being affected in sinus disease and resulting in a retro-bulbar neuritis.*

Not infrequently the sphenoidal sinus or a posterior ethmoidal air-cell may invade the roots of the lesser wing of the sphenoid, and even the wing itself. The nerve is then surrounded by air-cells.

(c) *In the Orbit* (Figs. 15, 278, 280).—At the optic foramen the nerve is surrounded by the origin of the ocular muscles, that of the superior and medial recti being closely adherent to the dural sheath. *It is this connection which gives*

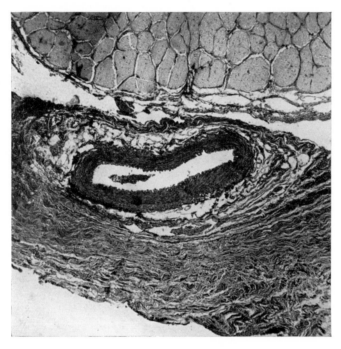

Fig. 293.—Transverse Section of Optic Nerve and Sheaths in the Optic Canal.
The ophthalmic artery is actually in the fibrous layer of the dura.

rise to the pain (in extreme movements of the globe) so characteristic of retro-bulbar neuritis.

Between it and the origin of the lateral rectus are the two divisions of the 3rd nerve, the naso-ciliary, the sympathetic, the 6th nerve, and sometimes the ophthalmic vein or veins (Fig. 261).

Farther forwards the muscles are separated from the nerve by orbital fat.

The naso-ciliary nerve, the ophthalmic artery, and the superior ophthalmic vein cross the nerve superiorly from lateral to medial.

The Ciliary Ganglion lies to the lateral side of the nerve between it and the lateral rectus (Figs. 278, 279).

The Long and Short Ciliary Nerves and Arteries gradually surround the nerve as it passes to the back of the eyeball.

The Arteria Centralis Retinæ, which comes off the ophthalmic near the optic foramen, runs forwards in or outside the dural sheath of the nerve, then with its accompanying vein *crosses the subarachnoid space* to enter the nerve on its under and medial aspect about ½ in. (12 mm.) behind the eye.   At the point of entrance

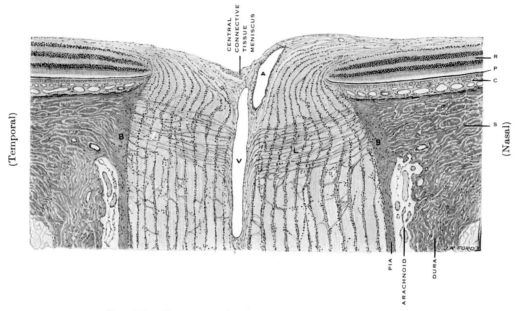

FIG. 294.—HORIZONTAL SECTION OF THE OPTIC NERVE HEAD.

A. = arteria   centralis.   V. = vena   centralis.   B. = border   tissue.   L. = lamina   cribrosa.
R. = retina.   P. = pigment epithelium and basal lamina.   C. = choroid.   S. = sclera.

of the vessels the nerve, instead of being round is oval or horseshoe-shaped, and if the vessels enter separately there are two oval regions (Kuhnt).

(d) *The Intraocular Portion.*—As the nerve passes into the eye its fibres lose their myelin sheaths, and at the same time there is diminution in the amount of supporting tissue.

This results in the optic nerve being 3 mm. in diameter at the back of the globe and only 1·5 mm. in its retinal portion.

The intraocular portion of the optic nerve passes through the sclera, the choroid, and finally appears inside the eye as the " papilla " optica, where it becomes continuous with the nerve fibre layer of the retina (Figs. 294 and 298).

We may thus subdivide the ocular portion of the nerve into **scleral, choroidal,** and **retinal** parts.

The junction between the medullated and non-medullated parts of the nerve is at the back of the lamina cribrosa (Figs. 295, 298)—at the distal end of the subarachnoid space—but this is not a sharp line, for some fibres lose their myelin sheath proximal and some distal to this point.

The Neighbouring Retina.—The layers of the *retina*, apart from the nerve fibres, end near the borders of the optic nerve, being separated from it, however, by a ring or partial ring of glial tissue called the *intermediary tissue of Kuhnt* (Figs. 298, 301). It is usually stated that the intermediary tissue of Kuhnt can be seen with the ophthalmoscope. This can hardly be true since neuroglia is transparent and also the tissue is covered by the whole thickness of the nerve fibre layer of the retina as it curves round to pass into the optic nerve. In the

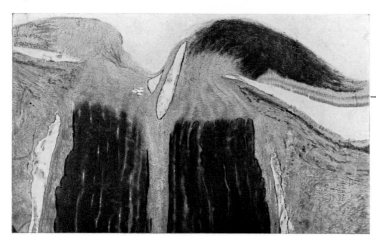

RETINA WITH MEDUL-
LATED NERVE FIBRES

Fig. 295.—Antero-posterior Section of the Optic Nerve to show Medullated (congenital) Nerve Fibres. (Weigert's Stain.)

Note that the normal medullation stops behind the lamina cribrosa, in which region the fibres are non-medullated.

(From a section kindly supplied by Mr. Percy Flemming.)

retinal portion the nerve fibres are in separate bundles, being separated from each other by columns consisting of neuroglial nuclei, fibres, and vessels. The individual fibres have extremely fine glial fibres around them.

The termination of the retina is usually oblique, but more so on the nasal than on the temporal side, where it may be vertical. The inner layers end before the outer. The rods and cones become smaller, maybe half their normal size, and cease altogether a little before the pigment epithelium which reaches almost up to the intermediary tissue. The basal lamina may come right up to the nerve fibres but is usually held away by glia.

The Neighbouring Choroid.—The posterior termination of the choroid will vary greatly as this portion of the scleral canal is widening or narrowing (see types of scleral canal).

Thus it may be pointed or straight.

Only the basal lamina, the two layers of which end almost together, reaches the aperture of entry of the nerve.   The pigment epithelium continues almost as far as the basal lamina, although the rods and cones have stopped earlier (Fig. 298).

The chorio-capillaris ends a variable distance from the end of the basal lamina, and earlier still the layer of smaller vessels (Figs. 298, 301).

The remaining layers of non-vascular stroma form a closely knit tissue containing numerous pigment cells.   Pigment cells of different types may thus come to lie on either side of the basal lamina.   The stroma lamellæ of the choroid do not reach right up to the edge of the nerve ; they are held away by the border

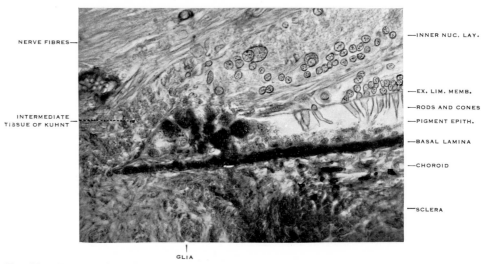

FIG. 301.—EDGE OF OPTIC NERVE (ANTERO-POSTERIOR SECTION).   COLLOID BODIES HAVE FORMED ON THE BASAL LAMINA (HYALOID MEMBRANE).

tissue.   The laminæ of the supra-choroidea usually have an oblique course between the sclera and the choroid proper, but near the optic nerve they become meridional and run parallel with the sclera.   Also pigmentation is dense as we approach the nerve.

The Neighbouring Sclera.—Near the optic nerve the innermost fibres of the sclera are meridional ; then meridional and circular, while the most superficial are circular.   These outer circular fibres as we approach the optic nerve interlace with the outer longitudinal fibres of the dura in the same manner as they do at the limbus with the cornea.   There is a great increase in the number of pigment cells as we approach the optic nerve.

The Marginal (Border) Tissue[1] (of Elschnig) (Figs. 298, 302–304) of the optic nerve is a ring of white fibrous tissue which separates choroid and sclera from the

[1] The marginal tissue is variously described.   Some hold that it belongs to sclera or choroid, while others believe it is a continuation forwards of the pia.

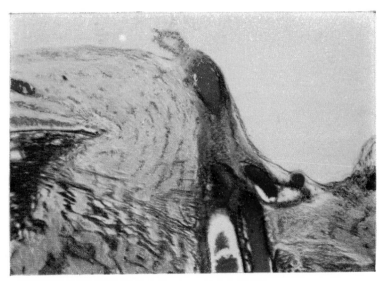

FIG. 296.—ANTERO-POSTERIOR SECTION OF OPTIC NERVE HEAD.   (MALLORY'S TRIPLE STAIN.)

Note red-staining glia lines physiological cup.   (Central connective tissue meniscus of Kuhnt.) Also remains of hyaloid artery (see Fig. 297).

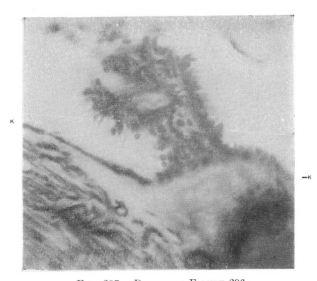

FIG. 297.—DETAIL OF FIGURE 296.

REMAINS OF HYALOID ARTERY CONSISTS OF GLIAL CELLS AND FIBRES.   SO-CALLED CONNECTIVE TISSUE MENISCUS OF KUHNT.   K = red-staining glia.

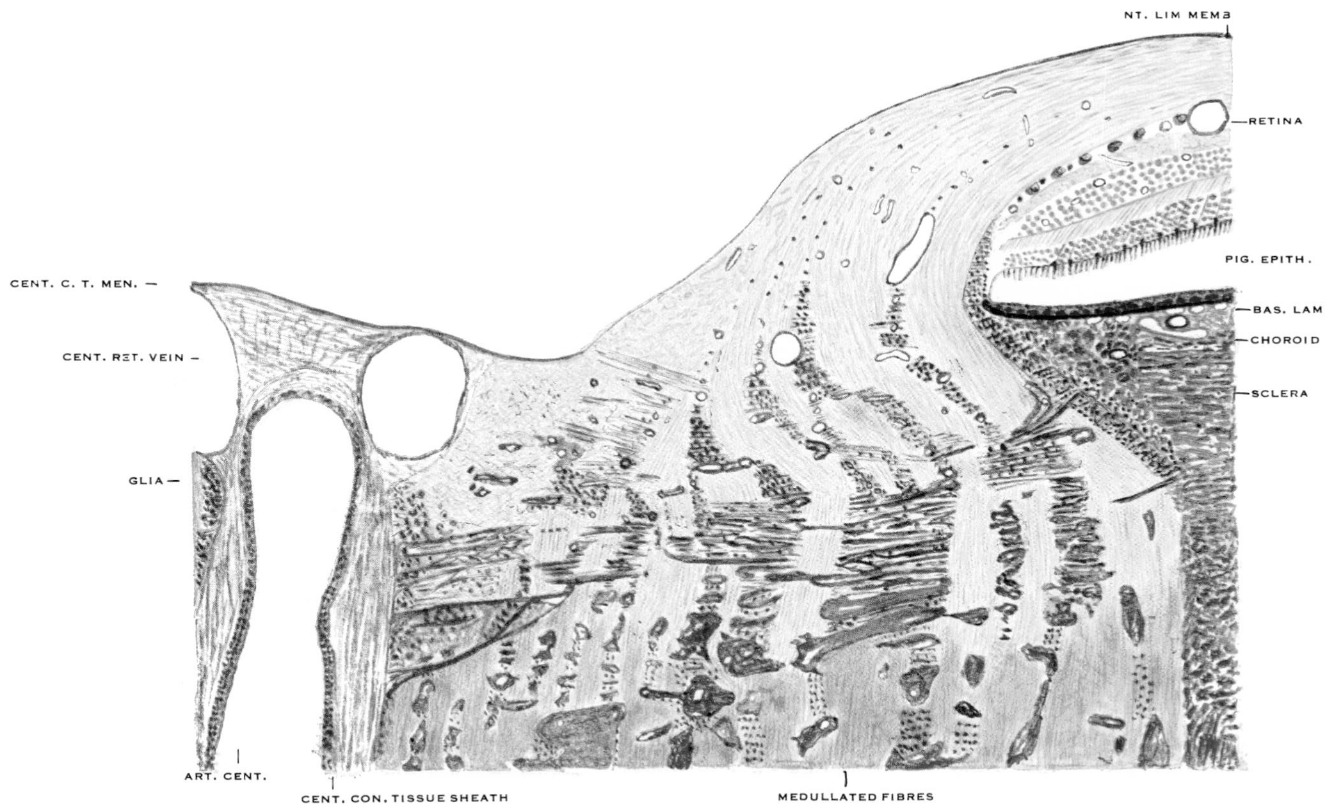

FIG. 298.—ANTERO-POSTERIOR SECTION OF THE OPTIC NERVE HEAD. (ZENKER. MALLORY'S TRIPLE STAIN.)

Connective tissue—blue.

Non-medullated nerve fibres, light red; medullated nerve fibres, darker red. Neuroglia still darker red. Note that the anterior portion of the lamina cribrosa is glial; the posterior consists of alternating layers of glia and connective tissue, but mainly the latter.

Glia separates the anterior portion of the sclera and the whole thickness of choroid from the nerve fibres and is continued anteriorly beyond the basal lamina (hyaloid membrane) and pigment epithelium to form the "intermediary tissue" of Kuhnt. This lies in the concavity of the nerve fibres as they sweep into the nerve.

(*Trans. Ophthal. Soc. U.K.*, 1938.)

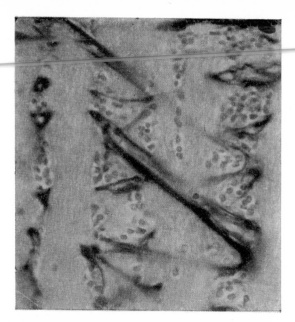

FIG. 299.—LONGITUDINAL SECTION OF OPTIC NERVE. (MALLORY'S TRIPLE STAIN.)
Note columns of glial nuclei and portions of septa (blue), some containing vessels.

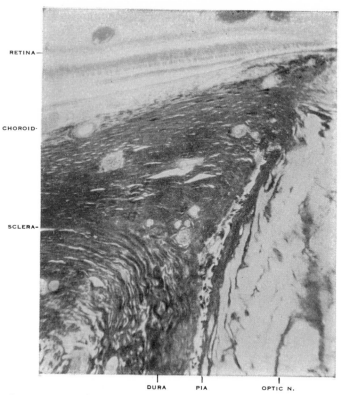

FIG. 300.—LONGITUDINAL SECTION OF EDGE OF OPTIC NERVE TO SHOW HOW THE DURA BECOMES
CONTINUOUS WITH OUTER THIRD OF SCLERA.

nerve fibres. With ordinary stains the border tissue differs but little from the sclera, although it can usually be distinguished from it. In longitudinal sections it appears as a strip of tissue which separates the sclera from the optic nerve, and is then continued forwards to delimit the choroid from the nerve fibres. It consists of dense collagenous tissue, in which are also found many glial and elastic fibres and some pigment (Salzmann). It is better marked on the temporal than on the nasal side.

Thus we see that none of the three tunics, except the basal lamina, reaches right up to the nerve, and even this is usually held away by neuroglia (Fig. 298).

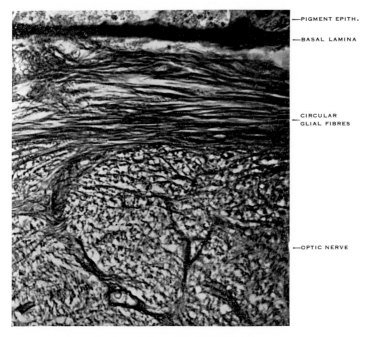

—PIGMENT EPITH.

—BASAL LAMINA

CIRCULAR GLIAL FIBRES

—OPTIC NERVE

FIG. 302.—TRANSVERSE SECTION OF EDGE OF OPTIC NERVE AT LEVEL OF BASAL LAMINA (HYALOID MEMBRANE). (ZENKER, MALLORY'S TRIPLE STAIN.)

The Scleral Canal is the canal through which the optic nerve passes to reach the retina. It is bounded by the border tissue, which separates the nerve fibres from the choroid and anterior third of the sclera proper. It is some 0·5 mm. long, and may run straight forward or be directed slightly nasally, temporally, or downwards.

As regards its shape, there are three types of scleral canal : (*a*) a cone with its narrowest point at the basal lamina ; (*b*) the canal narrows to the inner third of the sclera, the portion anterior to this keeping the same diameter ; (*c*) the canal narrows to the inner third of the sclera and then widens again, i.e. is X-shaped or double-funnel-shaped. In (b) and (c) a scleral ring is present and can be seen with the ophthalmoscope (Kuhnt).

The Lamina Cribrosa consists of a series of sieve-like membranes arranged transversely across the scleral canal, through the holes of which the fibres of the optic nerve pass (Figs. 298, 305, 306).

In order to understand its structure it is best to consider its development, which in its *posterior portion* is like that of the septa of the optic nerve (see p. 338).

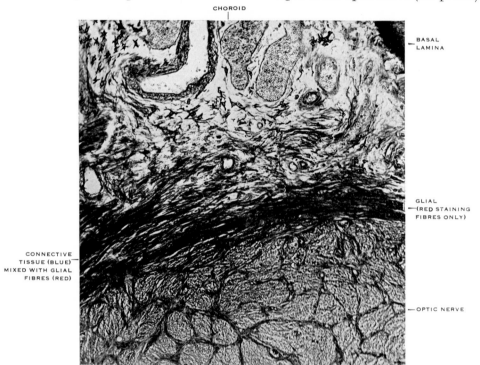

CHOROID

BASAL LAMINA

GLIAL (RED STAINING FIBRES ONLY)

CONNECTIVE TISSUE (BLUE) MIXED WITH GLIAL FIBRES (RED)

OPTIC NERVE

FIG. 304.—TRANSVERSE SECTION OF OPTIC NERVE A LITTLE BEHIND BASAL LAMINA (HYALOID MEMBRANE) (COMPARE FIG. 302). (ZENKER, MALLORY'S TRIPLE STAIN.)

The section is slightly oblique so that to the left, which is more posterior, there is still blue-staining connective tissue in the marginal tissue of the optic nerve.

Thus in its scleral portion each trabecula of the lamina cribrosa is essentially the result of the ingrowth of a vessel derived from the vascular circle of Zinn, which is accompanied by connective tissue and glia.

Each trabecula therefore has a vessel in its centre. This is surrounded by connective tissue containing a large number of elastic elements. This again is clothed by glia. Thus, in its posterior portion, in an antero-posterior section of the optic nerve, connective and glial tissues alternate (Fig. 298). The anterior or choroidal portion of the lamina cribrosa is quite different in structure. Here the trabeculæ consist of glial tissue only (Fig. 305).

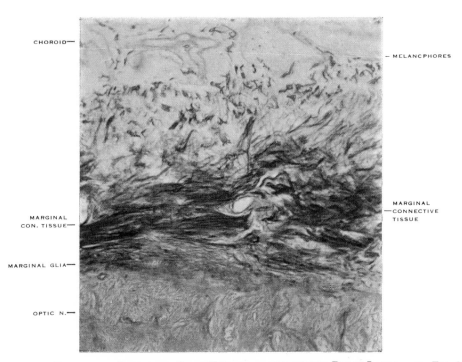

CHOROID—

— MELANCPHORES

MARGINAL
CON. TISSUE—

MARGINAL
—CONNECTIVE
TISSUE

MARGINAL GLIA—

OPTIC N.—

FIG. 303.—Transverse Section of Optic Nerve a little behind Basal Lamina and Fig. 302.
(Zenker.   Mallory's Triple Stain.)

Connective tissue is blue, glia is red.

The vessels from the vascular circle of Zinn, as they pass into the nerve, divide and reunite to form a network which fills the interval between the side wall of the scleral canal and the connective tissue around the central vessels.

The form of the lamina cribrosa on transverse section depends on this vascular network. It also forms a net of narrow meshes which are transversely oval (Figs. 305, 306).

In an antero-posterior section it is seen that three to eight dense trabeculæ of

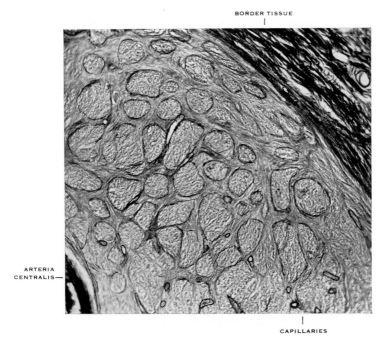

FIG. 305.—TRANSVERSE SECTION THROUGH THE ANTERIOR (GLIAL) PORTION OF THE LAMINA CRIBROSA. (ZENKER, MALLORY'S TRIPLE STAIN.)

Contrast with Fig. 306. The glial fibres are stained red and the only blue-staining connective tissue fibres are those round the vessels (shown here as dark rings and ovals).

(Wolff's preparation.)

hyaline appearance pass out of the side wall of the scleral canal. The most posterior run inwards and backwards (Fig. 298) to reach the central connective tissue a little in front of the outer limit of the sclera and make with the corresponding fibre of the opposite side a letter **V** with its concavity forwards. The more anterior ones run more directly inwards but are all slightly concave anteriorly. At the posterior boundary of the lamina cribrosa a very thick trabecula often passes out from the sclera (Fig. 298). It contains a correspondingly large artery which has a relatively strong muscularis and well-marked elastica. But in general the limits of the lamina cribrosa are not quite definite, for posteriorly it shades off into the framework of the optic nerve, and indeed some anatomists regard it as simply the continuation forwards of this framework.

THE NEUROGLIA OF THE OPTIC NERVE HEAD

The optic nerve head is extremely rich in neuroglia.   This is due to the fact that the peduncle of the optic vesicle is first transformed into neuroglia and it is only later that this neuroglial cord is traversed by nerve fibres (Redslob). Moreover, at a certain stage of development the arteria centralis gives off the

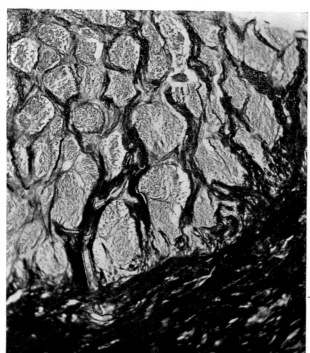

FIG. 306. — TRANSVERSE SECTION THROUGH THE POSTERIOR PORTION OF THE LAMINA CRIBROSA. (ZENKER, MALLORY'S TRIPLE STAIN.)

The trabeculæ are much denser and consist mainly of connective (blue staining) tissue. Note the contained vessel passing in from the sclera.   Contrast with Fig. 305.

(*Wolff's preparation.*)

—SCLERA

hyaloid artery.   The origin of this artery is surrounded by a conical bud of neuroglia.   Later the artery disappears and all that remains of the bud is a lamella of neuroglia which separates the central portion of the nerve head, including the connective tissue round the central vessels (central connective tissue sheath), from the vitreous (Figs. 296, 297, 298).

This lamella of neuroglia, called the *central connective tissue meniscus* of Kuhnt, replaces the internal limiting membrane, which is absent here, but is continuous with it at the periphery (Fig. 298).

Since there are no connective tissue fibres (except those in the walls of vessels) in the choroidal and retinal portion of the scleral canal, the supporting tissues are all neuroglial.   Thus the great majority of cells seen in this region, and forming the " nuclear columns " between the nerve fibre bundles, are glial.   According to Marchesani, they are astrocytes.

The glial fibres also form the net which constitutes the choroidal portion of the lamina cribrosa (Fig. 305).

Also radial neuroglial fibres become attached to the capillary walls by a sort of end plate (perivascularis gliæ).

Oligodendroglia is present (Lopez Enriquez) and is also interfascicular.   The cells of Hortega (microglia) are also found and occur here with irregular or rod-shaped bodies.

Not infrequently in infants a filamentary remnant of the hyaloid artery may be seen to enter the vitreous for 1–1½ mm., after a short intrapapillary course.

Rochon Duvigneaud describes the disc as the umbilicus of the eye for it is traversed in the embryo by an artery which later disappears.

There are no fibres of Müller in the disc and thus no material which binds the nerve fibres together at right angles to their course, as occurs in the retina generally.   They can thus be separated much more easily from each other and the tissue distended with œdematous fluid.   *This is no doubt the reason why the disc swells so easily in papillœdema while the neighbouring retina remains relatively flat.*

Neuroglia also lines the anterior portion of the scleral and the whole of the choroidal portion of the canal of entry of the optic nerve (Fig. 298, 302).

This neuroglia is continued anteriorly beyond the pigment epithelium where it forms the intermediary tissue of Kuhnt.   The neuroglia here forms a mass of nuclei and circularly-running fibres placed in the concavity of the nerve fibres of the retina as they curve round at the edge of the disc to enter the optic nerve (Figs. 298, 301).

As regards the lamina cribrosa, the choroidal portion is entirely glial.   In the scleral portion glial and connective tissue fibres alternate.   It is usually stated that the most posterior laminæ contain no glia but, while there is less glia than anteriorly, this tissue is always present.

The Sheaths of the Optic Nerve

The optic nerve in the cranial cavity is at first surrounded only by pia, but in the optic canal gets a covering of arachnoid as well.

At the optic foramen the cranial dura splits into two layers.   The outer becomes continuous with the periosteum of the orbit (periorbita), the inner forms the dural covering of the optic nerve.

Thus in the canal and in the orbit the nerve is surrounded by three sheaths, namely, **dura, arachnoid,** and **pia**.

Between the dura and arachnoid is the *subdural space* [1] ; and between the

---

[1] The subdural space often appears in ordinary microscopic sections to be as large as the sub-arachnoid (Fig. 160).   This is an artefact.   The subdural space here is capillary only, as it is in the cranial cavity.

arachnoid and pia is the *subarachnoid space.* Both these spaces communicate with the corresponding intracranial spaces ; thus fluid injected into the subarachnoid space in the cranial cavity easily passes into the subarachnoid space around the optic nerve.

The Dura consists of bundles of tough fibrous tissue which are larger than those of the sclera and composed of collagenous fibrillæ, in which are found numerous elastic fibres. The dura varies in thickness from 0·35 to 0·5 mm. It is thickest where it becomes continuous with the sclera.

The central dural fibres run for the most part circularly, the peripheral ones

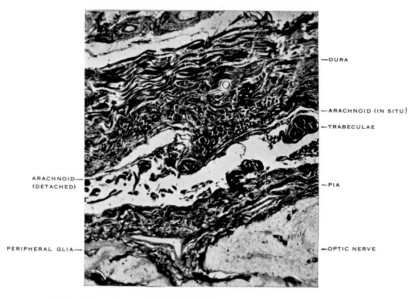

FIG. 307.—LONGITUDINAL SECTION OF OPTIC NERVE SHEATHS.

(i.e. those nearest the supravaginal space) tend to run longitudinally with oblique ones interspersed (Figs. 160, 307).

The outer longitudinal portion (or layer) is loosely knit and often divides up into two to five lamellæ. Between the lamellæ are spindle-shaped nuclei which tend to be more numerous in childhood. The nuclei belong to flattened oblong or star-shaped cells which are in close relationship with numerous elastic fibres.

The inner aspect of the dura is covered with a continuous endothelial lining, which very easily becomes detached as an artefact (Fig. 160), and which is reflected on to the trabeculæ which pass to the arachnoid and pia.

Where the ciliary vessels and nerves approach the sclera, the lamellæ become condensed, surround these, and eventually blend with the sclera. The ciliary ganglion sends numerous fine nerves with very thick epineurium along the vessels. These form a plexus in which ganglion cells may be present. The vessels have a very thick adventitia and a remarkably thick structureless subendothelial layer.

Around the dura is the supravaginal space of Schwalbe, who described it as a lymph space lined by endothelium. It has, however, the structure of loose connective tissue which is easily distensible with fluid (see p. 269).

The Arachnoid is a very thin membrane some 10 μ in thickness, which consists of a central core of, for the most part, non-nucleated collagenous tissue, which is covered on either side by endothelium. The outer endothelium (i.e. that facing the dura) has a tendency to proliferate and become several layers thick. (? villi – Shanthaveerappa and Bourne, *Exp. Eye Res.* 1964, **3**, 31). It may even form endothelial pearls (corpora amylacea) (Fig. 308).

From it numerous trabeculæ pass to the pia, and criss-crossing amongst themselves form a network in the subarachnoid space. Each trabecula consists of a central core of collagenous tissue surrounded by endothelium.

The Pia has a structure similar to the dura, only here the peripheral fibres tend to be circular and the innermost ones longitudinal.

Also the pia sends numerous septa into the optic nerve, which divide its fibres into separate bundles (Figs. 260, 312). Thus the pia is intimately connected with the optic nerve and only separated from it with difficulty. There are numerous vessels in the pia which lie for the most part between the longitudinal and circular fibres. The pia is thus much more vascular than the dura.

Traced anteriorly :

The Dura becomes continuous with the outer two-thirds of the sclera, usually without line of demarcation (Fig. 300). The outer fibres pass into the sclera and then bend outwards at an angle of about 110°. They do not run parallel with the scleral fibres, but interlace with them. The inner dural fibres pass in more obliquely.

The Arachnoid ends on a level

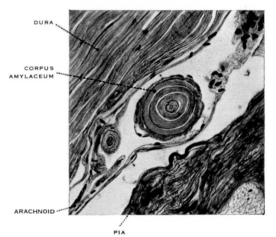

FIG. 308.—CORPORA AMYLACEA IN ARACHNOID.

with the posterior part of the lamina cribrosa by becoming continuous with the sclera (Figs. 294, 300).

The Pia, turning outwards, also becomes continuous for the most part with the sclera, but some fibres run into the choroid and some into the border tissue round the optic nerve. The pia increases in thickness as it approaches the bulb by the addition of more circular fibres. Its outer fibres pass outwards into the densely knit meridional fibres of the inner one-fifth or two-fifths of the sclera.

This union of the pia with the inner meridional fibres of the sclera and of the dura with the outer circular fibres gives this transition zone an extremely dense structure which can be made out macroscopically.

The innermost layers of the pia do not end as above described, but pass forwards to the basal lamina between the choroid and the nerve, becoming in fact continuous with the choroid (Key and Retzius).

Some circular pial fibres insinuate themselves between the fused lamellæ of the suprachoroid lamina, and some run into the border tissue of the nerve. All this tissue has the firm consistency characteristic of the border territories of the sclera.

This denser area of sclera forms a ring which is bounded by a line running

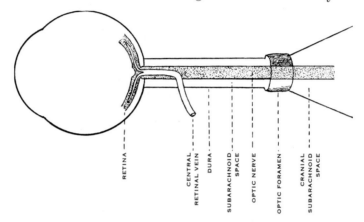

Fig. 309.—Diagram to show the Continuity between the Cranial Subarachnoid Space and that around the Optic Nerve.

Note how the central vessels cross the space and may be compressed if the intracranial pressure be raised and thus produce papillœdema.

from the hyaloid to the outer edge of the dura, and thus gets narrower as we trace it forwards (Fig. 300).

The Subarachnoid Space ends in a cul-de-sac which lies in the sclera and whose anterior extremity reaches the back of the lamina cribrosa (Fig. 294). It is widest anteriorly, where the optic nerve is thinnest, and in a temporally directed scleral canal is wider on the nasal side.

It will thus be seen that for the most part the dura is connected through the arachnoid to the pia by trabeculæ.[1]   In most places these tear easily, so that the dura can be made to slide backwards and forwards on the pia. (Normally in the movements of the eye a slight amount of this sliding probably also takes place.)

Close to the eyeball, however, the connection is stronger, and again in the optic canal the relationships of the various sheaths are of special interest.

[1] See Schwalbe (1870), *Arch. mikr. Anat.*, **6.**

Here the dura is so firmly united to the optic nerve that it is impossible to separate them (see p. 324).

This close union of the dura to the optic nerve is of importance, as the dura is itself firmly united to the bone.

This clearly forms a point of fixation for the nerve, which might otherwise be

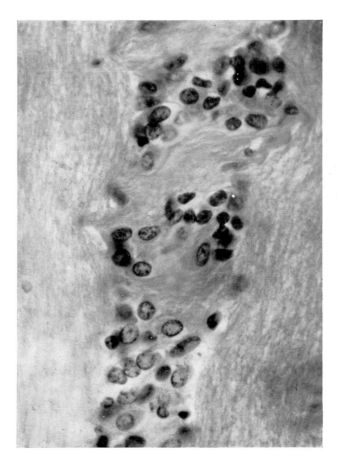

FIG. 310.—NORMAL OPTIC NERVE (× 220). (MASSON'S STAIN.)
Longitudinal section. Columns of glial nuclei. Note pale and dark types.

pushed into the cranium and thus be liable to injury in the canal (Schwalbe).

Structure of the Optic Nerve.—The optic nerve consists essentially of visual fibres, which are the axons of the ganglion cells of the retina, and which will synapse in the lateral geniculate body, superior colliculus, etc., after partially decussating in the chiasma (Fig. 126).

But the optic nerve contains other fibres besides the visual :

A.E.—22

1. Pupillary fibres.

2. Retino-motor fibres from the brain to the retina (Fig. 126).

3. Probably inter-retinal fibres = commissural fibres between the two retinæ.

4. Possibly trophic fibres.

If we examine a cross-section of the nerve, we find it is immediately surrounded by the pial sheath, and from this septa pass into the nerve and divide it into numerous (800–1,200) bundles (Fig. 160). There are about one million fibres in the optic nerve, which is 38 per cent. of the afferent fibres of all the cranial nerves put together. This makes vision by far the most important of the special senses.

The framework of the optic nerve is most dense in its most vascular portion, i.e. distal to the entrance of the central vessels and in the optic canal. Near the chiasma there is a well-marked glial septum which passes obliquely from above downwards and medially to or just beyond the centre of the nerve. This, as well as the trabeculæ, disappears in the chiasma. There are no trabeculæ in the optic tracts.

The Septa.—To understand the structure of the septa it is best to study their development. The developing optic nerve has a glial membrane surrounding it.

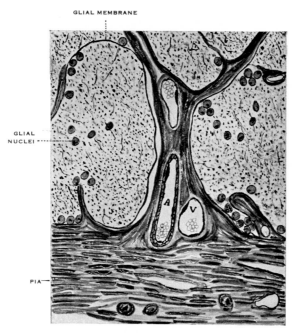

GLIAL MEMBRANE

GLIAL NUCLEI

PIA

As the septal vessels, carrying with them connective tissue cells, invade the nerve at about the fourth month of intra-uterine life, they invaginate this membrane. Thus each septum has a vessel in its centre; this is surrounded by connective tissue which in turn is bounded by neuroglia (Fig. 312). The vessels enter the nerve transversely (radially), divide dichotomously repeatedly and, anastomosing with neighbouring vessels, form a vascular net which reaches the centre of the nerve or the central vessels. The septal vessels also send branches anteriorly and posteriorly between the nerve bundles.

FIG. 312.—TRANSVERSE SECTION OF A SEPTUM OF THE OPTIC NERVE (ZENKER. MALLORY'S TRIPLE STAIN) TO SHOW THAT EACH SEPTUM CONTAINS A VESSEL (OR VESSELS); AROUND THIS IS CONNECTIVE TISSUE AND THEN A GLIAL MEMBRANE.

(*Wolff's preparation.*)

The septa pass into the cross-section of the nerve radially. There are some six to nine very thick primary septa which divide the nerve

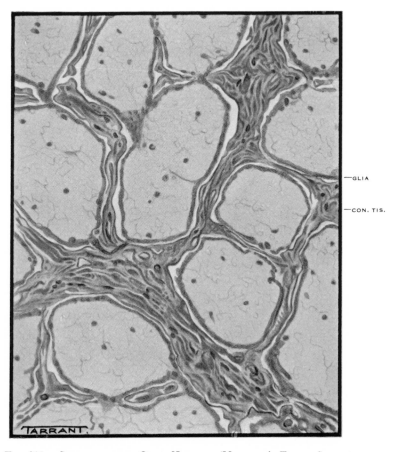

—GLIA

—CON. TIS.

TARRANT.

FIG. 311:—SECTION OF THE OPTIC NERVE.   (MALLORY'S TRIPLE STAIN.)

To show " open " and " closed " compartments.   Connective tissue is blue, glia is red.   " Closed " means closed by connective tissue.   If closed by glia only, it does not count for purposes of the definition.

into sectors, and between these a great number of thinner, secondary, septa, 1 mm. or less apart. These, as did the blood-vessels, divide repeatedly and dichotomously, and joining with neighbouring septa form meshes which divide the nerve into bundles. The spaces formed by the septa are round or polyhedral, but in man the angles are always rounded in contradistinction to that seen in most animals.

The antero-posterior branches of the septal vessels anastomose with each other and with the transverse branches to form a longitudinal vascular net around each nerve bundle. The septa formed on this scaffolding, therefore, surround the bundles in the form of a tube or cylinder. This tube, however, is not closed, for it is perforated to allow neighbouring nerve bundles to communicate with each other.

It thus comes about that in an antero-posterior section of the optic nerve the longitudinal septa are not continuous. The gaps in each septum correspond to the holes in the cylinder and are normally occupied by columns of glial cells (Fig. 270). There are two kinds of glial nuclei: (a) small, round, staining homogeneously and darkly with hæmatoxylin; (b) large, more oval, staining poorly and having a fine granular chromatin (Figs. 299, 310). Usually no cell body can be made out except by special stain (methylene-blue-Benda).

On transverse section also " incomplete " septa are seen. These are so called because they are not completely surrounded by connective (blue-staining) tissue. They are however completed by glia (Fig. 311).

The cross-section of each septum may be flattened or quadrilateral or prismatic, depending on the position of the septal vessels.

The structure of each trabecula is as follows :

In the centre is a vessel which in the case of the larger septa has a well-marked muscularis and elastica. Around this is a variable amount of loose connective tissue. This in turn is surrounded by dense connective tissue. Around this again are glial fibres and glial nuclei (Fig. 312).

The septa are continuous with the pia and this is the reason why the latter is only separated from the nerve with difficulty.

Generally speaking the septa are best developed where most movement is liable to take place : that is, directly behind the globe and just in front of the optic foramen, but with reference to the septa we may divide the optic nerve into five parts (Behr) :

1. The anterior 1 cm. shows a strong development of the septa with marked transverse fibres.

2. The middle intraorbital portion with narrower septa and only slight transverse bundles.

3. The posterior part of the intraorbital portion is like the anterior but the transverse bundles are more marked.

4. The anterior part of the intracranial portion : while generally the septa

are regularly distributed there is here a great difference between the peripheral and the axial portions where the papillo-macular bundle is placed. The septa are not only thinner but less numerous, so that larger bundles are enclosed by them. Probably the vascular arrangements, therefore, of the papillo-macular bundle are not so good as those of the other fibres (Behr).

5. In front of the chiasma the connective tissue septa disappear entirely and only glial septa remain.

Lining the pia is the " glial mantle " of Fuchs, which consists of a layer of

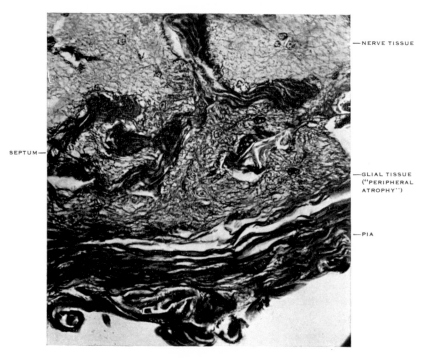

FIG. 313.—TRANSVERSE SECTION OF THE OPTIC NERVE (ZENKER. MALLORY'S TRIPLE STAIN) TO SHOW FUCHS' " PERIPHERAL ATROPHY " OR GLIAL MANTLE.

Note that this is normal glial tissue. This stains much more densely (redder with the triple stain) than the nerve tissue. The difference in texture can also be seen clearly.

glial tissue (Fig. 313). This also sends prolongations into the nerve, which not only line the septa, but also pass into the nerve bundles themselves. Glial cells lie scattered along the glial prolongations. The glial mantle varies in thickness but is generally quite thin. It is greatly thickened, however, in the floor of the third ventricle and, again, just behind the optic canal. This latter thickening lies at the upper and lateral part of the nerve.

From it an important oblique, somewhat triangular, glial (previously described as pial) septum runs from above downwards and medially and backwards, to end in a point a little in front of the chiasma. It sends spidery processes into the nerve which join with the trabeculæ. The septum divides the nerve fibres into a ventro-medial and a dorso-lateral portion, the former being the fibres which will cross over to the other side and the latter forming the temporal uncrossed bundle.

The glial septum marks the end of the septal systems of the optic nerve, which are therefore not found in the proximal part of the nerve. The absence of septa

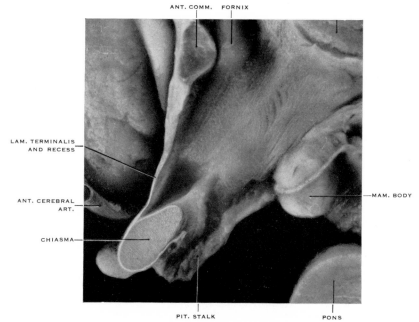

Fig. 314.—Sagittal Section of Third Ventricle.

here enables the unhindered course of those (anterior) loops formed by fibres which come from the opposite optic nerve (Wilbrand) (see p. 374 and Fig. 347).

Also, the end of the glial septum marks the actual beginning of the *physiological chiasma*, i.e. it marks the position where the crossed fibres first separate from the uncrossed, which therefore takes place above the *macroscopic chiasma*.

Sometimes spaces are seen between the septa and the nerve bundles. These are held to be lymphatic spaces, since they fill when the optic nerve is injected as in the experiments of Schwalbe and Key and Retzius.

But Salzmann holds that they are artefacts, and has never been able to make out an endothelial lining. Not infrequently one sees nodes of ill-staining tissue in the optic nerve. These constitute the fleck-form degeneration of Siegrist and are most probably artefacts due to bruising in removing the nerve post-mortem. Corpora amylacea are highly refractile bodies, showing concentric lamellation, found among the nerve fibres or in the glial tissues most commonly in old people or in atrophic eyes.

The Fibres of the optic nerve are of *two kinds*, fine and coarse, or more correctly fine and very fine, for they vary from 0·7 to 10 μ, whereas the diameter of a fibre from an ordinary peripheral sensory nerve is 20 μ.   The greatest number of the fibres is under 1 μ and the next greatest from 1 to 2 μ (Chacko).

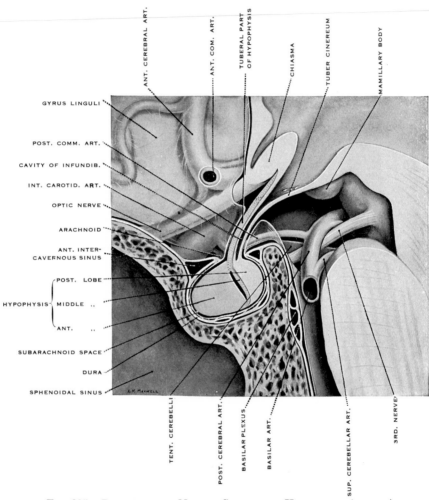

FIG. 315.—DIAGRAMMATIC MEDIAN SECTION OF HYPOPHYSIS (IN SITU).
(The existence of a subarachnoid space around the gland in the pituitary fossa is doubtful.
(From Cunningham's " Anatomy."

Electron Microscopy of the Optic Nerve.—Yamamoto[1] (1966) in normal human optic nerves confirms that the septa are composed of collagen fibres continuous with the pial sheath.   Blood vessels are found only in the septa, not in the nerve bundles.   Glial cells intrude into the bundles of nerve fibres.   Yamamoto suggests

[1] Yamamoto, T. (1966)   *Jap. Jour. Ophth.* **10,** 1, 40.

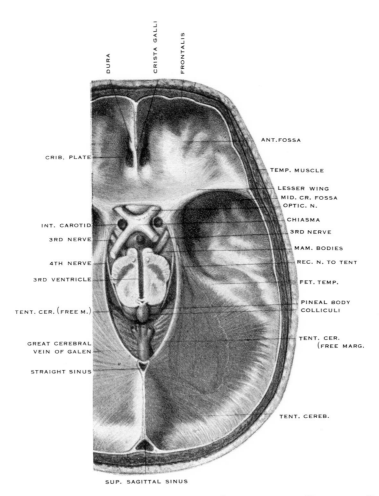

DURA

CRISTA GALLI

FRONTALIS

ANT. FOSSA

CRIB. PLATE

TEMP. MUSCLE

LESSER WING
MID. CR. FOSSA
OPTIC. N.

CHIASMA

INT. CAROTID

3RD NERVE

3RD NERVE

MAM. BODIES

4TH NERVE

REC. N. TO TENT

3RD VENTRICLE

FET. TEMP.

PINEAL BODY
COLLICULI

TENT. CER. (FREE M.)

GREAT CEREBRAL
VEIN OF GALEN

TENT. CER.
(FREE MARG.

STRAIGHT SINUS

TENT. CEREB.

SUP. SAGITTAL SINUS

FIG. 316.—SECTION OF CRANIUM JUST ABOVE THE OPENING IN THE TENTORIUM CEREBELLI.
(*From Hirschfeld and Leveillé.*)

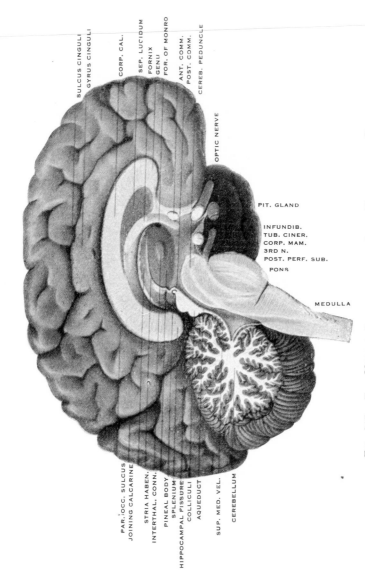

SULCUS CINGULI
GYRUS CINGULI
CORP. CAL.
SEP. LUCIDUM
FORNIX
GENU
FOR. OF MONRO
ANT. COMM.
POST. COMM.
CEREB. PEDUNCLE

OPTIC NERVE

PIT. GLAND

INFUNDIB.
TUB. CINER.
CORP. MAM.
3RD N.
POST. PERF. SUB.
PONS

MEDULLA

PAR. OCC. SULCUS
JOINING CALCARINE
STRIA HABEN.
INTERTHAL. CONN.
PINEAL BODY
SPLENIUM
HIPPOCAMPAL FISSURE
COLLICULI
AQUEDUCT
SUP. MED. VEL.
CEREBELLUM

FIG. 317. — THE MEDIAL SURFACE OF THE LEFT HALF OF THE BRAIN.

(From Hirschfeld and Leveillé.)

[A.E.—343

that oligodendrocytes are concerned with myelinization and astrocytes with nutrition of the avascular nerve bundles. He finds over 80 per cent of the nerve fibres to be less than 1 μ in diameter. The non-myelinated fibres run around the circumference of nerve bundles.

The fibres have a medullary sheath, but no sheath of Schwann (neurilemma). They thus resemble the fibres of the central nervous system. *Hence, perhaps, the reason why they do not regenerate when cut.* According to Ingvar, the pupillary fibres are older phylogenetically, are non-medullated, and run in the periphery of the nerve.

THE OPTIC CHIASMA

The Optic Chiasma is a flattened, oblong band some 12 mm. in its transverse diameter and 8 mm. from before backwards. It is placed at the junction of anterior wall and floor of the third ventricle, itself forming the floor of the recess which reaches almost to its anterior border (Fig. 314). Clothed in pia it lies obliquely with its posterior border higher than the anterior in the anterior part of the cisterna interpeduncularis over the diaphragma sellæ, above and behind the so-called optic groove on the sphenoid bone (Figs. 258, 315). It is thus suspended in and surrounded by cerebro-spinal fluid except at its posterior border.

In the majority [1] of cases (79 per cent.) it lies above the pituitary fossa in such a way that a part of the fossa shows in front of it. Only in 5 per cent. does it lie in the (so-called) optic groove.

In 4 per cent. it lies right behind the fossa, and in 12 per cent. a greater part of the fossa shows behind the chiasma than in front.

The chiasma is not in contact with the diaphragma sellæ, but is separated from it by 5 to 10 mm. It follows from this that a portion of the cisterna interpeduncularis lies deep to the chiasma (Fig. 315).

Relations.— *In front* are the anterior cerebral arteries and their anterior communicating branch.

Laterally, the internal carotid artery, as it passes upwards, after having pierced the roof of the cavernous sinus, lies on each side in contact with the chiasma in the angle between optic nerve and tract (Figs. 316, 353). Laterally, too, is the anterior perforated substance (Fig. 318).

Behind is the tuber cinereum. This is a hollow elevation of grey matter situated between the corpora mamillaria behind and the optic chiasma in front. Laterally it is continuous with the grey matter of the anterior perforated substance and anteriorly with the lamina terminalis. From its under-surface the infundibulum (or pituitary stalk), which is a hollow conical process, passes downwards *and forwards* and through a hole in the posterior part of the diaphragma sellæ to be attached to the posterior lobe of the pituitary body. The

[1] de Schweinitz, G., *Trans. Ophthal. Soc. U.K.*, 1923, **43**, 12.

infundibulum is thus in close contact with the lower and posterior part of the chiasma, which it joins at an acute angle (Figs. 258, 315, 353).

Above is the third ventricle, in the floor of which the chiasma makes a prominence which is continuous anteriorly with the lamina terminalis.

The medial root of the olfactory tract lies close above and to the lateral side of the anterior angle of the chiasma (Fig. 318).

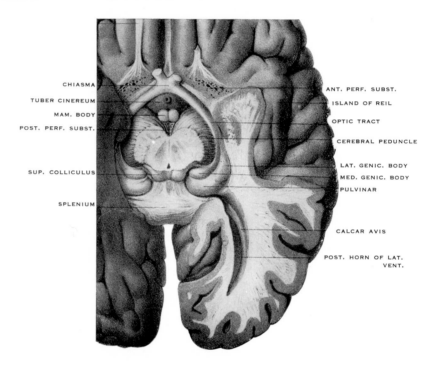

CHIASMA

TUBER CINEREUM

MAM. BODY

POST. PERF. SUBST.

SUP. COLLICULUS

SPLENIUM

ANT. PERF. SUBST.

ISLAND OF REIL

OPTIC TRACT

CEREBRAL PEDUNCLE

LAT. GENIC. BODY

MED. GENIC. BODY

PULVINAR

CALCAR AVIS

POST. HORN OF LAT. VENT.

FIG. 318.—VIEW OF BASE OF THE BRAIN.
(*From Hirschfeld and Leveillé.*)

Below is the pituitary body, and under the lateral edge of the chiasma is the cavernous sinus (with its contents), with the third nerve here the closest relation where it lies on the diaphragma before entering the sinus.

The arachnoid is spread like an apron between the optic nerves. It is attached to the tip of the temporal lobe and internal carotid at the sides and to the frontal lobes anteriorly (Fig. 257).

It closely surrounds the infundibulum, and in the angle between this structure and the chiasma a dense vascular network of pia-arachnoid is found. The chiasma is thus surrounded by a membrane which holds it up to the brain and which becomes densely matted and thickened in inflammatory conditions, notably syphilis (Traquair).

Hypophysis Cerebri (Pituitary Body)

The pituitary body consists of an anterior lobe derived from the stomodæum, cellular in structure, and a posterior lobe, formed as an outgrowth from the primary brain vesicle, the pars nervosa, having the structure of neuroglia, but containing also fine unmyelinated nerve fibres, and some colloid material coming from the anterior lobe. A cleft separates the anterior lobe from the pars intermedia which, although continuous with the pars nervosa, yet is derived from the anterior lobe.

The pituitary body, about the size of a hazel nut, is situated in the sella turcica (pituitary fossa) on the upper surface of the body of the sphenoid, about midway between the root of the nose and the posterior margin of the foramen magnum.

In front are the tuberculum sellæ and optic groove ; behind, the overhanging dorsum sellæ.

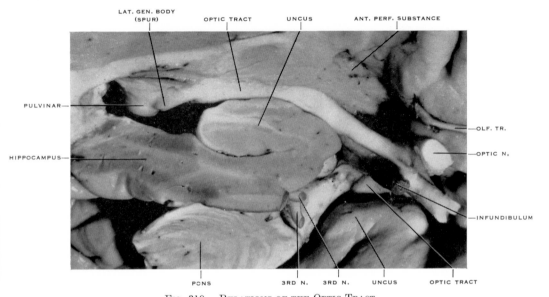

FIG. 319.—RELATIONS OF THE OPTIC TRACT.

The uncus and hippocampus have been divided vertically.

The roof of the pituitary fossa (diaphragma sellæ) is formed by dura mater (Fig. 315), perforated at its centre to allow the pituitary stalk or infundibulum to pass through. This connects the pituitary body with the third ventricle.

On either side the hypophysis is walled in by dura mater, which separates it from the cavernous sinus and the structures within it. In the lateral wall of the sinus from above downwards are the 3rd, 4th, and 1st and 2nd divisions of the 5th cranial nerves (Fig. 366).

In the sinus itself are the internal carotid artery and lateral to it the 6th nerve.

A glance at Fig. 260 will show why the 3rd and 4th nerves are more often affected in pituitary tumours than that weakling of the cranial contents, namely, the 6th, which is here protected by the internal carotid artery.

Joining the cavernous sinuses on either side, and situated in the floor of the sella turcica, is the so-called circular sinus (intercavernous plexus), which is usually represented by a plexus of veins.

In the body of the sphenoid and below the pituitary body is the sphenoidal air sinus (see p. 27) divided by a median septum, and having in its lateral wall the carotid buttress, a ledge of bone, which can often be made out in X-rays, and is an important landmark in approaching the pituitary by the nasal route (see p. 28).

The optic chiasma usually lies above the posterior part of the diaphragma sellæ. Only very rarely does it actually lie in the optic groove (see p. 343).

The circle of Willis lies above the pituitary fossa in such a way that an enlarging pituitary tumour may be encircled by it.

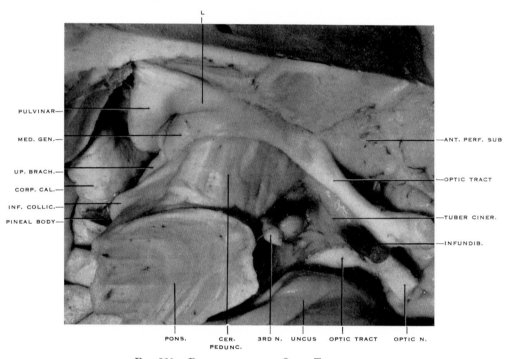

FIG. 320.—RELATIONS OF THE OPTIC TRACT, ETC.

A further stage in the dissection of Fig. 319. The uncus and hippocampus have been removed. L = lateral geniculate body (spur). Below this is the hilum and below this again is slight elevation (lateral geniculate body) produced by its medial portion.

Above this again is the cisterna chiasmatica.

The trigeminal ganglion lies on the apex of the petrous temporal bone to the lateral side of the cavernous sinus, and above this is the uncus, pressure on which by an enlarging pituitary tumour gives rise to olfactory hallucinations.

The meninges blend with the capsule of the hypophysis and cannot be identified as separate layers in the fossa (Gray).

The hypophysis receives its blood-supply from the internal carotid by upper and lower hypophyseal branches that anastomose with each other. These supply the stalk and posterior lobe, from the capillaries of which a portal system of vessels provides the major supply to the anterior lobe. The hypophyseal veins drain to the intercavernous plexus and cavernous sinuses (J. P. Stanfield (1960), *J. Anat.*, **94**, 2, 257).

THE OPTIC TRACTS

The optic tracts represent the last extracerebral portion of the visual pathway ; for behind them the visual fibres lie in the white matter of the brain itself.

Each **optic tract** is a cylindrical band, slightly flattened from above down, which runs laterally and backwards from the postero-lateral angle of the chiasma, between the tuber cinereum and the anterior perforated substance (Fig. 318). It forms the antero-lateral boundary of the inter-peduncular space.

Becoming more flattened and strap-like, it is closely applied to the upper part of the anterior then lateral surface of the cerebral peduncle, between the internal capsule and the basis pedunculi, i.e. close to the point of disappearance of the peduncle into the cerebral hemisphere (Fig. 320).

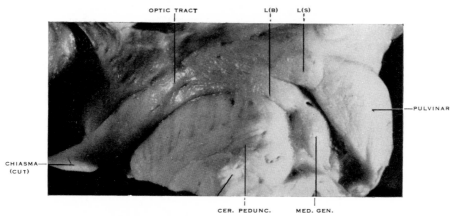

FIG. 321.—THE OPTIC TRACT, ETC., FROM BELOW.
Note two portions of lateral geniculate body with hilum between them.
L(S) = elevation produced by the lateral part of the lateral geniculate body.
L(B) = slighter elevation produced by the medial part of the lateral geniculate body.

Below and parallel to it runs the posterior cerebral artery. *But the satellite vessel is the anterior choroidal.* This arises from the internal carotid just beyond (lateral to) the origin of the posterior communicating artery, at the lateral side of the commencement of the optic tract (Figs. 352, 353, 357, 359). It runs backwards and medially, crosses the optic tract on its under surface, and comes to lie on the medial side of this structure. It maintains this relation to the anterior part of the lateral geniculate body. Here it turns abruptly laterally, recrosses the optic tract, and breaks up into a number of branches (see p. 410). The posterior communicating artery may at times cross below the beginning of the optic tract from lateral to medial.

At its commencement the tract lies free except on its medial side, where it is attached to the outer wall of the third ventricle by a narrow band. As it passes laterally, backwards, and a little upwards round the cerebral peduncle, it rotates outwards slightly on its own axis so that the band connecting it to the brain substance comes to lie at first dorso-medially and finally dorso-laterally, the free edge which was at first lateral becoming ventral (Roenne, Traquair). The dorsal fasciculi are partially surrounded by the commissures of Meynert and (?) Gudden (see later), while the ventral bundles are free and covered by thin pia mater. The surfaces are at first directed upwards and downwards, but round the cerebral peduncle they face upwards and medially, and downwards and laterally (Fig. 321).

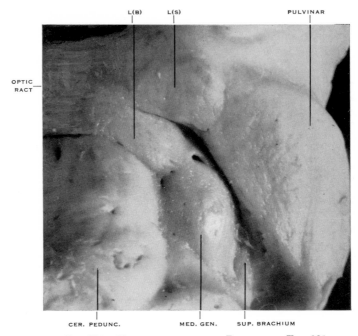

FIG. 322.—ENLARGED VIEW OF A PORTION OF FIG. 321.

To show especially the two portions of the lateral geniculate body, the medial elevation being unusually well developed. Note hilum between them. See legend to Fig. 321.

In the first portion of its course the optic tract lies superficial on the under aspect of the brain (Fig. 318). It runs above the dorsum sellæ [1] and crosses the third nerve from medial to lateral (Fig. 316). Above is the posterior part of the anterior perforated substance and the floor of the third ventricle, while medially is the tuber cinereum (Fig. 318).

In the middle portion of its course the tract lies hidden between the uncus and the cerebral peduncle. It is here also that the flattening commences to conform with the upper aspect of the uncus (Fig. 319). The optic tract here crosses the pyramidal tract which occupies the middle segment of the basis pedunculi. Nearby, just dorsal to the substantia nigra, are the lemnisci carrying sensory

[1] The exact relations here will depend on the varying position of the chiasma.

fibres.   It thus comes about that a single lesion here can affect vision and also the great motor and sensory tracts.

(As will be seen later, the optic radiations also cross and come close to the motor and sensory tracts in the posterior part of the internal capsule, so that here also a single lesion may affect all three.)

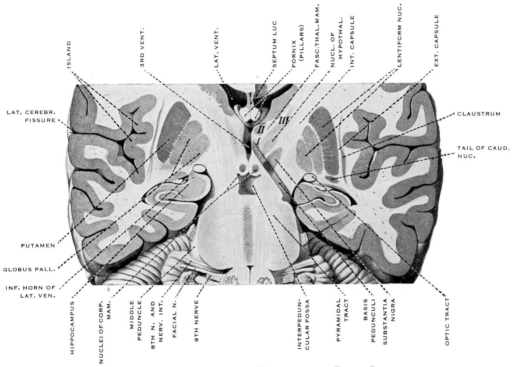

FIG. 323.—A SECTION OF THE BRAIN IN THE PLANE OF THE BRAIN STEM FROM IN FRONT.

On the left the section through the hemisphere is somewhat dorsal to that on the right.   I, II, and III indicate the anterior, medial, and lateral nuclei of the thalamus.

(*From Sabotta.*)

In the posterior part of its course the optic tract lies in the depths of the hippocampal sulcus close to the medial part of the roof of the inferior horn of the lateral ventricle.   It has the globus pallidus above, the internal capsule medially, and the hippocampus below (Figs. 323, 328).

In the posterior portion of its course also the tract is divided by a shallow furrow (which may be difficult to find) into its so-called medial and lateral roots.

The medial root was almost universally described as being the same as the commissure of Gudden and to have nothing to do with vision (see p. 350).   It was held to connect the two medial geniculate bodies by passing to the medial side of each optic tract and behind the chiasma, and to be an auditory commissure.

But the medial root although directed towards the medial geniculate body does not join it (Pfeifer) but penetrates the brain substance just in front of it to enter the medial part of the saddle that is the body of the lateral geniculate (Figs. 326, 327), which, indeed, not infrequently causes a slight elevation on the surface (Figs. 321, 322). The medial root is therefore also visual in function.[1]

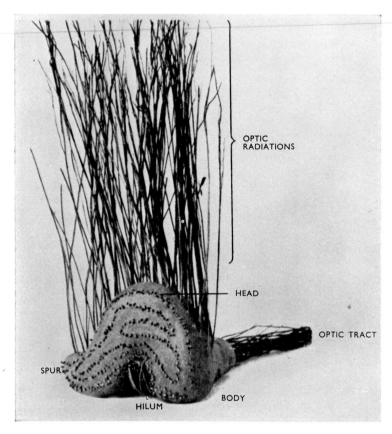

FIG. 324.—MODEL OF LEFT LATERAL GENICULATE BODY FROM BEHIND AND MEDIAL SIDE.
(*From Pfeifer in the Kurzes Handbuch.*)

The lateral root spreads over the lateral geniculate body, and for the most part ends in it. The groove between the roots runs into the hilum of the lateral geniculate body, which is always a definite cleft (Figs. 321, 322).

The fibres of the optic tract, coming from the ganglion cells of the retina, reach three major destinations :

(1) the lateral geniculate body for relay to the cortex—these are visual

(2) each pretectal nucleus—these are for pupil constriction to light

(3) the superior colliculus—these are for general reflex responses to light (movements of the eyeballs, face muscles, neck, trunk and limbs).

[1] See Wolff, E. (1953), *Brain*, **76,** 455.

The Commissures of Gudden and Meynert.—These are both *dorsal* commissures. The commissure of Gudden is called the postero-inferior commissure and is actually in the optic tract.

The commissure of Meynert is postero-superior and is outside the tract, but accompanies it. Meynert is a narrow bundle of coarse well-staining fibres and therefore easily demonstrated. It lies dorso-medial close to the lentiform nucleus. It has been demonstrated in man.

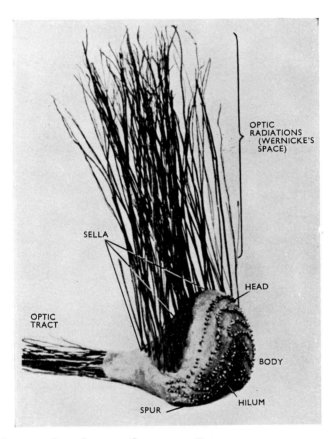

FIG. 325.—MODEL OF LEFT LATERAL GENICULATE BODY FROM BEHIND AND LATERAL SIDE.

The origin of the optic radiations from the anterior portion of the saddle (Sella) is seen. This is the stalk of the lateral geniculate body, or Wernicke's field, as it is also called.

(From Pfeifer in the Kurzes Handbuch.)

But the commissure of Gudden is but doubtfully present in the human : its presence is denied by Dejerine and Winkler. Gudden himself demonstrated it after removal of the eyes of a rabbit.

At any rate the ventrally placed medial root of the human optic tract obviously has nothing to do with Gudden's commissure (Pfeifer).

The Transverse Peduncular Tract arises from the optic tract, where it enters the mid-brain, passes round the ventral aspect of the cerebral peduncle, to enter the brain close to the exit of the oculo-motor nerve. This tract is better marked in the lower animals than in man, in whom it is found in only 30 per cent. of cases. It is said to atrophy when the eye is enucleated, but it is extremely doubtful that it has anything to do with vision.

The Tract of Darkschewitsch passes from the optic tract to the ganglion habenulæ, then through the posterior commissure to the oculo-motor nucleus. Darkschewitsch thought it carried pupillary impulses, but this is doubtful.

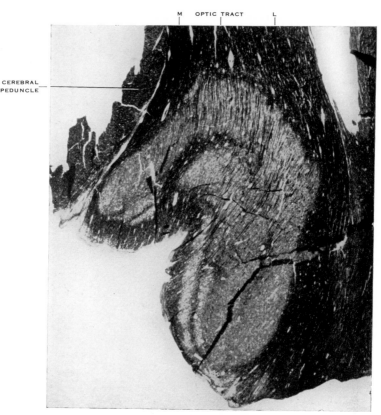

FIG. 326.—HORIZONTAL SECTION OF HUMAN LATERAL GENICULATE BODY WITH TERMINATION OF OPTIC TRACT. (STAINED WEIGERT-PAL.)

M = medial portion of tract.   L = lateral portion.

THE LATERAL GENICULATE BODIES

Each lateral geniculate body has, according to Pfeifer, the form of a Moorish saddle markedly raised posteriorly (Figs. 324, 325).

It is made up of the following. The *spur* (calcar) is inferior, lateral and anterior. The *body* (corpus) is inferior, medial and posterior. The *hilum*, which is ventral, lies between the spur and the body and is roofed over by the head (caput). There is an unnamed antero-inferior portion. This runs forward into the optic tract, which splits to enfold it.

The saddle is somewhat asymmetrical, the lateral portion (the spur) projecting farther downwards than the medial portion (the body) (Fig. 326).

It thus comes about that it is the lateral portion which causes the surface elevation known as the lateral geniculate body. This usually projects but little, forming a flattened oval elevation at the posterior end of the optic tract on the lateral portion of the inferior aspect of the pulvinar of the thalamus (to which both geniculate bodies belong).

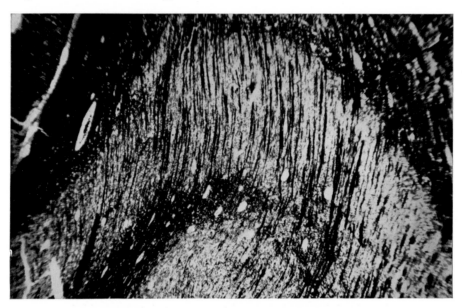

FIG. 327.—AS FIG. 326, BUT UNDER HIGHER POWER.

Note medullated fibres entering lateral geniculate from the tract. No line of demarcation between medial and lateral portion of the tract.

The medial portion of the saddle does not usually cause a surface elevation but may do so just in front of the medial geniculate body (Figs. 321, 322).

It will thus be seen that by far the greater portion of the lateral geniculate body lies hidden from a surface view, being enfolded by the pulvinar and only seen in vertical (Fig. 328) and horizontal sections of the region.

On coronal section the lateral geniculate body has the shape of an inverted heart. On horizontal section it is shown to be related anteriorly with the optic tract which ends therein; laterally with the retro-lenticular portion of the internal capsule; medially with the medial geniculate body; posteriorly with the hippocampal convolution, and postero-laterally with the inferior horn of the lateral ventricle. At a higher level the lateral geniculate body is part of the pulvinar which it penetrates (Fig. 328). Here it has anteriorly the pregeniculate grey matter flanked anteriorly by the temporo-pontine fibres of Türck and the posterior portion of the internal capsule, laterally the area of Wernicke (see below), and medially the medial geniculate body.

Structure.—On section it is seen to consist of alternating white and grey areas. The white areas are formed by the medullated fibres of the optic tract, alternating layers coming from opposite eyes, while in the grey areas are the cell bodies in which these terminate, and from which arises the new relay of visual fibres forming the optic radiation.

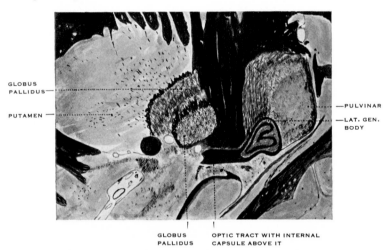

FIG. 328.—PARA-SAGITTAL (VERTICAL) SECTION OF THE BRAIN (WEIGERT).

Showing optic tract dividing to form capsule to lateral geniculate body; also its relation to the internal capsule.   (*After Lhermitte, slightly modified.*)

On sagittal section it is seen that the fibres of the optic tract divide into two layers (Fig. 328). The inferior of these forms the white layer of the hilum, the superior forms the dorsal portion of the saddle. Between these laminæ which form the capsule of the lateral geniculate body are alternating layers of myelinated fibres and cells which give the body its characteristic appearance (see also p. 377).

From the dorsal portion of the lateral geniculate body pass a mass of fibres (which form its peduncle) into the area of Wernicke. This is a small region of myelinated fibres enclosed by the thalamus medially, the internal capsule laterally, and the lateral geniculate body posteriorly. The main constituents of the area of Wernicke are the fibres of the optic radiation. It also contains the vertical temporo-thalamic fibres of Arnold.

The lateral geniculate body is connected to the superior colliculus by a slender band called the superior brachium (Figs. 269, 352).

THE SUPERIOR COLLICULI

The Superior Colliculi are small rounded elevations situated on the dorsal aspect of the mid-brain. They are separated from each other by an antero-posterior groove, in which lies the pineal body, while a transverse groove comes between them and the inferior colliculi which lie below (Fig. 269). Above each superior colliculus is the thalamus. The superior colliculus receives no *visual* fibres from the optic tract. The fibres it does receive from it most probably subserve photostatic reflexes. It is doubtful whether any pupillary fibres reach it. The two pairs of colliculi are together known as the *tectum*.

Structure.—The surface of the superior colliculus is covered by a thin stratum of *white* fibres (*the stratum zonale*), the majority of which are derived from the optic tract. Beneath this is a layer of *grey* matter (*the stratum cinereum*) which resembles a cap, and is thicker in the centre than at the margins. It consists of numerous small multipolar nerve cells embedded in a fine network of nerve fibres. Deep to this again is the *stratum opticum*, consisting mainly of fibres, in which are embedded large multipolar nerve cells.

The fourth layer, or *stratum lemnisci*, consists mainly of fibres derived from the lemniscus or fillet and *stratum opticum*, in which are embedded large multipolar nerve cells.

Afferent Fibres.—(1) From the optic tract viâ the superior brachium, which runs alongside the lateral geniculate body to the superior colliculus (Fig. 269).

(2) From the occipital cortex viâ the optic radiations (cortico-fugal fibres) to the lateral geniculate body, and thence viâ the superior brachium.

(3) From the spino-tectal tract, connecting it with the sensory fibres of the cord and medulla.

Efferent Fibres.—Of the fibres which arise from cells of the grey matter some cross to the superior colliculus of the opposite side, many, after undergoing decussation in the *fountain decussation of Meynert*, make connection with the ocular nuclei, and form the tecto-spinal tract which connects it with the spinal nerves.

No fibres pass from the superior colliculus to the cortex, i.e. it has no cortical projection.

The Thalamus

The thalami are two large ovoid ganglionic masses situated above the cerebral peduncles on either side of the third ventricle and reaching for some distance behind that cavity. Each measures about $1\frac{1}{2}$ in. (4 cm.) in length.

The anterior extremity of the thalamus is narrow, lies close to the mid-line, and forms the posterior boundary of the interventricular foramen of Monro (Fig. 317).

The posterior extremity is expanded and overlaps the superior colliculus. Medially it presents a well-marked angular prominence, the posterior tubercle or *pulvinar*, which is continued laterally with but a slight line of demarcation into *the lateral geniculate body*. Beneath the pulvinar, but separated from it by the superior brachium, is *the medial geniculate body* (Fig. 352).

Laterally the thalamus is separated from the *lenticular nucleus* of the *corpus striatum* by the posterior part of the *internal capsule* (Fig. 328).

It was generally held that the pulvinar of the thalamus was a relay station for the visual fibres on their way to the cortex. As the result of the work of Brouwer and Zeeman (1926), Minkowski (1913), and Henschen (1924), it would appear that the pulvinar is not one of the "lower visual centres."

The lateral geniculate body is, however, connected to the thalamus by the "tractus geniculo-thalamicus," in regard to which Wolff quoted from Professor Elliot Smith's Bowman Lecture (1928):

"Only in mammals does the lateral geniculate body emit an optic radiation which passes to the cortex. What becomes of the optic impulses to the lateral geniculate body in animals

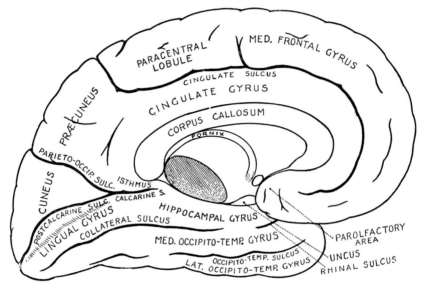

FIG. 329.—THE MEDIAL SURFACE OF THE LEFT CEREBRAL HEMISPHERE.
(*From Gray's Anatomy.*)

in which there are no optic radiations? It seems that the thalamus is the part of the brain which is responsible for the affective appreciation of experience, and therefore in the last resort determines the animal's behaviour. It is essentially the leading segment of the brain. The cerebral hemisphere is primarily a receptive apparatus for olfactory impressions. The part of the brain which determines what an animal will do in response to stimuli is the thalamus; it receives impulses coming from the skin, muscles and joints, and from every part of the body, which make the animal aware of what is happening in the world outside the surface of its skin and determines its affective state. It seems inconceivable that the lateral geniculate body which receives optic impressions and is actually spread out on the surface of the thalamus should not participate in this function of awareness. It is obvious to those who study the behaviour of fish, amphibian, reptile, bird or mammal that visual experience enters consciousness and plays a large part in determining the animal's behaviour. Therefore it seemed inconceivable that there should be no connection between geniculate body and the part of the brain which is responsible, in the last resort, for the shaping of the animal's feelings and determining what its behaviour shall be. Yet on looking through the literature I could find only three lines of reference to such a connection : it is in a paper by Dr. Chiao Tsai, published three years ago. He called attention to the fact that there was a small fibre tract connecting the lateral geniculate body with the sensory nuclei of the thalamus.[1] But he did not consider it important enough to give a name to the bundle.

" Prof. Le Gros Clark lent me sections of the brain of the jumping shrew (*Macroscelides*), which display the connecting bundle—which might be called ' tractus geniculo-thalamicus '

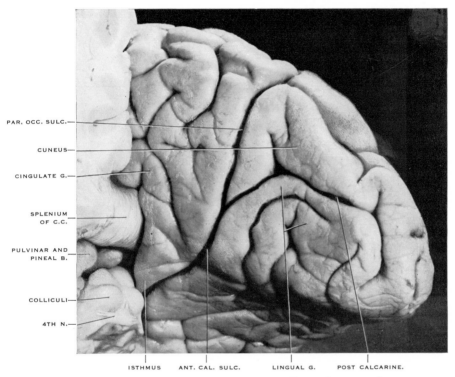

PAR. OCC. SULC.—
CUNEUS—
CINGULATE G.—
SPLENIUM OF C.C.
PULVINAR AND PINEAL B.
COLLICULI—
4TH N.—
ISTHMUS ANT. CAL. SULC. LINGUAL G. POST CALCARINE.

FIG. 330.—MEDIAL AND INFERIOR ASPECTS OF RIGHT OCCIPITAL LOBE, ETC.

—as a large bundle of fibres linking up the lateral geniculate body with the rest of the thalamus.

" A most striking demonstration of such a connecting bundle was given many years ago by Ramon y Cajal. In the preparation of the brain of a small mammal stained by the Golgi method and cut in horizontal section a thalamic nucleus is seen receiving fibres both from the medial lemniscus and from the lateral geniculate body. But neither in the drawing (of which this fibre-tract is the most obtrusive feature) nor in the text is any reference made to it. Such a centre for correlating ocular and articular impulses may represent the germ of that swelling which becomes highly developed in the thalamus of man and is known as the pulvinar. It is connected with the angular gyrus, and is supposed by some authorities

[1] It must, however, be stated that many still do not believe that geniculo-thalamic fibres exist in any mammal.

to be concerned with stereognosis.   Clinical observers, such as Winkler, of Utrecht, have been impressed with the possibility of the blending in the thalamus of impulses from the eyes with those coming from the joints and skin."

THE OPTIC RADIATIONS

The Optic Radiations (of Gratiolet) or geniculo-calcarine pathway, that is the fresh relay of fibres that carry the visual impulses to the occipital lobe, arise in the lateral geniculate body (and possibly, as some hold, from the pulvinar of the thalamus as well).

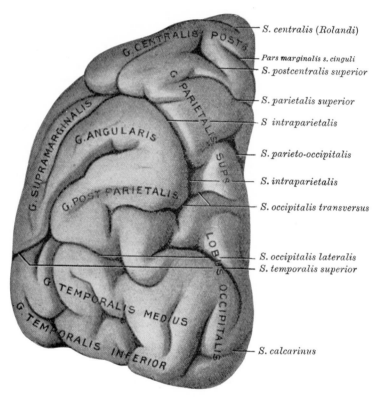

FIG. 331.—LEFT CEREBRAL HEMISPHERE FROM BEHIND.   NATURAL SIZE.
(From Quain's Anatomy.)

They pass forwards and then laterally through the area of Wernicke, forming the *optic peduncle* and lying anterior to the lateral ventricle, and in the retro-lenticular part of the internal capsule behind the sensory fibres and medial to the auditory tract.   The fibres spread out fanwise to form the medullary optic lamina. This is at first vertical but becomes horizontal near the striate cortex.

In their course posteriorly the optic radiations lie lateral to the temporal and occipital horns of the lateral ventricle.   In this part of their course they are found in the lateral sagittal stratum, which is separated from the cavity of the ventricle by the medial sagittal stratum and the tapetum of the corpus callosum (Fig. 333).

The ventral portion of the optic radiation instead of sweeping straight backwards plunges forwards into the temporal pole before passing backwards as an inferior longitudinal fasciculus (Meyer). Interference with this temporal loop[1] of the radiations gives rise to a superior homonymous quadrantic hemianopia.

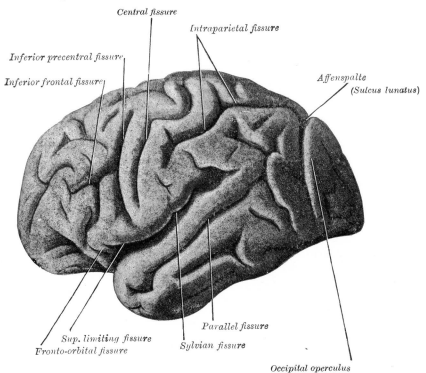

Central fissure

Intraparietal fissure

Inferior precentral fissure

Inferior frontal fissure

Affenspalte
(Sulcus lunatus)

Sup. limiting fissure
Fronto-orbital fissure

Parallel fissure

Sylvian fissure

Occipital operculus

FIG. 332.—LATERAL ASPECT OF LEFT CEREBRAL HEMISPHERE OF CHIMPANZEE.
Note Sulcus Lunatus.
(From Quain's Anatomy.)

The optic radiation as it passes back in the white matter of the cerebral hemisphere lies deep (approximately) to the middle temporal gyrus, so that tumours of this portion of the temporal lobe may give rise to visual defects.

The optic radiation ends in the occipital lobe in an extensive area of thin cortex [2] (1·4 mm. or less in thickness), in which is found the distinctive white line or stria first described by Gennari in 1776.

Apart from these cortico-petal fibres the optic radiations also contain fibres

[1] Although this is now the usual teaching, Androgue holds that the loop does not exist, and Traquair is rather of the opinion that the quadrantic hemianopia may be due to interference with the optic tract.

[2] See Smith, G. Elliot (1907), *J. Anat. and Physiol.*, **40**, 200.

that pass from the cortex to the lateral geniculate body, the thalamus, the superior colliculus, and oculo-motor nuclei.

The Calcarine Sulcus [1]

The calcarine sulcus lies for the most part on the medial aspect of the hemisphere. But its anterior end is on the under aspect, and the posterior portion may wind round the occipital pole and appear on the lateral surface.

The calcarine is a deep sulcus extending from near the posterior extremity of the brain, where it usually begins in a T-shaped fork, the lower limb of which is often grooved by the sagittal sinus (Fig. 302). From here the calcarine sulcus passes forwards, making a bend convex upwards, and ends below the splenium of the corpus callosum. The forked posterior extremity at the occipital pole is sometimes cut off from the rest of the sulcus and then appears as an independent sulcus. Sometimes, as stated above, the sulcus extends round the posterior pole on to the lateral surface, as the lateral calcarine sulcus, and then has the form of a shepherd's crook.

The calcarine sulcus usually runs just above the medial margin of the occipital lobe which is placed at the junction of the falx cerebri and tentorium cerebelli, but may be a varying distance above it.

The parieto-occipital sulcus joins the calcarine at an acute angle a little in front of its middle, dividing it into anterior and posterior portions and forming a Y-shaped figure.

If the lips of the parieto-occipital and calcarine sulci are widely separated, it will be seen that although on the surface they appear to be continuous they are separated from each other by a small buried vertical gyrus (gyrus cunei). The gyrus cunei may in fact at times

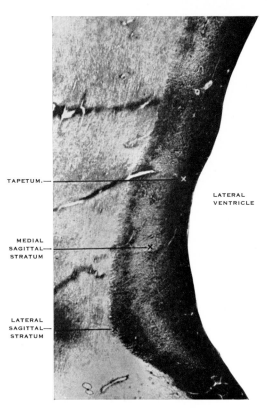

TAPETUM.—

LATERAL
VENTRICLE

MEDIAL
SAGITTAL—
STRATUM

LATERAL
SAGITTAL—
STRATUM

Fig. 333.—Strata Sagittalia.

(From Brouwer.)

[1] Classically the whole sulcus is called the calcarine, which is divided into anterior and posterior portions, a mode of description which will be followed here. According to modern nomenclature, however, the anterior portion is called the calcarine sulcus, the posterior, the postcalcarine sulcus.

come to the surface when it shuts off the continuity of the two fissures superficially also (Quain).

The posterior part of the calcarine is developed independently of the stem, which is a direct representative of one of the total fissures of the fœtal hemisphere, while the posterior part of the calcarine is formed much later by two depressions, which ultimately run together and into the true calcarine. The original independence of these parts is indicated by the existence of two annectent gyri (anterior and posterior cuneo-lingual) concealed within the posterior part of the calcarine: one at its junction with the stem of the Y, and the other near the hinder end (Quain).

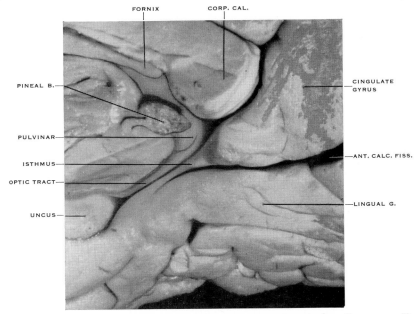

FIG. 334.—THE RELATIONS OF THE ANTERIOR PORTION OF THE ANTERIOR CALCARINE FISSURE. Further stage in dissection of Fig. 330.

The anterior calcarine sulcus crosses the infero-medial margin of the hemisphere to reach the inferior surface where it forms the infero-lateral boundary of the isthmus (Fig. 330) which connects the gyrus cinguli with the hippocampal gyrus. Sometimes the anterior calcarine passes into the so-called hippocampal sulcus as it does constantly in many of the quadrumana. As will be seen from Figs. 330 and 334, the anterior end of the calcarine sulcus may be fairly close to the colliculi and even to the pulvinar of the thalamus and lateral geniculate body, but its point of termination varies a good deal.

The Sulcus Lunatus [1] when present is situated just in front of the occipital pole. It is placed vertically with its concavity backwards. At times it forms a ⊢ with the calcarine fissure but is usually separate from it.

[1] From Gray and Elliot Smith (1930), *J. Anat.*, **64**.

The lips of the lunate sulcus, which is operculated in type, separate the striate from the peristriate area of the cortex, but the parastriate area is buried within the walls of the sulcus and intervenes between them. The lunate sulcus forms the posterior boundary of the gyrus descendens (Ecker), which lies behind the superior and inferior occipital gyri. Two curved sulci, named the superior and inferior polar sulci, are often present near the extremities of the lunate sulcus. The *superior polar sulcus* arches upwards on to the medial aspect of the occipital

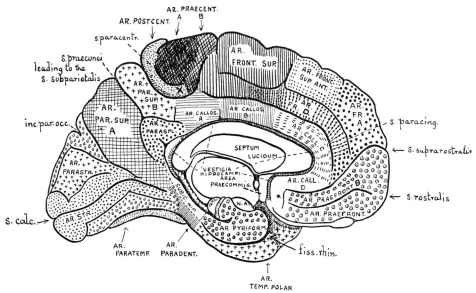

FIG. 335.—TOPOGRAPHICAL PLANS OF THE CORTICAL AREAS (MEDIAL SURFACE).
Note that there is area striata on both sides of the posterior calcarine sulcus, but only on the lower side of the anterior.
(*Elliot Smith.*)

lobe from the neighbourhood of the upper limit of the lunate sulcus ; the *inferior polar sulcus* arches downwards and forwards on to the inferior aspect from the lower limit of the same sulcus. These two polar sulci enclose semilunar extensions of the striate area and indicate the expansion of the visual cortex associated with the formation of its large macular area.

The lingual gyrus lies between the calcarine and collateral sulci. Posteriorly it reaches to the occipital pole. Anteriorly it is continuous with the hippocampal gyrus which itself (anteriorly) has the mid-brain medially (Fig. 329). Anteriorly also the hippocampal gyrus is continuous with the uncus which is recurved and hooklike and forms the postero-lateral boundary of the anterior perforated substance. The slit between the uncus and its parent hippocampal gyrus is at the tip of the inferior horn of the lateral ventricle, and here the anterior choroidal artery enters the choroid plexus of the lateral ventricle.

The lateral occipital sulcus runs forward to divide the lateral aspect of occipital lobe into superior and inferior gyri (Fig. 331).

Parieto-occipital Sulcus.—The parieto-occipital sulcus is best marked on the medial surface of the hemisphere where it appears as a deep cleft extending downwards and a little forwards from the margin of this surface some 5 cm. from the occipital pole to near the posterior extremity of the corpus callosum, where it

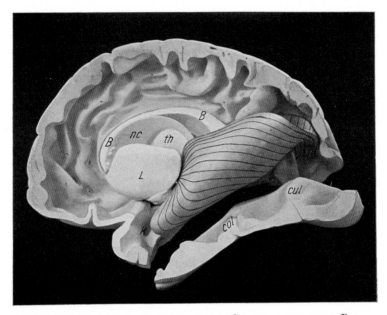

Fig. 336.—The Form and Position of the Geniculo-calcarine Pathway.

K = temporal bend of optic fibres. B = corpus callosum. L = lentiform nucleus. *nc.* = nucleus caudatus. *th.*= thalamus. *col.* = grey matter of collateral sulcus. *cul.* = highest level of grey matter of collateral sulcus.

(From Pfeifer in the Kurzes Handbuch, 1930.)

usually joins the calcarine fissure, the two together forming a Y which encloses a wedge-shaped portion of the occipital lobe, the cuneus. On the convex surface the upper end of the sulcus is continued transversely outwards for a variable distance, generally only a few millimetres (lateral part of the parieto-occipital sulcus). This fissure is here taken as the division between the parietal and occipital lobes. In Quadrumana the lateral portion of this fissure is concealed within a deep transverse cleft (Affenspalte), which intervenes between the parietal and occipital lobes, the cleft tending obliquely backwards, so that the occipital edge somewhat overlaps the parietal (occipital operculum) (Fig. 332) (Quain). The parieto-occipital sulcus is about on a level with the lambda or a little in front of the level of that spot : more so in the child than in the adult (Cunningham).

THE VISUAL CORTICAL AREA OR AREA STRIATA

The visual cortex is situated for the most part on the medial aspect of the occipital lobe in and near to the calcarine sulcus. A *variable* portion, however, may extend on to the lateral aspect of the occipital pole, and is limited there by a semilunar sulcus, the sulcus lunatus (of Elliot Smith [1]) or Affenspalte.

The visual cortex is characterised by the distinguishing *white line* or stria, of Gennari, which is visible to the naked eye, and is best seen on sectioning a fresh brain. Hence the region is called the *area striata*. The stria of Gennari is formed in the fourth layer of the cortex in part by the medullated fibres of the optic radiation but mainly by intracortical connecting fibres. The fibres run vertically, transversely and obliquely (Fig. 339).

The calcarine sulcus is divided at the point where the parieto-occipital sulcus cuts it into anterior and posterior parts, and while there is visual cortex on *both sides* of the posterior portion (Fig. 337), the stria is found only *below* the anterior (Fig. 335).

The upper boundary of the area striata is the sulcus cunei, which lies in the cuneus or region between the parieto-occipital and posterior calcarine sulci.

The lower boundary is the sulcus lingualis.

If the whole visual cortex be excised and flattened out, it will be found to present the form of an elongated ovoid some 3,000 sq. mm. in area. The narrow end of the ovoid lies close behind and below the splenium of the corpus callosum (see Fig. 335), while the rest of it expands backwards from this point to the occipital pole and beyond it on to its lateral aspect.

At about the sixth month of intrauterine life the area becomes folded along its axis. The fold so formed was called by Huxley the calcarine fissure, because its anterior part produces the prominence of the calcar avis in the interior of the posterior horn of the lateral ventricle.

The anterior part of the fissure is much deeper, more constant in form and position, and more precocious in development than the posterior. Phylogenetically, also, it is the older (Elliot Smith).

The calcarine fissure may be continued on to the lateral aspect of the occipital pole as the *sulcus calcarinus lateralis*.

As stated above, the area striata may extend on to the lateral surface of the occipital lobe, where it is bounded by the sulcus lunatus at or near which the white line of Gennari ends.

The position of the sulcus lunatus or Affenspalte is very variable, and depends on the development of the parietal and temporal association areas. If well developed these may push the sulcus lunatus and thus the visual area on to the medial aspect of the hemisphere, while in some brains it may be a large sulcus well on to the lateral aspect of the brain and resembling that found in apes (thus

[1] See Smith, G. Elliot (1907), *J. Anat. and Physiol.*, **40,** 200.

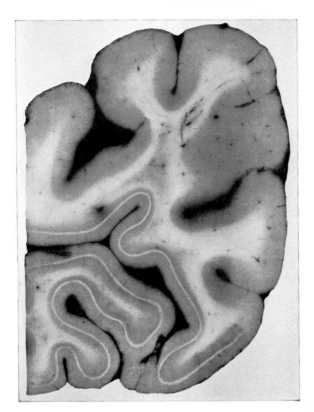

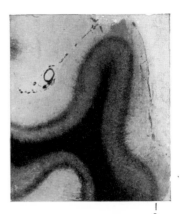

FIG. 338.—STRIA OF GENNARI (S.)
(WEIGERT'S STAIN).
Coronal section of portion of wall
of posterior calcarine fissure.

FIG. 337.—CORONAL SECTION OF OCCIPITAL LOBE TO
SHOW STRIA OF GENNARI IN BOTH WALLS OF POSTERIOR
CALCARINE FISSURE.

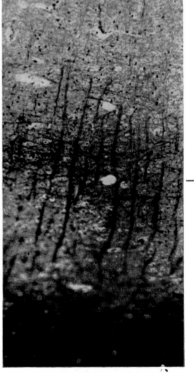

Affenspalte) (Fig. 332). *Hence the reason why,
in bullet wounds of the postero-lateral aspect of
the brain, some individuals show practically no
visual defect, while others show a great deal.*

The cellular structure of the visual cortex
is of the highly granular type associated elsewhere in the cortex with sensory function.
The outer and inner granular layers are made
up of small granular cells densely packed.

The fourth or granular layer of the visual
cortex (see Figs. 340, 342, 343) consists of small
granular cells and separates the layer of pyramidal cells superficially from the infra-granular
layers which lie deeper. It is probable that the

FIG. 339.—STRIA OF GENNARI (S.)
(WEIGERT'S STAIN).
(Portion of Fig. 338 enlarged.)

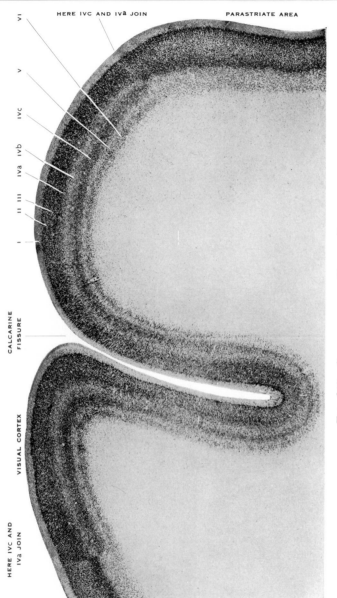

FIG. 340.—SECTION OF THE VISUAL CORTEX.

Lamination of the Visual Cortex.

According to Brodmann's classification there are six layers (*Journ. f. Psychol.*, 1903, Bd. 11, p. 137).

I. The *Lamina Zonalis* is the clear superficial layer. Next comes a thick dark layer which really consists of three portions : layers II, III and IVa.

II. The *Outer Granular Layer* is the outermost portion of the thick dark layer.

III. The *Lamina Pyramidalis* is the middle portion of this layer.

IVa. The *Inner Granular Layer* is the innermost portion of the thick dark layer.

IVb. The *Inner Granular Layer* (the stria of Gennari) is the clear layer that follows.

IVc. The *Inner Granular Layer* is the next dark layer.

V. The *Ganglion Layer* is the clear layer that follows.

VI. The *Lamina Multiformis* is the innermost dark layer.

Note that the stria of Gennari corresponds to IVb and that it is cut off from the parastriate area by the blending of IVa and IVc.

(*After* Vogt. *Journ. f. Psychologie*, 1902–4.)

fibres of the optic radiation arriving from the lateral geniculate body end predominantly if not entirely in the granular layer. A few collaterals may go to the infra-granular laminæ before they reach the granular cells.

Two main categories of fibre are found running up into the cortex :

(1) *Radial fibres*, probably associational from the neighbouring cortex, run vertically in discrete bundles.

(2) *Oblique fibres*, which form a diffuse plexus, are largely derived from the optic radiations (see Polyak and Clark).

" Each optic fibre undoubtedly ends in relation to a large number of granule cells, and this must result in an immediate amplification of the nervous impulses which arrive at the cortex. The subsequent destination of these impulses,

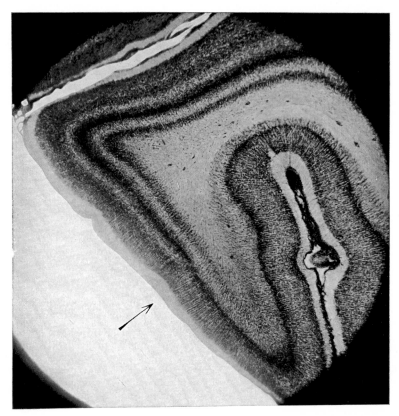

FIG. 341.—SAGITTAL SECTION THROUGH THE BRAIN OF A NEW-BORN CHILD. LOWER LIP OF THE CALCARINE FISSURE.

Note the sudden termination of the stria of Gennari. The area parastriata is to the right.

(From Pfeifer in the Kurzes Handbuch.)

however, depends on a diversity of connections through which the granule cells are linked with other cellular elements of the cortex. Some may be relayed directly to efferent neurones, leading to a discharge down to the mid-brain, whereby the visual cortex can exert an immediate influence on motor mechanisms of the brain stem. These efferent neurones are represented by certain large nerve cells which form a very conspicuous feature of the visual cortex of monkeys. They are found partly in that part of the granular layer traversed by the

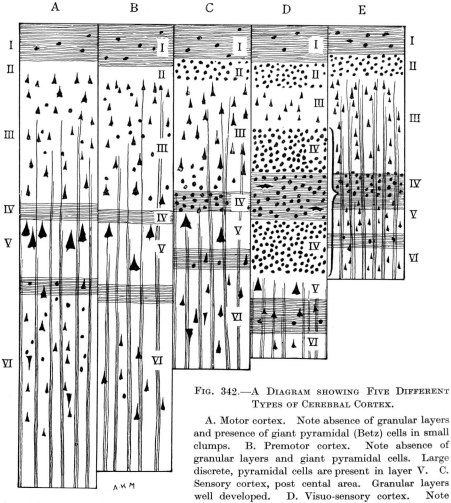

Fig. 342.—A Diagram showing Five Different Types of Cerebral Cortex.

A. Motor cortex. Note absence of granular layers and presence of giant pyramidal (Betz) cells in small clumps. B. Premotor cortex. Note absence of granular layers and giant pyramidal cells. Large discrete, pyramidal cells are present in layer V. C. Sensory cortex, post cental area. Granular layers well developed. D. Visuo-sensory cortex. Note reduction of layer III, and enormous increase of layer IV, which is traversed by the visual stria. Two large stellate cells, horizontally disposed, are seen in the visual stria. E. Visuo-psychic area. The granular layers are well developed, but large cells are absent from layer five. The relative depths of individual layers, and the relative depths of the whole cortex are approximately accurate.

(*From Gray's Anatomy.*)

'white line of Gennari,' and partly in the infra-granular layers. The latter are particularly striking cells, for they are unusually large. They are rather widely scattered, and possess horizontal dendrites which extend over relatively enormous areas. They are often known as the 'solitary cells of Meynert.' In the experiments on isolated areas of the visual cortex, we found that these cells undergo rapid atrophy when the connections of the cortex with subcortical centres are interrupted, and we suggested that they probably give rise to cortico-mesencephalic fibres. In order to test this supposition, I cut the cortico-mesencephalic fibres in one monkey at the level where they enter the mid-brain. This lesion led to quite definite signs of retrograde atrophy in the Meynert cells of the corresponding visual cortex, and thus established that they are the source of the fibres.

" It may be noted that in the monkey's brain the cells of Meynert are comparatively few—probably not more than about 1,300 in each hemisphere. On the other hand, by their widely spreading basal dendrites each cell is brought

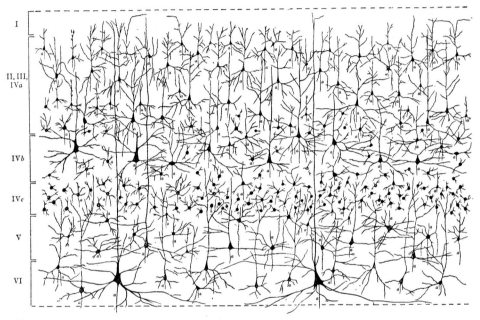

FIG. 343.—COMPOSITE DRAWING OF A SECTION OF THE VISUAL CORTEX OF A MACAQUE MONKEY, MADE FROM GOLGI MATERIAL. TWO MEYNERT CELLS ARE REPRESENTED IN THE LAMINA MULTI-FORMIS. THE APPROXIMATE EXTENTS OF THE CELL LAMINÆ ARE INDICATED ON THE LEFT. THE AXONAL PROCESSES OF THE CELLS ARE MARKED a. (LE GROS CLARK.)

into contact with a relatively extensive area of cortex. Indeed, not only does it appear that each cell provides an immediate focus of convergence for the activities of all the cortical laminæ with the exception of the pyramidal layer, but it is also estimated that its axon represents a ' final common path ' for a unit area of cortex of approximately $\frac{1}{2}$ mm. The Meynert cells are thus appropriately disposed to serve rapid ' mass reactions ' from the cortex, that is to say, reactions which rapidly reflect the gross activities of the cortex. It may be inferred that they are at least partly responsible for the functions which are commonly ascribed to the occipital oculomotor centre, such as the involuntary movement of the eye towards objects in the peripheral field of vision, the maintenance of fixation on a point, and so forth."—(Le Gros Clark (1942), *Trans. O.S.U.K.*, **52**, 241.)

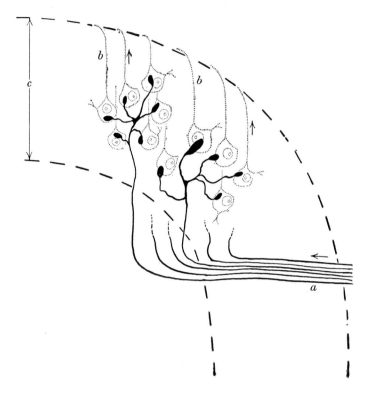

Fig. 344.—Diagram showing the Termination of Optic Fibres in relation to the Cells of the Lateral Geniculate Body in a Monkey.

A fasciculus of optic fibres (*a*) is shown entering the geniculate body from the right. From this fasciculus individual fibres turn out at right angles to enter their appropriate cell lamina (*c*). Each fibre ends in a spray of 5–6 branches, and each of these terminates in an end-bulb which lies in contact with the body of one geniculate cell. The axons of the geniculate cells (*b*) pass into the fibre laminæ of the nucleus and run through these to reach the optic radiations. (Glees and Clark, *Journ. Anat.*, 75, 1941.)

The distinguishing features of the visuo-sensory cortex are as follows :

(1) The white line of Gennari distinguishes it from all other portions of the cortex.

(2) It shares with the other sensory cortical areas a great increase in the number of granular cells. The outer and more especially the inner granular layers consist of a great number of small cells closely packed together. But the whole granular layer (IV) is wider here than in any other cortical area.

Hence the striate area contains approximately one-tenth of the total number of cells in the cerebral cortex (Gray).

(3) There are eight layers instead of the usual six. This is produced by a bifurcation of the granular layer into inner and outer leaving the white line between them ; and also by a duplication of the 6th (spindle-cell layer).

(4) Layer IVB (the stria) contains a few large cells horizontally placed (Fig. 342), which Cajal thought were the specific cells of vision.

(5) The ganglion layer (V) contains the large solitary cells of Meynert which are pyramidal in shape, measure about 30 μ, and are arranged in a single row widely spaced (see below).

(6) According to Flechsig, the striate area is myelogenetically a primordial region ; for it is already myelenated at birth.

The area striata is the true visual cortex, i.e. the true receptive centre for visual impressions. Around it is the parastriate area, and around this again the peristriate area.

These are the visual association areas (visuo-psychic or visual memory centres).

The evidence available from clinical observations indicates that in man the striate area or visual cortex is merely a perceptive centre. It is through it that all impulses from the retinæ must pass to reach consciousness. It also provides the physiological basis for the fusion of the two separate images received by it in binocular vision, for it is *only at this level that impulses from the two retinæ come together*.

Perception of colour, relative localisation, that is localisation of objects in space with reference to the direct line of vision, and recognition of form and discrimination of contour are all functions of the striate area.

Agnosia of letters, that is the inability to identify by vision symbols in the learning of which vision is predominantly concerned, is produced by a lesion involving the lateral and inferior surface of the occipital lobe close to the striate area (Holmes).

Injury to the *angular gyrus*, which caps the curled-up posterior end of the superior temporal sulcus, is said to lead to word blindness, i.e. the patient can see words but cannot grasp their meaning. Stimulation of the angular gyrus also is said to produce conjugate deviation of the eyes to the opposite side.

Visual attention may also be seriously influenced by lesions at or in front of the angular gyrus. When the disease is unilateral the patient fails to notice objects in the opposite halves of his fields of vision.

The motor centre for eye movements is in the posterior part of the middle frontal gyrus.

Stimulation of this area causes conjugate deviation of the head and eyes to the opposite side.

Connections of the Visual Cortex (Area 17).

(a) With the opposite visual cortex by commissural fibres which run in the splenium of the corpus callosum. It is probable, although the opposite view has been put forward by Polyak, Pfeifer and others, that no fibres (or only very few) from the striate area itself cross over in the corpus callosum to the striate area of the opposite side. But numerous fibres connect the peristriate areas of opposite sides. These anatomical findings were confirmed by the observations of von Bonin Garol and McCulloch, who elicited that stimulation of one striate area by strychnine never excites changes in (electric) potentials in the opposite hemisphere, while application of strychnine to the peristriate area " fires off " symmetrical areas on the other side.

(b) With the visual memory and word centres.

(c) With the auditory and speech centres by association fibres.

(d) With the lower visual centres.

(e) With the ocular nuclei and other motor nuclei by descending fibres which run in the optic radiations.

It is usually accepted that each spot in the visual cortex is directly connected with other parts of the visual cortex and with the frontal, parietal and temporal lobes by abundant association fibres. These are held to integrate the activity of the visual cortex as a whole and to provide an anatomical basis for visuo-tactile, visuo-auditory, and other associative functions.

But le Gros Clark points out that no association fibres extend for more than 5 mm. from a lesion in the visual cortex to adjacent parts of this area, and as regards other parts of the cerebral cortex, fibres can only be traced as far as the immediately contiguous cortical area (area 18). It seems, therefore, that on their arrival at the cortex, visual stimuli can only be propagated to distant cortical areas by a process of diffusion through relays of short association fibres.

LOCALISATION IN THE VISUAL PATHS [1]

It is of great importance for the localisation of lesions to know that the fibres in the visual pathway are not arranged anyhow but assume a definite orderly arrangement.

(a) **In the Retina.**—The nerve fibres converge towards the disc. On the temporal side is the important papillo-macular bundle. There is no overlap between the upper and lower halves of the fibres of the peripheral parts of the retina (Fig. 137).

In the retina the line dividing nasal from temporal fibres (in the sense of those that will cross in the chiasma and those that will not) passes through the centre of the fovea. Hence the temporal macular fibres remain on the same side, while the nasal ones cross.

[1] See Brouwer and Zeeman.

The upper temporal retinal fibres (and some of the nasal portion as well) are separated from the lower by the macular fibres, an arrangement which holds throughout the central visual pathway.

There is still dispute as to how the nerve fibres from the various portions of the retina arrange themselves at the optic nerve head. It is generally held that the fibres from the periphery of the retina pass to the centre of the nerve, while those arising close to the disc occupy the periphery of the nerve. But it would

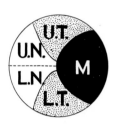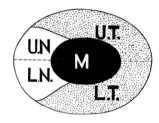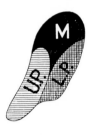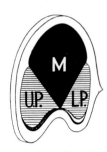

| A. In the optic nerve (distal). | B. In the optic nerve (proximal). | C. In the optic tract. | D. In the lateral geniculate body. |

The crescents below U.P. and L.P. are the uniocular fibres.

M. = macular.   U.T. = upper temporal.   L.T. = lower temporal.   U.N. = upper nasal.
L.N. = lower nasal.   U.P. = upper peripheral.   L.P. = lower peripheral.

(*After Brouwer and Zeeman.*)

FIG. 345.—DISTRIBUTION OF THE VISUAL FIBRES.

(Note that in Fig. D, Le Gros Clark and Penman hold that the macular area only occupies the posterior two-thirds of the geniculate body.)

now appear that the nerve fibres coming from the periphery of the retina lie deep in the nerve fibre layer and peripheral at the nerve head (see Wolff and Penman, 1950, also Loddoni, 1930) (Fig. 346).

(*b*) **In the Optic Nerve.**—(1) *In the distal portion* (Fig. 345, A).—Behind the eye the peripheral fibres are distributed exactly as in the retina ; those from the temporal side are lateral in the nerve, those from the nasal side medial. The macular fibres, which constitute almost one-third of the whole nerve (whereas the macular area is only one-twentieth of that of the retina), are laterally placed in the nerve, occupying a wedge-shaped area ; but as we approach the chiasma they insinuate themselves among the peripheral fibres, so that (2) *near the chiasma* they are centrally placed (Fig. 345, B).

(*c*) [1] **In the Chiasma** (Fig. 320).—The *nasal fibres*, constituting about three-quarters of all the fibres, cross over to run in the optic tract of the opposite side. But they do not do this by the shortest route, i.e. along the diagonals.

In the proximal part of the optic nerve the nasal fibres, which hitherto have kept to an orderly arrangement and run parallel with the optic nerve, spread out

[1] See Wilbrand.

so that in a horizontal section they occupy the whole width of the nerve and anterior portion of the lateral part of the chiasma.

The most medial of these, representing the fibres from the lower and medial quadrant of the retina, bend medially into the anterior portion of the chiasma and after decussating cross over to the opposite side. The fibres that lie most anterior in the chiasma now form loops convex forwards in the terminal part of the opposite optic nerve, and then having reached the temporal border, pass backwards to the medial and lower part of the tract. *It is because of these anterior loops that a lesion at the termination of the optic nerve may affect both fields.* It is probable that these fibres, i.e. those coming from the lower and medial quadrant of the retina, in

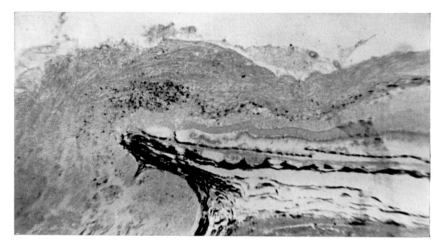

Fig. 346.—Edge of Nerve-head and Adjacent Retina of a Rabbit with a Peripheral Retinal Wound made One Month Previously. (Stained Marchi.)

The degenerate fibres as shown by the Marchi granules are deep in the nerve-fibre layer and peripheral at the nerve-head.

(*Wolff and Penman*, 1950.)

crossing over in the chiasma lie next its under-surface, i.e. nearest the pituitary body ; for they are first affected in tumours of this body as shown by the early loss of the upper temporal field. The *anterior loops* are crossed at right angles by those fibres in the optic nerve which are still running parallel to its axis, and thus is produced a characteristic basketwork of interlacing fibres (Korbgeflecht of Wilbrand) in the terminal part of the nerve.

The upper medial fibres coming from the upper and medial quadrant of the retina pass to the lateral side in the terminal portion of the nerve and mingle with the uncrossed bundle. They pass backwards here for varying distances. The most lateral ones actually form loops convex backwards in the beginning of the optic tract before crossing over in the chiasma to the supero-medial portion of the tract of the opposite side. The *posterior loops* formed by fibres before their crossing are less prominent than those formed by the crossed medial fibres in the terminal portion of the optic nerve.

The actual decussation takes place in the middle of the chiasma, the anterior fibres crossing each other at more acute angles than the posterior. The fibres cross over not only from left to right but from above downwards as well.

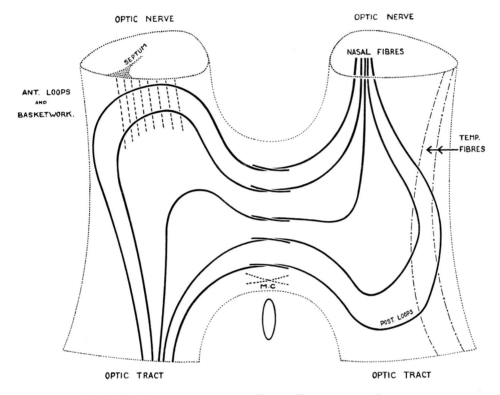

FIG. 347.—THE CROSSING OF THE VISUAL FIBRES IN THE CHIASMA.

To avoid confusion only the fibres from one side (except at the actual decussation) are shown.
M.C. = macular crossing.
Note that the most medial of the temporal fibres come much nearer the centre of the chiasma than is shown in the figure.

The Uncrossed Fibres.—Just anterior to the chiasma the uncrossed bundle forms a compact fasciculus which occupies almost the whole of the upper and lateral quadrant of the nerve.

These temporal fibres run directly backwards in the lateral portion of the chiasma, those coming from the upper part of the retina being above those from the lower. They pass into the tract lying here in the dorso-lateral part.

In the chiasma, however, the uncrossed fibres do not form a closed fasciculus, but with them mingle not only the nasal fibres of the same side which have passed laterally before crossing over to the opposite side but also those nasal fibres from the opposite side which form loops in the terminal portion of the optic nerve.

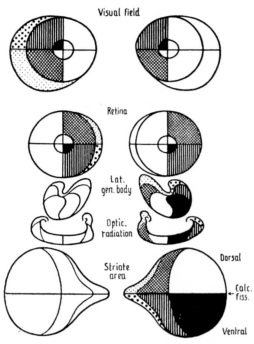

FIG. 348.—DIAGRAM OF THE PROJECTION OF THE DIFFERENT PARTS OF THE RETINA IN THE LATERAL GENICULATE BODY, THE OPTIC RADIATION AND THE STRIATE AREA.

(From Brodal, after Polyak, 1933.)

This intermixture of fibres is so marked that in a case of unilateral atrophy of the optic nerve horizontal sections of the chiasma do not reveal the position of the uncrossed bundle. Only in coronal sections can the atrophic area, i.e. the position of the uncrossed bundle, be made out. It then appears in the lateral part of the chiasma as a kidney-shaped area with its hilum medially.

The Macular Fibres.—In the posterior portion of the intracranial optic nerve the papillo-macular bundle is central and keeps this position in the anterior part of the lateral portion of the chiasma. Then the crossed fibres separate from the uncrossed ones and pass as a bundle obliquely backwards and upwards to decussate with the macular fibres of the opposite side in the most posterior portion of the chiasma, i.e. in the floor of the recess of the third ventricle. Lesions here will therefore cause a central temporal hemianopic scotoma (Wilbrand).

(d) **In the Optic Tract.**—In the chiasma crossed and uncrossed fibres are intermingled, and when they reach the optic tract they are rearranged to correspond with their position in the lateral geniculate body, i.e. the macular fibres (crossed and uncrossed) occupy an area of the cross-section dorso-laterally; the fibres from the lower retinal quadrants are lateral, those from the upper are medial.

The fibres from the peripheral portions of the retinæ lie more anteriorly.

(e) **In the Lateral Geniculate Body.**—The fibres from the upper part of the retina go to the medial part of the geniculate body, those from below to the lateral part. The macular area is somewhat wedge-shaped, involves all the laminæ, and is confined to the posterior two-thirds of the nucleus, broadening towards the caudal pole. It is probable that the peripheral areas farther away from the disc are represented, as in the retina, in the more anterior levels of the geniculate body (Le Gros Clark and Penman). (See below.)

(f) **In the Optic Radiation.**—The fibres originating in the medial portion of the geniculate body, and representing the upper portions of the retina, form the upper portion of the radiation going to the upper lip of the calcarine fissure ; those coming from the lateral portion of geniculate body form the lower portion of the radiation. The macular fibres, as in the geniculate body, continue in the radiation to separate the fibres representing the upper portions of the retina from those representing the lower. This accounts for the fact that one may get a quadrantic visual field defect with a sharp horizontal border.

There is a definite " point-to-point " localisation of the retina in the lateral

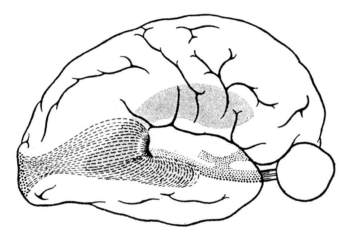

FIG. 349.—DIAGRAMMATIC REPRESENTATION OF THE COURSE OF THE FIBRES OF THE OPTIC RADIATION.

The geniculo-calcarine fibres are seen to swing from the geniculate body (not visible) around the lateral ventricle to reach the striate area.

(*From Brodal, after Cushing*, 1922.)

geniculate body with no bilateral (double) representation even of the macula. The body is split up into laminæ, six in number at its centre, which receive fibres alternately from the retina of the same side and the opposite side.

In the human lateral geniculate body, as in that of monkeys and apes, six well-defined layers of cells sharply separated throughout most of their extent by medullary laminæ are found. These cells may be conveniently numbered 1–6 from the surface of the brain. The first two layers consist of conspicuous large cells, and the remaining four of smaller cells closely packed together. The crossed retinal fibres end in laminæ 1, 4 and 6, while the uncrossed go to 2, 3 and 5 (Fig. 350). The localisation in the lateral geniculate body amounts practically to a point-to-point projection.

Crossed and uncrossed retinal fibres go to alternating layers of the lateral geniculate body, but in such a way that those fibres from corresponding parts of the two retinæ end in neighbouring parts of the different layers. When the fibres enter the lateral geniculate body, crossed and uncrossed fibres are not yet segregated.

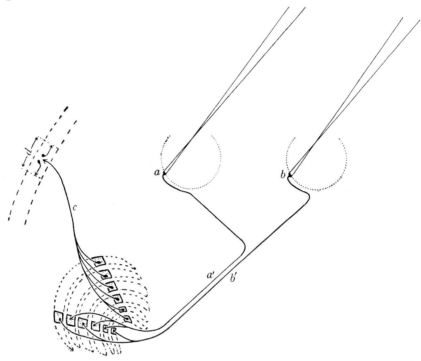

Fig. 350.—Diagram illustrating Certain Points in the Central Representation of the Retina.

Impulses from equivalent spots (*a, b*) in the two retinæ pass back in the optic tract to the same region of the lateral geniculate body. Crossed impulses (*b*) terminate in laminæ 1, 4 and 6 and uncrossed impulses (*a*) in laminæ 2, 3 and 5. Thus the *receptive unit* in the lateral geniculate body with respect to each retina is a band of cells radiating from the hilum of the nucleus, and involving three laminæ. On the other hand, the *projection unit* of the lateral geniculate body on to the visual cortex is a band of cells involving all six laminæ. (Clark (1941), *J. Anat.*, **75**.)

The optic fibres end in the lateral geniculate body in specialised ring formations called " terminal boutons." Each optic fibre ends within its appropriate lamina by dividing into five or six terminal branches, and each of these branches establishes connection with one cell only, which makes for great precision. This is in great contrast with the motor cells of the spinal cord, which may have as many as a thousand terminal boutons in relation to them. Also in the lateral geniculate body of the cat, Glees found 30–40 terminal boutons related to each geniculate cell, which probably makes for a high degree of sensitivity even at low intensities of illumination.   These findings allow a conclusion of some interest.   When the crossed and uncrossed optic fibres end in alternating layers of the lateral geniculate body, and each cell receives one terminal only from the optic fibres, this implies that the lateral geniculate body must function as a pure relay station.   The more complicated processes in visual perception, such as the fusion of the two retinal images, must be assumed to take place in the cerebral cortex (Brodal).

There is no fusion of crossed and uncrossed impulses at the level of the lateral geniculate body.   This takes place only in the cortex.   Also there are no intercalated neurones between the lateral geniculate and the area striata, and probably no cortico-geniculate fibres exist (Clark).

The smallest retinal lesion causes atrophy in all the three layers belonging to that eye ; hence, the conducting unit in the optic nerve is a three-fibre unit. The smallest lesion of the visual cortex, on the other hand, causes atrophy in six layers of the lateral geniculate body, and the conducting unit in the optic radiations is probably a six-fibre one.   The point-to-point projection of the retina to the lateral geniculate is also carried from the latter to the visual cortex.

(g) **Localisation in the Visual Cortex.**—*It is only in the striate area that the impulses originating from corresponding parts of the retinæ meet.*   Following a lesion of the striate area all laminæ of the lateral geniculate body are affected, which shows that the impulses entering its alternate layers and derived from corresponding parts of the two retinæ pass to the same cortical region.   There is a geographical projection or point-to-point localisation of the retina in the cortex ; that is, each point in the retina is sharply represented in a corresponding point of the visual cortex.

All visual stimuli which impinge upon the homonymous halves of the retinæ (e.g. both right halves) are ultimately transmitted to the lateral geniculate body of the same side, and finally to the homolateral striate area.   All light waves coming, for example, from the left will fall on the right halves of both retinæ, i.e. the temporal half of the right and nasal half of the left.   The fibres from the right eye pass without crossing to the right optic tract, those from the left eye cross to continue in the right optic tract.   Both sets of fibres reach the right lateral geniculate body and the right striate area.   Consequently the right striate area is concerned in the perception of objects situated to the left of the vertical median line in the visual fields.   This is in line with the fact that the right cerebral hemisphere is concerned in the motor and sensory activities of the left half of the body (Brodal).

The striate cortex may be described as the " cortical retina " because there a true copy of the retinal image is formed (Henschen).

For the rest, " the retinal projection on the cortex may be represented by picturing one half of the retina spread over the surface of the striate area, the macular region being placed posteriorly, the periphery anteriorly, the upper margin along its upper edge and the lower on its inferior border " (Holmes).[1]

Thus the upper and lower portions of the retina are localised above and below the calcarine sulcus respectively. The periphery of the retina along the vertical meridian corresponds to the upper and lower limits of the visual area, while the portions which lie next the horizontal meridian are projected in the depth of the calcarine sulcus.

The periphery of the retina along the horizontal meridian is represented in the anterior part of the visual cortex, and as we go centrally in the retina the corresponding area of cortical localisation will be farther back along the calcarine fissure.

The most anterior part of the striate area represents the extreme nasal periphery of the retina which corresponds to the temporal crescent in the visual fields, where vision is monocular.

The maculæ are represented posteriorly ; but while there is some degree of localisation of macular representation in the posterior part of the calcarine fissure and extending on the lateral surface of the occipital pole (Holmes, 1918), at the same time there seems little doubt that macular fibres are spread over the whole visual area much like the representation of the hand in the post-central gyrus.

The macular area is relatively much larger in proportion to the whole striate area than is the macular region in proportion to the whole retina. Because the macula is concerned with the most acute vision and its visual cells are more densely packed than elsewhere, it is more extensively represented in the striate area than the peripheral portion.

With regard to the localisation of the macula, Professor Elliot Smith (*Journ. of Anat.*, **64**, 1930, p. 478) writes : " In a horizontal section through the posterior pole of a human cerebral hemisphere the area striata, distinguished by the presence of the stria of Gennari, is seen to undergo a sudden change in character a short distance behind its midpoint. The thickness of the stria is reduced and the dark band (which is found on its inner side in the part representing the peripheral retina) disappears. The macular cortex begins at this place and extends around the pole on to the lateral surface of the hemisphere to end at the lip of the lunate sulcus. As this lateral part of the area striata is much broader than the medial part, exact measurements reveal the fact that the macular part is at least as extensive as the whole peripheral part. It is possible to identify the macular part of the area striata in many human brains by simple observation of the morphological features of the surface of the cerebral hemisphere. Looking at the posterior aspect of the hemisphere, three semilunar sulci—lunatus, polaris superior, and polaris inferior—may often be seen arranged in a trefoil or shamrock-leaf pattern (grouped around the calcarine sulci in the axis of the area

[1] Holmes, G., (1918), *Brit. J. Ophthal.*, **2**, 353, 449, 508 ; (1919) *Brit. med. J.*, **2**. Holmes, G., and Lister, W. T., (1915), *Brain*, **39**, 34.

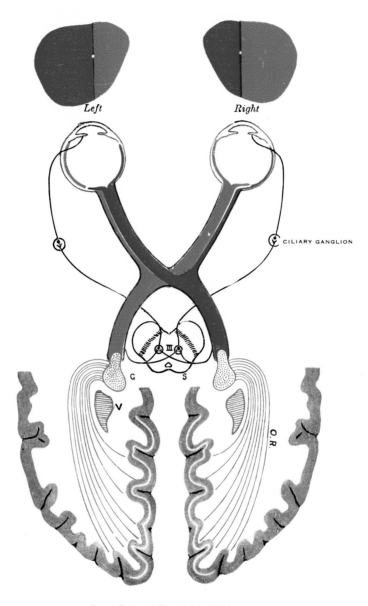

Left   Right

CILIARY GANGLION

G = Lateral Geniculate Body.
S = Superior Colliculus.
III = Third Nerve Nucleus.
V = Posterior Horn of Lateral Ventricle.
O.R. = Optic Radiations.

FIG. 351.—TO SHOW THE COURSE OF THE VISUAL AND PUPILLARY FIBRES AND THE CORRESPONDING
FIELDS OF VISION.

The cell station in the pretectal nucleus is not shown (see Fig. 363).

striata).   The rapid expansion of the lateral part of the area striata to afford cortical representation of the macula is responsible for the formation of three opercula bounded by these three semilunar sulci.   Hence the presence of this cortical shamrock pattern affords definite evidence of the position and extent of the macular area.''

It used to be held that each macula had a double representation, that is that each point in the macula was represented in both occipital poles ; but most observers now agree with Holmes and Lister who, as a result of their observations on soldiers with gunshot wounds of the occipital region came to the conclusion that each point in each macula had a unilateral representation only.   They explain the well-known phenomenon that in cases of thrombosis of the posterior cerebral artery the resulting homonymous hemianopia spares the macula (the scotoma falling short of the fixation point by 10°) by the fact that the occipital pole is the border-line territory between the distribution of the middle and posterior cerebral arteries (Fig. 359) and that the former artery will be able to supply the macular area if the latter is blocked.

With regard to this question Brodal says : '' There has been much discussion concerning this ' macular sparing ' frequently observed in these lesions.   Some authors have maintained that the macula is represented bilaterally in the striate area, in contrast to the rest of the retina.   This, of course, would explain the macular sparing.   Most of the adherents to this view assume that some fibres join the optic radiation on the other side, reaching this through the posterior part of the corpus callosum.   There would thus be a second crossing of some of the fibres in the optic system.   This view is, however, based on anatomical investigations of cases of lesions in the temporal and occipital lobes, and it is practically impossible to be sure in such cases that all fibres have been interrupted or that the entire striate area has been functionless.   In monkeys in which the entire area has been destroyed, all cells of the lateral geniculate body disintegrate, as was mentioned previously, a fact which clearly demonstrates that crossing fibres of the type assumed to be present in man cannot exist in these animals (monkeys and apes).   It appears reasonable that conditions should be essentially similar in man.   In investigations aiming especially at tracing the fibres of the optic radiation in man, crossing fibres have not been ascertained (Putnam, 1926). Human cases have also been described, in which a total ablation of the occipital lobe was not followed by any macular sparing (e.g. Halstead, Walker, and Bucy, 1940 ; however, they found macular sparing in another case).   Following unilateral occipital lobectomy, no cellular degeneration has been observed in the contralateral lateral geniculate body (German and Brody, 1940).   It should be remembered that it is extremely difficult to ascertain a moderate sparing of macular vision, and that some investigators are inclined to assume that a certain degree of shifting of the fixation point occurs normally.   A factor of some importance in this connection is that the macular representation in man occupies a very large proportion of the striate area, and probably even extends anteriorly in the depth of the calcarine fissure. The macular sparing might therefore be explained on this basis as being due to preservation of these regions in some cases which have been reported. In spite of the interest in the studies devoted to explain the macular sparing in lesions of the striate area, the problem is not yet solved. As Putnam and Liebman (1942) have emphasised in a review of this

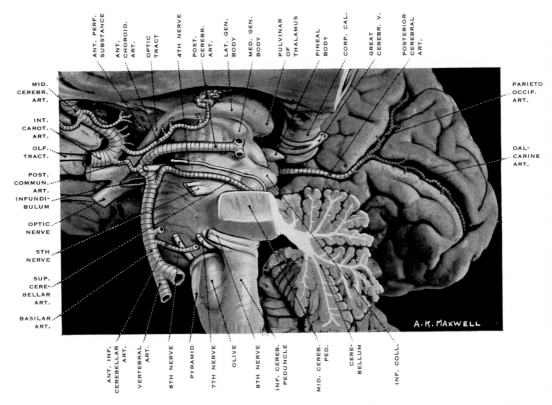

FIG. 352.—DISSECTION TO SHOW THE BLOOD-SUPPLY OF THE OPTIC PATHWAY AND THE RELATIONS OF THE VESSELS TO THE OCULAR NERVES.

From the side.

(*Wolff's preparation.*)

problem, "what is most urgently needed is a minute anatomical control of relevant cases which have been examined with exact methods during life"

Verhoeff explains the sparing of the macula by suggesting that there is a constant physiological shift of fixation so that an object in the hemianopic field may be brought into view and that a new fixation point is formed within the preserved field (*Archiv. Ophth.*, Oct. 1943).

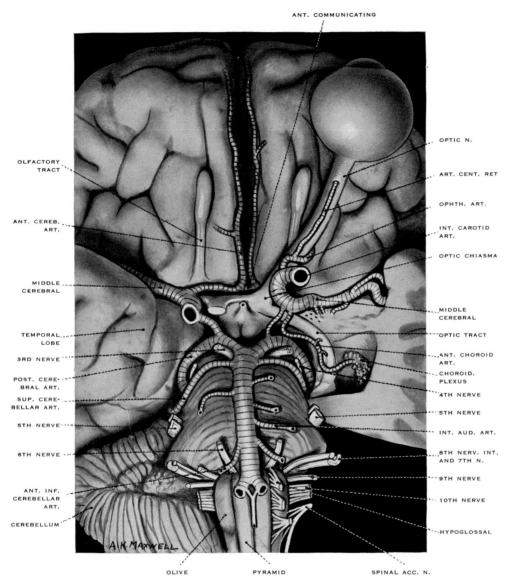

ANT. COMMUNICATING

OLFACTORY TRACT

ANT. CEREB. ART.

MIDDLE CEREBRAL

TEMPORAL LOBE

3RD NERVE

POST. CERE-BRAL ART.

SUP. CERE-BELLAR ART.

5TH NERVE

6TH NERVE

ANT. INF. CEREBELLAR ART.

CEREBELLUM

A.K.MAXWELL

OPTIC N.

ART. CENT. RET.

OPHTH. ART.

INT. CAROTID ART.

OPTIC CHIASMA

MIDDLE CEREBRAL

OPTIC TRACT

ANT. CHOROID ART.

CHOROID. PLEXUS

4TH NERVE

5TH NERVE

INT. AUD. ART.

8TH NERV. INT. AND 7TH N.

9TH NERVE

10TH NERVE

HYPOGLOSSAL

OLIVE   PYRAMID   SPINAL ACC. N.

FIG. 353.—DISSECTION TO SHOW BLOOD-SUPPLY OF OPTIC PATHWAY AND RELATIONS OF VESSELS TO OCULAR NERVES.
From below.
(*Wolff's preparation.*)

THE UNIOCULAR VISUAL FIELDS

It would appear that the fibres which subserve the uniocular and binocular visual fields run separately.

Brouwer and Zeeman found that in the rabbit the binocular field (which in this animal is only 20 degrees) occupies a very small area in the lateral geniculate body, while nearly the whole of the remainder is taken by the uniocular.

In man it is the other way round.

The uniocular field, that is the part seen by one eye only, is represented by the extreme temporal field. The retinal fibres involved are the most nasal. They form the nasal half-moon to the medial side of the crossed bundle and then go to a small strip on the ventral part of the lateral geniculate body (Fig. 345, D).

In the visual cortex the uniocular field is localised anteriorly in the lower lip of the calcarine sulcus.

The importance of all this clinically is that it is possible to have a lesion of the optic radiation, for instance, affecting one field only.

THE CORTICAL OCULO-MOTOR CENTRES

1. Frontal.
2. Occipital.
3. Angular Gyrus.

1. The frontal centre lies in the posterior part of the middle frontal gyrus. It controls voluntary movements. Stimulation of this area results in conjugate deviation of the eyes to the opposite side, stimulation above the centre results in conjugate deviation downwards, and stimulation below in conjugate deviation upwards.

Paralysis of this centre does not stop reflex movements due to labyrinthine or retinal impressions.

The path of the fibres from the cortical centre to the ocular nuclei is not known, but it probably runs with the pyramidal tract. There is a complete decussation of fibres of opposite sides.

2. The occipital centre probably has to do with the fixation reflex, i.e. with bringing on to the macula the image of an object which has " interested " the periphery of the retina. Stimulation of the visual area causes conjugate deviation of the eyes.

3. Conjugate deviation of the eyes has been produced in animals by stimulation of the angular gyrus, but not in man, in whom operative removal of the area has not resulted in any oculo-motor defect.

The blood-supply to these centres comes from the middle cerebral for the frontal and angular gyri and from the posterior cerebral for the occipital centre.

THE BLOOD-SUPPLY OF THE VISUAL PATHWAY

The blood-supply of the *retina* has been discussed on p. 145.

The Blood-supply of the Optic Nerve.—The optic nerve, an outgrowth from the brain, has its vascular supply modelled on that organ. The resemblance is great, but not absolute, for here we have no grey matter and no nerve cells. The optic

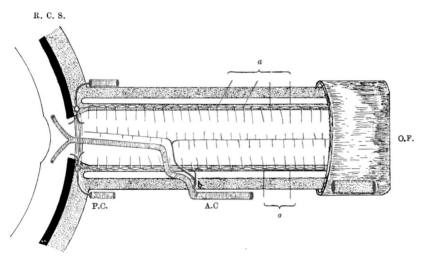

R. C. S.

a

O.F.

P.C.

A.C

b

a

FIG. 354.—SCHEMATIC LONGITUDINAL SECTION OF THE OPTIC NERVE TO SHOW ITS ORBITAL BLOOD-SUPPLY.

A.C., Arteria centralis; P.C., Posterior ciliary artery; O.F., Optic foramen; R., Retina; C., Choroid; S., Sclera; *a.*, Group (*a*) to pial plexus; *b.*, Group (*b*).

Note that the post-central artery supplies the macular bundle in this portion of its extent (p. 387).

nerve, chiasma, and tracts are covered with pia mater identical with that of the brain.   Only those portions of the chiasma and tracts adherent to the base of the brain are bare of pia.

All the arteries which will eventually supply the nerve tissue do so through the pial network of vessels (Figs. 354, 355).   This network is rich and fine and extends to the back of the globe.   In the intracranial portion of the nerve it is situated on the surface of the pia ; in the orbital portion in its thickness, between the longitudinal and circular fibres.

As in the case of the cerebral convolutions there are actually two networks, one inside the other.   The outer is the larger and formed of arterioles of fair size ; the other, lying within the first, consists of vessels so small that a loupe is necessary to see them.   The network is supplied by arteries which probably anastomose slightly in the network, but not before they reach it.

When the vessels pass into the nerve they take with them a coat of pia and also a covering of glia, which constitute the septa.   In fact, the distribution of the septa is exactly that of the blood-vessels.   Also the thickness of each septum is proportional to the size of the contained vessel.   While this is obvious in the orbital portion of the nerve, it is more difficult to make out in the tract and chiasma.   In the most posterior portion of the optic nerve (where the septa gradually disappear), in the chiasma, and in the optic tract even the larger vessels are surrounded by only a slight covering of connective tissue which gets less with the smaller vessels and seems to disappear entirely in the capillaries.   They are, however, always separated from the nerve tissue by the perivascularis gliæ.

There is a striking contrast between the great vascularity of the pia and the relatively few vessels in the dura (Magitot).   The pial network acts as a distributing centre which provides for a regular supply of blood to the nerve.   As the vessels pass into the nerve in the septa they divide dichotomously as these do and send branches anteriorly and posteriorly.

The vessels which join it eventually come from the internal carotid and, since the eye has grown out from the brain, its vessels have followed it.   This explains why the vessels to the chiasma are short and those to the globe relatively long (Magitot, *Thèse de Paris*, 1908).

The intracranial portion.—As in the case of the chiasma, the principal vessels are the anterior cerebral and the internal carotid—the former for the superior, the latter for the inferior aspects.   The ophthalmic artery and the anterior communicating may help.   The feeding vessels pass to the pial network and thus into the nerve.

A cross-section of the nerve shows that the septal network here has a special appearance—whereas in other parts of the nerve the thickness of the septa is fairly constant, in the axial part of the intracranial portion they are not only thinner but the meshes are wider.   Hence smaller vessels supply a large number

A.E.—25

of nerve fibres.   Thus any interference with the blood-supply would, according to Behr, affect first and most markedly the central papillo-macular bundle.

The whole of the remaining portion of the nerve and also the whole of the globe is supplied by the ophthalmic artery.

The intracanalicular portion is supplied by the ophthalmic, but differs from the orbital portion in that the pial network is relatively poor.

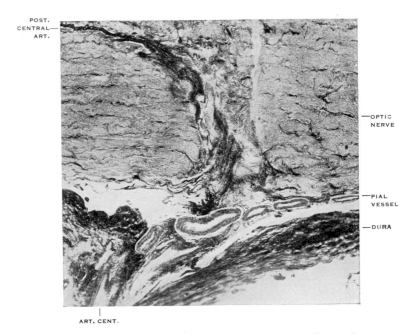

FIG. 355.—LONGITUDINAL SECTION OF THE OPTIC NERVE, SHOWING A LARGE BRANCH FROM THE ARTERIA CENTRALIS PASSING FORWARDS IN THE SUBARACHNOID SPACE TO THE PIAL PLEXUS ; ALSO A POST-CENTRAL ARTERY PASSING BACKWARDS.
(*Wolff's preparation.*)

The orbital portion is supplied by two groups of vessels :

(A) Those that pierce the dura behind the entrance of the central vessels.

(B) Those that enter the nerve or join the pial network at the site of entry of the central vessels.

Group A.—In approximately the posterior half of the orbital portion of the optic nerve some six to a dozen small vessels, derived from the ophthalmic and its branches (including the arteria centralis), pierce the dura on various aspects, but mainly above and at the sides.   The least pass in from below since this portion is supplied by recurrent branches from Group B.

Having pierced the dura these vessels pass across the subarachnoid space either at right angles or obliquely and, clothed in a portion of dura and arachnoid as is the central artery in like position, reach the pial network.

Group B.—At about the point where the central artery pierces the dura, it gives off one or more branches which diminish its diameter by about one-third. Some of these immediately enter the pia (Figs. 354, 355), dividing into branches which go forwards, backwards, and circularly and, joining the pial network, send branches into the nerve. Others pass into the nerve with the central artery running parallel with it. Although extremely well described by Kuhnt in 1879, these important vessels have often been forgotten in subsequent works and this has led to a great deal of confusion. To emphasise the fact that they do exist one would suggest the name of central collateral arteries (arteriæ collaterales centralis retinæ) (Figs. 162, 354).

One of these vessels larger than the rest runs with the central artery to the lamina cribrosa. The collateral vessels send branches into the nerve and hence get narrower as they pass anteriorly. At the point where the central artery bends forwards at the centre of the nerve, a branch of the collateral artery (not of the central artery itself (Magitot) passes backwards towards the optic foramen (Figs. 354, 355). This branch, the post-central artery, is accompanied by the posterior vein of Kuhnt *and supplies the macular fibres in this portion of their course.*

While, as we have seen, the collateral arteries get finer as we trace them forwards, the central artery remains much the same size from its point of penetration to its bifurcation. This is due to the fact that, in this portion of its course, the arteria centralis has no branches of any size.

The injections by Beauvieux and Ristitch of the arteria centralis *alone* appear to show that the region of the *lamina cribrosa* is supplied by the arterial circle of Zinn only. According to Leber, however, small branches do pass from the arteria centralis into the lamina cribrosa and form a capillary " anastomosis " with branches coming from the circle of Zinn. My own preparations[1] agree with this latter view (Fig. 163).

The *nerve head* is supplied by the central artery and the circle of Zinn which also sends branches into the neighbouring retina. The number and size of these branches to the retina are variable, but more evident on the temporal side. Here we find all grades up to what is known as a cilio-retinal artery (see p. 149).

The Blood-supply of the Chiasma.—The chiasma gets its main blood-supply from the anterior cerebrals and internal carotids. The posterior communicatings, which are near its under-surface and the anterior choroidals, may help, as also the anterior communicating when it is present. Thus it will be seen that, if

---

[1] According to Behr, the arteria centralis from its point of entry into the optic nerve to its bifurcation gives off no branches. Hence in this portion of its course it takes no part in the nutrition of the nerve. I subscribed to this view in an article in the *Trans. O.S.U.K.* for 1939. But since writing that paper I have been fortunate in obtaining normal material and thus been able to make serial sections of the lamina cribrosa region. These showed that the arteria centralis does give small branches (Fig. 140) to this region, which agrees with Leber's view. These branches, however, do not alter the clinical fact that a block of the artery anywhere in its intraneural course leads to blindness (Eugene Wolff).

we include the vessels on either side with the median anterior communicating, nine arteries may take part in the supply of the chiasma ; or, if with Abbie we count the middle cerebrals apart from the internal carotids, eleven arteries. It is thus extremely unlikely that a block of any one vessel will have any marked effect on the visual fibres. The anterior cerebrals supply most of the superior aspect while the internal carotids are mainly responsible for the under-surface. The feeding vessels again pass to the pial network and thence into the chiasma.

The Blood-supply of the Optic Tract.—The optic tract is also supplied through the pial network of vessels. This is continuous anteriorly with that of the

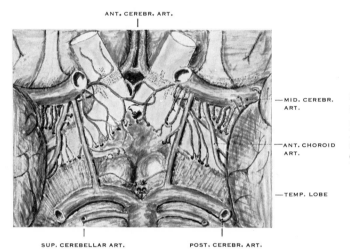

FIG. 356.—THE INTER-PEDUNCULAR SPACE AND CIRCLE OF WILLIS (MODIFIED AFTER JAYLE), SHOWING THE BLOOD-SUPPLY TO THE CHIASMA, OPTIC NERVE AND TRACT.

chiasma. The feeding vessels come partly from the posterior communicating but mainly from the anterior choroidal artery (Figs. 352, 353, 356, 357, 359).

Generally the latter artery gives several branches to the tract, but the largest of these pass completely through it to enter the base of the brain and supply, among other structures, a portion of the optic radiation.

According to Shellshear, these perforating vessels enter the tract between the crossed (which are the older fibres phylogenetically) and the uncrossed fibres. Sometimes they wind round the tract before entering it. (In this case it is thought that pressure on the tract may disturb nutrition by obstructing the arteries rather than by direct pressure on the nerve fibres themselves.) There is considerable mutual interchange between the anterior choroidal artery and the posterior communicating, and occasionally one or other predominates to the complete exclusion of its fellow (Abbie).

Injection investigations (François, 1959) have shown the optic tract supplied mutually by the anterior choroid arteries and by branches of the middle cerebral, overlapping and intermingling, but not anastomosing. That is, each individual artery is a true end artery, but the amount of overlap explains the absence of hemianopia after occlusion of the anterior choroidal.

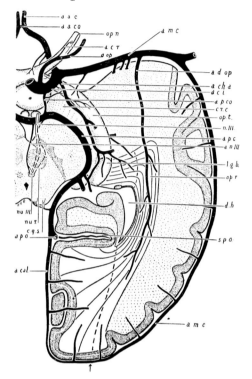
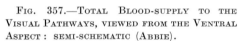

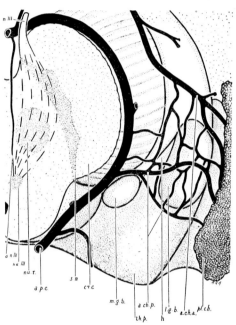

FIG. 357.—TOTAL BLOOD-SUPPLY TO THE VISUAL PATHWAYS, VIEWED FROM THE VENTRAL ASPECT : SEMI-SCHEMATIC (ABBIE).

Note the different sources of supply to the optic radiation. The arrow at the bottom of the figure marks the point of anastomosis between the calcarine and middle cerebral arteries.

FIG. 358.—THE ARTERIAL NETWORK OVER THE LATERAL GENICULATE BODY (SIMPLIFIED) (ABBIE).

Note its derivation from the anterior and posterior choroidal arteries. The specific end-artery from posterior cerebral to the oculo-motor nucleus is indicated.

ABBREVIATIONS EMPLOYED IN THE FIGURES.—a.a.c., anterior cerebral artery ; a.a.co., anterior communicating artery ; a.b., basilar artery ; a.c.i., internal carotid artery ; a.c.r., central artery of the retina ; a.cal., calcarine artery ; a.ch.a., anterior choroidal artery ; a.ch.p., posterior choroidal artery ; a.d.op., deep optic branch of the middle cerebral artery ; a.m.c., middle cerebral artery ; a.n.III, artery to oculo-motor nucleus ; a.op., ophthalmic artery ; a.p.c., posterior cerebral artery ; a.p.co., posterior communicating artery ; a.p.o., parieto-occipital artery ; b.ol., olfactory bulb ; c.a., anterior commissure ; c.c., corpus callosum ; c.q.s., superior colliculus ; cr.c., cerebral peduncle ; f., fornix ; h., hilum of lateral geniculate body ; h.a., hilar anastomosis ; l.g.b., lateral geniculate body ; m.g.b., medial geniculate body ; n.III, oculomotor nerve ; nu.III, oculomotor nucleus ; nu.r., red nucleus ; op.ch., optic chiasma ; op.n., optic nerve ; op.r., optic radiation ; op.t., optic tract ; pl.ch., choroidal plexus ; po., pons ; s.cal., calcarine sulcus ; s.lun., lunate sulcus ; s.n., substantia nigra ; s.p.cal., posterior calcarine sulcus ; s.p.o., parieto-occipital sulcus ; t.p., temporal pole ; th.p., pulvinar thalami.

The Blood-supply of the Lateral Geniculate Body.—It used to be held that the lateral geniculate body was supplied by the posterior cerebral artery and thus had a different vascular supply from the optic tract. This has been shown by Abbie and others to be incorrect. In fact, in the human, while the main supply, and especially that to the postero-medial aspect, comes from the posterior cerebral, the anterior and lateral aspects are supplied almost entirely by the anterior choroidal artery (Figs. 358, 359).

The region of the hilum is nourished through a rich anastomosis from both sources.

The anterior choroidal supplies the fibres coming from the inferior homonymous quadrants of the retinæ, while the posterior cerebral supplies those coming from the superior homonymous quadrants. The intervening region which radiates dorsally from the hilum and contains the macular fibres is supplied by both vessels.

Within the lateral geniculate body the terminal twigs from the penetrating vessels end chiefly in the individual cell laminæ ; some pass beyond into the commencement of the optic radiation (Abbie).

The Optic Radiations.—The blood-supply falls into three parts (Abbie) :

1. While the radiations are passing laterally over the roof of the inferior horn of the lateral ventricle, they are supplied by perforating branches of the anterior choroidal artery.

2. In their posterior course—lateral to the descending horn of the ventricle— they are supplied by the deep optic branch of the middle cerebral artery which enters the brain through the anterior perforated substance with the lateral striate arteries (Figs. 357, 359).

3. As the radiations spread out to reach the striate cortex, they are supplied by perforating cortical vessels, mainly from the calcarine branch of the posterior cerebral, but also from the middle cerebral artery. It is said that of these perforating vessels those which supply the radiations are independent of those which supply the cortex.

François *et al.* (1959) put some finishing touches to the above general account. In the first part of the radiation, where the fibres are passing *forwards* from the lateral geniculate body (the *carrefour*), the middle cerebral and even the posterior cerebral overlap the anterior choroid without anastomosis. They confirm the well-known fact that while there are surface anastomoses between the posterior and middle cerebral arteries, all *perforating* branches are end arteries. The optic radiation itself receives few arterioles ; these branch on its surface and enter the radiation as non-anastomosing pre-capillaries. The vascular network so formed is completely separate from the vascular network of the cortex.

The Visual Cortex is supplied mainly by the posterior cerebral, especially viâ its calcarine branch (Figs. 352, 357, 359). The middle cerebral helps at the anterior end of the calcarine sulcus, and on the lateral surface near the posterior pole there is, according to Shellshear, a fairly well-marked anastomosis between

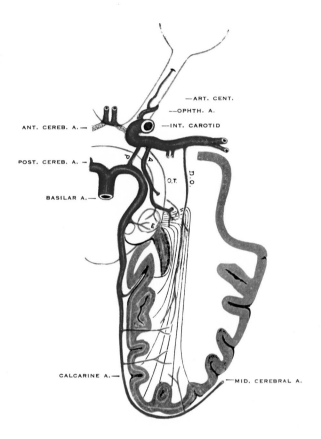

ART. CENT.

OPHTH. A.

ANT. CEREB. A. —

INT. CAROTID

POST. CEREB. A. —

O.T.

D.O.

BASILAR A. —

E

CALCARINE A. —

MID. CEREBRAL A.

O.T. = Optic Tract.
E = Lateral Geniculate Body.
A = Ant. Choroidal Artery.
P = Post. Communicating Artery.
D.O. = Deep Optic Artery.

FIG. 359.—THE BLOOD-SUPPLY TO THE VISUAL TRACT, SEEN FROM BELOW.
(In part, after Abbie.)

posterior and middle cerebrals, *which may account for the sparing of the macula in cases of thrombosis of the posterior cerebral.*

Smith and Richardson (1966) give further details of normal variations of vascular pattern, and relate specific arterial branches to their respective areas in the visual fields.

These vessels form a rich network in the pia, from which short branches pass to the grey matter, while larger branches pierce this to reach the white matter. The latter vessels are end arteries, communicating by capillaries only. Thus we may have localised areas of softening in the white matter.

The Blood-supply of the Lower Centres.—The tectum of the mid-brain is supplied from a network of vessels coming from the posterior cerebral and superior cerebellar arteries, but the former vessels provide the main supply to the superior colliculi.

According to Alezais and D'Astros, the oculomotor and trochlear nuclei are supplied by specific end arteries which arise from the posterior cerebral artery and enter the mid-brain through the posterior perforated substance (Fig. 356). (Stopford, however, states that these nuclei are supplied from the basilar artery.) The abducens nucleus is supplied by a specific end artery which comes from the basilar (Stopford). Very rarely the anterior spinal helps (Shellshear).

The Venous Return is partly by the cortical veins and partly by the basal vein which runs close to the posterior cerebral artery and has been divided in approaching a pineal tumour (see Harris and Cairns, *Lancet*, 1932, p. 3).

These veins are also practically end veins, so long as they are in the brain substance, but intercommunicate in the pia. A thrombosis of the veins is less likely to lead to as permanent damage as a corresponding lesion of the artery.

Practical Considerations

1. Division of one optic nerve results in blindness of that eye and a dilated pupil which does not react to light directly, but does consensually. The vision of the other eye is unaffected ; its pupil reacts to light directly, but not consensually. A glance at the diagram (Fig. 362) will make it clear that the reflex can get to the sphincter centre of the affected side, when light is thrown on to the good eye, either through the chiasma or through the posterior crossing in the mid-brain.

The affected pupil will, of course, react to convergence, but does not come under the category of the Argyll Robertson pupil (*q.v.*).

2. Sagittal section of the chiasma results in bitemporal hemianopia (a condition most commonly, but by no means invariably, seen in pituitary tumours). It abolishes neither the direct nor the consensual pupil reactions.

Theoretically, at any rate, a modified Wernicke (see later) ought to be present, i.e. the pupil ought to react when the light falls on the temporal (i.e. seeing) halves of the retina only. Division of the uncrossed fibres of the chiasma gives rise to binasal hemianopia. This was noted in a case of Knapp's, and was found on post-mortem to be due to calcified internal carotid arteries.

3. Behind the chiasma complete unilateral division of the visual pathway in any part of its course will result in a contralateral hemianopia, e.g. if the left pathway is divided, there results loss of the right halves (temporal of the right side and nasal of the left) of the visual fields.

4. Division of the optic tract produces a contralateral homonymous hemianopia, and, while it abolishes neither the direct nor the consensual pupil reaction, it gives rise to Wernicke's hemiopic pupil reaction, i.e. the pupils do not react when a narrow pencil of light is thrown on the blind halves of the retinæ, but do react if it falls on the seeing portions. It may not be out of place here to state that, owing to the scattering of light by the media of the eye, the test is exceedingly difficult to perform. A lesion of the optic tract may however be distinguished from a lesion of the optic radiation by the following facts. There is often slight ptosis of the same side and inequality of the pupils, the larger one being on the side of the hemianopia. Also the macula is not usually spared and optic atrophy sets in after a time.

5. Since the pupillary and visual fibres part company in the posterior third of the tract, behind this point they are usually affected separately. This accounts for the fact that the Wernicke's hemiopic pupil reaction differentiates a tract lesion from a lesion of the visual pathway behind the point of separation. (See, however, above.)

6. Destruction of the lateral geniculate body gives rise to a contralateral homonymous hemianopia (Henschen, Brouwer and Zeeman).

While this is the view which is now becoming generally accepted, one must state that von Monakow and others hold that the pulvinar of the thalamus must be involved as well to produce it.

7. Le Gros Clark (*J. Anat.*, **75**, 1941) has correlated the fact that a minute lesion of the retina always causes transneuronal atrophic changes in three corresponding laminæ of the lateral geniculate body, with the Young-Helminholtz theory of colour vision.

It is suggested that the three-fibre unit in the optic nerve and the three laminæ correspond to the three fundamental colours red, green, and violet. In favour of this is the fact that whereas the laminæ are clearly defined in the central part of the nucleus which is concerned with central vision, they tend to merge in the parts of the nucleus concerned with peripheral vision : perception of colours being probably wholly a function of the macular area.

8. It is now generally held that destruction of the superior colliculi has on effect on vision. It is still disputed how many (if any) pupillary fibres reach

them. Brouwer and Zeeman say that if any do they must be non-myelinated, and Levinsohn finds that destruction of a superior colliculus in rabbits has no effect on the pupillary reaction.

9. Destruction of the optic radiation or visual cortex on one side, as occurs in thrombosis of the posterior cerebral artery, gives rise to a contralateral homonymous hemianopia. The pupils are unaffected and the macula is spared.

If the hemianopia is accompanied by hemiplegia or hemianæsthesia, the lesion is in the posterior limb of the internal capsule behind the lentiform nucleus. Destruction of that portion of the geniculo-calcarine fibres, which passes forwards into the temporal lobe, results in a superior quadrantic hemianopia.

10. The visual pathway extends from the eyeball to the occipital pole of the brain. Hence, it may be affected by a great many lesions and thus help in diagnosis.

11. The definite localisation throughout the optic system explains the fact that even circumscribed lesions in tract, radiation, or striate area may produce sharply delimited scotomata in corresponding places in the visual field of the two eyes.

12. In general, a complete hemianopia is much more likely to occur where the visual fibres are tightly packed in a relatively narrow structure such as the optic tract. In the radiations and occipital cortex where the fibres are more widely spread partial defects are more likely developed in the form of a partial homonymous field defects, and quadrantic or smaller scotomata (Brodal).

THE MEDIAL LONGITUDINAL BUNDLE

The Medial Longitudinal Bundle is a well-marked band of fibres which runs close to the mid-line through the midbrain, pons, and medulla. Above, it establishes intricate connections with the region immediately above the mesencephalon, below it is continuous with the fasciculus anterior proprius of the medulla at the decussation of the pyramids.

In the mid-brain it lies ventral to the central grey matter and below this directly beneath the floor of the fourth ventricle. It closely interconnects the nuclei of the 3rd, 4th, and 6th nerves and the vestibular nucleus (Figs. 258, 262, 263). The nuclei of the oculomotor and trochlear nerves are closely applied to its medial and dorsal aspect, while that of the abducens lies on its lateral side.

" It would appear, therefore, that one of the most important functions of the strand is to bind together those nuclei, and thus enable them to act in harmony one with the other." [1]

Thus, in looking to the right, for instance, the lateral rectus of the right side is enabled to work with the medial rectus of the left.

" The most important element in the medial longitudinal bundle, however,

[1] Elliot Smith in Cunningham's *Anatomy*.

consists of fibres coming from the vestibular nucleus which proceed to the ocular group of nuclei of both sides as well as to both accessory nuclei in the medulla oblongata. By means of these connections, movements of the fluid in the semicircular canals can reflexly move the eyes and the head.

" It is evident that it is a brain tract of high importance from the fact that it is present in all vertebrates, and further that its fibres assume their medullary sheaths at an extremely early period. In fishes, amphibians, and reptiles it is one of the largest bundles of the brain stem. In man, its fibres medullate between the sixth and seventh months of fœtal life and at the same time as the fibres of the fasciculus anterior proprius of the spinal medulla with which it stands in connection."

BIBLIOGRAPHY

ABBIE, A. A. (1938): *Med. J. Aust.*, **2**, 199.
ARNOLD (1851): Handbuch der Anatomie des Menschen, *Freiburg*.
BADAL (1882): *Ann. Oculist.*, **45**, 241.
BEHR, C. (1935): *v. Graefe's Arch. Ophthal.*, **134**, 227.
BLUM (1913): *Dtsch. med. Wschr.*, **39**, 1588.
BRODAL, A. (1950): Neurological Anatomy, *Oxford*.
CARPENTER (1911): *Folia neuro-biologica*, **5**, 738 (Bibliography).
CHACKO, L. W. (1948): *Brit. J. Ophthal.*, **32**, 457.
CLARK, W. LE G. (1928): *Brain*, **52**, 334.
CLARK, W. LE G., and PENMAN (1934): *Proc. Roy. Soc.*, B., **114**, 129.
CUNEO (1904): " Les nerfs craniens," in Poirier-Charpy, Traité d'Anatomie Humaine, 2nd ed., *Paris*.
CUSHING (1904): *Bull. Johns Hopk. Hosp.*, **15**, 213.
DEJERINE (1914): Sémiologie des Affections du système Nerveux, *Paris*.
DELBERT, PIERRE (1887): *Arch. Ophtal.*, *Paris*, **8**, 485.
DEYL, J. (1896): *Anat. Anz.*, **11**, 687.
ECONOMO and KOSKINAS (1925): Die cytoarchitektonik der Hirnrinde des erwachsenen Menschen. *Wein u. Berlin*.
FLECHSIG, P. (1927): Meine Myelogenetische Hirnlehre, *Berlin*.
FRANÇOIS, NEETENS and COLLETTE (1959): *Brit. J. Ophthal.*, **43**, 394.
GIRI (1913): *Ophthalmoscope*, **11**, 390.
GASKELL (1899): *Brain*, **22**, 329.
—— (1920): Involuntary Nervous System, *London*.
HOVELACQUE, A. (1927): L'Anatomie des Nerfs Craniens et Rachidiens, 2 vols., *Paris*.
HOVELACQUE and REINHOLD (1917): *Rev. anthrop.*, **27**, 277.
KRAUSE, W., and TELGMAN, J. (1869): Les Anomalies dans le parcours des nerfs chez l'homme, *Paris*.
LAWRENCE (1894): See *J. Anat. Physiol.*, 1894, **28**; *Proc.*, **18.**
LODDONI (1930): *Ann. Ottalm.*, **58**, 468.
MECKEL, J. F. (1748): De quinto pare nervorum cerebri, *Göttingen*.

NATHAN and TURNER (1942): *Brain*, **65,** 343.

NEAL (1914): *J. of Morphol.*, **25,** 1.

PFISTER (1890): *v. Graefe's Arch. Ophthal.*, **36,** Abt. I, 83–93.

PRINCETEAU (1908): *Congr. franç. Chir.*, 781–805.

ROUVIÈRE (1914): *Bibliogr. Anat.*, **24,** 92.

SCHWALBE (1887): Lehrbuch der Anatomie der Sinnesorgane, *Erlangen.*

SMITH, C. G. and RICHARDSON, W. F. G. (1966): *Am. J. Ophthal.* **61,** 1391.

TESTUT: *Lyon méd.*, **130,** 1216.

TRAQUAIR (1946): Clinical Perimetry, 5th ed., *London.*

WALLIS (1917): *Practitioner*, **98,** 41.

WILBRAND, H. (1929): Der Faserverlauf durch das Chiasma, *Berlin.*

WILLIS (1664): Cerebrii Anatome, cui accessit nervorum descriptio et usus.

WOLFF and PENMAN (1950): *Proc. Int. Congr. Ophthal.*, London, **2,** 625.

See also Bibliography to Comparative Anatomy, 487.

CHAPTER VII (*continued*)

THE NERVES

THE AUTONOMIC NERVOUS SYSTEM

THIS consists of two parts, the sympathetic and the parasympathetic systems. Generally the viscera are supplied by each system, and in such cases the sympathetic and parasympathetic systems exercise opposite effects.

The **sympathetic nervous system,** like the central, has sensory (receptor) connector, and motor (excitor) elements, but in the former the excitor elements have left the central nervous system to form the various ganglia. The sensory elements have remained in the same position as those of the central system, i.e. in the posterior root ganglia, and connect by means of the sensory root with cells of the connector elements, which have remained in the central nervous system. The connector fibres have passed out as white rami communicantes to reach the motor excitor (or effector) elements which may have wandered to the lateral chain ganglion, or to a peripheral ganglion such as the cœliac.

Hence the cell in the lateral chain ganglia is homologous with the anterior horn cell of the somatic system, and the lateral horn cell is homologous with the cell of the (intercalated) connector neurone of the somatic system (Fig. 360).

The collaterals of the sympathetic system make connection with many neurones. Hence movements produced by the sympathetic nervous system are primitive, i.e. *en masse* (cf. protopathic sensation).

To Summarise.

Central System.—*Sensory* (*receptor*) neurones, both spinal and cranial, their cell bodies in the posterior root ganglion or its homologue (e.g. trigeminal ganglion).

Motor (*effector*).—Neurones whose cell bodies are in the central nervous system.

Connector (*intercalated*).—Neurone also in the central nervous system.

Sympathetic System.—Sensory neurone, cell body in the posterior root ganglion.

The motor (effector) neurone, cell body in the lateral chain ganglia, or in the peripheral ganglion.

The connector neurone starts in the lateral horn of the thoracic region, and leaves the cord by the white rami communicantes.

They are thus *medullated* pre-ganglionic fibres. The post-ganglionic fibres are non-medullated.

The **parasympathetic system** is in two parts, cranial and sacral. It is built on the same three-neurone plan. The *connector neurone* is in the nucleus of a cranial nerve or in the grey matter of the sacral part of the spinal cord (segments 2, 3 and sometimes 4). The *effector neurone* generally is on the wall of the viscus that is being innervated. There is an exception to this in the case of part of the cranial outflow, where ganglia are established for relay of the connector neurone on to the effector cell body. These ganglia are the ciliary, pterygo- (spheno-) palatine, submandibular and otic. Only parasympathetic relay occurs here. All four ganglia transmit both sensory and sympathetic fibres to share in the peripheral distribution of the branches, but none of these fibres relay in the ganglia (Fig. 364).

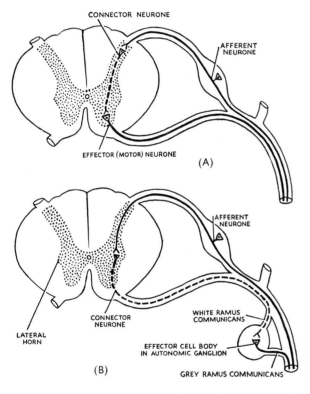

Fig. 360.—(A). The Three Neurones of a Spinal Reflex.

(B). The Same Three Neurones Comprise an Autonomic Reflex but the Site of the Cell Bodies is Different. The connector cell body lies in the lateral grey horn and the effector (motor) cell body lies in an autonomic ganglion. The connector axis cylinder (white ramus) leaves the spinal nerve distal to the posterior primary division. The grey ramus usually joins the spinal nerve *proximal* to the white ramus.

(From Last's "Anatomy: Regional and Applied," by permission. J. & A. Churchill Ltd.)

There are thus four outflows of fine medullated nerves to peripheral motor ganglion cells.

1. Prosomatic or mid-brain .   .   . } cranial parasympathetic.
2. Bulbar .   .   .   .   .   . }
3. Thoraco-lumbar .   .   .   .   . sympathetic system.
4. Sacral (nervi erigentes) .   .   .   . sacral parasympathetic.

1. **The Mid-brain Outflow** of connector fibres probably arise in the nucleus of Edinger-Westphal, pass out with the 3rd nerve to the ciliary ganglion, where they make connection with motor cells. From here post-ganglionic *medullated* fibres

pass in the ciliary nerves to the sphincter pupillæ and ciliary muscles. The medullation may be associated with the fact that these muscles are striated in birds. Acetylcholine has no effect on this outflow.

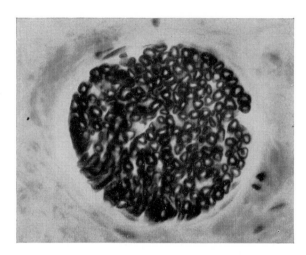

FIG. 361.—SECTION OF POSTERIOR CILIARY NERVE OF RHESUS MONKEY JUST BEHIND THE GLOBE TO SHOW MEDULLATED FIBRES. (WEIGERT'S STAIN.)

There is reciprocal innervation of antagonists. Thus stimulation of the 3rd nerve contracts the sphincter and inhibits the dilatator, and likewise the sympathetic is motor to the dilatator, and inhibitor to the sphincter.

2. **The Bulbar Outflow** of connector fibres (corresponding to the white rami of the thoracic region) arises in the nucleus intercalatus of Staderini, which consists of small cells in the dorsal nucleus of the vagus in the floor of the fourth ventricle.

The following are the cranial nerves which contain fibres corresponding to white rami and belonging to the bulbar outflow :

(1) **Superior salivatory nucleus,** secretomotor fibres leave in nervus intermedius for two destinations : (*a*) viâ greater (superficial) petrosal nerve to relay in pterygo-palatine (spheno-palatine) ganglion for lacrimal gland and glands of nose, paranasal sinuses and palate, (*b*) chorda tympani to submandibular ganglion for relay to sublingual, anterior lingual and submandibular salivary glands.

(2) **Inferior salivatory nucleus,** secretomotor fibres leave in 9th nerve, and by local relay in mucous membrane supply glands of oro-pharynx. In tympanic branch of 9th secretomotor fibres run in lesser (superficial) petrosal nerve, for relay in otic ganglion to supply parotid gland.

(3) Dorsal nucleus of vagus, motor fibres destined to relay in wall of viscus concerned (heart, lung, gut).

The **Sympathetic Fibres** which pass to the eye are discussed on p. 401.

THE SEGMENTAL VALUE OF THE OCULAR NERVES [1]

In some of the lower vertebrates, especially the elasmobranchs, there are at least nine segments included in the constitution of the head. In the higher vertebrates it is difficult to be sure which nerve belongs to which segment, but the following is a commonly accepted view.

The 3rd nerve belongs to the 1st head segment. It includes a large-fibred medial somatic efferent part distributed to the orbital muscles derived from the 1st somite, and a small-fibred splanchnic efferent part, passing to the ciliary ganglion.

[1] See Thane in Quain's *Anatomy*, 10th edition.

The lateral somatic efferent fibres are perhaps represented as suggested by Gaskell by the upper (ocular) facial, which is held to be derived from the oculo-motor nucleus. The ophthalmic division of V appears to be the afferent nerve of this segment. In the elasmobranchs, Hoffmann finds the ramus ophthalmicus profundus, which corresponds to our nasociliary nerve (Ewart), is developed independently of the rest of the 5th, and in close relation to the 1st somite.

Gaskell, however, considers that the afferent fibres of the 1st segmental nerve, with their stationary ganglion, have undergone degeneration and are now represented only by the vestigial structures on the roots of the 3rd nerve, and his view receives support from the observation of Martin that, in the early embryo of the cat, the 3rd nerve is provided with a dorsal root which subsequently disappears ; a ganglionated dorsal root to the oculo-motor nerve has been described by Kupfer in Ammocetes and by Froriep in Torpedo.

The 4th nerve supplies the superior oblique, the muscle of the 2nd somite.

The 5th nerve, excluding the ophthalmic division, also belongs to this segment (Hoffmann), of which the motor root is the lateral somatic efferent.

The pterygo- (spheno-) palatine and otic ganglia belong to this segment.

The 6th, 7th, and 8th cranial nerves belong to the 3rd segment.

The 6th and 7th are the medial and lateral somatic efferent respectively. The great superficial petrosal and a part of the nervus intermedius (that to submandibular ganglion) constitute the splanchnic efferent, while the geniculate ganglion belongs to the splanchnic afferent.

The somatic efferent is the 8th, with its acoustic ganglion.

The 4th segment is suppressed ; possibly it is represented by the nervus intermedius.

The 9th nerve belongs to the 5th segment.

The 10th nerve belongs to the 6th and 7th segments, but the medial somatic efferent of the 7th segment is in the hypoglossal, which is composed of the medial somatic efferent parts of the last three or more cephalic (originally 1st spinal) segmental nerves.

The Path of the Light Reflex

Two main views are expressed with regard to the origin of the light reflex.

1. Hess (1908 and 1922), in his experiments with diurnal birds which have yellow oil globules between the inner and outer portions of the rods, and nocturnal birds which have none, showed that visual and pupillary reactions to light stimuli of varying intensity and under different conditions of adaptation ran parallel, and came to the conclusion that the outer portion of the rods and cones are the receptor organs—both for vision and for the light reflex. This is the view most widely accepted.

2. Schirmer (1894) believed that the light reflex started in the inner nuclear layer, especially in the amacrine cells. For in diseases of the outer retinal layers, sight is affected much more than the pupil reflex. But Von Hippel points out that these cells are absent just in the macular area where the light reflex is most easily obtained.

It is probable that the light reflex can be obtained from any portion of the retina up to the ora serrata, and not as Hess thought from the macular area only. But it is certainly much more easily elicited when light falls on the central area ; while strong illumination is necessary to produce it from the peripheral retina.

The Afferent Tract.—Here again two views are expressed as to whether the visual and pupillary fibres are different or identical. That they are probably different is shown by the fact that in certain cases of complete blindness the pupillary reflex was obtained. Also, as Parsons pointed out, if the fibres had two functions it would controvert Müller's law of specificity of nerve conduction.

Much, however, may be said for the view expressed by Ingvar and Lenz that the pupillary fibres are non-medullated and run in the periphery of the optic nerve.

Current views are that the reflex fibres in the superior brachium are collateral branches of the visual axons.

The pupillary fibres run in the optic nerve ; for its division abolishes the direct but not the consensual light reflex. *The pupillary fibres partially cross in the chiasma, as do the visual, a portion going over to the opposite side, while the remainder pass on in the optic tract of the same side.* We know that the pupillary fibres cross in the chiasma, because division of one optic tract abolishes neither the direct nor the consensual pupil reaction. Experimental division of the chiasma abolishes neither the direct nor the consensual light reflex. *Hence there must be a posterior crossing as well.*

The pupillary fibres do not pass from the chiasma to the floor of the third ventricle, for experimental separation of the chiasma (Trendelenburg and Bumke, 1911) from this structure has no effect on the light reflex. *The pupillary fibres run in the optic tract,* division of which causes Wernicke's hemiopic pupil reaction.[1]

They leave the visual fibres at the posterior part of the tract, do not form a cell station at the lateral geniculate body, but run superficially in the superior brachium conjunctivum to the lateral side of the superior colliculus. Division of both superior brachia abolishes the pupil reactions to light on both sides (Karplus and Kreidl, 1913).

It is probable that the fibres which enter the superior colliculus have nothing to do with the pupillary reflex, for as Levinsohn has shown, destruction of this body down to the aqueduct has no effect on the pupillary reflex.

The pupillary fibres pass into the mid-brain to the lateral side of the superior colliculus to reach the pretectal nucleus (which is an ill-defined collection of small cells under cover of the lateral margin of the superior colliculus), where they make a cell station. The new relay of fibres partially crosses in the posterior commissure and also ventral to the aqueduct, and thus reaches the sphincter centre of the same and opposite side viâ the medial longitudinal bundle.

The Sphincter Centre is certainly in the anterior part of the 3rd nerve nucleus, in the small-celled paired nucleus of Edinger-Westphal.

[1] See experiments by Karplus and Kreidl, 1913. Case of Marie and Chatelin, *Revue Neurologique,* 1915.

To Sum Up.

The probable course of the afferent pupillary fibres is as follows (Figs. 362, 363) :

They start in the rods and cones—pass through the retina to reach the optic nerve ; partially cross in the chiasma like the visual fibres ; accompany the visual fibres in the tract to its posterior third, where they leave the tract as a separate bundle of fibres to enter the superior brachium conjunctivum ; pass into the mid-brain lateral to the superior colliculus to reach the pretectal nucleus ; partially cross to reach the anterior part of the 3rd nerve nucleus (Edinger-Westphal) of the same and opposite side viâ the medial longitudinal bundle.

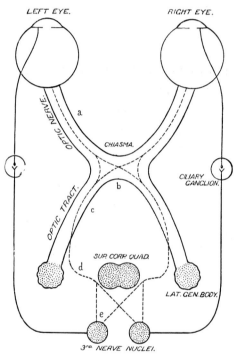

FIG. 362.—SCHEME OF THE PUPILLARY PATH (INTERRUPTED LINES).

Section at (a), i.e. of the left optic nerve, causes blindness of the left eye, abolition of the direct reaction to light of the left eye with retention of the consensual, and abolition of the consensual reaction of the right eye with retention of the direct.

At (b), i.e. of the chiasma, causes bitemporal hemianopia ; abolishes neither the direct nor the consensual pupil reaction.

At (c), i.e. of left optic tract, causes contra-lateral (i.e. right) homonymous hemianopia ; Wernicke's hemiopic pupil reaction.

At (d), i.e. of the superior brachium on *both* sides, causes Argyll Robertson pupils.

At (e), i.e. both afferent fibres coming to left nucleus ; unilateral (left) Argyll Robertson pupil.

At (e), on both sides causes bilateral Argyll Robertson pupils.

N.B.—*The cell station in the pretectal nucleus (see Fig. 363) is not shown.*

We see therefore that there is a double crossing—namely, in the chiasma and in the midbrain.

The Efferent Tract.—From the sphincter nucleus, the fibres pass into the 3rd nerve, then along its branch to the inferior oblique to reach the ciliary ganglion viâ its short root. Here they make a cell station. Then viâ the *medullated* short ciliary nerves they pierce the globe round the optic nerve, occupy a position between the choroid and sclera, and so reach the sphincter pupillæ.

The Pupillo-dilator Fibres.—The dilator centre (centrum-cilio-spinale of Budge) lies in the lateral column of the spinal cord at the junction of its thoracic and cervical regions. The dilator fibres leave the cord viâ the white rami communi-

A.E.—26

cantes of the 1st and 2nd thoracic nerves. They pass up the cervical sympathetic trunk to reach the superior cervical ganglion, where they form a cell station. From here the *post-ganglionic* fibres run upwards with the sympathetic plexus around the internal carotid artery,[1] which they leave to join the trigeminal ganglion. They pass into the orbit viâ the naso-ciliary nerve and enter the eye viâ the long ciliary nerves and so reach the dilatator muscle.

A Higher Centre for the Dilator Path.—Although dilatation of the pupil results almost invariably from stimulation of the cerebral cortex, there is no cortical dilator centre. Parsons (1904) provisionally placed it in the mesencephalon near the third nucleus, but Karplus and Kreidl (1912) showed that it was higher than this in the medial and frontal portion of the hypothalamus close to the optic tract. The descending tracts pass through the cerebral peduncles and cross partially before reaching the centre of Budge.

With regard to the homologies between the sphincter and dilator systems, the centrum-cilio-spinale of Budge corresponds to the sphincter centre in the mid-brain, and the ciliary ganglion to the superior cervical ganglion.

The Path of the Accommodation Reflex

The accommodation reflex is initiated by the necessity to get a clear image of a near object. It is usually accompanied by fixation, which consists essentially of a converging movement of the eyeballs, and by diminution in the size of the pupils.

The afferent path of the whole reflex is probably along the visual pathway to the occipital cortex. From here to the peristriate area, whence it is carried to the premotor area of the frontal lobe. Thence viâ the corona radiata and internal capsule it reaches the oculomotor (including Edinger-Westphal) nucleus, bypassing the pretectal nucleus. Next it passes by the 3rd nerve directly to the medial rectus or viâ the ciliary ganglion to the ciliary muscles and sphincter pupillæ.

Some, however, believe that the *convergence part* of the reflex has a different path and does not involve the occipital cortex. It is held to start in proprioceptive impulses in the medial recti. Hence, via the 3rd nerve or 1st division of the 5th to the mesencephalic nucleus of the 5th. From here to the constrictor centre of the 3rd nerve nucleus. Hence, via the 3rd nerve for an unknown distance. Then leaving the 3rd nerve it misses the ciliary ganglion and makes a cell station in an accessory ganglion (see p. 311), whence it passes to the sphincter pupillæ.

Practical Considerations

1. The results on the pupillary reactions of division of the optic nerve, the optic chiasma, the optic tract, and the visual pathways behind the point of separation of the pupillary fibres have been discussed on p. 391.

---

[1] Sympathetic ganglion cells have been found in the internal carotid plexus. These should not be forgotten when considering the effects of extirpation of the superior cervical ganglion (Sunderland and Hughes).

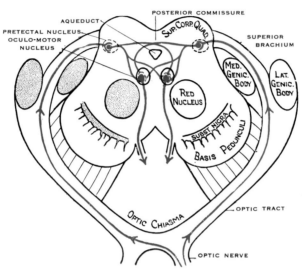

FIG. 363.— DIAGRAM OF SECTION THROUGH MID-BRAIN AND OPTIC CHIASMA TO SHOW PATH OF
PUPILLARY CONSTRICTOR FIBRES.

Note especially the pretectal nucleus

(*From Cunningham's Anatomy, after Ranson and Magoun.*)

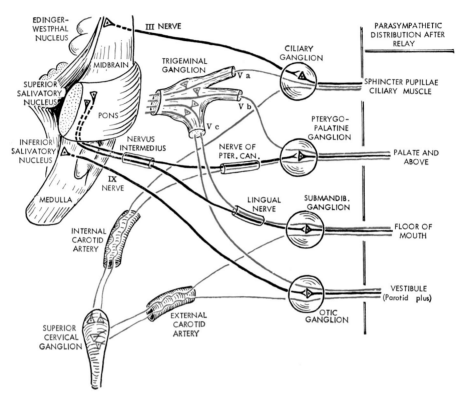

FIG. 364.—PLAN OF CONNEXIONS OF THE CRANIAL PARASYMPATHETIC GANGLIA.

The otic ganglion lies high up near the skull base but by its connexions and branches it is actually the most caudal of the four.

1. Only the parasympathetic roots (black) *relay* in the ganglia. They come from three nuclei, one each in midbrain, pons and medulla. The pontine nucleus (superior salivatory nucleus) relays in the middle two ganglia.

2. The sensory roots (blue) come from the trigeminal ganglion, where their cell bodies lie. The third division (V c) sends branches through the last two ganglia.

3. The sympathetic roots (red) come from cell bodies in the superior cervical ganglion and travel along the internal and external carotid arteries, two on each, to reach their respective ganglia.

(From Last's "Anatomy : Regional and Applied", by permission, J. & A. Churchill).

2. Division of both brachia conjunctiva results in loss of the light reflex with retention of the reaction to convergence (Argyll Robertson pupil).

3. For the relation of the superior colliculus to the light reflex, see p. 400.

4. Division of all the pupillary fibres in the mid-brain before they reach the sphincter centre results in bilateral loss of light reflex with retention of the reaction to convergence (Argyll Robertson pupils).

5. If the direct and crossed fibres going to one sphincter centre only are divided a unilateral Argyll Robertson results. The pupil does not react directly or consensually. The reason for this is easily seen from the diagram, for the sphincter centre of the affected side cannot be reached from either eye. The pupil on the sound side reacts directly and consensually (Fig. 363).

6. Total pupillary paralysis, that is, failure to react to light and convergence, may be due to : (a) a supra-(extra)nuclear lesion ; (b) a nuclear lesion ; (c) a lesion of the 3rd nerve ; (d) a lesion of the ciliary ganglion ; (e) a lesion of the short ciliary nerves. It is probable that the fixed pupil in acute glaucoma is due to pressure on the short ciliary nerves as they lie between choroid and sclera. The mydriatics (atropin, etc.) act on the post-ganglionic fibres of the parasympathetic, in this case the third nerve fibres in the short ciliary nerves ; (f) a lesion of the ciliary and sphincter muscles ; (g) one ought to add here that loss of reaction to light and convergence may be due to mechanical causes—most commonly posterior synechiæ. It should be noted that (apart from (g)) the larger the pupil the more complete the paralysis.

7. *The Anatomy of the Argyll Robertson Pupil.*—There are three main possibilities for the site of the lesion [1] :

(a) That it is on the afferent side of the reflex arc just before the pupillary fibres reach the sphincter centre. This is probably the most generally accepted view. The difficulty about accepting this, and indeed all the other theories, is that it is based on practically no pathological evidence. Current views incline strongly to the belief that the lesion is in the pretectal nucleus (Adler, 1959).

(b) That it is on the afferent side, the lesion being in the superior brachium conjunctivum. Lenz and Ingvar believe that the pupillary fibres run superficially in the optic nerve and superior brachium. They hold that the spirochætal (or other) toxin is in the cerebro-spinal fluid, and will therefore affect the fibres nearest the subarachnoid space, i.e. pupillary fibres. It will be remembered that Karplus and Kreidl produced the Argyll Robertson pupil by dividing the superior brachia.

(c) That it is on the *efferent* side in the ciliary ganglion (Marina). While the pupillary fibres are certainly more vulnerable than those which have to do with convergence, it is difficult to see how, if the lesion were in so small a body as the

---

[1] In trying to fix a site for the lesion, it is very important to remember that in the unilateral Argyll Robertson pupil, the pupil on the affected side does *not* react to light directly or consensually, while the pupil on the sound side reacts to light both ways.

ciliary ganglion, the Argyll Robertson pupil may be present for years and the reaction to convergence not be diminished but actually increased. Cameron (1959) answers this objection by suggesting that only the light-reflex fibres, and not the near-vision fibres, of the third nerve synapse in the ciliary ganglion.

There is very little to be said for Reichardt's view that the lesion is in the spinal cord. Argyll Robertson himself argued that the lesion must be in the cilio-spinal (i.e. sympathetic) pathways, thus explaining the contracted pupil.

8. *The Sympathetic Pathway.*

Division of the cervical sympathetic results in Horner's syndrome or Horner's triad : ptosis, small pupil, and enophthalmos.

The affected pupil does not dilate in the dark or after the instillation of cocaine or after pinching the neck (cilio-spinal reflex). In bright light both pupils contract and their inequality disappears.

The affected side of the face d˙es not flush or sweat, and the ear feels colder than on the normal side. The area of absence of sweating includes the whole of the upper limb (Purves Stewart, Sherren[1]).

According to Levinsohn the ocular symptoms are more pronounced if the superior cervical ganglion is destroyed than if the cervical sympathetic cord forming the pre-ganglionic fibres is cut.

Injury to the cervical sympathetic may result from wounds, accidental or operative, and involvement in growths, etc. The pupillary fibres may also be affected in the lower-arm type of brachial birth palsy (Klumke's paralysis), and in injuries to the spinal cord.

Stimulation of the cervical sympathetic results in exophthalmus, widening of the palpebral fissure, dilatation of the pupil, and often flushing and sweating. It results from pressure by aneurysms, tumours, apical tuberculosis, etc.

THE RÔLE OF THE SUPERIOR COLLICULUS

Receiving non-visual fibres (? collaterals) from the optic tract, the cell bodies of the superior colliculus are connected by tecto-bulbar and tecto-spinal tracts with the motor nuclei of the ocular, neck, trunk, and limb muscles. Thus are mediated reflex effects of light—eyeball movements, face (e.g. screwing up the eyes), trunk and limbs (e.g. turning the neck and body, throwing up the hands, jumping, etc.). These subcortical pathways do not, of course, depend upon seeing. The inferior colliculi have parallel connections with sound pathways, independent of hearing.

BIBLIOGRAPHY

ADLER, F. H. (1959) : Physiology of the Eye, *St. Louis, U.S.A.*
BEHR (1924) : Die Lehre von den Pupillenbewegungen, *Berlin.*
BUMKE and TRENDELENBURG (1911) : *Klin. Mbl. Augenheilk.*, **49** (2), 145.

[1] See Sherren in Choyce's *Surgery.*

FUCHS (1907) : *Arb. neurol. Inst., Wien,* **15,** 1.

HESS (1908) : *Arch. Augenheilk.,* **58,** 182.

—— (1922), *Med. Klin.,* **18,** 1214.

INGVAR, S. (1923) : *Acta med. Scand.,* **59,** 696.

—— (1928) : *Bull. Johns Hopk. Hosp.,* **93,** 363.

KARPLUS and KREIDL (1909-10) : *Pflüger's Arch. ges. Physiol.,* **129,** 401; **135,** 138.

—— (1913), *Wien. Klin. Wschr.,* **83.**

—— (1912) : *Klin. Mbl. Augenheilk.,* **1** (1), 586.

—— (1913) : *Neurol. Zbl.,* **82.**

LENZ (1924) : *Klin. Mbl. Augenheilk.,* **72,** 769.

MARIE and CHATELIN (1915) : *Revue Neurologique,* **22.**

MARINA (1899) : *Dtsch. Z. Nervenheilk.,* **14,** 356.

—— (1901) : *Dtsch. Z. Nervenheilk.,* **20,** 369.

PARSONS (1904) : *Ophth. Hosp. Rep.,* **16,** 1, 20.

—— (1924) : *Trans. Ophthal. Soc. U.K.,* **44,** 1.

ROBERTSON, ARGYLL (1869) : *Edin. Med. Jour.,* **14,** 696 ; **15,** 491.

CHAPTER VIII

THE VESSELS

THE OPHTHALMIC ARTERY

THE ophthalmic artery arises as a vertical branch (Fig. 291), from the medial side of the convexity of the fifth bend of the internal carotid, just after this vessel has left the cavernous sinus by piercing the dura forming its roof. At its origin (Figs. 276, 277, 291), the ophthalmic artery is medial to the anterior clinoid process and inferior to the optic nerve. After a very short course upwards (Fig. 291) it bends forwards at a right angle. It runs directly forwards for a few millimetres under the *medial* side of the nerve, then bends laterally. Usually the origin of the artery lies under the middle of the nerve, but since its course here is antero-posterior and that of the nerve laterally as well as forwards, it may appear at the *medial* border of the nerve before eventually passing laterally (Figs. 272, 353).[1] The nearer the origin of the artery is to the optic foramen, the nearer the medial side of the nerve is it placed, and vice versa.

It passes through the optic canal within the dural sheath of the nerve, at first lying under the nerve ; then passing to its lateral side, it pierces the sheath near its entrance into the orbit. It will be seen that the internal carotid artery is anchored to the dural sheath by its ophthalmic branch ; and it is also indirectly attached to the optic nerve by the adherence of the sheaths and by branches to the nerve from the ophthalmic artery (see p. 324). (Figs. 292, 293.)

In the posterior part of the orbit it lies in the cone of muscles, with the ciliary ganglion and the lateral rectus to its lateral side and the optic nerve medial Fig s. 278, 280).

The artery ascends, crosses over the nerve and below the superior rectus to reach the medial wall of the orbit in company with its satellite naso-ciliary nerve (Fig. 278). It passes forwards between the medial rectus and superior oblique towards the maxillary process of the frontal, behind which it ends by dividing into dorsal nasal and supratrochlear branches.

The ophthalmic artery and its branches are markedly tortuous.

Summary of Distribution.—The ophthalmic artery supplies the orbit and beyond. One branch transcends all the others in importance—the central artery of the retina. This is an end artery and its loss (e.g. from embolism) results in complete and irrevocable blindness. Beyond the orbit the ophthalmic artery supplies the forehead to the vertex, and the lateral wall of the nose. Here, especi-

---

[1] Fawcett (1896), *J. Anat. Physiol.*, **30**, N.S., x, 49–53.

ally in the scalp, exists the field of anastomosis between external and internal carotid arteries.

Branches.—Convention dictates that these should be named, but great variation exists and some or other of the branches are commonly incapable of being demonstrated in a dissection of the orbit. The significant branches of the ophthalmic artery are as follows :

1. The central artery of the retina (arteria centralis retinæ).
2. Posterior ciliary arteries.
3. The lacrimal artery.
4. Recurrent branches.
5. Muscular branches.
6. Supraorbital.
7. Posterior ethmoidal.
8. Anterior ethmoidal.
9. Superior and inferior medial palpebral.
10. Dorsalis nasi (Nasal) ⎱
11. Supratrochlear (Frontal) ⎰ terminal.

1. **The Central Artery.**—Its terminal branches have no anastomosis except a slight one with the circle of Zinn or Haller around the entrance of the nerve into the eye (see p. 149).

2. **The Posterior Ciliary Arteries** come off as two trunks, while the ophthalmic artery is still below the optic nerve. These divide into some 10 to 20 branches which, running forwards, surround the nerve and pierce the eyeball close to it. The majority, called the *short ciliary arteries*, enter the choroid coat of the eye. Two branches—*the long posterior ciliaries*—however, pierce the sclera to the medial and lateral sides of the nerve respectively (Fig. 278). They run forwards between the sclera and choroid to supply the ciliary body, and then, anastomosing with the *anterior ciliary* arteries to form the *circulus arteriosus iridis major* (see p. 94), supply the iris.

3. **The Lacrimal Artery** arises from the ophthalmic to the lateral side of the optic nerve. It runs forwards at the upper border of the lateral rectus muscle in company with the lacrimal nerve (*q.v.*) to the lacrimal gland, which it supplies. Having passed through or to the lateral side of the gland, it supplies the conjunctiva and eyelids (Figs. 277, 278).

Branches.—(*a*) The *recurrent meningeal* branch passes backwards through the superior orbital fissure or through a small foramen in the greater wing of the sphenoid to anastomose with the middle meningeal artery, a branch of the maxillary, which in turn comes off the external carotid. This anastomosis is therefore one between the internal and external carotids, i.e. between the primitive dorsal and ventral aortæ. At times it may be quite large and replace the ophthalmic or middle meningeal in part.

(*b*) *The temporal and zygomatic* (*malar*) *branches* accompany the corresponding branches of the second division of the 5th nerve, and anastomose with the anterior deep temporal and transverse facial arteries respectively.

(*c*) *The lateral palpebral* branches form arcades in the lids by anastomosing with the corresponding *medial palpebral* branches of the ophthalmic artery.

4. **Small Recurrent Branches** pass back through the superior orbital (sphenoidal) fissure to join similar branches from the internal carotid. Others run back in the dural sheath of the optic nerve.

5. **The Muscular Branches** are usually given off as two main branches, *lateral* and *medial*, with a varying number of smaller twigs. These latter come from the main artery and also from the lacrimal and supraorbital. The lateral branch supplies the lateral and superior recti, the levator and superior oblique. The medial branch is the larger of the two, and supplies the inferior and medial recti and the inferior oblique. The muscular branches give off the *anterior ciliary arteries* (see p. 91).

6. **The Supraorbital Artery** (Figs. 274, 278) comes off where the ophthalmic lies above the optic nerve. It lies at first medial to the superior rectus and levator, and then above the latter muscle and under the roof of the orbit. It meets the nerve of the same name at the junction of the posterior and middle thirds of the orbit, and then accompanies it through the supraorbital notch or foramen, and with it crosses the areolar tissue deep to the frontalis (the danger area), and so reaches the scalp, where it anastomoses with the superficial temporal and supratrochlear arteries. It supplies the upper eyelid, the scalp, and also sends twigs to the levator, the periorbita, and the diploë of the frontal bone.

7. **The Posterior Ethmoidal Artery** (Fig. 278) is a small vessel which enters the posterior ethmoidal canal in company with the posterior ethmoidal nerve (nerve of Luschka) when this is present. It supplies the mucous membrane of the posterior ethmoidal air-cells and upper part of the nose.

8. **The Anterior Ethmoidal Artery** (Figs. 277, 278) is larger than the preceding. It comes off where the ophthalmic lies between the superior oblique and medial rectus. It accompanies the anterior ethmoidal nerve through the anterior ethmoidal canal to appear in the anterior cranial fossa. It enters the nose by a slit in the anterior part of the cribriform plate, occupies the groove on the deep surface of the nasal bone, and eventually appears on the face between the lateral nasal cartilage and the nasal bone.

It gives the *anterior meningeal branch* to the dura mater of the anterior fossa ; and it also supplies the mucous membrane of the front part of the nasal cavity, the anterior ethmoidal air-cells, and the skin of the nose.

9. **The Superior and Inferior Medial Palpebral Branches** come off near the front of the orbit. They pass above and below the medial palpebral ligament to reach the upper and lower lids respectively (Fig. 214). Here they lie in a plane

between the orbicularis and the tarsal plate, where they anastomose with the corresponding branches of the lacrimal, to form the arterial arches or arcades of the lids (see p. 199).

The medial palpebral arteries also send twigs to the conjunctiva, the caruncle, and lacrimal sac.

10. **The Dorsalis nasi (Nasal) Branch** pierces the septum orbitale above the medial palpebral ligament to supply the skin of the root of the nose and the lacrimal sac. It anastomoses with the angular and nasal branches of the facial artery.

11. **The Supratrochlear Artery** (Figs. 214, 274) pierces the septum orbitale with the supratrochlear nerve which it accompanies. It passes upwards, round the medial end of the supraorbital margin about $\frac{1}{2}$ in. (1·25 cm.) from the mid-line, and supplies the skin, muscles, and periosteum of the medial part of the forehead. It anastomoses with the supraorbital and with its fellow of the opposite side.

VARIATIONS IN THE OPHTHALMIC ARTERY [1]

1. The ophthalmic artery in 15 per cent. of cases crosses beneath instead of over the optic nerve.

2. It may enter the orbit through the superior orbital fissure.

3. The lacrimal often, and the ophthalmic rarely, may arise from the middle meningeal—by an enlargement of the recurrent lacrimal artery which joins the lacrimal to the middle meningeal (that is, marks a union between primitive ventral and dorsal aortæ).

4. The lacrimal may be reinforced by the anterior deep temporal.

5. The branches of the ophthalmic artery show great variation. The supraorbital and posterior ethmoidal are both inconsistent, and there are often accessory ciliary trunks. The dorsal nasal branch may replace the facial in part.

THE CEREBRAL ARTERIES (Figs. 352 and 353)

The Anterior Cerebral Artery arises from the internal carotid close to the anterior perforated substance, crosses above the optic nerve, and approaching its fellow of the opposite side is joined to it by *the anterior communicating* vessel, which is, as a rule, about 4 mm. long. It then curls round the front or *genu* of the corpus callosum, on the upper aspect of which it runs to the splenium, where it anastomoses with the posterior cerebral.

It supplies the front of the caudate nucleus by branches which enter the anterior perforated substance ; the corpus callosum ; the medial aspect of the hemisphere as far back as the parieto-occipital sulcus ; a small strip on the upper part of the lateral surface, and the medial portion of the under-surface of the frontal lobe.

So far as vision is concerned the anterior cerebral artery supplies the upper aspects of the chiasma and intra-cranial portion of the optic nerve.

Blocking of this vessel may give rise to no symptoms ; but hebetude and dullness of intellect may result (Osler).

The Middle Cerebral Artery is the largest branch of the internal carotid, of which it appears to be the direct continuation. It runs laterally into the lateral sulcus, and breaks up into branches on the insula, which supply the lateral aspect of the hemisphere, except for a strip near its upper border (anterior cerebral), and a strip along the lower border (posterior cerebral).

[1] See F. Mayer (1886), *Morph. Jahrb.*, **12**.

It also sends the **medial** and **lateral striate** arteries through the anterior perforated substance.

The *medial striate arteries* pass through the medial part of the lentiform nucleus, which they supply, and also send branches to the caudate nucleus.

The *lateral striate arteries* pass between the lentiform nucleus and the external capsule. The largest of these was called by Charcot the " artery of cerebral hæmorrhage." Abbie, however, emphasises the fact that all branches of the middle cerebral artery have become crowded into a small space at the base of the external capsule in the human brain ; this is the anatomical basis for the clinical observation that this situation is the commonest site of origin for cerebral hæmorrhage.

So far as vision is concerned the middle cerebral supplies twigs to the under and lateral aspects of the chiasma and anterior portion of the optic tract.   Viá the deep optic branch it supplies the optic radiations, while its terminal branches anastomose with the calcarine branch of the posterior cerebral to supply a small portion of the striate cortex, probably contributing to the macular area (see p. 390).

The Deep Optic Artery is an artery of medium size which arises from the middle cerebral with the lateral striate vessels and passes posteriorly, partly through the substance of the putamen, to reach the fibres from the infra-lenticular and retro-lenticular parts of the internal capsule, thus supplying the auditory *and optic radiations immediately after they leave the capsule* (Abbie).   (Figs. 357, 359.)

The Posterior Communicating Artery arises from the internal carotid close to where it becomes the middle cerebral ; in fact, Testut calls this vessel, the anterior choroid and the anterior cerebral its terminal branches.

It passes horizontally backwards and a little medially to join the posterior cerebral, which is a branch of the basilar, at the superior border of the cerebral peduncle.

It is thus an anastomosis between the internal carotid and vertebral system of vessels.

In its course posteriorly it crosses the under-surface of the postero-lateral angle of the chiasma or the beginning of the optic tract from lateral to medial (Figs. 352, 353, 356). Near the cerebral peduncle it crosses above the oculomotor nerve from medial to lateral (Fig. 258).

The posterior communicating supplies the genu and about the anterior third of the posterior limb of the internal capsule.   It also sends branches to the globus pallidus and thalamus.

So far as vision is concerned it sends twigs to the under-surface of the chiasma and supplies the anterior third of the optic tract.

There is considerable mutual interchange between the anterior choroidal and posterior communicating (in fact between most of the vessels of the interpeduncular space).

Thus occasionally one or other predominates to the almost complete exclusion of its fellow, and rarely either of these vessels may usurp the stem of the posterior cerebral artery which then arises from the internal carotid and takes over the whole of the supply to the posterior cerebral field (Abbie).

The Anterior Choroidal Artery arises from the internal carotid just beyond (lateral to) the origin of the posterior communicating at the lateral side of the commencement of the optic tract (Figs. 352, 353, 357, 358).

It runs backwards and mediaily, crosses the optic tract on its under-surface and comes to lie on the medial side of this structure.   It maintains this relation to the anterior part of the lateral geniculate body.   Here it turns abruptly laterally, recrosses the optic tract and breaks up into a number of branches, which enter the inferior horn of the lateral ventricle to reach the antero-inferior part of the choroid plexus.

During its passage backwards the anterior choroidal gives off branches which either pierce the tract or wrap themselves round either its medial or its lateral aspect (Aitken).

Next to the internal carotid the anterior choroidal artery, by means of these branches, is the most important source of blood to the internal capsule, of which it supplies rather more than the posterior two-thirds of the posterior limb. It supplies in addition the whole of the infra-lenticular and retro-lenticular portions of the internal capsule containing the auditory and optic radiations. The anterior choroid also gives branches to the middle third (pyramidal portion) of the cerebral peduncle, to the tail of the caudate nucleus, to the thalamus and the globus pallidus.

So far as vision is concerned it gives twigs to the pial network supplying the chiasma and is the main source of supply to the optic tract (posterior two-thirds); it also supplies the anterior and lateral aspect of the lateral geniculate body, and by means of branches which pierce the tract, the commencement of the optic radiations (Fig. 359). The supply to the tract is mainly viâ the pial plexus (p. 388).

Blocking of the middle cerebral—" the artery most commonly involved—results in permanent hemiplegia from softening of the internal capsule, if plugged before the central arteries are given off. Blocking of the branches beyond this point may be followed by hemiplegia, which is more likely to be transient, involves chiefly the arm and face, and if the lesion be on the left side associated with aphasia. There may be plugging of the individual branches passing to the inferior frontal gyrus (producing typical motor aphasia if the disease be on the left side), to the anterior and posterior central gyri (usually causing total hemiplegia), to the supra-marginal and angular gyri (giving rise—if the thrombosis be on the left side, probably without exception—to the so-called visual aphasia, and usually also to right-sided hemianopia), or to the temporal gyri (in which event with left-sided thrombosis word-deafness results) " (Osler).

The Circle of Willis (Figs. 258, 353, 356) is an anastomosis between the two internal carotids and the basilar. *It is the most important reason why ligature of one or other common or internal carotid does not always produce cerebral softening.* It lies in the subarachnoid space, and surrounds the structures in the interpeduncular cistern.

It is formed as follows : behind, the basilar divides into the two posterior cerebrals ; these are united to the internal carotids by the posterior communicatings. From the internal carotid, running forwards and medially, are the anterior cerebrals, and uniting these is the anterior communicating.

The Basilar Artery is formed by the union of the two vertebrals at the lower border of the pons. It runs upwards near the median groove of the pons on the base of the skull, and at its upper border bifurcates into the two posterior cerebral arteries.

Blocking of the basilar artery may produce " bilateral paralysis from involvement of both motor paths. Bulbar symptoms may be present ; rigidity and spasm may occur. The temperature may rise rapidly. The symptoms, in fact, are those of apoplexy of the pons " (Osler).

BRANCHES (BILATERAL)

Pontine.—Several on each side to the pons.

Labyrinthine (Internal Auditory) runs with the 7th, 8th, and nervus intermedius into the internal acoustic meatus, and is distributed to the internal ear.

The Anterior Inferior Cerebellar usually crosses the 6th nerve on its ventral aspect (Figs. 260, 352, 353), but it may pass between it and the pons, or through its fibres. The author [1] has seen the nerve pressed into the substance of the pons by an arterio-sclerotic vessel. The artery supplies the anterior and inferior surfaces of the cerebellum.

The Superior Cerebellar comes off close behind the posterior cerebral. It winds round the cerebral peduncle, having the 3rd and 4th nerves between it and the posterior cerebral. It supplies the upper surface of the cerebellum.

The Posterior Cerebral Artery.—Each posterior cerebral artery is formed by the bifurcation of the basilar at the upper border of the pons, and winds round the inferior border of the cerebral peduncle of its own side (Figs. 352, 353, 356, 357, 358).

It runs below and parallel to the optic tract which is at the upper border of the brain stem. Also above it are the uncus and hippocampal gyrus.

Below and parallel to the posterior cerebral is the superior cerebellar artery, and between the two arteries are the third and fourth nerves. The posterior cerebral passes anterior to or through the rootlets of origin of the oculomotor while it is alongside the trochlear at the side of the midbrain (Figs. 352, 353).

The posterior cerebral, continuing backwards above the free margin of the tentorium cerebelli, passes under the splenium of the corpus callosum and enters the anterior part of the calcarine sulcus. Here it divides into branches which run in the parieto-occipital and posterior part of the calcarine sulci respectively.

The *calcarine branch* of the posterior cerebral runs posteriorly in the depths of the calcarine sulcus (Fig. 352). Then it turns around the occipital pole, in the lateral calcarine sulcus if one is present, to reach the lateral surface of the hemisphere. Arterial twigs emerge between the lips of the sulcus and extend above and below to the limits of the striate area. On the lateral surface of the hemisphere the calcarine artery supplies all the striate cortex except the peripheral fringe, where the supply is taken over by small anastomosing twigs from the middle cerebral (Shellshear, Rubino, Abbie).

The calcarine artery also sends perforating branches to the posterior portion of the optic radiation as this spreads out to reach the cortex.

The posterior cerebral thus supplies : (*a*) the medial surface and the posterior part of the lateral surface of the occipital lobe ; (*b*) the posterior portion of the optic radiation ; (*c*) the whole of the tentorial surface of the hemisphere except the anterior part of the temporal lobe; and also (*d*) central branches to the thalamus, internal capsule, red nucleus, geniculate bodies, tela chorioidea and choroid plexus of the lateral ventricle.

So far as vision is concerned the posterior cerebral supplies the postero-medial aspect of the lateral geniculate body, almost the whole of the visual cortex, and is the main supply to the posterior portion of the optic radiation.

[1] Eugene Wolff.

A block of the right posterior cerebral artery causes :

(*a*) *Destruction of the visual fibres from the right side of each retina, that is, from the left fields—and hence produces a left homonymous hemianopia.*

(*b*) *Sensory aphasia.*

(*c*) *Sometimes hemianœsthesia from involvement of the posterior part of the internal capsule.*

Very often the posterior cerebral of one side thromboses with the middle cerebral of the other, and produces the most pronounced cases of apraxia (Osler).

THE VEINS

The orbit is drained by the superior and inferior ophthalmic veins. They and their tributaries are curious in having no valves, being markedly tortuous and having many plexiform anastomoses. They communicate, moreover, with the veins of the face, with the pterygoid plexus, and with the veins of the nose. They drain into the cavernous sinus.

THE SUPERIOR OPHTHALMIC VEIN

The Superior Ophthalmic Vein is formed near the root of the nose by a communication from the angular vein soon after it has been joined by the supra-orbital.

It passes into the orbit above the medial palpebral ligament, and then accompanies the ophthalmic artery across the optic nerve and under the superior rectus to the superior orbital fissure, by which having, as a rule, been joined by the inferior ophthalmic vein, it leaves the orbit to enter the fore-part of the cavernous sinus.

Its position in the superior orbital fissure is usually above the cone of muscles, but it may pass between the two heads of the lateral rectus, or occupy the lowest compartment of the fissure.

Tributaries

(*a*) The inferior ophthalmic vein usually (*vide infra*).

(*b*) Anterior ethmoidal
(*c*) Posterior ethmoidal
(*d*) Muscular   correspond to the arteries of the same name.
(*e*) Lacrimal
(*f*) Central vein of retina

(*g*) Anterior ciliary.

(*h*) (Two of the) venæ vorticosæ or posterior ciliary veins.

The Central Vein of the Retina leaves the optic nerve close to the central artery, but usually nearer the bulb (Vossius). As a rule it opens directly into the cavernous sinus, but may end in the superior ophthalmic vein, to which, as Sesemann showed, it always gives a well-marked anastomotic branch. This is of some practical importance.

Graefe thought that papillœdema was due to venous stasis produced by pressure on the cavernous sinus and then back along the vena centralis. Sesemann's observation negatived this theory.

The Anterior Ciliary Veins accompany the arteries of the same name. They pierce the sclera near the cornea, and then, having received some branches from the conjunctiva, join the muscular veins (see also p. 92).

The Inferior Ophthalmic Vein commences as a plexus near the front of the floor of the orbit. It runs backwards on the inferior rectus to enter the cavernous sinus either after having joined the superior ophthalmic vein or separately.

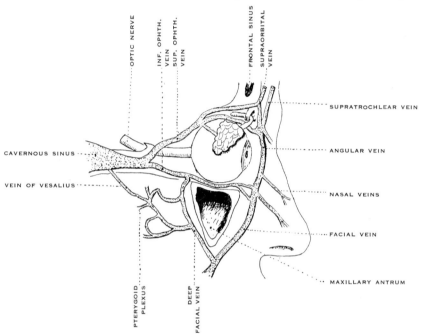

FIG. 365.—SCHEME OF THE VEINS OF THE ORBIT.
(Slightly after Allen Thomson.)

In the latter case, it passes through the superior orbital fissure either between the two heads of the lateral rectus or occupies the lowest compartment.

The inferior ophthalmic vein communicates with the pterygoid plexus through the inferior orbital (spheno-maxillary) fissure ; with the anterior facial vein over the inferior orbital margin and with the superior ophthalmic vein. It also gets tributaries from the lower and lateral ocular muscles, the conjunctiva and lacrimal sac, and receives the two inferior vorticose veins.

THE ANGULAR VEIN

The angular vein is situated at the junction of the veins of the forehead, orbit, and face. It is formed by the union of the supraorbital and supratrochlear veins, and runs down at the side of the nose lateral to the angular artery, across the nasal edge of the medial palpebral ligament some 8 mm. from the medial canthus (Fig. 221). It is subcutaneous, and visible (as a dark blue ridge) through the skin here, and above and below this point till it pierces the orbicularis. The angular vein (or one of its palpebral branches) is one of the bugbears in approaching the lacrimal sac from the front. It communicates freely with the beginning of the *superior ophthalmic vein*, and is continuous below with the *facial vein*.

Tributaries.—(*a*) **The Supraorbital Vein** runs transversely along the orbital margin deep to the orbicularis, which it pierces under the medial end of the eyebrow to join the supratrochlear and form the angular vein. It communicates with the superior ophthalmic vein through the supraorbital notch, at which point it receives a vein from the frontal sinus and the diploë.

(*b*) **The Supratrochlear Vein** runs down the forehead, accompanying the supratrochlear artery.

(*c*) **The Superior and Inferior Superficial Palpebral Veins.** *One of the upper veins not infrequently crosses the medial palpebral ligament between the angular vein and the medial canthus, where it, too, can be made out through the skin.*

(*d*) **Superficial Nasal Branches**—from the side of the nose.

The Facial Vein runs obliquely downwards and backwards across the face. It is lateral to and more superficial than its accompanying artery. It crosses the mandible, and joins the retromandibular (posterior facial) vein to form the common facial vein, which opens into the internal jugular.

The (anterior) facial vein communicates with the pterygoid plexus of veins (Fig. 338), and thus establishes a second communication with the cavernous sinus (*q.v.*), the first being viâ the angular and superior ophthalmic veins.

The flow of blood from the frontal region is naturally into the angular and facial veins. But in such a low pressure system it is easy to occlude the facial vein (e.g. lying face down on even a soft pillow) and then blood from the forehead flows via the angular vein into the ophthalmic veins. Hence the danger of septic spots on the forehead and face, which may result in cavernous sinus thrombosis.

The Cavernous Sinuses

Like the other intracranial venous sinuses, the cavernous sinuses are venous channels formed by the splitting of the dura mater (Fig. 366).

They extend on each side of the pituitary body and body of the sphenoid from the medial end of the superior orbital (sphenoidal) fissure to the apex of the petrous part of the temporal bone.

They are traversed by numerous fibrous trabeculæ, which give them on section the appearance of cavernous tissue, and from this fact they derive their name.

In each sinus is found the internal carotid artery, and lateral to it the 6th nerve. Both these structures receive an investment from the endothelium lining the sinus.

The internal carotid artery enters the sinus by passing upwards from the termination of the carotid canal at the medial end of the foramen lacerum, between the lingula and the petrosal process of the sphenoid (Figs. 10, 260). It then runs forwards in its groove on the body of the sphenoid (*q.v.*) to the medial side of the anterior clinoid process, where it turns upwards and pierces the roof of the sinus between the optic and oculo-motor nerves (Fig. 258).

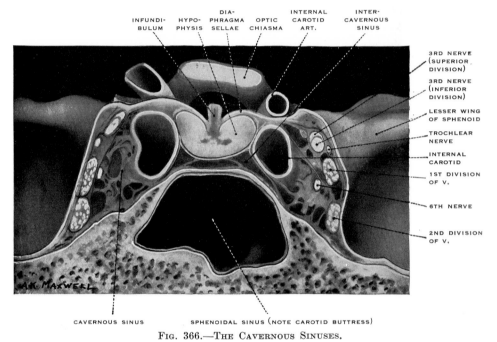

FIG. 366.—THE CAVERNOUS SINUSES.

(From Professor Elliot Smith's Textbook of Anatomy. Drawn from a dissection in the Moorfields Pathological Museum.)

While in the sinus it is surrounded by filaments of the sympathetic.

It is the presence of the artery in the sinus which explains how arterio-venous aneurisms may arise in fracture of the base of the skull.

In the *lateral wall* of the sinus from above down are the 3rd, 4th, and first and second divisions of the 5th cranial nerves. They are passing forwards to the superior orbital fissure and foramen rotundum respectively. At the anterior end of the sinus the 4th nerve crosses to lie above the 3rd (see p. 288).

To the lateral side of these again, and in contact with the lateral wall of the sinus, are the trigeminal ganglion (Fig. 272) and the temporal lobe of the brain.

Tributaries.—*In front*, the ophthalmic veins and the spheno-parietal sinus, which lies along the lesser wing of the sphenoid. *On the roof*, the superficial middle cerebral vein.

Veins of Exit.—The superior and inferior petrosal sinuses, and emissary veins through the foramen ovale and the foramen of Vesalius.

Communicating Veins.—The intercavernous plexus.

The Ophthalmic Veins communicate with the angular vein on the face. *This is the reason why a small septic spot on the nose, for instance, may produce thrombosis of the cavernous sinus.*

The spehno-parietal sinus drains from the side wall and vault of the skull.

The Superficial Middle Cerebral Vein drains the cortex alongside the lateral sulcus. Retrograde thrombosis from the cavernous sinus may involve this vein.

The Superior Petrosal Sinus runs along the upper border of the petrous temporal in the attached margin of the tentorium cerebelli. It crosses above the 5th and 6th nerves and drains from the cavernous sinus into the transverse. It is usually small.

The Inferior Petrosal Sinus is placed in the groove between the petrous temporal and basi-occipital (Fig. 270). It is often penetrated by the 6th nerve and receives veins from the internal ear. It drains the cavernous sinus into the beginning of the internal jugular vein below the base of the skull.

The petrosal sinuses *explain how thrombosis in the cavernous sinus may spread to the transverse, and finally also produce a swelling behind the ear through the mastoid emissary vein.* This passes through a foramen in the mastoid part of the temporal bone, and unites the sigmoid sinus with the posterior auricular vein. The fact that the auditory veins open into the inferior petrosal sinus marks the route *by which infection of the labyrinth may produce cavernous sinus thrombosis.*

The Emissary Vein that passes through the foramen of Vesalius drains into the pterygoid plexus ; so also do the veins that pass through the foramen ovale and foramen lacerum.

Moreover, there are indirect communications with the pterygoid plexus viâ the deep facial vein which unite it to the anterior facial vein, the continuation of the angular, and viâ the branch which the inferior ophthalmic vein sends to the plexus, through the inferior orbital (spheno-maxillary) fissure (Fig. 365).

The pterygoid plexus of veins corresponds to the second and third parts of the maxillary artery and covers both surfaces of the lateral pterygoid muscle and also the deep surface of the medial pterygoid.

Thus we have the anatomical explanation of how a thrombosis of the cavernous sinus may spread to the pterygoid plexus and produce an abscess so often found post-mortem in this condition in the tonsillar region (Percy Flemming).

The Intercavernous Plexus connects the two cavernous sinuses across both the roof and the floor of the pituitary fossa. This explains *how thrombosis of the cavernous sinus in the majority of cases becomes bilateral.*

Lymphatics of the Orbit

There are no lymph nodes in the orbit. The eyelids and conjunctiva drain for the most part to preauricular lymph nodes, though from alongside the medial canthus a few lymphatics accompany those from the bridge of the nose to the submandibular group of lymph nodes. From the depths of the orbit lymph vessels leave the inferior orbital fissure and cross the infratemporal fossa to reach lymph nodes buried in the parotid gland.

BIBLIOGRAPHY

Festral, A. F. (1887) : Recherches anatomiques sur les veines de l'orbite, *Thése méd. Paris.*

Gurwitsch, M. (1883) : *v. Graefe's Arch. Ophthal.*, **29.**

Sesemann, E. (1869) : *Arch. Anat. Physiol. wiss. Med.*, **154.**

CHAPTER IX

THE DEVELOPMENT OF THE EYE

THE central nervous system is derived from a thickening in the ectoderm, called the *neural* or *medullary plate*. This is converted into a groove and then into a canal which becomes separated from the surface ectoderm and is called the *neural tube*. The ectodermal cells lining the neural tube are known as neural ectoderm. The cranial end of the neural tube expands to form the three primary brain vesicles.

The eye is partly mesodermal, partly ectodermal in origin. The ectodermal portion is derived from that region of the neural tube (neural ectoderm) which goes to form the fore-brain and also from the ectoderm of the surface of the body. The *neural ectoderm* gives rise to all the layers of the retina, to the fibres of the optic nerve, and to the smooth muscle of the iris. *The surface ectoderm* provides the lens and the corneal and conjunctival epithelium, with the lacrimal and tarsal glands. *Mesoderm* provides the remaining structures : cornea and sclera, choroid, iris and ciliary muscle, the vitreous and the " endothelial " cells lining the anterior chamber (p. 458).

There are three stages in the early development of the *retina* and *optic nerve* :

1. The optic groove.

2. The primary optic vesicle.

3. The secondary optic vesicle or optic cup.

The optic grooves appear on either side of the mid-line in the cranial end of the neural plate at a time when the neural plate at this end of the embryo has been converted into a groove, but before its closure to form a canal (the anterior neuropore). The primordium of the retina,

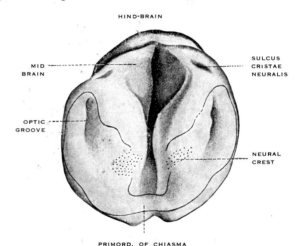

FIG. 367.—MODEL OF CRANIAL END OF A HUMAN EMBRYO OF TWELVE SOMITES. × 75.

The eye primordium is surrounded by a black line. Laterally it is continuous with the surface ectoderm ; to the medial side is the anterior end of the neural crest ; centrally the areas of opposite sides are joined by a narrow zone—the foremost part of the primitive brain—which later becomes the chiasma.

(*Fischel, after Bartelmez-Evans.*)

419

in other words, appears very early ; in fact, it is already seen in a 2·2 mm. embryo.

The areas of opposite sides are joined by a narrow zone which later becomes the chiasma (Fig. 367).

On the closure of the neural tube the optic grooves deepen and appear as hollow symmetrical, hemispherical outgrowths at the side of what is now the fore-brain vesicle. The growth is affected by cell division, the mitoses taking

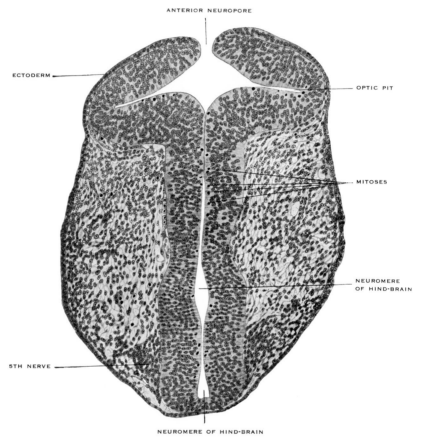

Fig. 368.—Horizontal Section through the Fore- and Hind-brains of a Human Embryo of Eighteen Somites. × 133.
Note that the ocular outgrowth lies lateral to the anterior neuropore.
(*Fischel.*)

place almost entirely on the inner aspect next the cavity of the primary optic vesicle (ventricular mitoses). The epithelium of the optic vesicle is high columnar. At first the nuclei are arranged in many layers ; later there are many layers of cells.

The cavity of the hollow outgrowth or primary optic vesicle naturally communicates with that of the fore-brain vesicle (Fig. 369). The outgrowths are relatively large, and since the optic vesicle is an evagination of the brain itself, it may be described as an ophthalmencephalon and its cavity as the optic ventricle (Fischel). As development proceeds, the breadth of the head increases and so does the distance between the brain and the surface ectoderm, with which the optic vesicle remains in contact. As a result of this, the optic vesicle becomes separated from the fore-brain by a constriction, its pedicle or stalk, which is best marked dorsally (Fig. 369). Meanwhile, the fore-brain has developed

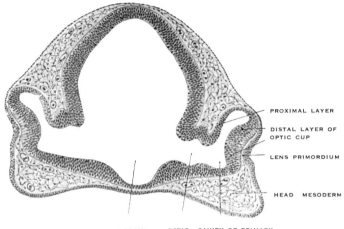

FIG. 369.—TRANSVERSE SECTION THROUGH THE FORE-BRAIN OF A 5-MM. HUMAN EMBRYO.

(From Seefelder, in the Kurzes Handbuch.)

PROXIMAL LAYER

DISTAL LAYER OF OPTIC CUP

LENS PRIMORDIUM

HEAD MESODERM

FORE-BRAIN   OPTIC   CAVITY OF PRIMARY
              STALK   OPTIC VESICLE

into the telencephalon (cerebral hemispheres) and diencephalon and the optic stalk arises from the lower portion of the side wall of the latter. The cavity of the diencephalon, i.e. the future third ventricle, is continued into the cavity of the optic stalk at the recessus opticus. The optic stalk is directed mainly laterally with a slight inclination cranially and dorsally. In the 4 mm. embryo the optic vesicle presses on the ectoderm causing an elevation of the surface which is thus placed laterally (Fig. 375).

The optic vesicles thus, unlike the condition in the adult, lie laterally, being separated from each other by the broad fronto-nasal process (Fig. 405). In a 19-mm. embryo the direction of growth makes an angle of 65° with the mid-sagittal plane, whereas in the adult the corresponding angle made by the optic nerves is 40°.

Opposite the distal end of the primary

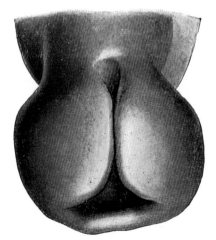

FIG. 370.—OPTIC CUP OF 7-MM. HUMAN EMBRYO. VENTRAL VIEW. × 100.

(From Seefelder, in the Kurzes Handbuch d. Ophth., 1930.)

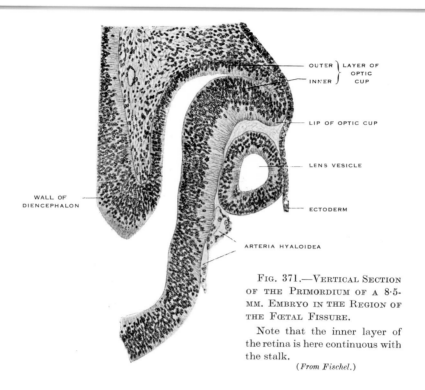

OUTER ⎱ LAYER OF
INNER ⎰ OPTIC CUP

LIP OF OPTIC CUP

LENS VESICLE

ECTODERM

WALL OF
DIENCEPHALON

ARTERIA HYALOIDEA

FIG. 371.—VERTICAL SECTION
OF THE PRIMORDIUM OF A 8·5-
MM. EMBRYO IN THE REGION OF
THE FŒTAL FISSURE.

Note that the inner layer of
the retina is here continuous with
the stalk.

(*From Fischel.*)

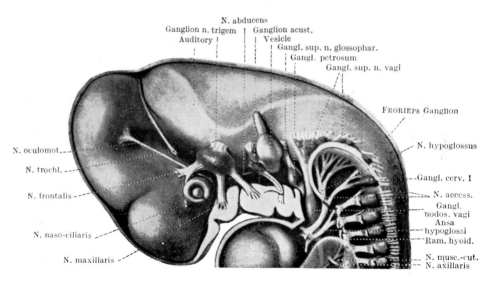

N. abducens
Ganglion n. trigem Ganglion acust.
Auditory Vesicle
Gangl. sup. n. glossophar.
Gangl. petrosum
Gangl. sup. n. vagi

FRORIEPS Ganglion

N. oculomot.

N. hypoglossus

N. trochl.

Gangl. cerv. I

N. frontalis

N. access.
Gangl.
nodos. vagi
Ansa
hypoglossi
Ram. hyoid.

N. naso-ciliaris

N. maxillaris

N. musc.-cut.
N. axillaris

FIG. 372.—RECONSTRUCTION OF THE CEREBRO-SPINAL NERVES OF A 10-MM. HUMAN EMBRYO. × 10.
Note the close relation of the naso-ciliary nerve to the eye.

(*From Fischel, after Streeter.*)

422

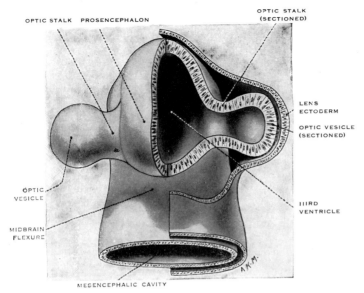

OPTIC STALK PROSENCEPHALON

OPTIC STALK
(SECTIONED)

LENS
ECTODERM

OPTIC VESICLE
(SECTIONED)

OPTIC
VESICLE

IIIRD
VENTRICLE

MIDBRAIN
FLEXURE

A.K.M.

MESENCEPHALIC CAVITY

Fig. 373.—Schematic Representation of the Cranial Aspect of the Forebrain (Prosen-
cephalic) and Optic Vesicles in a 4-mm. Human Embryo.

(*From Hamilton, Boyd, and Mossmann, after Mann.*)

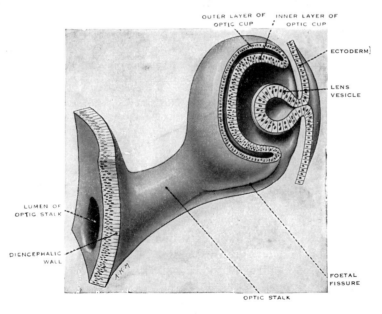

OUTER LAYER OF   INNER LAYER OF
OPTIC CUP   OPTIC CUP

ECTODERM

LENS
VESICLE

LUMEN OF
OPTIC STALK

DIENCEPHALIC
WALL

A.K.M

FOETAL
FISSURE

OPTIC STALK

Fig. 374.—Schematic Representation of the Optic Cup and Stalk in a 7·5-mm. Human Embryo.

(*From Hamilton, Boyd, and Mossmann, after Mann.*)

optic vesicle, but separated from this by a reticulum of protoplasmic [1] fibrils, there is a thickening of the surface ectoderm, which represents the first stage of the development of the lens (Fig. 369).

With the conversion of this thickening first into a groove and then into the lens vesicle, the primary optic vesicle is first flattened, and then as it were

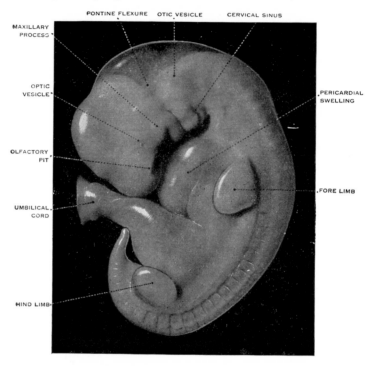

FIG. 375.—THE LEFT SIDE OF A 6·2-MM. CROWN-RUMP LENGTH HUMAN EMBRYO.
(Estimated age, 36 days.)
(From Hamilton, Boyd, and Mossmann's Human Embryology.)

" invaginated " from its distal aspect and below. Thus the two-layered optic cup is produced.

In the mechanism of production of the optic cup it used to be taught that the lens actually pushed in the distal wall of the primary optic vesicle, as one might push in the wall of a toy balloon with one's fist. Its formation is, however, due to the fact that the distal and ventral portions of the vesicle stop growing, while the margins of these areas continue to develop. Thus the lips of the vesicle grow round the developing lens at the sides and dorsally, but not ventrally.

Since the apex of the vesicle, which was originally convex, stops growing,

---

[1] I.e. the embryonic supporting tissue of von Szily. Similar tissue will be seen to exist later between the lens and the inner layer of the optic cup and there form what is known as the primary vitreous (see p. 452).

and as it is in contact with the lens, it first appears flattened and then becomes concave. Thus the lumen of the vesicle is reduced to a slit (Fig. 374).

Since growth stops below, this area remains depressed, while its margins continue developing and thus is formed the **foetal, ocular, or choroidal fissure.** (Of these names, " Foetal " fissure is official, though there is no " foetus " yet, but only an " embryo ".)

The function of the foetal fissure, apart from allowing the entrance of meso-derm into the eye, is to provide the shortest route by which the nerve fibres from the ganglion cells can reach the optic stalk and brain. Otherwise, with the formation of the optic cup, they would have to travel round the edge of the cup. For the optic stalk is at first directly continuous with the outer or pigment layer.

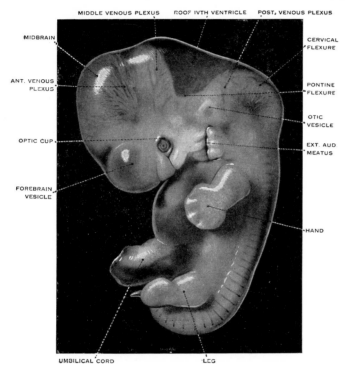

FIG. 376.—THE LEFT SIDE OF A 12·2-MM. CROWN-RUMP LENGTH HUMAN EMBRYO.
(Estimated age, 43 days.)
From Hamilton, Boyd, and Mossmann.

The direct continuity of the inner or nervous layer with the optic stalk is only made possible at the floor of the foetal fissure where it becomes continuous with the floor of the fissure on the stalk (Fig. 371).

[In early embryos (between 7·7 and 17·1 mm. (Lindahl)), the rim of the optic cup may present small *accessory notches.* Their significance is doubtful. Possibly they are made by vessels.]

Hence it comes about that as the lens pit is converted into a little pouch or sac, the optic cup also deepens and surrounds it more and more. Also the opening of the cup is gradually differentiated into a laterally directed rounded portion, the primitive pupil, and a ventrally directed part, the fœtal fissure (Fig. 370). The fœtal fissure extends back along the optic stalk. As soon as it is formed, the fissure becomes filled with embryonic connective tissue which contains the hyaloid artery (future arteria centralis). With the pigmentation of the outer layer of the cup the cleft also is visible through the surface ectoderm.

The optic cup is thus composed of two layers which are continuous with each other at the margin of the cup and at the fœtal fissure. The inner layer is much

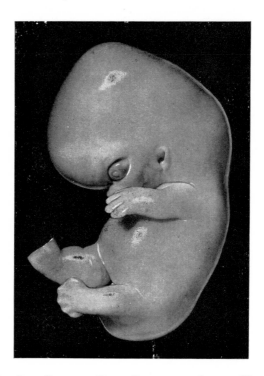

Fig. 377.—The Left Side of a 17-mm. Crown-rump Length Human Embryo.
(Estimated age, 47 days.)
(*From Hamilton, Boyd, and Mossmann.*)

thicker than the outer, and will form the nervous portion of the retina, while the outer layer gives rise to the pigment epithelium only.

The nervous portion of the retina consists of the pars optica and the pars cæca, which in turn is made up of the pars ciliaris retinæ and the pars iridica retinæ.

The cavity of the primary optic vesicle is potential only, but pathologically can be reconstituted into a real cavity. This happens in detachment of the retina, when fluid collects between the pigment layer (which remains adherent to the choroid) and the rods and cones.

Similarly in the separation of posterior synechiæ the posterior of the two layers of the ectodermal part of the iris becomes separated from the anterior and remains adherent to the lens. This separation re-forms the anterior part of the cavity of the primary optic vesicle or ring sinus of von Szily, which indeed may also take place as a senile change

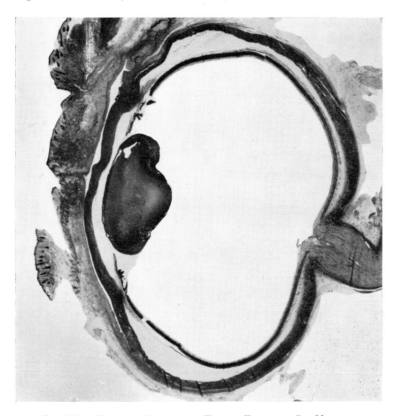

FIG. 378.—VERTICAL SECTION OF EYE OF FŒTUS OF SIX MONTHS.

The fœtal fissure closes by its lateral walls growing towards each other and eventually fusing. This fusion begins at the centre at the fifth week (15-mm. stage) and extends forwards and backwards, to be completed at about the 17-mm. stage.

Distally a small notch remains before the fusion completes the primitive pupil, making it round. At the proximal end of the fissure the fusion is complicated by the fact that the inner layer of the cup grows more rapidly than the outer. It thus comes about that there is a slight eversion of the inner layer (Fig. 379), which prevents the pigmented layer from fusing and results in a pale area below the disc. In man,[1] however, this pale area soon becomes pigmented, and usually no trace is left of the fissure except at its extreme posterior end, which remains as the site of entry of the central vessels.

Non-closure of the cleft results in colobomata.

With the closure of the cleft the portion of the mesoderm which has made its way into the eye through the cleft is cut off from the surrounding mesoderm, and gives rise to the hyaloid system of vessels.

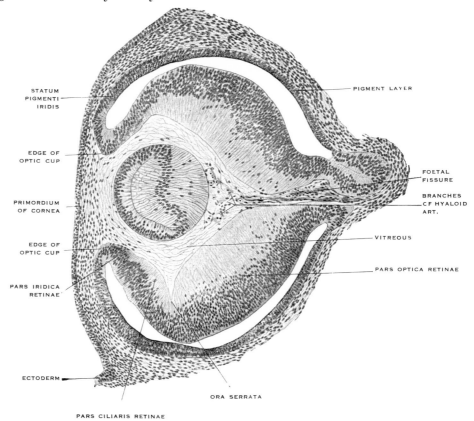

STATUM PIGMENTI IRIDIS

PIGMENT LAYER

EDGE OF OPTIC CUP

FOETAL FISSURE

BRANCHES OF HYALOID ART.

PRIMORDIUM OF CORNEA

VITREOUS

EDGE OF OPTIC CUP

PARS OPTICA RETINAE

PARS IRIDICA RETINAE

ECTODERM

ORA SERRATA

PARS CILIARIS RETINAE

Fig. 379.—Section through the Eye and Fœtal Fissure of a 13·5-mm. Human Embryo. × 157.

Note the eversion of the inner layer of the optic cup at the posterior (proximal) end of the fœtal fissure.

(*From Fischel.*)

While these changes are taking place, the lens has developed and the mesoderm around the eye forms the primordium of the choroid and sclera. Thus with the closure of the fœtal fissure the eye possesses all its essential parts and forms what may be termed the "embryonic eye."

[1] In birds it develops into the cauda (see p. 482).

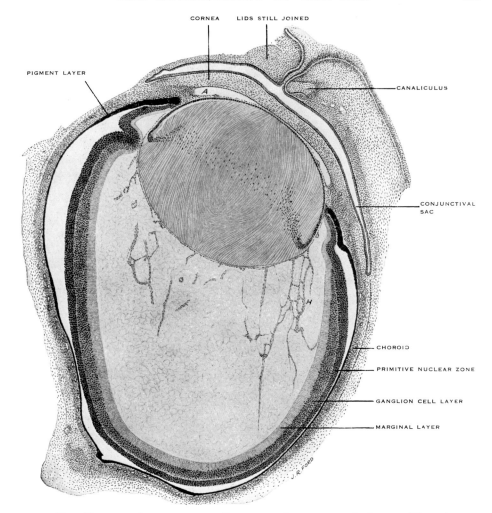

FIG. 380.—VERTICAL SECTION OF THE EYE OF AN EMBRYO OF $2\frac{3}{4}$ MONTHS (38 MM.).
A = anterior chamber (artefact).   H = hyaloid vessels.

(Wolff's preparation from a specimen supplied by Dr. A. G. Gilchrist.)

THE DEVELOPMENT OF THE RETINA

The development of the retina may be divided into three stages (Magitot), which are, however, not sharply separated :

1. The epithelial stage.
2. The stage of differentiation.
3. The stage of growth.

The primordium of the nervous portion of the retina is the distal wall of the primary optic vesicle, and consists at first of a single layer of cylindrical epithelium.

The nuclei soon divide and become arranged in several layers. Later there are several layers of cells. These cells are at first all alike. The mitoses take place at the side next the future pigment layer (ventricular mitoses), so that the oldest cells get pushed towards and lie nearest the future vitreous (Fig. 382).

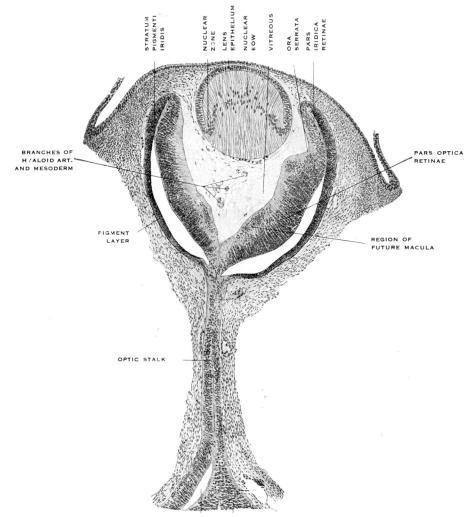

FIG. 381.—LONGITUDINAL SECTION THROUGH THE EYE AND OPTIC STALK OF A 17-MM. HUMAN EMBRYO × 76.

From Fischel.)

By differentiation is meant the different changes which, in view of their different future functions, the different portions of the retina and their contained cells undergo. This stage may also, therefore, be called the stage of specialisation.

The first change in the differentiation of the retina is the appearance, first in the macular region towards the side of the future vitreous of a clear, almost anuclear zone which is like that which occurs in C.N.S. This change later affects the more peripheral portions of the retina and also the pars cæca up to the pupillary margin, although here the clear zone is narrower. Thus as the retina rapidly increases in thickness it becomes divided into a **nuclear zone** and a zone containing at first no nuclei—the **marginal layer of His** (Figs. 380, 381). This is formed by anastomotic protoplasmic processes of the retinal cells, and is the primordium of the supporting tissue of the retina—namely, the neuroglia. At the time of the formation of the optic cup the marginal layer is well developed, as are also the internal and external limiting membranes. The retina remains in this primitive condition until the closure of the fœtal fissure (17-mm. stage).

The Ganglion Cells and the Nerve Fibre Layer.—The ganglion cells are formed from the innermost cells of the *nuclear zone* which invade the *marginal zone* at about the fifth week (in embryos of 11·3 to 13 mm.). This latter takes place first in the region of the future macula. These young neuroblasts have a small round nucleus and practically no protoplasm. Later the nuclei grow larger, stain less deeply, and are then easily distinguished from the deeper staining nuclear zone (Fig. 382). No sooner have the ganglion cells invaded the marginal zone than the nerve fibres grow out from them, run parallel to the surface of the retina to find the shortest way to the optic stalk, and thence to the brain.

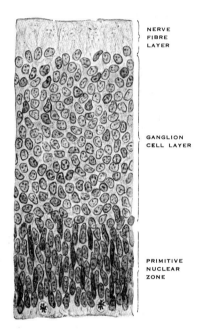

Fig. 382.—Section of the Retina (near the Posterior Pole) of a 31-mm. Human Embryo.
(*From Seefelder, in the Kurzes Handbuch.*)

The differentiation of the retina proceeds from the posterior portion of the eye anteriorly.

With the formation of dendritic processes from the outer aspect of the ganglion cells, a clear non-nuclear zone is produced between these and the remaining cells, and thus is formed the beginning of the **inner molecular layer.** Later are added the branching processes of the inner horizontal and bipolar cells.

The Nuclear Layers and Outer Molecular Layer.—The separation of the two nuclear layers also takes place first in the central area and about the same time as the formation of the inner molecular layer, while from the primitive nuclear zone a single layer of the outermost cells separates to form the future cones and rods

(Fig. 383). Between these cone cells and the remaining cells is a clear zone containing Müller's fibres only.

The outer molecular (plexiform) layer is developed about the end of the fifth month at first by processes of the middle cell layer.

In the inner nuclear layer Müller's fibres are first developed, then the bipolar cells, then the inner horizontal cells (amacrines), and lastly the outer horizontal cells.

Probably no new retinal cells are produced after the sixth month. Thus the relative size of the pars optica of the retina to the whole bulb is much greater in

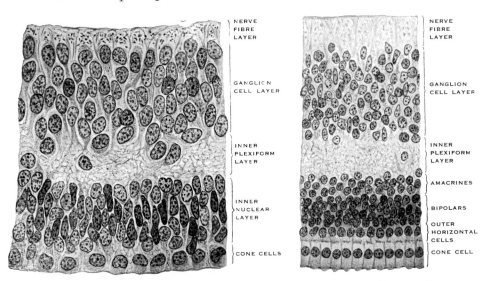

FIG. 383.—MACULAR REGION OF A 65-MM.
HUMAN EMBRYO.
(*From Seefelder, in the Kurzes Handbuch.*)

FIG. 384.—THE MACULAR REGION IN
A FŒTUS OF FIVE MONTHS.
(*From Seefelder, in the Kurzes Handbuch.*)

the embryo, where it reaches to the cornea, than in the adult, where it ends at the equator.

Thus mitoses cease first in the central area, so that growth goes on longer at the periphery of the retina. Then new cells are found only in the pars cæca, and finally only at the pupillary margin.

The Rods and Cones.—Up to the middle of the second month, the outer aspect of the inner layer of the optic cup presents only a border made up of tiny cilia which are little apparent and often stuck together. This border is like the surface of the cerebral ventricles and the ependyma of the canal of the spinal cord, whose cavity is homologous with the interparietal cavity of the retina : it is the ciliated border of the ependymal epithelium. Many embryologists held that it is these cilia which form the outer members of the rods and cones, but this is probably not the case (Dejean, Bach and Seefelder).

The rods and cones are developed from a single row of cells which separate from the primitive nuclear zone (Fig. 383). The diplosomes which lie in the outer side of these primitive cells play an important part in their development (Fig. 386).

The young cone cells have a small round deeply staining nucleus and a fair amount of protoplasm which lies next the outer limiting membrane. Later the protoplasm and the diplosomes break through this, and the cone cells become cylindrical and more like epithelial cells. Threads pass outwards from the

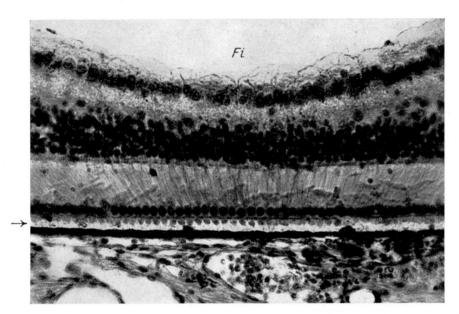

FIG. 385.—FOVEA OF THE NEWBORN.

Extensive foveal depression Fi. The transitory layer of Chievitz has disappeared, the outer nuclear layer is thinned and the ganglion cells reduced to a single row. The cones are still very immature (arrow) (this applies only to the foveal cones) while at the periphery the stumpy form has long since changed.

(From Pfeifer, after Wolfrum.)

diplosomes which, becoming surrounded by a soft protoplasmic material, form the outer portion of the cones. The rods are developed in a similar way.

The Macular Area and Fovea Centralis.—In the third month a marked thinning is seen in the retina of the postero-lateral quadrant. All layers are affected. *This, however, does not constitute the macula.* The appearance of the macular area is shown by a thickening of the ganglion cell layer at about the fifth month (fœtus of 122 mm. according to Seefelder) between the above area and the papilla.

In the fifth month there is developed in the central area an additional fibre

A.E.—28

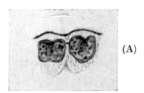
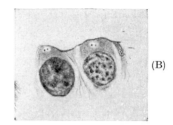

CONE CELLS FROM THE CENTRAL AREA OF A 65-MM. FŒTUS.

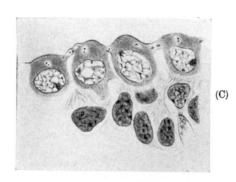

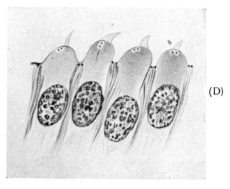

CONE CELLS FROM THE CENTRAL AREA of a 80-MM. FŒTUS.

CONES FROM PARA-CENTRAL AREA OF 345-MM. FŒTUS.

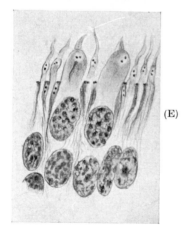

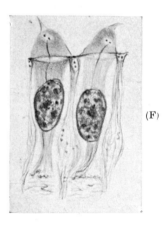

RODS AND CONES FROM THE PARA-CENTRAL AREA OF A 345-MM. FŒTUS.

CENTRAL CONES OF A 420-MM. FŒTUS.

FIG. 386.—STAGES IN THE DEVELOPMENT OF THE RODS AND CONES.
(*From Bach and Seefelder.*)

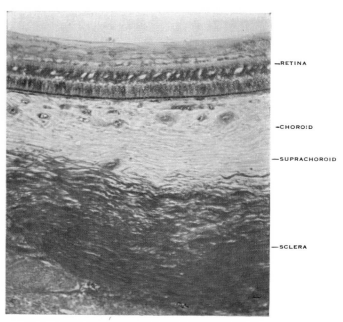

—RETINA

—CHOROID

—SUPRACHOROID

—SCLERA

FIG. 388.—COATS OF EYE OF FŒTUS OF SIX MONTHS.

The choroid appears as a reticulum in which the vessels are enmeshed.

layer, namely the transitory layer of Chievitz, which disappears only after birth. Its significance has not yet been decided. It is formed through the inner horizontal cells (amacrines), separating from the remainder of the inner nuclear layer (Fig. 387).

The development of the fovea commences at the end of the sixth month by a thinning of the ganglion cells, which move away to leave a central shallow depression. This is deepened by a thinning of the outer layers, except of course the outer nuclear layer, which remains as before, one layer thick. Up to the time of the formation of the fovea the development of the macula precedes the remainder of the retina, but after this it falls behind, especially with regard to the neuro-epithelium. Thus in the macular region the cones appear later than in the remaining portions of the retina and at birth the foveal cones are still very plump

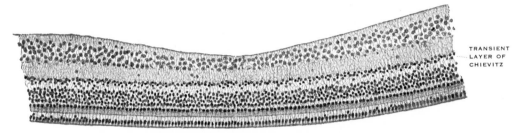

TRANSIENT
LAYER OF
CHIEVITZ

FIG. 387.—THE FOVEA CENTRALIS OF A FŒTUS AT THE END OF THE SIXTH MONTH.
(*From Seefelder, in the Kurzes Handbuch.*)

structures (Fig. 385), about 5 μ in diameter and only 8 μ in height, and it is only when the child is several months old that the cone gets its definitive form, and only then can the central area show its superiority over the remainder of the retina. Hence also the reason for the absence of central fixation at birth. It is remarkable that the fovea centralis is as far away from the nerve head at its formation as in the adult.

The thickening of the outer cell layer in the region of the fovea arises after birth, and results from the fact, as pointed out by Druault, that as the limbs of the cones get thinner they are more crowded together and therefore also their nuclei.

From the fourth to the eighth month of fœtal life, as was first pointed out by von Ammon and confirmed by Treacher Collins and others, the retina may be thrown into folds which, however, disappear completely.

THE OUTER RETINAL LAYER (PIGMENT EPITHELIUM)

With the " invagination " of the primary optic vesicle the two layers of the secondary optic vesicle which have at first the same epithelial structure start differentiating.

The cells of the outer layer are at first high cylindrical, occupy its whole thickness, and have their nuclei arranged in two or three rows.

Pigmentation of the cells starts in embryos of from 6 to 7 mm. at about three weeks and these appear before any other pigment in the body. Yellowish granules appear which rapidly become darker and eventually appear black. They are formed for the most part in that portion of the cell nearest the retina. The anterior portion is pigmented first and then the process passes backwards. This pigmentation makes the vesicle visible through the surface ectoderm.

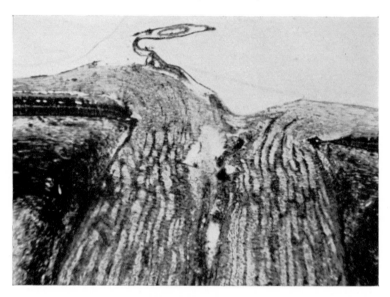

FIG. 389.—OPTIC NERVE-HEAD OF FŒTUS OF SIX MONTHS.
Note hyaloid artery.

By the time the embryo has reached 10 mm. the whole of the outer layer is pigmented.

As development proceeds the pigment cells become flatter, i.e. cubical with the nuclei arranged in a single row, probably because they have to line a larger area.

[1] The pigment is formed in the cell itself. Probably there is a colourless precursor of the melanin pigment, of the nature of dioxyphenyl-alanine (dopa) which is converted to melanin by a peroxidase enzyme.

The continuation forwards of the pigment epithelium of the retina forms the stratum pigmenti ciliaris and the stratum pigmenti iridis.

THE OPTIC NERVE

The optic nerve is developed from the optic *stalk* or *pedicle*. Its cavity communicates on the one hand with the cavity of the diencephalon, and on the other with the primary optic vesicle (Fig. 368).

[1] Miescher (1922), *Die Pigment Genese. Arch. mikrosk. Anat.*, **97**.

After the formation of the optic cup the fœtal fissure extends back on the optic stalk, which also becomes " invaginated " from ventrally. Hence a transverse section of the optic stalk resembles that of the optic vesicle, with a thick inner wall and a thinner outer one (Fig. 390).

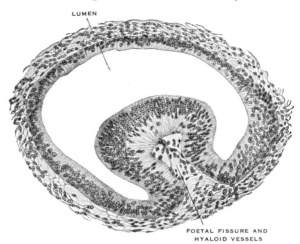

FOETAL FISSURE AND
HYALOID VESSELS

FIG. 390.—TRANSVERSE SECTION OF THE OPTIC STALK OF A 9-MM. HUMAN EMBRYO. DISTAL PORTION.

(*From Fischel*, 1929.)

As development proceeds the distance between the diencephalon and the surface ectoderm increases more and more, and this necessitates a lengthening of the optic stalk which is at first short, broad and wide. A new piece is drawn out of the side wall of the diencephalon. The optic stalk thus comes to consist of a distal primitive portion which is grooved by the fœtal fissure and a proximal portion, added later, which is not (Figs. 370, 373).

The closure of the continuation backwards of the fœtal fissure converts the optic stalk into a rounded cord. The cavity of the stalk is closed by the development of the nerve fibres which grow towards the brain from the ganglion cells.

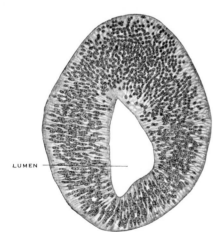

LUMEN

FIG. 391.—TRANSVERSE SECTION OF THE OPTIC STALK OF A 9-MM. HUMAN EMBRYO. PROXIMAL PORTION.

(*From Fischel.*)

Nerve fibres first appear in the ventral and lateral portions of the stalk, so the cavity becomes half-moon shaped (Fig. 392), and at first displaced dorsalwards ; later when the dorsal fibres grow it is displaced ventralwards and disappears about the third fœtal month.

The epithelial cells forming the walls of the stalk develop into the glial system of the nerve.

At the third month the glial cells become arranged in rows parallel to the long axis of the optic nerve and between these the nerve fibres run.

Glial tissue also develops round the hyaloid artery and around the periphery of the nerve. The glial tissue or glial mantle around the hyaloid artery at its entrance into the vitreous forms a protruding mass (glial cushion or Bergmeister's papilla[1]), which not only clothes the artery and some of its branches, but fills the physiological excavation of the optic nervehead as well (Figs. 413, 414). With the regression of the hyaloid artery this glial mantle disappears also.

The fibrous (mesodermal) septa of the optic nerve are developed from the mesoderm of the vessels which invade the nerve at the middle of the third fœtal month, and which have the form and position of the future septa (see p. 338). The mesodermal lamina cribrosa is only formed in the last fœtal months, and then has not the strength of the previously existing glial lamina (Seefelder).

The nerve sheaths are derived from the head mesoderm, and develop concurrently with the posterior part of the sclera. At the fifth month dura, arachnoid, and pia can be distinguished from each other.

Medullation of the nerve fibres takes place from the brain distally, and reaches the lamina cribrosa just before birth. The so-called "congenital" nerve fibres, seen not infrequently near the disc (Fig. 295), are therefore not really congenital at all, since they are medullated after birth. At six weeks the optic fibres penetrate the under-surface of the fore-brain ; at about seven and a half weeks the chiasma has been formed by partial decussation of the fibres and at nine and a half weeks the optic tract is plainly present.

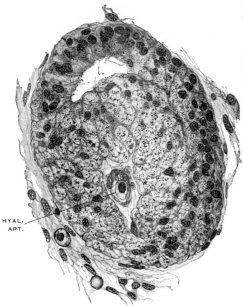

HYAL.
ART.

FIG. 392.—TRANSVERSE SECTION OF THE OCULAR END OF THE OPTIC NERVE OF A 19-MM. HUMAN EMBRYO.

(From Seefelder, in the Kurzes Handbuch.)

THE DEVELOPMENT OF THE LENS

Stages :

(a) Lens plate.

(b) Lens pit.

(c) Lens pouch or sac.

(d) Lens vesicle.

[1] **Bergmeister's Papilla.**—As the optic nerve fibres pass from the ganglion cells to the optic stalk they have to traverse the remainder of the retina. As they do this they cut off a cone-shaped mass of glial cells at the centre of the disc, which is known as Bergmeister's primitive epithelial papilla. This becomes vascularised by the hyaloid artery, and supplies this vessel and its branches with their sheaths (Seefelder 1910, von Szily 1921–2). Later, with the disappearance of the hyaloid system the papilla also atrophies, the amount of atrophy determining the depth of the physiological cup.

Remains of the papilla are always found in the glial sheaths of the vessels and the glial tissue which separates the optic cup from the vitreous (the central connective tissue meniscus of Kuhnt). (Figs. 297, 298.)

At the 4·5-mm. stage the surface ectoderm opposite the distal part of the primary optic vesicle is thickened by the cells assuming a high [1] columnar form, and their nuclei, which show mitotic figures, are arranged in several layers. This thickening is called the *lens placode* (Fig. 369). A groove or pit appears in this. The pit deepens into a pouch which closes and forms a *vesicle* at about four and a half weeks. The *lens vesicle* moves away slightly from the surface ectoderm, being connected to it, however, by a protoplasmic reticulum, the embryonic supporting tissue of von Szily.

With the formation of the lens vesicle the primary optic vesicle is " invaginated " to form the optic cup. At this stage the optic cup is almost completely filled by the lens. (Fig. 371).

The mitoses subserving the growth of the lens occur posteriorly, in the cells towards the free surface of the placode and later towards the cavity of the vesicle. The proliferation of cells (in the human) is so rapid that some cells are thrown off into the lens pit and into the vesicle. They mix with the fluid in the vesicle and soon degenerate, but Schwalbe believes they later go to form the thin layer of amorphous substance beneath the anterior epithelium. While the vascular capsule is present the lens grows very quickly. Hence it is almost full-grown in fœtal life.

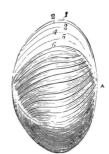

FIG. 393.—To ILLUSTRATE THE COURSE OF THE FI-BRES IN THE FŒTAL CRYSTALLINE LENS.

A = anterior pole.
P = posterior pole.
(*After Allen Thomson, from Quain's Anatomy.*)

The cells of the posterior part of the vesicle become columnar and eventually elongate to fill the lens vesicle. These primitive lens fibres run from the front to the back of the lens ; *later none do*. The lengthening of the cells first takes place in the centre of the posterior wall, which therefore bulges convex forwards into the cavity of the vesicle. This lengthening is the first sign of transformation of the cells into lens fibres and is associated with the loss of power of multiplication which stops when the cells are about 0·18 mm. long (Fischel).

The nuclei of the lens fibres pass anteriorly, and at the equator form a line convex forwards (the nuclear bow) (Fig. 380), which is continuous laterally with the equatorial nuclei of the cells of the anterior epithelium which will form all except the first fibres.

The new lens fibres formed from the equatorial cells are laid down concentrically round the filled-in lens vesicle, and thus the lens gets its laminated structure. Also the new fibres are laid on tangential to the equator ; hence on equatorial section the lens shows radial lamellæ. At three months there are

---

[1] According to Rabl (*Über den Bau und die Entwicklung der Linse*, 1899), the cells forming the lens plate in mammals are high, very narrow and closely packed, but always arranged in a single layer like that of birds and reptiles. The appearance on section of several layers is given by the nuclei being situated at different levels in different cells, or by obliquity of the section.

1,474 radial lamellæ and 2,250 in the adult, numbers characteristic for the human (Fischel).

As pointed out above, none of the fibres run from the front to the back of

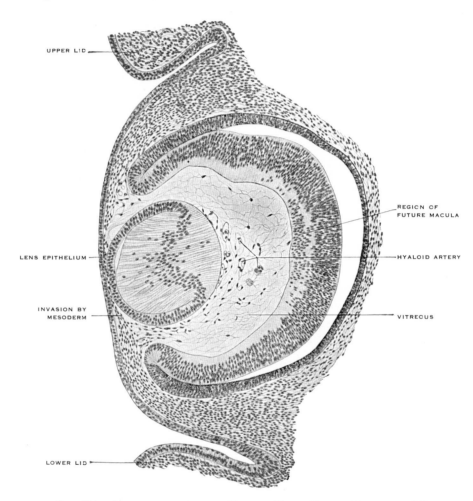

FIG. 394.—SECTION THROUGH THE EYE OF 17-MM. HUMAN EMBRYO. × 148.

(*From Fischel.*)

the lens. At the two surfaces of the lens mass the thicker ends of the fibres end in sutures, later to become the so-called lens stars.

The first indication of the sutures is seen in the second month, but only becomes really plain in the fourth month. Their formation comes about from the fact that as the new-formed lens fibres pass in a bow round the primitive ones, and being of equal length, the nearer the axis they end anteriorly the further away they end posteriorly, and vice versa (Fig. 393). At first the lens fibres end in a vertical suture anteriorly and a horizontal one posteriorly (Fischel). Later these become Y-shaped, vertical anteriorly, inverted posteriorly (Fig. 232).

The fibres formed later, for instance the superficial ones of the adult lens, start and finish in the more complicated stellate figures, conforming, however, to the above rule (see also p. 165).

Within the lens vesicle and later in the lens itself, there is a not inconsiderable tension which plays an important part in the regular growth of the lens fibres.

The lens grows very rapidly so long as it is supplied by its vascular capsule. It thus comes about that at birth it has already acquired its definitive antero-

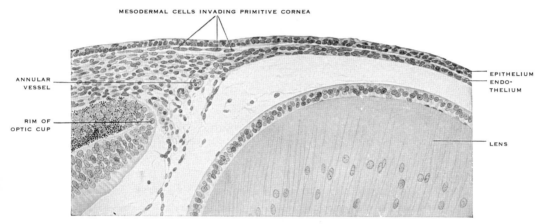

FIG. 395.—ANTERO-POSTERIOR SECTION OF A 23-MM. HUMAN EMBRYO.
From Seefelder, in the Kurzes Handbuch.)

posterior diameter and two-thirds of the equatorial. It is more or less spherical at birth. The antero-posterior flattening of the adult is brought about by the method of laying on of the lens fibres and the pull of the suspensory ligament.

The Lens Capsule.—At the 13-mm. stage the lens epithelium secretes its hyaline capsule.

THE CORNEA

After the formation of the lens vesicle mesoderm cells grow into the proto-plasmic [1] fibrillæ (the so-called anterior vitreous) between the lens and the

---

[1] Many years ago Kölliker (1861) noted that in birds at a very early period a thin structureless ectodermal membrane is laid down, which apparently formed the scaffolding on which the cornea is built. Hagedoorn (1928) holds that such a directing membrane (" Richtungshäutchen ") exists in the anterior vitreous of all vertebrates. Mesoderm grows in firstly as the endothelium behind this membrane and secretes Descemet's membrane, and secondly as a wedge-shaped mass which forms the substantia propria between the epithelium and the primary cornea.

See also Laguesse (1926), *Arch. d'Anat. Micros.*, **22**; Seefelder (1926), *Arch. f. Augen.*, **97**; Mann (1931), *Trans. Ophthal. Soc. U.K.*, **51**, 63.

surface ectoderm. They become arranged in a single row parallel to the surface and go to form Descemet's endothelium (Fig. 395).

Into the space between Descemet's endothelium and the surface ectoderm there grow more mesodermal cells from the region of the edge of the optic cup. These form the substantia propria of the cornea. The differentiation of these cells into the corneal fibrillæ takes place from behind forwards. The surface ectoderm forms the epithelium of the cornea.

Descemet's membrane is produced about the fourth month by a secretion from the endothelial cells, whereas Bowman's membrane is simply a condensation of the anterior corneal fibrillæ (Seefelder).

As development proceeds the cell content of the cornea diminishes. Wandering cells appear about the fourth month.

The cornea is transparent from the first as is all early embryonic tissue.

THE SCLERA

The sclera arises through a condensation of the mesoderm round the optic cup. The anterior portion is formed first—no doubt associated with the insertion of the eye muscles. The limbus is at first much farther back, lying over the ciliary body, but gradually shifts forwards.

Elastic fibres appear about the third month, like the collagenous elements, as an intraprotoplasmic formation.

The *fascia bulbi* (Tenon's capsule) is developed in the same way as the sclera, but somewhat later, and again the anterior portion is differentiated before the posterior.

THE PUPILLARY MEMBRANE

Of the mesoderm which invades the anterior vitreous, i.e. the protoplasmic reticulum between the surface ectoderm and the lens, the anterior portion is non-vascular, and, as we have seen, forms the main portion of the cornea.

The posterior portion in which vessels develop goes to form the irido-pupillary lamina (of Jeannulatos) (Figs. 400, 401, 450).

The peripheral portion of this unites with the rim of the optic cup to form the iris, while the central portion is the pupillary membrane (Figs. 400, 404).

The pupillary membrane is thus developed in the mesoderm at the same time as, and behind, Descemet's membrane. It consists of numerous anastomosing vessels and a fibrillary tissue between them. It forms, in fact, the anterior part of the tunica vasculosa lentis, with the remainder of which it is continuous under the rim of the optic cup. As the edge of the pupil grows forwards, however, this continuity is broken. The pupillary membrane is nourished, as is the iris, by the long posterior ciliary arteries, and is thus entirely independent of the hyaloid system and continues to develop when the latter is regressing.

The pupillary membrane is at first attached to the edge of the pupil, but later comes to arise from the front of the iris. This is due to a split in the mesoderm between the sphincteric portion of the iris and the pupillary membrane. After the eighth month the pupillary membrane begins to disappear. Remains of it may, however, frequently be seen in the new-born babe and sometimes persist throughout life (Fig. 450). They arise from the *anterior* aspect of the iris in the region of the circulus iridis minor (collarette) (see p. 247).

THE ANTERIOR CHAMBER

The Anterior Chamber commences peripherally as a slit in the mesoderm between the cornea and iris, which gradually travels centrally. It is probable that this happens quite late in fœtal life.

According to Cirincione, who used the freezing method for making his sections, an earlier date for the appearance of the anterior chamber is probably erroneous, the result of artefacts due to fixation (as in Fig. 380).

At birth the anterior chamber is still very shallow.

The region of the future angle is at first filled with loose mesodermal tissue (uveal framework of H. Virchow), which later disappears, except for the portion at the extreme periphery. The sinus venosus scleræ is present at three months, and from the first carries blood corpuscles (Seefelder) (Fig. 398).

THE UVEAL TRACT

The choroid, ciliary body, and iris are partly mesodermal, partly ectodermal in origin. They are formed from the anterior portion of the optic cup and the mesodermal and vascular covering of the whole cup.

The mesodermal portion of the uveal tract depends for its development on the optic cup, especially on its pigment layer (von Hippel). Normally, it covers the optic cup from the stalk to the pupillary margin, and should any portion of the cup be missing the mesoderm does not develop and a coloboma results.

As soon as the lens vesicle has become detached from the surface ectoderm, mesoderm grows between the lens and the optic vesicle on the one hand and the surface ectoderm on the other. Thus the optic cup and lens become embedded in a common mass of mesoderm which is pierced by the optic nerve. From this mesoderm is developed the choroid, the ciliary body, the stroma of the iris, as also the sclera and non-epithelial portions of the cornea. Peripherally this mesoderm gradually passes into that of the side-wall of the head, from which are derived the fascia bulbi, the episcleral tissue, and the orbital fat ; anteriorly it becomes continuous with the mesoderm of the skin, i.e. of the future eyelids. The septum orbitale is also genetically the boundary between the connective tissue of the skin and that around the optic vesicle. All this connective tissue is originally quite homogeneous. But soon it divides into two portions which are differentiated by the relative density of their packing and the shape of the cells. That portion round the pars optica is invaded by vessels.

The epithelium of the pars cæca is at first high columnar with the nuclei arranged in several layers. Later there are several layers of cells. A small clear marginal zone which reaches to the pupillary margin forms as in the pars optica. With the general increase in size of the eye and the formation and forward growth of the iris, these cells are converted into a single layer of cubical cells which become lower as we go towards the pupillary margin.

The Iris is formed from the anterior portion of the optic cup, i.e. the stratum pigmenti iridis and the pars iridica retinæ and the mesoderm, which covers it.

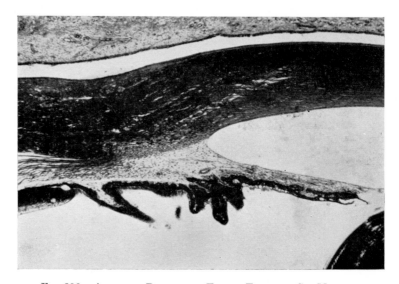

FIG. 396.—ANTERIOR PORTION OF EYE OF FŒTUS OF SIX MONTHS.

Note how the true ligamentum pectinatum iridis which is present in the human at this stage fills the future angle of the anterior chamber. It passes forwards to the end of Descemet's membrane.

The neural ectoderm gives rise to the sphincter and dilatator pupillæ and to the posterior epithelium; the mesoderm forms the stroma and the vessels.

Up to the end of the third month of embryonic life there is no true iris, and the margin of the optic cup extends but a little way beyond the equator of the lens (Fig. 380). The retinal and mesodermal portions are continuous with those of the ciliary body without line of demarcation, and, moreover, the mesodermal portion is not delimited from the pupillary membrane. The development of the iris as such commences about the middle of the fourth month by a forward growth of the rim of the optic cup with its overlying mesoderm. It is preceded by a spur-like process of mesoderm (Fuchs), to which is attached the pupillary membrane. The iris thus bcomes more or less differentiated from the ciliary body and pupillary membrane.

At this period a space, *the ring sinus of von Szily,* is present between the two

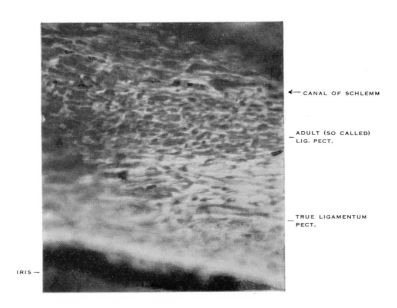

← CANAL OF SCHLEMM

_ ADULT (SO CALLED)
_ LIG. PECT.

_ TRUE LIGAMENTUM
PECT.

IRIS —

FIG. 398.—DETAIL OF FIGURE 396. ANGLE OF ANTERIOR CHAMBER OF FŒTUS OF SIX MONTHS
Canal of Schlemm (sinus venosus scleræ) contains blood.

layers of ectoderm forming the rim of the optic cup. It is at first small, but increases in size up to about five months, when it gets smaller, to disappear at seven months. It represents the last trace of the cavity of the primary optic vesicle. The sphincter pupillæ is developed at this period from the pigment epithelium of the rim of the optic cup. *It is thus curious, as Nussbaum first pointed out, in being a muscle derived from ectoderm.* At the 10-mm. stage there is a proliferation of the cells of the stratum pigmenti iridis at the pupillary margin and a mass of cells grows backwards towards the ciliary border. The slight amount

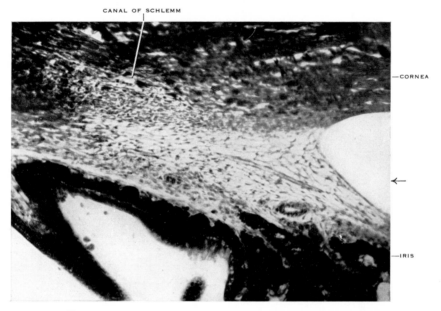

Fig. 397.—Detail of Figure 396. Angle of Anterior Chamber filled by True Ligamentum Pectinatum as occurs in Lower Animals. (Compare Fig. 49.)

Deep to canal of Schlemm is the primordium of the adult (so called) ligamentum pectinatum (corneoscleral trabeculæ). Canal of Schlemm (sinus venosus scleræ) contains blood.

of contained pigment disappears and the cells are differentiated in plain muscle cells. These cells become limited peripherally by a ridge of pigment known as Michel's spur. At about the sixth month the sphincter begins to separate from the cells that gave it origin, passes into the mesodermal portion of the iris and is invaded by vessels. Numerous connections with the pigment epithelium, however, always persist, and Michel's spur represents the most peripheral of these. Pigment cells, derived from the anterior portion of the optic cup, pass through the sphincter and into the iris stroma to form *the clump cells* (Figs. 25, 77, 78). At birth the sphincter pupillæ is still closely adherent to the epithelial cells of the pupillary border. The dilatator pupillæ is also derived from the same ectodermal cells at the end of the sixth month. The nuclei of the cells of the stratum pigmentum, first in the ciliary zone, wander from their anterior to their posterior portions in which also the pigment collects. The anuclear portions become drawn out and arrange themselves radially to the pupil ; then muscle fibrillæ form in them and thus the dilatator is formed. Thus whereas a whole cell of the anterior layer goes to form a muscle fibre of the sphincter pupillæ, only part of it forms a fibre of the dilatator. The anterior epithelium already contains pigment when the iris commences to form. Pigmentation of the posterior epithelium commences at the pupillary margin, and reaches its base at about the sixth month. The iris develops in width more slowly than the rest of the eye ; so the pupil gets wider up

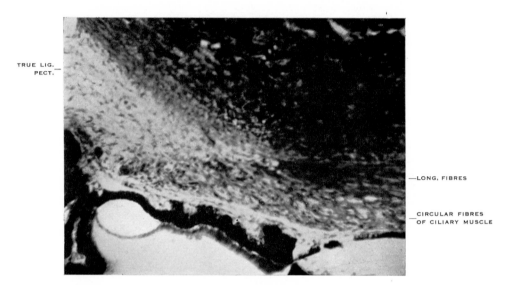

TRUE LIG. PECT.

LONG. FIBRES

CIRCULAR FIBRES OF CILIARY MUSCLE

FIG. 399.—DETAIL OF FIGURE 378.

Note how far back true ligamentum pectinatum passes at this stage. Circular fibres of ciliary muscle can be readily distinguished.

to the beginning of the seventh month. At five months the iris is hidden by the limbus and resembles the condition of aniridia.

After the eighth month the pupil becomes smaller, due to the development of the sphincteric portion of the iris. With the disappearance of the pupillary membrane changes take place in the front of the iris with the formation of iris crypts. At about this time the *anterior border or limiting layer* can be recognised. It is formed by several rows of star-shaped cells which anastomose with each other and which may at times contain pigment cells at birth. The pigmentation of the stroma usually takes place in the first years after birth, and appears to be under the control of the sympathetic system. Also the pattern of the anterior surface of the iris is produced during the first year, and generally the iris is not fully formed till twelve months after birth.

The Ciliary Body.—The neural ectoderm, i.e. pars ciliaris retinæ and the stratum pigmenti ciliaris, forms the epithelium of the ciliary body, while the mesoderm is responsible for the stroma, the ciliary muscle, and the vessels.

The junction of the pars optica with the pars cæca, i.e. the future ora serrata, can be made out quite early owing to the sudden diminution of thickness at this point (Fig. 379). But the ciliary body is further demarcated from the true retina by the formation of the ciliary folds at the beginning of the third month. Vessels sink into these folds and form what is for the most part a venous net. At the sixth month the ciliary arteries have formed the circulus iridis major and given

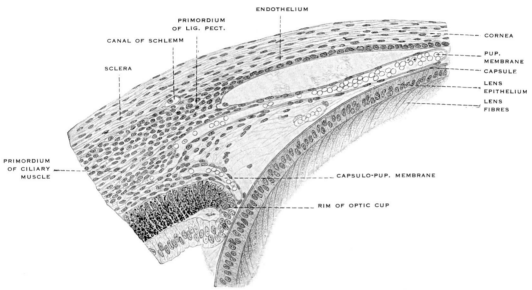

Fig. 400.—Region of the Angle of the Anterior Chamber in an 88-mm. Human Embryo.
(*From Seefelder, in the Kurzes Handbuch.*)

off branches to the pupillary membrane, the stroma of the iris, and the ciliary region.

During fœtal life the most anterior of the ciliary folds lie behind the peripheral portion of the iris and then gradually move backwards. The longitudinal portion of the ciliary muscle is formed from the mesoderm next the sclera at the fourth month, while the circular portion develops at the end of the sixth month. The anterior portion of the ciliary muscle and the ligamentum pectinatum are developed from a continuous mass of mesodermal cells in the neighbourhood of the future angle of the anterior chamber (Fig. 400).

By the fourth or fifth month of intra-uterine life the tendinous fibres of the ciliary muscle are well differentiated, and can be followed directly into the fibres of the ligamentum. The essentially circular fibres of the scleral spur condense round some of the tendinous fibres, leaving a variable number to continue beyond the tip of the spur directly into the ligament. Thus the adult relationships are established.

At first only the corona ciliaris is present. The orbiculus ciliaris is formed at the fifth month by the limit of the true retina, i.e. of the pars optica moving backwards towards the equator. By this, too, the original small teeth of the ora serrata are lengthened.

The Choroid.—The primitive choroid is developed in the mesoderm round the primary optic vesicle, which it clothes as a vascular venous net. It is thus a

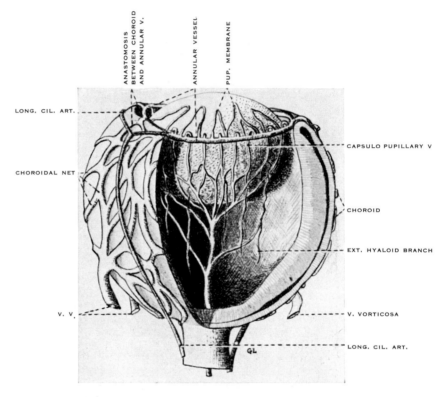

Fig. 404.—Scheme of the Vessels of the Embryonic Eye.
From Traité d'Ophtalmologie. Tome 1, p. 96. G. Leplat.)

very early formation (Figs. 380, 404). It is at first very cellular but gets less so as time goes on. It gradually divides into two and then more layers of vessels. By the fifth month all the layers of the choroid can be recognised. By the sixth month the elastic lamina is present. The time of pigmentation of the choroid varies. The pigment is developed in the melanoblasts or fixed cells of the choroid somewhere towards the end of fœtal life, and first in the neighbourhood of the posterior ciliary arteries.

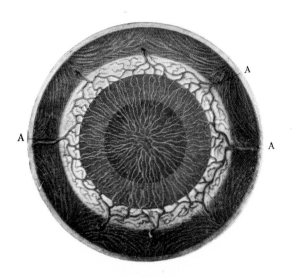

FIG. 401.—THE PUPILLARY MEMBRANE OF A FŒTUS OF ABOUT 3½ MONTHS.
The ciliary arteries (A) have been injected.
(*From Hirschfeld and Leveillé.*)

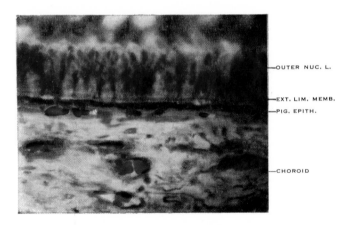

FIG. 402.—DETAIL OF FIGURE 388.

ORBICULARIS   GLANDS OF WOLFRING   CORNEA

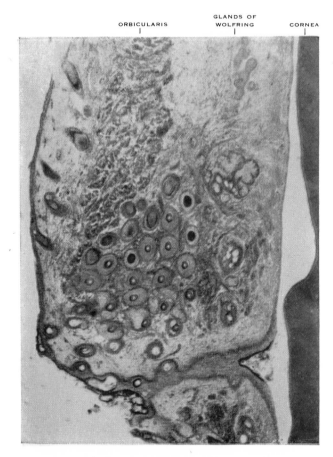

Fig. 403.—Vertical Section of Fused Eyelids in a Fœtus of Six Months.
Note tarsal glands, hair follicles, and ciliary muscle of Riolan are easily distinguishable.

A E.—449

The final anatomical relationships between the three coats of the eye are determined by function rather than by embryonic origin.

Thus the corneo-sclera and the uveal tract derived from the same mass of mesoderm are separated from each other in the adult eye anteriorly by the anterior chamber and posteriorly by the suprachoroidal space. They are only attached where the ciliary muscle arises from the scleral spur and at the optic nerve. On the other hand, the uveal tract is closely connected with the inner coat. Thus the pigment layer of the retina derived from the outer layer of the optic cup rarely separates in the living from the choroid and never from the ciliary

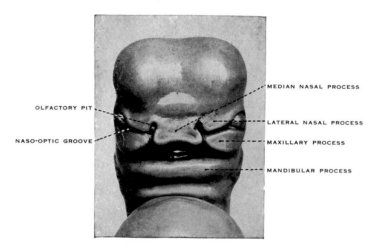

OLFACTORY PIT

NASO-OPTIC GROOVE

MEDIAN NASAL PROCESS

LATERAL NASAL PROCESS

MAXILLARY PROCESS

MANDIBULAR PROCESS

FIG. 405.—MODEL OF THE FACE OF AN EMBRYO (RECONSTRUCTION BY HIS) TO SHOW THE PROCESSES WHICH FORM IT. THE TWO MANDIBULAR PROCESSES HAVE FUSED AT THIS STAGE. (The clefts between the maxillary and nasal processes are diagrammatic—no actual clefts exist, but merely surface grooves.)

From Whitnall, Anatomy of Human Orbit.)

body. Thus also the anterior layer of the pars iridica retinæ is inseparably connected with the iris, as are also the sphincter and dilatator pupillæ which are derived from it.

THE LIDS

The embryonic eye lies at the side of the head covered only by a thin transparent layer of ectoderm. At the beginning of the second month a circular fold forms around and at some distance from the eye. The palpebral fissure is therefore at first round with no angles and relatively wide. The upper and lower portions of the fold grow towards each other and so angles are formed and the upper and lower eyelids demarcated from each other. The eyelids meet and unite loosely at two and a half months (Figs. 380, 406), union taking place from the edge towards the middle. At about the fifth month they start separating again through keratinisation of the cells of the united edges, separation being completed at the seventh or eighth month.

A.E.—29

The **Tarsal Glands** are developed about the end of the tenth week by the ingrowth of a regular row of solid columns of ectodermal cells from the lid margins directly behind the posterior row of cilia. These later acquire a lumen and begin secreting at the end of the fifth month.

Moll's and Zeis's Glands are developed as outgrowths from the follicle of the cilia (16-cm. stage).

The **Tarsus** is formed as a condensation of the mesoderm around the tarsal and Zeis's glands.

The first hairs of the eyebrows make their appearance when the lids unite. They are the first hairs of the embryo (Contino).

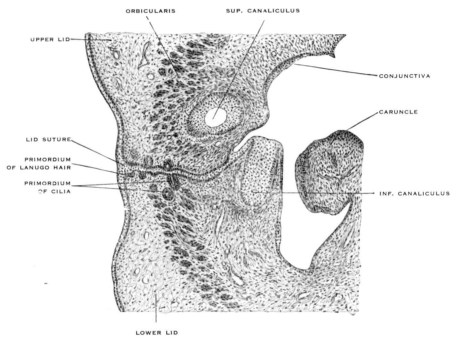

FIG. 406.—SECTION OF THE JOINED LIDS OF AN EMBRYO OF 14 CM. × 45.

(*After Fischel.*)

The **cilia** appear a little later, first in the upper lid and then in the lower. They develop as epithelial buds from the lid margins soon after their union. Two or three rows, one behind the other, are formed. As the follicles of the cilia and the tarsal glands grow into the embryonic connective tissue, they split the ciliary muscle (of Riolan) from the remainder of the orbicularis.

The **Lacrimal Gland** is developed by about eight wedge-shaped epithelial buds which grow towards the end of the second month from the upper and temporal side of the conjunctival sac (Fig. 407) and repeatedly divide. With the development of the levator and the fascia bulbi, the gland is divided into orbital and palpebral portions. The full histological differentiation does not, however, take place till after birth, so that tears are not produced till about the beginning of the third month.

The conjunctival (Krause's) glands are developed as growths of the basal cells of the upper conjunctival fornix and to a slight extent from the lower fornix at about six months.

The Lacrimal Sac.—The primordium of the lacrimal sac lies in a solid column of cells which, derived from the surface ectoderm, sinks into the furrow between the lateral nasal and maxillary processes at about the 10-mm. stage. At the 15-mm. stage it is free from the ectoderm and grows upwards into the lids to form the canaliculi and downwards into the nose to form the naso-lacrimal duct.

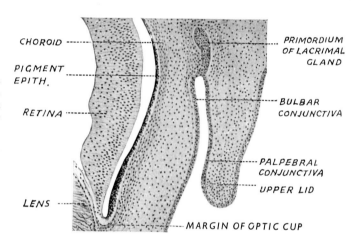

FIG. 407.—SAGITTAL SECTION OF THE LATERAL PORTION OF THE UPPER LID OF AN EMBRYO OF 34 MM.

(*From Poirier, after Cirincione,* 1908.)

CHOROID

PIGMENT EPITH.

RETINA

LENS

PRIMORDIUM OF LACRIMAL GLAND

BULBAR CONJUNCTIVA

PALPEBRAL CONJUNCTIVA

UPPER LID

MARGIN OF OPTIC CUP

The lower canaliculus is the thinner of the two and grows farther laterally than the upper. Hence the lower punctum is lateral to the upper.

Errors in development, such as multiplication of the canaliculi or puncta and abnormal diverticula, arise from abnormal division or outgrowths of the primitive solid column of cells.

Canaliculisation of the solid columns of cells takes place by a degeneration and shedding of the central cells (Fig. 409), first in the region of the lacrimal sac, at about the third month. It reaches the nose at six months and the puncta at seven months. The debris of these cells may cause blocking of the nasal duct, *and give rise to a mucocele, not uncommon in the first few weeks of life.*

The Conjunctiva is developed from the ectoderm lining the lids and that covering the globe (Figs. 380, 407).

The Lacrimal Caruncle.—According to Ask, the caruncle is developed by the cutting off of a portion of the lower lid with its contained cilia, sebaceous and sweat glands, by the ingrowth of the lower canaliculus.

The Semilunar Fold develops from the conjunctiva at about five and half weeks.

The Development of the Vitreous

The primordium of the vitreous is present at the earliest stage of the primary optic vesicle, between this vesicle and the surface ectoderm (Fig. 410).

Dejean has shown that the material which lies between these two structures is constituted by the basement membranes of the ectoderm and the lens, thickened and hypertrophied at the pole of the vesicle. These basement membranes are indistinct with ordinary stains, but show up well with collagen stains : Mallory, picro-naphthol black, light green of Prenant, trichrome of Masson, etc. Fig. 410 shows a primary optic vesicle of an embryo sheep 7·5 mm. in length stained with picro-naphthol black. The vesicle is surrounded by a fine blue line which represents a section of the basement membrane. This line is thickened in the region of that part of the surface ectoderm which will form the lens.

As to the nature of these membranes, Redslob believes they are ectodermal. But Dejean thinks they consist of collagen, that is of mesoderm which has in-

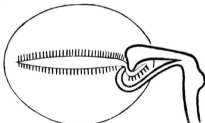

Fig. 408.—Development of the Lacrimal Caruncle (Embryo of 170 mm.).

Note how the lower canaliculus cuts off a piece of the lid margin which forms the caruncle. Actually the eyelids are fused at this stage, but are drawn separated to show the developing tarsal glands (vertical lines).

(*From Ask.*)

sinuated itself between the surface and neural ectoderm in the earliest stages of development.

At any rate, the presence of a collagen-like membrane covering the retina from the earliest stages puts out of court the theory that the vitreous is an outgrowth from the retina.

As the lens separates from the retina these membranes are drawn out, fibrillated, and converted into a network which fills the space between them. It will be noted that the reticulum stains the same way as the basement membranes.

The primitive vitreous is vascular, the vessels being formed in the first place by vaso-formative cells which are present from the earliest stages. Then it is invaded by the hyaloid artery and its branches.

Formation of the Definitive Vitreous.—When the primitive vitreous with its vessels fills the whole vitreous cavity there appears on the surface of the retina a dense layer. This will form the definitive vitreous and arises like the primitive vitreous from the basement membrane of the retina (but not from the optic disc). It enlarges rapidly, pushing the primitive vitreous and its vessels before it. It is at first homogeneous but soon becomes lamellar. It is characterised by being avascular and fine-meshed.

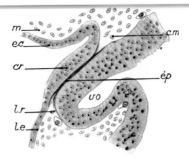

Fig. 410.—Section of the Eye of a Sheep Embryo of 7·5 mm. at the Stage of the Primary Optic Vesicle. (Stained Picro-black-naphthol.)

e.c. = head ectoderm ; m. = mesoderm ; v.o. = optic vesicle ; c.r. = lens thickening ; l.e. = basement membrane of ectoderm ; l.r. = basement membrane or limitans of optic vesicle ; e.p. = their thickening forming the retino-lenticular material of union ; c.m. = wedge of mesoderm.

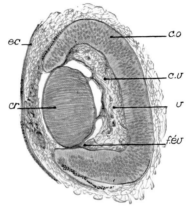

Fig. 411.—Section of the Eye of a Sheep Embryo of 20 mm.

c.o. = optic cup ; e.c. = head ectoderm ; c.r. = lens ; c.v. = primitive vitreous   v. = its vessels ; f.é.v. = fan-like fibres or faisceau isthmique.

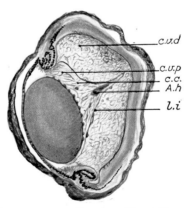

Fig. 412.—Section of the Eye of a Sheep Embryo of 90 mm.

c.v.d. = definitive vitreous ; c.v.p. = primitive vitreous filling hyaloid canal of Cloquet ; l.i. = intervitreous condensation ; A.h. = hyaloid artery ; c.c. = primitive vitreous.

(From Dejean in the Traité d'Ophtalmologie, 1939.)

[A.F.—453

The primitive vitreous is then pushed behind the lens, into the ciliary region and to the central axis, where it surrounds the trunk of the hyaloid artery.

The Intervitreous Condensation.—This is a lamellar-like condensation between the primitive and definitive vitreous. It runs forwards from the disc to the back of the lens, then bends round to reach the ora serrata. It forms the walls of the hyaloid canal and the anterior limiting layer of the vitreous (Fig. 412).

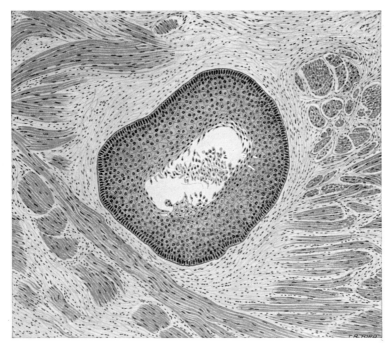

Fig. 409.—To show the Formation of the Lumen in the Lacrimal Canaliculus of a Fœtus of about Eight Months.

The debris of the central cells may at times cause the mucocele, not uncommon in the first weeks of life. Around are fibres of the orbicularis.

(*Wolff's preparation.*)

The Ciliary Zonule.—The zonule is developed from that portion of the primitive vitreous which has been pushed into the ciliary region, i.e. the region of the future zonule by the rapidly growing definitive vitreous, and by fibres derived from the basement membrane of the ciliary body. The primordium of the zonule is of the same structure as the rest of the primitive vitreous, i.e. it is wide-meshed and supplied with vessels. It is separated from the definitive vitreous by the intervitreous membrane (Fig. 412).

But the zonule is not derived from the primitive vitreous only. Numerous fibres, for the most part fine, derived from the basement membrane of the ciliary body invade the primitive vitreous. Then the structure of the primitive vitreous alters and fibres make their appearance. These—straight, rigid, and directed towards the lens—gradually increase in number and in thickness till the adult condition is produced.

The Internal Limiting Layer of the Retina.—The essential part of what we have called the internal limiting layer of the retina (see p. 131) is derived from

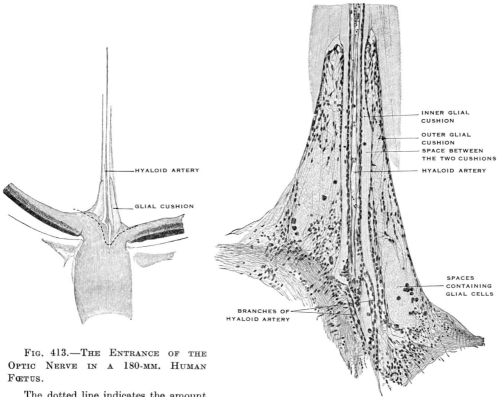

FIG. 413.—THE ENTRANCE OF THE OPTIC NERVE IN A 180-MM. HUMAN FŒTUS.

The dotted line indicates the amount of atrophy to form the normal physiological cup.

(*From Seefelder in the Kurzes Handbuch.*)

FIG. 414.—THE REGION IN FIG. 413 ANTERIOR TO THE DOTTED LINE, ENLARGED.

(*From Bach and Seefelder, in the Kurzes Handbuch.*)

the basement membrane of the retina, which, as we have seen, is present from the earliest stages of development. It thus has the same origin as the vitreous and stains the same way. At about the 11-mm. stage the feet of the fibres of Müller reach it and form the irregularities on its retinal aspect.

POST-NATAL DEVELOPMENT OF THE VITREOUS

At birth the hyaloid canal extends horizontally backwards from a point a little below and to the nasal side of the posterior pole of the lens.

The extreme anterior end of the main trunk of the hyaloid artery extends horizontally backwards from the lens capsule along the first part of the canal. After birth the remains of the artery curl up like a corkscrew and hang down behind the lens. The walls of the hyaloid canal become very lax and hang down, moving with the movement of the eye and head (Mann); its attachment to the back of the eye probably remains as the arcuate line.

The Hyaloid System of Vessels

At the stage of the optic cup two sets of vessels can be made out : one inside the cup, the other on its surface (Fig. 404) :

(a) The hyaloid artery, a branch of the ophthalmic, *enters* the optic cup viâ the fœtal fissure, and drains anteriorly into the annular vessel. It also anastomoses with the vessels of the optic stalk.

(b) A second set ramifies *on the surface* of the optic cup and will eventually form the choroid (q.v.). The most anterior part of this plexus forms the annular vessel round the rim of the cup.

Fuchs called it the *annular artery*, but although it is impossible at this stage to differentiate arteries and veins structurally, it is most probably a vein since the hyaloid artery drains into it.

The circulus iridis major is later developed in the same position as the annular vessel, but is not derived from it.

The hyaloid artery divides repeatedly, and gradually forms a network of vessels covering the back of the lens (the tunica vasculosa lentis). Other branches of the artery practically fill the vitreous chamber at this stage and reach their greatest development at the middle of the third month (vasa hyaloidea propria) (Fig. 353).

The hyaloid artery at first emerges from the middle of the nerve head (Figs. 413, 414, 415), but later is shifted more and more to the nasal side. It at the same time becomes smaller and smaller, while the arteria centralis grows larger. Eventually the hyaloid artery appears to be a twig arising from the central retinal artery.

The hyaloid system of vessels disappears first at the peripheral parts of the vitreous (about the fifth month), and concurrently with this the point of division of the main hyaloid artery shifts farther forwards and its attachment to the lens farther medial.

The venous return of the whole system is viâ the capsulo-pupillary membrane, which covers the lens from its equator to the edge of the pupil.

The Blood-supply of the Optic Nerve and Retina

At first the optic nerve and retina have no vessels, as the hyaloid system supplies the developing lens and the vitreous only. At two and a half months with the invasion of the septal vessels a plexus of veins forms round the hyaloid artery while it is still in the optic nerve. In this, two vessels can be distinguished early, and these unite near the nerve head to form the vena centralis retinæ. After this, at about three and a half months, the retinal arteries are developed as two buds from the hyaloid artery which grow into the nerve fibre layer of the retina and later become canaliculised. Similar buds form the retinal veins.

The vessels gradually grow out towards the ora serrata, and at the eighth month the vascular arrangements of the retina are complete.

That portion of the hyaloid artery enclosed in the optic nerve becomes the arteria centralis.

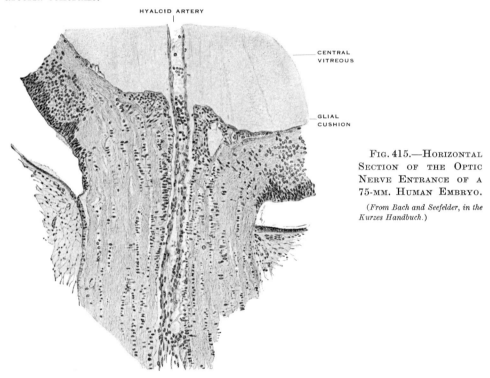

HYALOID ARTERY

CENTRAL VITREOUS

GLIAL CUSHION

Fig. 415.—Horizontal Section of the Optic Nerve Entrance of a 75-mm. Human Embryo.

(*From Bach and Seefelder, in the Kurzes Handbuch.*)

THE ORBIT

The orbit is formed in the mesoderm around the eye. This mesoderm is, however, derived from several sources :

1. Above, from the mesodermal capsule of the fore-brain.
2. Below and laterally, from the maxillary process.
3. Medially, from the fronto-nasal process ; and
4. Behind, from the pre- and orbito-sphenoids.

The optic vesicle at first lies at the side of the head between the head fold and the maxillary process (Fig. 405). As the maxillary process grows forwards and forms the floor and lateral wall of the orbit, the eye passes forwards too. The fronto-nasal process divides into two lateral and two medial nasal processes.

Each lateral nasal process goes to form the medial wall of the orbit (including the fronto-nasal process, the lacrimal and ethmoid bones) of its side and eventually unites with the maxillary process.

The roof of the orbit is formed from the capsule of the fore-brain.

The optic nerve passes into the eye between the two roots of the orbito-sphenoid, which are attached to the orbito-nasal septum.

All the bones of the orbit (including the greater wing of the sphenoid) are

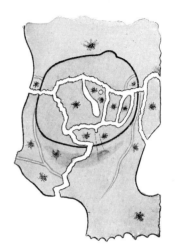

Fig. 416.—Diagram to show the Approximate Position and Number of Centres of Ossification in the Bones which form the Orbit.

The centres appear between the sixth and eighth weeks of fœtal life, and, except for the sphenoidal, have fused into component bones before birth (6th to 7th month). In very rare cases one of the secondary centres may remain ununited.

(*From Whitnall's Anatomy of Human Orbit.*)

membrane bones, but the pre- and orbito-sphenoids belonging to the base of the cranium are developed in cartilage.

As it is formed round the eye, the orbit is at first much more of a sphere than in the adult, and also the orbital opening is more circular.

The eye at first grows faster than the orbit, whose margin at six months only reaches to the equator.

THE EXTRINSIC MUSCLES

The extrinsic muscles of the eye are developed by a condensation of the mesoderm round the eye. At first (at 7 mm.) they form one mass which Lewis (1910) found was supplied by the 3rd nerve only. Later (at 9 mm.) when the 4th and 6th nerves enter, this mass divides into separate muscles. The levator does not separate from the medial part of the superior rectus till the 55-mm. stage.

According to Seefelder, the muscles grow from behind forwards, which accounts for the numerous variations in their insertions and constancy of origin.

Surface Ectoderm gives rise to :

Lens.

Epithelium of cornea.

Epithelium of conjunctiva, (and hence) lacrimal gland.

Epithelium of lids and its derivatives, and cilia, the tarsal glands, and the ciliary and conjunctival glands.

Epithelium lining lacrimal apparatus.

Neural Ectoderm gives rise to :

Retina with its pigment epithelium.

Epithelium covering ciliary processes.

Pigment epithelium covering posterior surface of iris.

Sphincter and dilatator pupillæ muscles.

The optic nerve (neuroglial and nervous elements only).

Associated Paraxial Mesoderm gives rise to :

The blood-vessels, i.e. the choroid, the arteria centralis retinæ, ciliary vessels, and other vessels of the orbit which persist, as well as the hyaloid artery, the vasa hyaloid propria, and the vessels of the vascular capsule of the lens which disappear before birth.

The sclera.

The sheath of the optic nerve.

The ciliary muscle.

The substantia propria of the cornea, and the endothelium of its posterior surface.

The stroma and anterior epithelium of the iris.

The extrinsic muscles of the eye.

The fat, ligaments, and other connective tissue structures in the orbit.

The upper and medial walls of the orbit.

The connective tissue of the upper lid.

Visceral (Mesoderm of Maxillary Process) below the eye gives rise to :

The lower and lateral walls of the orbit. The structures lying behind and below the eye (i.e. the alisphenoid, zygomatic, and orbital plate of maxilla).

The connective tissues of the lower lid.

A list of age-length relationships at representative stages is added for reference (crown-rump length in mm.) :

4 weeks (28 days)	.	.	.	7·8 mm.	11 weeks (77 days) .	.	.	59·2 mm.
5 „ (35 „)	.	.	.	12·2 „	12 „ (84 „) .	.	.	70·5 „
6 „ (42 „)	.	.	.	17·6 „	18 „ .	.	.	130·0 „
7 „ (49 „)	.	.	.	24·0 „	24 „ .	.	.	190·0 „
8 „ (56 „)	.	.	.	31·3 „	30 „ .	.	.	250·0 „
9 „ (63 „)	.	.	.	39·6 „	36 „ .	.	.	310·0 „
10 „ (70 „)	.	.	.	49·0 „	39 „ .	.	.	340·0 „

PRINCIPAL LANDMARKS IN OCULAR GROWTH

The following table from Ida Mann (1957) shows in italics the changes of greatest moment in the production of developmental abnormalities :

Period	Structures undergoing change	Approx. size of embryo at end of period	Approx. age at end of period
	Organogenetic period		
1	*Optic pit changes into optic vesicle.* Lens plate forms	3 mm.	3–4 weeks
2	Lens pit and vesicle appear. *Optic vesicle invaginates to form optic cup.* Pigment appears in outer layer of optic cup	7 mm.	End of 4th week
3	*Fœtal fissure closes.* Lens separates from surface and *primary lens fibres form.* Retinal differentiation begins. Tunica vasculosa lentis begins	14 mm.	6th week
	Neo-fœtal period		
4	Secondary lens fibres begin. Tunica vasculosa lentis fully formed. Lid folds develop. *Ectodermal layers of iris begin*	70 mm.	3 months
	Fœtal period		
5	The following appear : Arteria centralis retinæ, ciliary muscle, sphincter and dilator of pupil, sclera, ciliary body and outer layer of choroid. *Posterior vascular capsule of lens begins to retrogress*	110 mm.	4 months
6	*Pupillary membrane retrogresses.* Pars plana begins. Medullation of optic nerve begins	250 mm.	7 months
7	*Hyaloid artery disappears.* Medullation reaches lamina cribrosa	300 mm.	9 months
	Neo-natal period		
8	*Macula lutea finally differentiates*	—	4–6 months after birth
	Post-natal or adolescent period		
	Further formation of *secondary lens fibres.* Growth of whole eye	—	25 years

THE EYE AT BIRTH

The eye at birth is less of a sphere than in the adult.   This is due to the bulge of the postero-lateral quadrant.

Its antero-posterior diameter varies from 12·5 to 15·8 mm., and the vertical diameter from 14·5 to 17 mm.   To offset the comparative shortness of the eye which would make it exceedingly hypermetropic, the media are more highly refractive than in the adult, the seat of the excess of refractivity being in the lens (Fuchs [1]).

The cornea is relatively large, its diameter (10 mm.) being three-fifths that of the antero-posterior axis.

[1] Weiss, however, gives the following measurements for the antero-posterior, vertical, and transverse diameters respectively, 16·4, 15·4, 16 mm. Sorsby and Sheridan (*J. Anat.*, 1960, **94,** 192) found the full-term measurements to be respectively 17·9, 17·3 and 18·4 mm.

It is more curved at the periphery than at its centre, i.e. just the opposite of the condition in the adult (Merkel and Orr).

The medial rectus is very close to the cornea.

The corneal stroma contains more nuclei than in the adult.

The stroma of the uveal tract has no pigment except possibly posteriorly near the optic nerve.

The pigmentation of the anterior border layer of the iris commences in the first few days of life.

The pupil is small and does not dilate fully.

The anterior chamber is shallow and its angle is narrow.

The ligamentum pectinatum is still somewhat fœtal in character, i.e. it still fills the angle to a large extent.

The ciliary processes are still in contact with the iris.

The stroma of the ciliary body is very cellular, but the various types of muscle can be recognised.

The ridges of the ciliary processes are as dark as the valleys between them.

The macula is as far from the disc as in the adult. A depression in it is just visible. The cones are still short and stumpy.

The teeth of the ora serrata are just visible (Hess), and the retina passes much more gradually into the pars ciliaris. The two nuclear layers fuse, and are continued into the ciliary epithelium.

A fold of the retina at the ora serrata is often found (Lange's fold), but this must be regarded as an artefact.

The orbiculus ciliaris is very short, so that the retina lies just behind the ciliary muscle.

The nerve fibres behind the lamina cribrosa are still not medullated.

The lens is rounder than in the adult, and on account of its anterior bulging the anterior chamber is shallow.

Post-natal Growth and Changes in the Eyeball

The eye grows rapidly in the first years of life, the vertical diameter growing faster, so that the eye becomes more nearly spherical. The rate then decreases till puberty, when it again becomes more rapid till the early twenties (Weiss).

There is a distinct parallel between the growth of the eye and that of the brain. Thus, from birth to adult life, the eye grows 3·25 times and the brain 3·76. The body, on the other hand, increases 21·36 times.

The increase in size during the first years of life affects mainly the anterior segment, i.e. the cornea and the sclera up to the insertions of the muscles.

Thus the cornea reaches adult size at about two years or earlier.

The later growth affects mainly the posterior segment, but the distance between the fovea and optic nerve remains the same as at birth.

Medullation of the optic nerve is completed in the first three weeks after birth, and seems to be hastened by exposure to light. Thus a premature baby will have its medullation farther advanced by the time it reaches the ninth month than a newly born full-term child.

The fovea is not properly developed till one month after birth.

There is little difference between the ciliary and pupillary zones of the iris at birth. This can be made out at about six months.

The colour of the iris changes in the first few years of life, depending on the amount of stroma pigment laid down.

The Ciliary Body.—As the retina recedes, so there is an increase in the size of the orbiculus ciliaris. The line of demarcation between the retina and

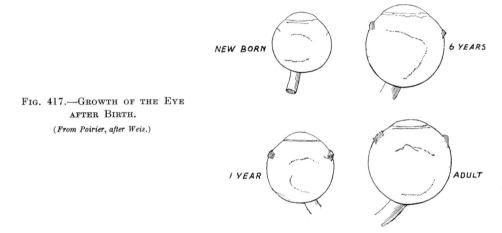

FIG. 417.—GROWTH OF THE EYE
AFTER BIRTH.
(From Poirier, after Weis.)

ciliary body is well marked, but does not reach adult relationships till about seven years.

As the ciliary processes are displaced backwards the angle of the anterior chamber widens to adult size between two and four years.

There is no muscle of Müller at birth (Fuchs). It is only after the fifth year that the ciliary muscle, and thus the whole ciliary body, takes on a triangular form.

The lens grows rapidly in the first years of life and becomes flatter, owing to being pulled on by the ever-widening circle formed by the ciliary body. The lens continues growing throughout life (p. 166).

The eye of the new-born child is normally hypermetropic. The increase in axial length would, however, render it myopic were it not for this flattening of the lens.

The eyes get farther apart and the orbits enlarge especially anteriorly, so that their temporal borders are more widely separated. As the eyes separate they also tend to diverge, since the separation makes the lateral rectus act to greater and the medial rectus to less advantage than before (Fuchs).

SIGNS OF AGE IN THE EYEBALL

The cornea flattens with age, but more in the vertical than in the horizontal meridian. This gives rise to an astigmatism against the rule. *Hence the onset of astigmatism against the rule in emmetropes after about forty years may be regarded as normal, and, further, for the same reason, astigmatism with the rule tends to lessen and that against the rule tends to increase with age.*

The arcus senilis is a manifestation of the fatty degeneration which tends to take place with age throughout the fibrous tunic of the eye.

It starts above and below as two grey crescents, close to and parallel with the corneal margin. The crescents eventually fuse and become whiter and more opaque. The ring so formed is thicker above than below. There is always a portion of clear cornea between it and the limbus. It is sharply defined peripherally, but fades more gradually into clear cornea centrally.

The fatty degeneration affects first the superficial layers of the stroma and Bowman's membrane. Peripherally it is limited by a line passing from the end of Bowman's membrane obliquely outwards for a varying distance into the sclera.

The sclera becomes thicker and more rigid. There is a tendency for the deposition of fat, which changes the colour from white to yellowish.

In the uveal tract there is a great increase in the amount of connective tissue. The ciliary body, therefore, thickens and the circumlental space is diminished. Senile myosis and rigidity of the sphincter pupillæ are also due to increase in the amount of connective tissue in its neighbourhood.

The various glass-like membranes become thicker, and there is a great tendency to wart formation seen specially at the periphery of Descemet's and in the basal lamina (membrane of Bruch).

The warts on the basal lamina are secreted by the pigment epithelium which covers them, but thins over the summits of the elevations. They, therefore, appear with the ophthalmoscope as yellowish-white spots surrounded by a narrow pigmented border. The spots in Tay's choroiditis are of this nature.

The pigment epithelium tends to show areas of atrophy, especially round the disc.

BIBLIOGRAPHY

The classical work on the development of the human eye is BACH & SEEFELDER (1911–12) Entwicklungsgeschichte des menschlichen Auges, *Leipzig.*

The most complete account in English is I. C. MANN's Development of the Human Eye, 2nd edition, *London,* 1949.

OTHER STANDARD WORKS

DRUAULT (1912) : " Appareil de la Vision," in Poirier, Traité d'Anatomie Humaine, **5**.
FISCHEL, A. (1929) : Lehrbuch der Entwicklung des Menschen, *Berlin*.
LEPLAT and DEJEAN (1939) in Traité d'Ophtalmologie, *Paris*, **1**.
MANN (1957) : Developmental Abnormalities of the Eye, 2nd Ed., B.M.A., *London*.
SEEFELDER (1930) in Schieck & Brückner, Kurzes Handbuch der Ophthalmologie, **1**.

HAGEDOORN (1928) : *Brit. J. Ophthal.*, **12,** 479.
LEWIS (1910) in Keibel & Mall, Manual of Embryology, 2 vols., *Philadelphia*.
MANN (1927) : *Trans. Ophthal. Soc. U.K.*, **47**, 172.
MAWAS and MAGITOT (1912) : *Arch. Anat. micr.*, **14,** 41.
NUSSBAUM (1901) : *Arch. mikr. Anat.*, **58,** 199.
SZILY, A. VON (1921) : *v. Graefe's Archiv. Ophthal.*, **106,** 195.
—— (1903) : *Anat. Anz.*, **24,** 417.
—— (1908) : *Anat. Hefte*, **35,** 649.

CHAPTER X

COMPARATIVE ANATOMY

RESPONSE to the light stimulus does not in itself indicate an organ of vision. We know that many inorganic substances react to light. One of the most remarkable examples of this is seen in the photographic plate. Also, as is well known, a colourless solution of eserine goes pink when exposed to light.

Plants, too, respond to light. Thus the portions above ground as a rule grow towards the light (positive phototropism) while the roots grow away from it (negative phototropism). Also the formation of chlorophyll, the hæmoglobin of plants, depends on the presence of light ; but we do not postulate an organ of vision.

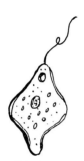
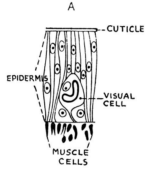
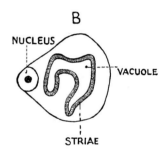

FIG. 418.—EUGLENA VIRIDIS (A FLAGELLATE) WITH ITS "EYE-SPOT."

FIG. 419.—VISUAL CELL AND EPIDERMIS OF THE WORM STYLARIA LACUSTRIS.

(From Bütschli, after Hesse.)

FIG. 420.—THE VISUAL CELL UNDER GREATER MAGNIFICATION.

In the unicellular animals (amœbæ, infusoria) the animal usually reacts as a whole in its response to light ; thus the amœba crawls away from a beam of light thrown on it. On the other hand, *Paramœcium bursaria*, which contains algæ, swims towards the light which is necessary for its symbiotic chlorophyll-containing partners to build up starch and sugar. But even in the protozoa there may be some specialisation. Thus Engelmann found that the anterior portion of *Euglena viridis*, an infusorian, is much more sensitive to light than the posterior. In this anterior portion he described an " eye-spot " which at first he thought was the most primitive eye. But later he found that the area most sensitive to light was in front of this. In stentor, another protozoon, the anterior end also is especially susceptible. When light falls on this part, the animal turns away and seeks a shady corner.

In the multicellular animals (metazoa) there is further specialisation.   In the earthworm, for instance, there are specialised visual cells first described by Hesse in 1895 and since found in many other animals.   Each cell is shorter and wider than the other epithelial cells among which it is placed ; also, the protoplasm is

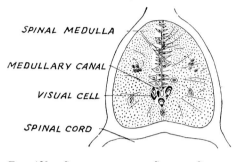

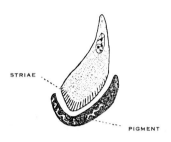

FIG. 421.—SECTION OF THE SPINAL CORD
OF AMPHIOXUS.

(From Poirier, after Hesse.)

FIG. 422.—VISUAL CELL OF
AMPHIOXUS.

clearer and contains vacuoles ; at its proximal end it is continued into a filament, probably a nerve fibril (see also p. 472).

Earthworms are sensitive to bright light and crawl away from it.   They come out of their burrows before dawn to feed, but, at break of day, they return.

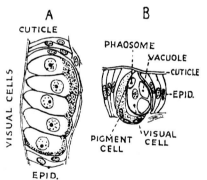

FIG. 423.—THE EYE OF STYLARIA
LACUSTRIS.

A = on transverse section.
B = on horizontal section.

(From Bütschli, after Hesse.)

The return to the burrow is an expression of negative phototropism.

In passing up the animal scale, we find that to arrive at true vision we pass through three stages :

(*a*) **Phototropism.**—The animal as a whole moves either towards or away from the source of light (positive or negative phototropism), as we saw in the *Paramœcium bursaria* and amœba.

(*b*) **Sensation.**—Here the animal receives the light stimulus by a special mechanism, but does not recognise it as light.   As an example of this, we saw how the earthworm avoids sunlight.   Also the tubeworm rapidly withdraws its feathery tentacles (each of which is possessed of an " eye ") when the light falling on it is shaded.   This " shading reaction " (an expression of negative phototropism) is present in many sluggish and sessile shore creatures.   It is obviously protective.   A fish in search of food casts a tell-tale shadow.   This shadow will cause barnacles to close, sea squirts to contract up into gelatinous blobs, and burrowing bivalves to withdraw their soft protruding syphons into the sand. On the other hand, a sudden shading of the light will cause the sea urchin to bristle up its spines. Thus, this " shading reaction " enables the invertebrate to hide or arm itself at the approach of its enemies.

(c) **Specific Sensation.**—Here the animal, owing to the development of the central nervous mechanism of vision, recognises the light as light. It is only animals which have the last type of vision which really *see* in the true sense of the word.

CLASSIFICATION OF THE TWO BIG GROUPS OF VISUAL ORGANS

A. **The epithelial eye of invertebrates** developed from the skin.

- Simple eye :
  - 1. Single epithelial cell.
  - 2. A collection of epithelial cells :
    - (a) Flat.
    - (b) Cup-shaped.
    - (c) Vesicular.
- Compound or faceted eye.

B. **The cerebral eye of vertebrates** developed from the central nervous system.

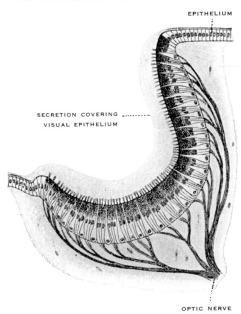

EPITHELIUM

SECRETION COVERING
VISUAL EPITHELIUM

OPTIC NERVE

FIG. 424.—THE EYE OF PATELLA—A MOLLUSC (STILL WIDE OPEN ON TO THE SURFACE).

The visual epithelium consists of pigmented visual cells and non-pigmented secretory cells.

(*From Hesse.*)

A. The most rudimentary " eye " is the visual cell. This, as we have seen, is an epithelial cell, but slightly differentiated and well seen in worms.

In the next stage we find a mantle of pigment associated with the cell (Fig. 422). The pigment is there to absorb the light and to convert it into heat and possibly other forms of energy. In amphioxus these visual cells lie deep next the medullary canal (Fig. 421). A further stage is seen in the worm, *Stylaria lacustris*, in which a number of these cells have become grouped together (Fig. 423). Such a rudimentary eye, whether consisting of one or more cells, is called an ocellus (= little eye).

Cup-shaped Eyes.—In these the visual cells of the surface epithelium have sunk in so as to line a fossa or cup. Thus there is a greater crowding together of visual elements and a better orientation of the incident light. They have (as we say in certain cases of cataract) fair projection (*yeux à direction*).

These eyes, although superior to the flat eyes, and although they have arrived at a certain degree of differentiation, consist almost exclusively of visual cells. They form a simple depression, open widely on the surface (Fig. 424). A further advance is seen where the opening is more or less closed, the " eyes " then opening on the surface by a small hole or " pupil " only (Fig. 427). These latter are formed on the principle of the pin-hole camera—i.e. a dark chamber with a small hole leading into it.

A further stage is seen where, apart from the visual cells, a kind of lens formed by the cuticle is present, and between the lens and the retina a kind of vitreous

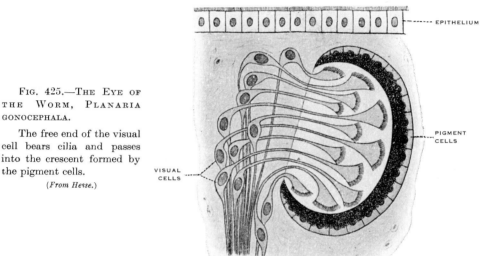

FIG. 425.—THE EYE OF THE WORM, PLANARIA GONOCEPHALA.

The free end of the visual cell bears cilia and passes into the crescent formed by the pigment cells.

(*From Hesse.*)

substance. This is formed by secretory cells placed among the visual cells (Fig. 429).

Cup-shaped eyes are seen in the arthropods and molluscs.

Vesicular Eyes.—This is a further stage in development. Here, the opening in the depression is closed so that the eye forms a vesicle, which sinks in from the surface and becomes covered over by surface epithelium (Figs. 430, 431).

Such eyes are seen in the ocelli of spiders and scorpions and in cephalopods, which have the most differentiated invertebrate eye. Nautilus, a cephalopod, however, still has a simple cup-shaped eye which opens on the surface (Fig. 427).

In the cephalopods (Fig. 433) the eye is partially contained in a cartilaginous orbit. The proximal (deepest) part of the vesicle forms the retina, the distal part is responsible for the posterior portion of the lens. The surface ectoderm becomes thickened to form the anterior portion of the lens (which joins the posterior part), and is so folded that it forms a kind of iris, pupil, cornea, and anterior chamber which is open at one point to the surrounding fluid in which the animal lives. The mesoderm between the optic vesicle and the ectoderm forms two laminæ of cartilage (equatorial and iridic), and outside these is formed the silvery membrane or tunic which passes forwards to the pupil. Ciliary and iridic muscles are also found, so that accommodation and pupillary movements are provided.

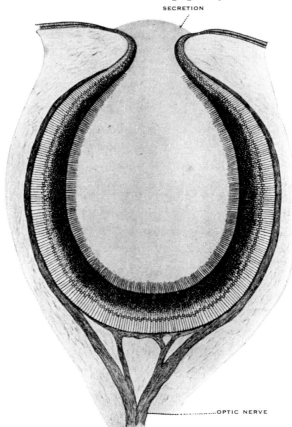

FIG. 426.—THE EYE OF THE SNAIL HALIOTIS.
(The opening is much narrower than in Fig. 424.)
(*From Hesse.*)

The Compound or Faceted Eye is found in the arthropods, especially in the crustaceans and insects. It is formed by the union of a number of modified ocelli. Each ocellus, which goes to form such an eye, is called an ommatidium (resembling an eye). The number of ommatidia varies from one to many thousands.

An ommatidium usually consists of the following : the dioptric apparatus is formed by a corneal facet and a lens cone. Behind this are the retinal elements, usually four to eight to each corneal facet forming a *single* unit, from which a single nerve fibre passes to a collection of nerve cells, the optic ganglion.

It is the fact that in the ommatidium a number of retinal elements are structurally and functionally united to form a single unit *the retinule*, which distinguishes it from the ordinary ocellus.

The whole eye usually forms a portion of a sphere and on section is fan-shaped.

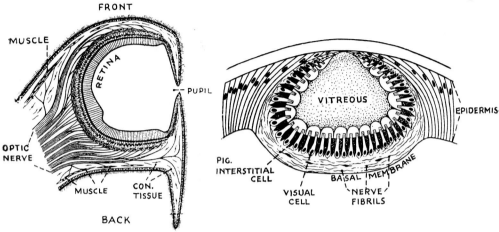

FIG. 427.—THE EYE OF NAUTILUS, A
CEPHALOPOD.
(*From Bütschli.*)

FIG. 428.—THE EYE OF THE CARNIVOROUS WORM,
NEREIS CULTRIFERA.
(*From Bütschli, after Hesse.*)

The surface, which is formed by the corneal facets united together, appears smooth to the naked eye, but under the loupe or microscope it forms a mosaic.

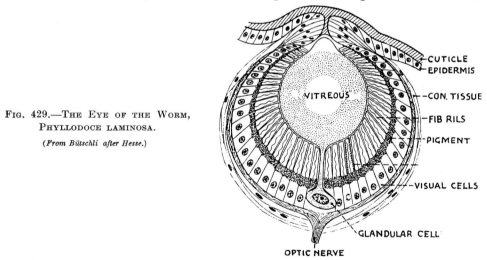

FIG. 429.—THE EYE OF THE WORM,
PHYLLODOCE LAMINOSA.
(*From Bütschli after Hesse.*)

The facets are hexagonal in the insects, quadrilateral in crustaceans, and convex in butterflies.

B. **The Vertebrate or Cerebral Eye.**—Unlike that of the invertebrate, the vertebrate eye is remarkable for the uniformity of its development and general structure.

Generally speaking, the cerebral eye consists of a retina, a dark chamber, and a dioptric apparatus.

There are, however, exceptions, such, for instance, as in the cyclostomes, *Proteus anguineus*, amphioxus, ascidia, the mole, and others.

In the cyclostomes generally the eye is a simple vesicle under the skin ; only in the adult lamprey is it more developed, and one finds traces of a lens, cornea,

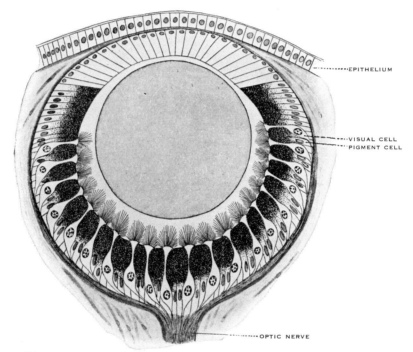

Fig. 430.—The Eye of the Snail, Helix pomatia (completely cut off from the surface).

(*From Hesse.*)

The visual cells have cilia.   The space between the lens and retina is filled with secretion.

and iris.   In the larva of this animal the lens is still a vesicle.   The myxinoids have no lens.

The Proteidæ or amphibian urodeles are cave-dwellers.   In them the eye is also a simple vesicle under the skin and does not contain a differentiated refracting apparatus.   The eye has no orbital cavity (Configliachi and Rusconi), and is practically hidden in the masseter muscles.   It is very rudimentary, about 0·5 mm. in diameter, and seen with difficulty as a dark shadow under the skin.

In the mole the eye is more differentiated, but is still very small, being about 2 mm. in diameter.   It is practically covered by the skin, in which there is always, however, a small hole (Ciaccio).   This varies from 0·125 to 0·975 mm. in the *seeing* mole (*Talpa Europa*), to 0·50 to 0·20 in the blind mole (*Talpa cœca*).

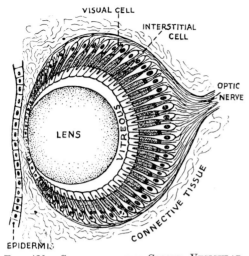

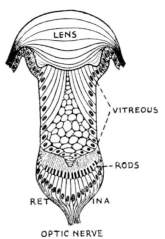

FIG. 431.—SCHEME OF THE CLOSED VESICULAR EYE OF A GASTROPODE MOLLUSC.

(From Bütschli.)

FIG. 432.—SECTION OF THE OCELLUS OF THE SPIDER, SAL-TICUS.

(From Bütschli, after Grenacher.

At any rate, in the latter type the hole is too small for vision, and as was already realised by Dante, the mole sees through its skin.

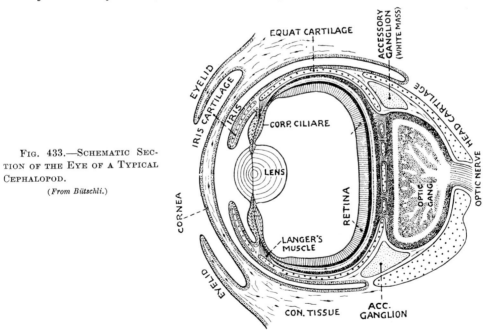

FIG. 433.—SCHEMATIC SEC-TION OF THE EYE OF A TYPICAL CEPHALOPOD.

(From Bütschli.)

Then there is the *Lancelet (amphioxus)*, belonging to the acraniate fishes, which really lies between the invertebrates and vertebrates. Its " eyes " are unicellular ocelli, which are placed next the medullary canal (Figs. 421 and 422) and thus far from the surface. The light can reach the eyes because the animal is small and transparent.

The " eyes " of amphioxus, too, are said to lie between the invertebrate and vertebrate types. Here the eyes have sunk into the depths, but have not grown back to the surface as do the cerebral eyes.

In the larva of ascidia, also, a rudimentary eye is attached to the medullary canal.

Thus in the genesis of the vertebrate eye there are three stages :

(*a*) Development of the eye from the surface ectoderm (epithelial eye of invertebrates).

(*b*) The eye sinks in to lie next the medullary canal (amphioxus, larva of ascidia (sea-squirt)).

(*c*) The eye grows out again to the surface (cerebral eye of vertebrates).

In the epithelial eye of the invertebrates as a rule [1] the light strikes the retinal cells before the nerve and the retina is called a verted or converse retina.

In the cerebral eye of vertebrates, the retina being produced from the anterior " invaginated " portion of the optic vesicle, the light strikes the nerve fibres first, and the retina is said to be of the inverted type.

THE COMPARATIVE ANATOMY OF THE RETINA

The Retina of the Invertebrates.—The invertebrate retina consists of visual cells and their processes. In the vertebrate retina to these are added the bipolar, the ganglion cells, and supporting fibres.

The visual cells of the invertebrate are of two main kinds :

(*a*) A cell with a ciliated border or a striated zone (" Stiftchensaum " of Hesse).

(*b*) A rod-like cell.

The latter is the only form that obtains in the vertebrate retina. A third type of visual cell is one with a phaosome or phaosphere, i.e. a large vacuole which undergoes changes when exposed to the light (Fig. 423, B).

(*a*) CELLS WITH A STRIATED ZONE

The single cell constituting the primitive eye may be ciliated. Often the cells contain large vacuoles round which the striæ are arranged (e.g. in the leech) (Figs. 422, 434).

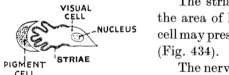

VISUAL CELL

NUCLEUS

PIGMENT CELL   STRIAE

FIG. 434.—EYE OF TREMATODE WORM (TRISTOMUM PAPILLOSUM).

(*From Bütschli, after Hesse*)

The striated portion is often enlarged to increase the area of light reception, and, to the same end, the cell may present digitations as in *Tristomum papillosum* (Fig. 434).

The nerve fibre leaves the cell opposite the striated region and, indeed, according to Hesse, is continuous through the cell with the cilia.

[1] Exceptions are seen in the shell-fish, pecten, and in spiders (Fig. 438).

(b) Rod-like Cell

These are found in many worms, in the ocelli of arthropods and in the eyes of molluscs.

These visual cells also form the neuro-epithelium of the vertebrate retina and are usually arranged in a single layer. But in the mollusc (*Pecten jacobeus*) there are two layers of cells between which are the nerve fibres, and behind the proximal visual cells there is a layer of epithelial cells rich in pigment (Fig. 439). In the cephalopods the visual cells are rod-like and form a single layer resting on the choroidal cartilage.

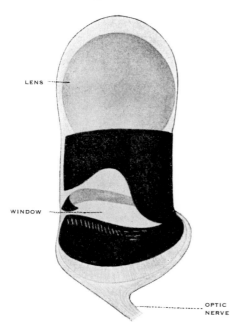

Fig. 435.—The Telescopic Eye of Pterotrachea coronata. a Mollusc.

(*From Hesse.*)

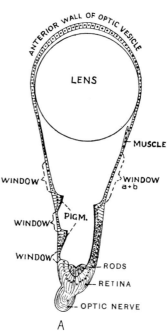

Fig. 436.—Telescopic Eye
of Pterotrachea coronata, on
Section.

(*From Bütschli, after Hesse.*)

The nerve fibres leave the eye posteriorly by several holes in the cartilage.

Generally speaking, the nerve fibres pass into a ganglion which may be directly behind the eye or in the central nervous system.

The Retina of the Vertebrates is generally more complex than that of the invertebrates. Here we find three neurones. The neuro-epithelium is nearest the sclera.

Rods and cones are found in all classes of vertebrates except in certain rudimentary forms. Amphioxus is of course an exception, having only unicellular " eyes " (Fig. 421).

Some have more cones, others more rods.

As we pass up the animal scale, we find more and more rods and cones per sq. mm.   Thus Mann (1928) found in a strip of retina 1 mm. long and 0·1 mm.

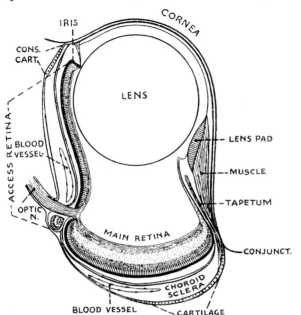

Fig. 437.—The Telescopic Eye of a Deep-sea Bony Fish, Disomma anale.

(From Bütschli, after Brauer.)

wide 100 cones in the lamprey, 125 in the frog, 327 in the hen, while at the human macula there were 652.

Generally speaking, there are the same layers as in the human.

The Pigment Epithelium is much the same in all classes of vertebrates, but it may contain, apart from pigment, oil droplets in great variety, and crystals of guanine.

The pigment is morphologically different from that of the choroid.

In the choroid it is almost entirely amorphous, in the retina crystalline (Greeff).   In the retina the pigment is epithelial in origin, in the choroid mesodermal.

In those animals which have a tapetum the retinal pigment in the region of the tapetum is absent.

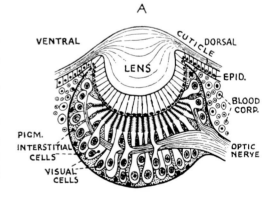

Fig. 438.—The Inverse Eye of the Spider, Tegenaria domestica.

(From Bütschli, after Widman.)

In the outer nuclear layer one finds in certain vertebrates the fibres (massues) of Landolt.   These are filaments ending in knobs towards the outer limiting membrane and probably derived from the bipolar cells (inner nuclear layer).

The Area Centralis.—In all vertebrates there is found an area where the visual cells are narrower and more closely packed—an area of more acute vision than the rest of the fundus.

Such an area has even been described in some invertebrates ; for instance, Hess found it in some cephalopods, and a trace of it is seen in certain plathelminths (flat worms), and also in many insects. Now, while these areas result in some advance in visual acuity over the rest of the fundus, it can be nothing like the specialisation first really seen in tarsius. In man and in many monkeys the area is characterised by a yellow pigment, hence the name macula lutea (see p. 142). In the centre of this is found the fovea centralis.

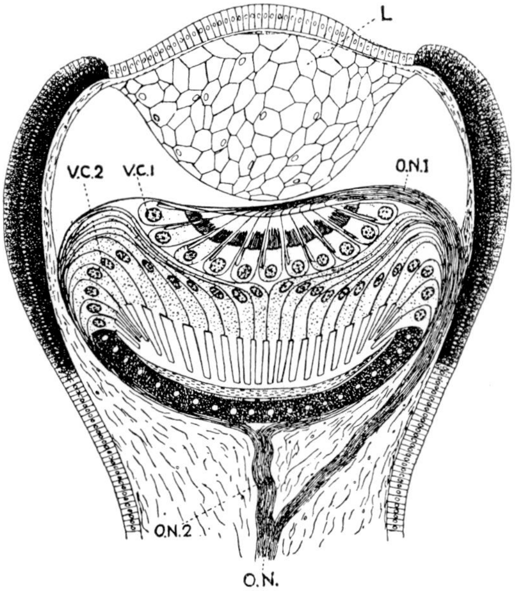

The Retina of Fishes is complex, and differs much in the different species. In general, however, it resembles that of the mammals.

The pigment epithelium is often characterised by numerous granules of guanine (Kühne), especially in the cyprinidæ, perch, and bream.

Fig. 439.—The Eye of the Mollusc, Pecten Jacobeus.
(*From Hesse.*)

L. = lens. V.C.1 = first layer of visual cells. O.N.1 = nerve fibres from this layer. V.C.2 = second layer of visual cells. O.N.2 = nerve fibres from this layer. O.N. = optic nerve.

These granules may be brilliant white or reddish yellow in colour. They were first described in 1836 by Della Chaie, who called them ophthalmoliths.

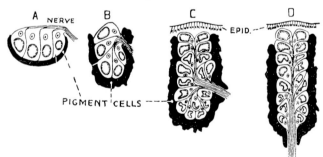

Fig. 440.—Schematic Representation of Stages in the Change from the Inverse Eye of Clespine (A) and Nephelis (B) to the Converse Eye of the Leech (Hirudo) (D).
(*From Bütschli, after Hesse.*)

They are abundant, especially in the upper part of the eye, and, from the reflex to which they give rise, have been mistaken for a tapetum.

The rods and cones are very long, so that, especially in the bony fishes, the neuro-epithelium may occupy one-third to one-half the whole thickness of the retina (Max Schultze). The rods and cones often resemble each other very closely, and Greeff and Max Schultze doubted the existence of the latter in selachians (shark).

The largest cones are found in the perch, where they are often double (Fig. 441, B). Usually there are no oil droplets, but M. Schultze found colourless ones in the sturgeon between the outer and inner segments of the cones. A kind of membrane or cloak is often seen round the rods and cones.

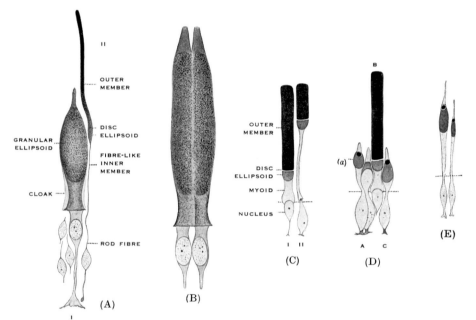

FIG. 441.—(A) ROD (II) AND CONE (I) OF THE PERCH. (B) LARGE DOUBLE (OR TWIN) CONE OF THE PERCH. (C) RED (I) AND GREEN (II) RODS OF THE FROG. (D) VISUAL CELLS FROM THE RETINA OF A FROG WHICH HAS BEEN IN STRONG LIGHT (A = double cone, one part (a) of which has an oil droplet. B = rod. C = cone with oil droplet). (E) CONES OF THE SPARROW (note oil droplets). (After Greeff.)

The outer nuclear layer has four rows usually, but there are six in the bream and one in the lamprey. Many medullated nerve fibres are found.

Area Centralis.—It used to be believed that there was no area centralis in fishes, but Carrière showed it in hippocampus and W. Krause in syngnathus, belonging to the lophobranchs. Hesse found it in cephalopods, in selachians (scyllium), and in the bony fishes, red mullet and the minnow.

THE RETINA OF AMPHIBIANS

Rods and cones are found, the former being usually more numerous.

They are much larger than in the human, the smallest being double the size of ours.

The pigment cells are very large, covering eight to fifteen visual cells in the frog. They contain numerous oil droplets. The frog has two kinds of rods :

(a) Violet-red, the larger and more numerous.

(b) Green.

The intercalated disc which lies between the inner and outer segments of the rods is better marked than in other animals (Fig. 441, C and D). Oil droplets are found between the two segments of the cones. They may be colourless or slightly yellow.

The visual cells all end in a ramifying footpiece. (Generally speaking, the cones end in this way and the rods in a knob.) Cajal describes double cones and rods.

The fibres of Landolt are more numerous than in any other vertebrates.

According to Nicati the nerve fibres from the right side of the retina go to the left side of the disc and vice versa. The author's (Wolff's) own preparations would corroborate this.

In *Proteus anguineus* and *Axolotl* (cave-dwellers), which belong to the urodele amphibians, the retina is primitive and little differentiated, and fills practically the whole bulb.

The Retina of Reptiles

The retina is generally characterised by the predominance of the cones over the rods. The crocodile and gecko are exceptions.

The pigment epithelium is like that of the vertebrates generally except in the crocodile, where in the upper part of the retina it contains guanine crystals as well as pigment.

The cones often contain oil droplets. They are abundant and coloured in the tortoise, fewer and almost colourless in the lizard.

The outer nuclear layer consists of two rows of large cells like those of the amphibians.

Both the rod and cone fibres end in a ramifying footpiece, and since this is the usual termination of the cone fibres, it was believed that only cones were present. *Rods and cones are, however, best distinguished by their connections rather than by the type of termination.* (Also by their staining reactions, see p. 113.)

[1] The inner nuclear layer is very wide. In the crocodile a horizontally striated area centralis is found. In the reptiles the cells of the pars ciliaris retinæ are very large.

The Retina of Birds

The retina of diurnal birds contains many cones and few rods. In the fowl and pigeon, however, in a certain area, coloured yellow in the former and red in the latter, the rods are more numerous.

In the nocturnal birds the rods are much more numerous.

The neuro-epithelium is especially distinguished by the *oil droplets*, which are more abundant here than in any other vertebrate. The oil droplets are situated

---

[1] See also I. C. Mann (Jan. 1933), *Brit. Ophthal.* Re macula of Sphenodon.

between the inner and outer segments of rods and cones, but more numerous in the latter (Fig. 441, E).

In the diurnal birds the droplets are of varied and bright colours. Most usually they are red, but there are different shades of yellow, green, and blue. In the nocturnal birds the droplets tend to be yellow.

The pigments producing these colours were called chromophanes by Kuhne.

In the postero-superior quadrant of the retina in fowls the yellow droplets predominate and give this area its yellow colour. The same quadrant in the pigeon is red, giving rise to the red area in these birds. The remaining portion of the fundi appears slightly red in fowls and slightly yellow in the pigeon, owing to predominance of these colours in the oil droplets.

The fibres of Müller are narrower, and in the distal portion of the inner granular layer break up, like those of the reptiles, into a brushwork of fibres.

Area Centralis and Fovea.—Birds have an area centralis, often two. A fovea is often present, and in some, including the pigeon and sparrow, H. Müller found two in each eye.

According to Rochon Duvigneaud the insect and grain-eating birds which have their eyes more or less lateral and whose visual axes make an angle of 120° or more with each other have a single fovea more or less central. The nocturnal birds of prey and the swallow have a double fovea, one central, the other lateral—the latter being placed behind and below the former.

In some birds a band-shaped area of acute vision may be associated with the macula. Where two maculæ are present, these may be joined by such a band (see Casey Wood, 1917).

The Retina of Mammals

A central area is present in practically all mammals, although it is said to be absent in the mouse, rat, and sheep. Only man and some monkeys have a true macula and fovea centralis subserving binocular and stereoscopic vision.

In tarsius, the sole surviving representative of a group between lemurs and monkeys, there is a great crowding together of the rods in the macular region, but there is no spreading apart of the various layers so that light may fall directly on the neuro-epithelium. This takes place first in the marmoset (Woollard, 1926).

Medullated Nerve Fibres in the Retina

What occurs as a rarity in man is normally present in a number of animals.

The rabbit has a well-marked horizontal band of opaque nerve fibres on either side of the disc (Fig. 443).

Johnson found medullated nerve fibres in the retina of perameles lagotis and other marsupials.

In the dog (Fig. 459) the nerve fibres of and all round the disc are medullated and Kolmer saw them in dentex and lophias.

THE CHOROID

The choroid is seen only in the vertebrate eye ; it is usually ½ mm. in thickness, but in the whale and seal may be greater than 1·5 mm.

The pigment is most abundant near its outer part, that is, in the suprachoroidal lamina, but is absent here in birds and fishes. Thus in the latter the *silvery membrane* (argentea), which is placed between the lamina suprachoroidea and the layer of large vessels, shows through.

Sattler in 1876 described in the human (in the macular region) a cellular membrane with elastic fibres which he believed was homologous with the tapetum of mammals.

The Silvery Membrane (argentea) of the choroid of fishes (especially of the bony fishes) is placed between the suprachoroidea and the large vessels. It extends over the whole choroid and also over the iris.

It is formed of crystals of guanine which give the membrane its brilliant white appearance, and are responsible for the metallic lustre of the iris of fishes and cephalopods.

The Choroidal Gland.—The choroid of fishes is thicker than that of other vertebrates, and has a spongy structure. It is very vascular, especially in its posterior part. The retina thus appears to rest on a vascular cushion. To this posterior thickened portion the name of choroidal gland has been given. It is particularly well developed in certain ganoid fishes such as amia, and in some bony fishes, for instance the angler fish (lophius).

The Tapetum is seen in most mammals. It is responsible for the green reflex seen in the cat's eye and the emerald green in that of the dog. It is best seen in the carnivores, ruminants, horse, cetaceæ, seals, and dolphin. One also finds it in fishes, but not in rodents, reptiles (except the crocodile), and amphibians.

The (Choroidal) Tapetum may be cellular or fibrous. It may occupy the whole fundus, but more often only the upper and back portion. It is found in the mammals and in certain cartilaginous fishes (skate, shark).

Among birds, only in the ostrich is there a rudiment of the tapetum, but even here it is covered by pigment. The bright reflex from the ostrich eye is (according to Sattler) produced by the basal lamina on the inner surface of choroid, which is especially thick in this animal.

The tapetum is placed just deep to the chorio-capillaris, and is visible because this and the retina are devoid of pigment.

Among the carnivores the tapetum is usually cellular, consisting of several layers of flattened cells.

Among the herbivora and dolphins the tapetum is fibrous, i.e. composed of fine fibres, also in several layers. The tapetum reflects the light strongly, and on account of its stratified structure diffracts the light and gives rise to the different colours seen in the fundus.

In the horse the tapetum is extensive ; in the lamb and ox it extends especially on the temporal side ; in the goat it is quadrilateral and symmetrical round the posterior pole. It is triangular in the roebuck, the dog, and the cat.

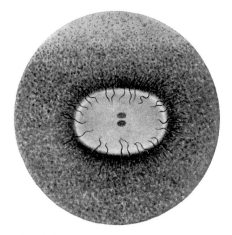

FIG. 442.—THE FUNDUS OF THE HORSE.

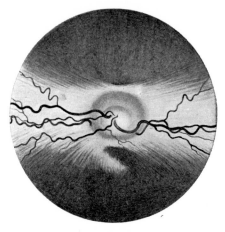

FIG. 443.—THE FUNDUS OF THE RABBIT.

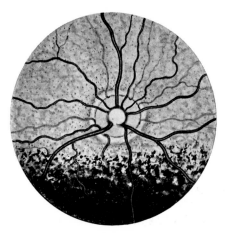

FIG. 444.—THE FUNDUS OF THE DOG.
The pale area above is the tapetum.

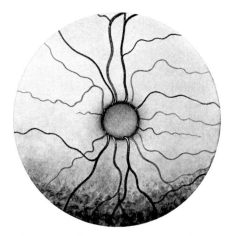

FIG. 445.—THE FUNDUS OF THE CAT.
The pale area above is the tapetum.

In the dog it is usually entirely above the disc, in the cat it reaches a little below this area. It is brighter in the carnivores than in the herbivores, and is thickest in the ox.

In some animals there is also what is called a *retinal tapetum*. It is formed of crystals of guanine, and occurs in certain bony fishes, especially the perch and cyprinoids (gold-fish). It is typical of the bream, and in the crocodile it is of the same nature. In the crocodile [1] the upper portion of the fundus is brilliantly white but becomes redder in the dark.

We must not forget, however, that in the higher molluscs (cephalopods) and in the bony fishes there is a silvery membrane (argentea), so called because the crystals which it contains give it a silvery brightness.

But this is not a tapetum, for it is placed outside the layer of large vessels and, being covered by pigment, is not seen from the interior of the eye (Ovio).

THE FUNDUS [2]

The Colour.—In those animals which have no tapetum the colour of the fundus comes from the blood in the choroid modified by the density of the pigment epithelium. Otherwise, it is the tapetum which is responsible for the colour.

A red colour in the fundus is seen in primates (including man, but excluding some lemurs), and also in some insectivores.

A yellow colour (principally) is seen in the prosimians, chiroptera, in some cats, elephants, and squirrels.

A green colour is the least frequent ; it is seen in some carnivora and in the ruminants, except the goat and camel, in which it is red.

In the ox the disc is pink and transversely oval. It has no physiological cup, and often remains of the hyaloid artery are seen on it. The retina is well vascularised. The fundus generally is red, but there is a large blurred green tapetum below the disc. The fundi of the other ruminants are similar, but the disc is round in the goat, semilunar in the sheep, and the tapetum is absent in the pig.

In the horse (Fig. 442) the disc also is transversely oval, and has no physiological cup. From it numerous small vessels run for a short distance only into the fundus (paurangiotic). The tapetum is greenish blue and above the disc. Generally the fundus is reddish grey, but varies with the colour of the animal. Myelinated fibres are often seen.

In the marmot and squirrel the disc forms a longish horizontal band. It is kidney-shaped in the wolf, jackal, and fox. It is white in lemurs, bats, rodents, edentates, marsupials, echidna ; bright red in the hedgehog and mole ; black or green in the galagos and loris. In the carnivores it may be white, grey, brown, maroon, or red.

In the guinea-pig the disc is small, round, greyish white and placed in a dark grey retina, which is almost devoid of vessels.

In the rabbit the disc is pale pink, transversely oval, and deeply excavated. It is continued at the sides into bands of medullated nerve fibres, to which the vessels are confined (Fig. 443). There are no retinal vessels on the rest of the fundus, but in the albino rabbit the choroidal vessels show through.

[1] Abelsdorff (1905), *Archiv. f. Augen.*, **53.**
[2] See Lindsay Johnson (1901), *Phil. Trans.*, Ser. B., **194,** 1–82.

A.E.—31

In the dog the disc is round or triangular. It is characterised by a well-marked venous ring (Fig. 444). The arteries are small, cilio-retinal, and leave the disc at its periphery. The tapetum is yellowish green, and for the most part in the upper part of the fundus. Remains of the hyaloid artery are not infrequently seen.

In the cat the disc is grey and round, and since the vessels leave it peripherally, it looks something like a glaucoma cup (Fig. 445). The bright reddish-green tapetum surrounds the disc and occupies the upper part of the fundus. Remains of the hyaloid artery are often seen.

In birds the fundus is difficult to see, owing to the fact that the pupil is small and does not dilate under atropin (Ovio). The disc is hidden by the pecten which is attached to it and its continuation downwards, which is known as the cauda.

In the pigeon the two foveæ are seen as dark spots.

In reptiles the disc is difficult to see owing to the small pupil. The hyaloid circulation is visible. In the crocodile the disc is black (Hirschberg, Abelsdorf).

In amphibians the circulation is visible in the hyaloid system owing partly to the great magnification produced by the lens and partly to the large size of the blood corpuscles.

In the frog the disc forms an oblique streak (see Hirschberg).

In fishes.—In the minnow the entrance of the optic nerve is marked by a round disc not well defined, which has a wing-like prolongation upwards and medially. The vessels converge on the disc and some project into the vitreous.

In the eel a disc is not seen, but the nerve entrance is marked by the point of convergence of the whitish nerve fibre bundles and the retinal vessels.

In the pike there is a worm-like streak provided with pigment, from the middle portion of which the nerve fibres radiate. No retinal vessels are seen.

The selachians have no hyaloid or retinal vessels.

Among the bony fishes many have a hyaloid network which Virchow divides into three types :

(*a*) The hyaloid artery and vein enter at the ora serrata (ganoids).

(*b*) The artery enters at the disc, and the vein leaves at the ora serrata (gold-fish).

(*c*) Both enter at the disc (eel).

In the cephalopods there are many discs, as the optic nerve enters through a number of holes (Fig. 433).

THE CILIARY BODY

In the human eye and that of the higher apes we find the ciliary body formed of two portions :

(*a*) Muscular.

(*b*) Ciliary processes (essentially vessels).

There is an analogous organ in the cephalopods, in which a structure similar to the iris is also seen (Fig. 433), but apart from this a ciliary body is only found in the vertebrates, in which, however, it varies greatly. The muscular portion is the more constant.

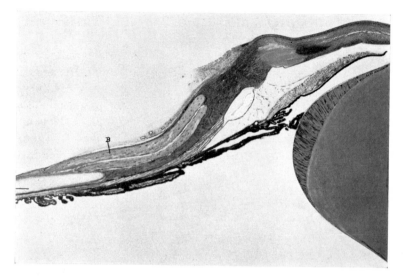

FIG. 446.—NORMAL FOWL'S EYE. ANTERO-POSTERIOR SECTION.

Note especially the normal adhesion of the ciliary process to the lens pad, which largely takes the place of our suspensory ligament, the large sinus venosus scleræ, and the bone and cartilage in the sclera.

The Ciliary Processes are absent, or practically so, in fishes and amphibians. In birds their number may be 200 as compared with 70 in man.

They may be so large as to leave an impression on the lens. In the human

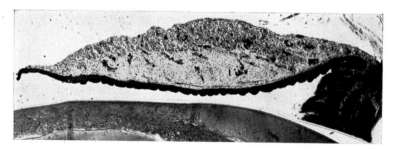

FIG. 447.—DETAIL OF FIGURE 446. IRIS AND LENS OF FOWL.

Note sphincter of iris is anterior. Note also adhesion of ciliary process to lens (in place of suspensory ligament). Compare human embryo at three months (Fig. 353).

the ciliary processes do not touch the lens (0·5 mm. away), nor are they in contact with the iris. But in some animals such as the rabbit they are in contact, a condition which obtains in the human embryo up to the last months.

The Ciliary Muscle.—In mammals there are two portions :

(*a*) Peripheral = muscle of Brücke.

(*b*) Central = muscle of Müller.

In birds there are three portions, the two above and an anterior portion known as Crampton's muscle, which is striped.

This passes from the deepest layers in the cornea to the anterior part of the sclera. The size of the ciliary body depends on the amount of accommodation and not on the amount of intraocular fluid. Thus in man the ciliary muscle is more developed than in other mammals. In the ass the amplitude of accommodation is 16D, in the dog 2·5 to 3·5D, and in the cat only 1D (Hess and Heine). It is feeble in herbivora and rodents, who have little power of accommodation, but well developed in diving birds and those that fly swiftly ; for instance, the swallow.

In birds (and reptiles) the contraction of the ciliary and Crampton's muscles raises the pressure in the vitreous. This pushes on the lens, which, being held peripherally by the iris, can only bulge forward axially. In most birds, except the nocturnal species, the power of accommodation is very great. Hess found 40 to 50D in the cormorant.

In the bony fishes, in which there is only a rudiment of a ciliary body, there is hardly a trace of ciliary muscle. In fact some authors deny the existence of a muscle and describe a ciliary ligament which binds the ciliary body to the corneosclera.

Fishes whose eyes are normally fixed for near vision have to accommodate for distance. This is done by the retractor lentis muscle which pulls the whole lens backwards. In some amphibians a high degree of miosis takes the place of accommodation, while in others the lens is pulled forwards by the protractor lentis (Hess).

The ciliary muscle and that of the iris in birds and reptiles (sauropsida) are striated, while in mammals they are smooth.

The Iris

Arthropods.—When we speak of the iris of the arthropod we mean the pigment and iridic tapetum. Each facet of the compound eye when looked at with the microscope appears to have a pupil surrounded by pigment.

Cephalopods have a real iris with pigment and a double sphincter and dilator. The pupil in the cephalopods is horseshoe-shaped, and in some species on contracting it forms a straight or curved line, which, however, remains open at the extremities. This type of dumb-bell-like pupil is also seen in scyllium.

Vertebrates always have an iris. It is, however, rudimentary in some deepsea fishes with telescopic eyes.

In fishes the iris has a metallic lustre owing to the crystals of guanine in the silvery membrane which extends into the iris. The same applies to the iris of cephalopods. Here the membrane is partially covered by chromatophores which give the iris its special colours.

The amphibians and reptiles have similar reflexes, but it is doubtful whether these are due to crystals of guanine, although they are present in the crocodile and chameleon.

Among birds the iris is brown in the singing varieties, yellow in the birds of prey. The heron, parrots, and pheasants have reddish irides, due to oil droplets of different refractions rather than to micro-crystals. Almost always the iris of birds has a black edge which may make the pupil appear larger than it really is.

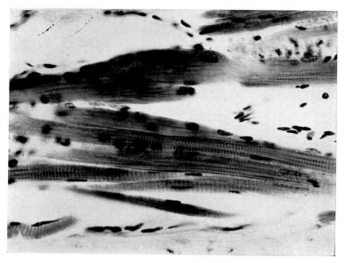

FIG. 448.—STRIPED CILIARY MUSCLE FIBRES OF FOWL.
(*McDonagh and Wolff, Brit. Journ. Ophth.*, 1939.)

The musculature of the iris, like that of the ciliary body, is striped in the sauropsida (birds and reptiles) and smooth in all other vertebrates.

In the fishes, amphibians, and cephalopods the muscles are rich in pigment.

In the lower animals there are no iris crypts, and the anterior epithelium is well marked.

The pupil, when constricted, is not always round ; when dilated it is always more or less circular. It is round as in the human in birds, except the owl, in many reptiles and fishes, and even in some amphibians.

The pupil is oval with the long axis horizontal in the horse, ox, goat, kangaroo, and in certain fishes ; oval with long axis vertical in the seal and alligator ; vertical slit in the cat, fox, and owl.

In nocturnal selachians, such as scyllium, torpedo, etc., it is a slit.

There is a pupillary operculum in the skate, and in pleuronectes (sole, etc.), which swim on their sides near the bottom of the sea, the pupil not only closes completely, but the upper part hangs over the lower. This is possibly analogous to the nodules of pigment (flocculi or corpora nigra) seen at the edge of the pupil of the horse and also to ectropion uveæ, which is met with as a congenital anomaly in man.

In the sauropsida the pupil is often displaced nasally and downwards (corectopia) ; in the amphibians downwards, and in the salamander upwards. Gecko has a vertical slit with irregular borders.

In some animals the pupil extends beyond the lens so that an aphakic portion is present, as obtains after iridectomy in the human. This is especially seen in some bony fishes.

It would seem that the essential structure of the adult iris in the different species of animals is determined by the embryonic ocular circulation, especially the presence or absence of a pupillary membrane and the number and position of the branches of the hyaloid artery.

The pupillary membrane exists only in mammals, who alone possess the arterio-venous anastomosis of the lesser circle. The vascular pattern of the iris is necessarily different in submammalian species. The degree of pigmentation and the shape of the pupil, however, are at any rate in part determined by function or habitat (see Mann, I. (1931), *Trans. Zool. Soc.*, Part 4 and *Developmental Abnormalities of the Eye*, 1957).

THE DIOPTRIC APPARATUS

In the most primitive eyes, such as that of the worm, *Stylaria lacustris* (Figs. 419, 423), the light acts directly on the epithelial cells of which it is composed, without first passing through a dioptric apparatus.

But soon a rudimentary refractive mechanism appears. It may be a simple transparent mass secreted by the epithelial cells, or it may be the cuticle covering the eye which becomes thick and transparent, or it may be the visual cells themselves which become differentiated into bodies refracting the light so as to focus it on the visual cells proper.

In the cephalopods there is a cornea-lens. This consists of two half-spheres in contact with each other.

A transparent mass, the primitive vitreous, always fills the cavity of the eye. Generally it is secreted by the indifferent cells which lie between the visual cells.

In *Phillodoce laminosa* there is only one of these secretory cells, but it is very large (Fig. 429).

In the compound or faceted eyes each " eye " has a small transparent cornea behind which is a cone-shaped lens.

THE CORNEA

Vertebrates.—*The cornea* is constant in vertebrates. It is generally larger in mammals and fishes, and, relative to the bulb, smaller in birds and reptiles, larger in nocturnal than diurnal birds.

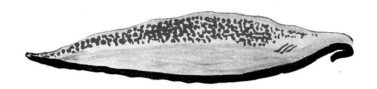

FIG. 449.—IRIS OF FOWL, STAINED WITH SUDAN III, TO SHOW FAT IN THE SPHINCTER MUSCLE
WHICH IS HERE PLACED ANTERIORLY (SEE FIG. 447).

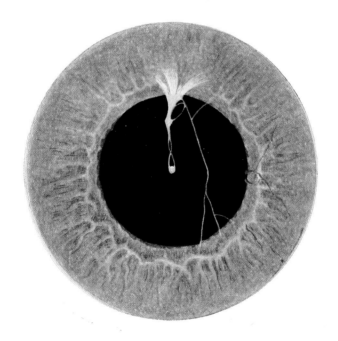

FIG. 450.—PERSISTENT PUPILLARY MEMBRANE AND TWO CAPSULO-PUPILLARY VESSELS.
(*From Mann: Developmental Abnormalities of the Eye, 2nd edition. British Medical Association. After Quarry Silcock.*)

In the cat and rabbit it is one-third of the bulb, in the bat and mouse one-half of the bulb.

It is more or less flat in fishes, acuminate in nocturnal birds. In several species of parrot it forms a keratoconus, while it is also prominent in the mole. In the whale and seals there is a high degree of astigmatism. In the horse the cornea is pear-shaped, being larger on the temporal side. Generally the astigmatism is greater in eyes with an oval or slit-like pupil.

The corneal epithelium is very thick in fishes and lies almost loose and not smooth as in the human. In some terrestrial animals the superficial layers are keratinised. Tetrophthalmus swims on the surface of the water with half its cornea out of the water and half in. Here only the upper half is keratinised. In man the epithelium has 5 layers (Virchow) (6 according to Ciaccio), the horse 20 (Virchow), amphibians 2–4, the ox 8–10, the rabbit 6.

In the calf, sheep, guinea-pig, chimpanzee, and in many birds and fishes, the corneal epithelium is so pigmented that this can be seen with the naked eye. With the microscope, pigment can be found in most corneæ.

In some cyprins (gold-fish) the cornea is vascularised, in others only during embryonic life.

In man the cornea is never vascularised except in disease.

In fishes and aquatic mammals the cornea is many times thicker at the periphery than at the centre.

The substantia propria in the lower vertebrates consists of regular lamellæ throughout. In man and the higher vertebrates this obtains in the central area only. Elsewhere it is broken up by the " fibrous cordage " superficially, and by elastic fibres in the deeper parts. The cornea is a powerful lens, but only in those animals which live in the air. It loses its refractive power in water. Gullstrand says the cornea in man has a refractive power of 43D and the lens 19D, i.e. more than double.

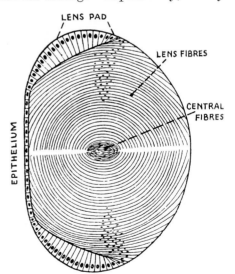

FIG. 451.—THE LENS OF LACERTA (LIZARD).
(*From Bütschli, after Rabl.*)

THE LENS

Generally speaking, as we pass up the vertebrate scale the lens becomes less and less spherical, but in fishes it is nearly round and often protrudes anteriorly to be almost in contact with the cornea. This is due to the fact that the cornea has no refractive power and the lens has to make up for it. In amphibians it forms a sphere, but is flattened anteriorly. Not

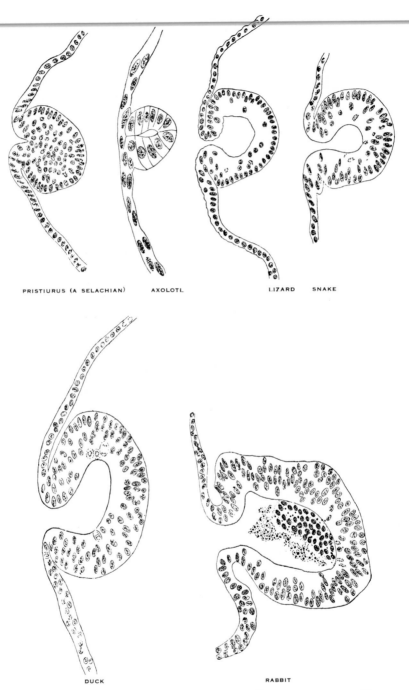

PRISTIURUS (A SELACHIAN)　　AXOLOTL　　　　LIZARD　　SNAKE

DUCK　　　　　　　　　　　　RABBIT

FIG. 452.—THE PRIMORDIUM OF THE LENS AT THE SAME STAGE IN DIFFERENT VERTEBRATES

Note that the debris of cells inside the saccule is found only in the mammal.

(*From Rabl.*)

infrequently one finds a lenticonus anterior or posterior. This is seen especially in the falcon and finch.

Among mammals the mouse and rat have a spherical lens. In the carnivores the lens is more convex anteriorly; in the herbivores and primates it is the posterior surface which is more convex.

As regards size, the nocturnal animals have a large lens, but in the owl it is small. In some fishes it is very big (moon-fish and whiting).

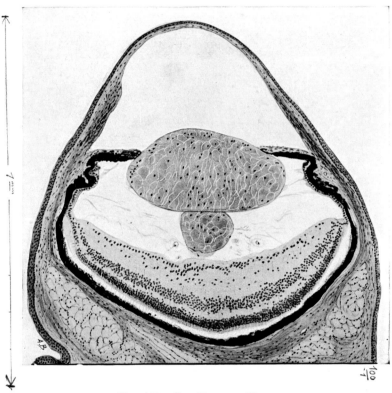

FIG. 453.—THE EYE OF A MOLE.

This presents a conical cornea with thinning of the central portion and a very deep anterior chamber. There is a curious hernia of lens substance which almost touches the retina.

(*From Rochon-Duvigneaud.*)

The nuclear zone in sauropsida (birds and reptiles) develops in a peculiar way to form the soft lens pad (Fig. 451). This is well developed in the chameleon and lizards and is huge in birds. It probably has to do with the amplitude of accommodation.

The general structure of the lens is the same in all vertebrates. In some animals (horse) the capsule is very thick and composed of many layers.

Lens Sutures

There are three types of suture (Rochon-Duvigneaud).

(1) *A Punctiform* central suture like a little (non-depressed) umbilicus with irregular borders. It is seen in birds, some bony fishes, and reptiles, and is produced by a great tapering of the lens fibres from the equator backwards and forwards so that the ends are so small that they can be accommodated in the small round suture (Fig. 454a).

(2) *A Straight Line* often quite short. This type of suture is seen in many selachians, bony fishes, and in the rabbit, etc. It is produced by the fact that although they taper somewhat the ends are too large to end in a point suture and so they have to be accommodated on a line (Fig. 454b).

(3) *Star-shaped Suture.* This type of suture is seen in mammals and especially in man. Here the ends, although there is *always* some tapering, are wider still and require more room than could be furnished by a straight line, which therefore

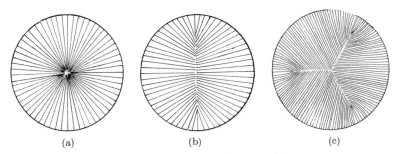

(a)   (b)   (c)

Fig. 454.—Different Types of Lens Suture.

(a) Lens of a pigeon, showing the sutures terminating anteriorly in a central point.
(b) Lens of oxyrhina spallanzani with a simple linear suture.
(c) Lens of a guinea pig with a triradiate suture.

(From Rochon-Duvigneaud.)

bifurcates, producing a star with three branches (Fig. 454c). More branches are often necessary.

It will thus be seen that the usual description of the lens fibres as bands with parallel borders is incorrect. They must taper in varying degrees from the equator towards the two poles.

The multiplication of sutures—there may be six or even nine in the human—is brought about by a large number of short fibres ; these stop short and create a number of secondary sutures which complicate the primary three of the newborn.

Suspensory Apparatus

The lens is held in position by the ciliary zonule of Zinn in all vertebrates. In birds the zonule, although less extensive, is much stronger than in mammals, and much more like a ligament between the lens and the ciliary processes (Figs.

446 and 447).   In fishes it is reduced to a triangular band consisting of strong fibres which are attached to the upper pole only of the spherical lens.

Fishes and amphibians have muscles in connection with the lens.

Fishes have the muscle of the campanule or retractor lentis.   It runs from the falciform process, and is attached to the back of the lens below and to the nasal side of its centre.   It pulls the lens laterally and backwards and is associated with accommodation.

In amphibians there is a protractor lentis.   In the urodeles it is a filament which runs from the summit of a ciliary process to the corneo-scleral junction. It is in relation with the foetal fissure, and appears to be of ectodermal origin. It pulls the lens forwards.

In the frog there are two protractor lentis muscles, one ventral, the other dorsal.

In some fishes, too, a retractor lentis arises from the region of the choroidal fissure.

Anterior Chamber

In cephalopods the anterior chamber is very large, reaching to the back of the bulb, and since in these animals the cornea is perforate, it is filled with the fluid in which the animal lives.

But in those whose cornea is not perforate (cuttle-fish, octopus) it is filled with a fluid analogous to our aqueous.

The anterior chamber is very large in birds and small in fishes.   In some birds it may be 8 mm. deep.

In the cat it is 2·5 times greater than in man.

The Vitreous

The vitreous is not entirely analogous to the primitive vitreous which fills the eye of invertebrates and which is a simple secretion (see p. 486).

Organs of Protection

In fishes the cornea may be considered as such, for, being submerged in water, it takes no part in the refraction of the eye ; so also the chitinous cornea of the ocellus and faceted eyes.   Primitive eyes are protected by their position because they are covered by the epithelium forming the surface covering of the body.

Much more protected are the eyes of amphioxus which are found close to the medullary canal.

Orbit

The invertebrate eye is more or less buried in ectoderm.   Only in the cephalopods is there a rudimentary cartilaginous orbit.

The orbit is constant in vertebrates, but varies in size, in completeness, and in the distance apart.   In relation to the size of the bulb the sea horse (*Trichechus*) has a large orbit, while in the owl the eyes are, as it were, walled in.

In man and monkeys 7 bones go to form the orbit.   The inferior orbital fissure is narrowest in man and monkeys. It is much larger in other vertebrates; so large, in fact, that the lateral wall may be absent and then the orbit opens into the temporal fossa and even, in the case of the amphibia, into the pharynx. In the horse the superior orbital fissure is a long canal (Nussbaum), and in ruminants, rodents, and some other mammals it is joined to the optic foramen.

In man the lateral wall is shorter than the medial, while in other vertebrates this wall, although membranous, is the longer.

The two bones always present are frontal and sphenoid. The ethmoid, on the other hand, does not take part in the orbit in the common mammals and often the palatine does not either.

In fishes the orbital cavity, much reduced, has accessory bones. The frontal is often divided into several parts.

In fishes the roof of the orbit is formed by 1 to 6 bones.

In pleuronectes (flat fish) the two orbits are asymmetrical and of different sizes. When young, these fishes resemble ordinary fishes, and have their eyes symmetrically placed. Later, when they come to lie on one or other side at the bottom of the sea, the lower eye, which is the left in the sole and the right in the turbot, makes its way through a hole in the frontal bone to come to lie next its fellow. They thus have what is known as a *migratory eye*.

In the lower vertebrates the lacrimal bone is little developed and really only makes its appearance in reptiles (Kober).

In ornithorhynchus, echidna, the marsupials, and edentates it is a simple plate perforated by the nasal canal. In the quadrumanes it is limited to the orbit, and does not reach the surface of the face.

In the bird, lizard, crocodile, and tortoise the orbits are close together. In the camel and hare there is one optic foramen for the two orbits. In man, monkeys, and nocturnal birds the orbits are anterior, in the dog and cat they are slightly lateral. In fishes, birds, ruminants, and carnivores they are lateral. In rodents, amphibia, and in some fishes they tend to be above.

The relative sizes of eye and orbit are interesting. According to Dexler:

Pig	1 : 2·4
Ewe	1 : 1·6
Goat	1 : 1·8
Horse	1 : 3
Ox	1 : 6

In the elephant the orbit is very large in relation to the eye (Virchow).

An Aponeurosis more or less extensive and containing muscle fibres is present in the orbital cavity. These muscle fibres in the frog help to move the bulb and the lower lid, in birds the lower lid only.

According to O. Burkard, this musculature is continuous with the maxillary musculature, which is in direct communication with the orbit, which opens laterally in most vertebrates. In amphibians, reptiles, and birds, the muscle tissue is striped. In the frog, salamander, and lizard it forms real muscles, which are attached to the globe and more especially the lower lid.

The more the outer wall of the orbit is closed, the more the tendency for this musculature to be unstriped.

Sharks have a cartilaginous peduncle which passes from the back of the globe to the back of the orbit. It is expanded anteriorly, and prevents the globe from being drawn back too far—a function taken over in the higher mammals by the fascia bulbi (capsule of Tenon) and the orbital fat.

THE SCLERA

In the most rudimentary ocellus the cup of pigment alone forms the outer covering of the eye ; but most of the ocelli are surrounded (besides this) by the basement membrane of the sensory epithelium or even by a connective tissue capsule.

A true sclera is present only in the vertebrates. It is fibrous in mammals, partly cartilaginous, partly bony, in the other classes of vertebrates. It is strengthened by a cartilage in birds, reptiles, and fishes, and in some amphibia. Traces are also found in some lower mammals (monotremes). The cartilage has the form of a cup perforated by the optic nerve.

In bony fishes and birds (Figs. 446, 457) the sclera is strengthened by cartilage and bone. In fishes there are usually two lateral lamellæ of bone, but these may be joined and form a ring (as in the tunny-fish and sword-fish).

In birds there is a posterior bony cup and an anterior intrascleral ring.

LIDS

Lids are found only in vertebrates. *Fishes*, owing to the fact that they live in water, have no, or only rudimentary, lids, which are in any case immobile. Among the sharks, the lids are more developed. The upper is the larger, while the nictitating membrane does the work of the lower (Harman). In *reptiles* there are many varieties of lids.

In *chelonians* they are thick and only slightly mobile, in *lizards* thin, and usually only the lower one is mobile. In the chameleon they are well developed, but joined so as only to leave a small circular orifice between them.

In the slow-worm, and other *scinquoidae*, the lower lid is transparent at the centre, and is the only mobile one.

It is also transparent in the geckos, but here it is adherent to the upper lid, as in serpents.

In the serpent the eye is covered by the lower lid, which is transparent, and forms a " lunette " or window, through which the animal sees. Hence arose the idea that the serpent had no lids, and it is also responsible for the " fixed stare " of these animals.

In *birds* the lower lid is by far the more mobile.

In *amphibians* Maggiore found special glands associated with the upper lid. while the lower lid and nictitating membrane were well developed. Lunettes somewhat like that of serpents are found in certain fishes, such as the eel and lamprey, but here the " lids " are not true lids, being a direct continuation of the skin and adherent to the front of the cornea.

The Tarsus.—In the higher animals the lids are strengthened by a tarsal plate, consisting not of cartilage but of dense connective tissue. Even in the dog it is only slightly marked ; in birds and lizards it is formed only in the lower lid, and is entirely absent in the parrot, duck, tortoise, alligator. In the iguana and lizard, Elizabeth Cords found traces of hyaline cartilage.

The Palpebral Opening varies in size and shape. It is generally, relative to the size of the animal, smaller than the human. Only in the elephant is it relatively larger. The smallest (relatively) are found in the camel and seal.

The Tarsal Glands, which are modified sebaceous glands of the skin, are little developed in other mammals.

It has been suggested that they represent a row of lashes which have disappeared in man, but may reappear in the condition of distichiasis when the tarsal glands are said to be absent.

In the camel they appear to be absent (Richiardi). They are replaced by the sebaceous glands in the huge caruncle of this animal, which fills the whole of the medial canthus.

In birds, only traces are found and they have the appearance of sebaceous glands of the skin, with the hairs of which they are still often found associated.

Lashes

Lashes are well developed, not only in primates, but also in the dog and pig. They are absent in the cat. Traces are found in the ostrich and vulture, where they are formed of rudimentary feathers. In the horse they are absent in the central portion of the upper lid.

Eyebrow.—The eyebrow is found not only in man, but in the higher apes. In the cat it is represented by a few long hairs, and in the camel there is a similar formation below the lower lid.

The Palpebral Muscles

Lid movements are usually accomplished by the orbicularis and levator palpebræ superioris. But in sharks, batrachians, and serpents there is no orbicularis. In the elephant there is a depressor palpebræ inferioris (Virchow). In the aquatic mammals there is a muscle in the form of a tube which is distributed all round the lids (Stannius, Virchow) ; in fact, a dilator rimæ palpebrarum.

Unstriped muscle was found by H. Müller in human lids, and also across the inferior orbital fissure, here mixed with elastic fibres. In other mammals it is much better developed, forming an orbital muscle which may act as antagonist to the retractor bulbi. All these are supplied by the sympathetic. The orbital muscles are striped in the lower animals, unstriped in the mammal, but appear to have a common origin from the periorbital aponeurosis (Groyer).

The palpebral or tarsal muscles of Müller which are unstriped in man are striped in the aquatic mammals. These arise with the recti, which divide into two —a part going to the eye, the other to the lids. But in most mammals the lid portion is unstriped.

In mammals, too, part of the tarsal muscles goes to the nictitating membrane. If unstriped they are supplied by the sympathetic, if striped by the nerves that go to the corresponding bulbar muscles.

Lashes, unlike ordinary hairs, have no arrector pili muscles as a rule, but Zietschmann found traces in the horse and pig.

The orbicularis is considered a cutaneous muscle, but in man it is independent of the other facial muscles, while in lower animals its common origin with these is more evident. In the lower animals the orbicularis hardly extends beyond the orbital margin.

In birds (Riehl, 1908) the orbicularis, levator, and depressor of the lids are unstriped.

The Conjunctiva

The conjunctiva in fishes is cutaneous. Lymphoid follicles are present in the calf, dog, and pig (Marano). The horse has many papillæ.

Physiologically no true papillæ or follicles are present in the human conjunctiva, although rudimentary forms of both are found.

Sweat glands have been described in the bulbar conjunctiva of the goat, pig. and ox.

The utricular glands of Manz at the limbus have been seen in the pig, ox, lamb, and fox, and have also been described in man.

Visible Pigmentation of the conjunctiva near the corneal margin is present in many animals. H. Müller found ramifying pigment cells which appeared possessed of remarkable contractile powers.

In the Japanese and Chinese (Steiner), the bulbar conjunctiva is always more or less pigmented. This pigmentation increases with age and in those who are much exposed to bright sunlight.

The Nictitating Membrane, or third eyelid, is conjunctival in origin. It is best marked in mammals, especially the herbivora, and in sauropsida, and batrachians.

Generally speaking, one finds this membrane less developed, as the hand is more able to wipe the eye (Ovio). Thus it is well developed in the solipeds, but less in the cat. In man and many monkeys it is absent, but some, as, for instance, the chimpanzee, have one. In man it is represented by the semilunar fold. Usually it is placed at the medial angle of the eye, and extends vertically. It passes laterally somewhat obliquely in front of the eye. In the frog and the selachians the nictitating membrane is below, and passes upwards in front of the eye, like the curtain of the ancient Greek theatre (Hirschberg).

In bony fishes and some others the nictitating membrane is on the temporal side.

The nictitating membrane in many animals contains a plate of cartilage, which is especially big in the large herbivora.   Traces of this have been seen in man, more especially in the dark races (Giacomini).

Elastic fibres are very abundant in the nictitating membrane.   The margin is often pigmented, and consists of a special band of elastic tissue, the limbus

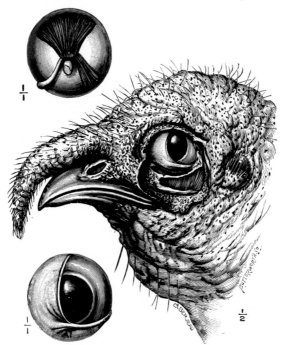

FIG. 455.—HEAD OF TURKEY.

The insets show the pyramidalis and quadratus, also the termination of the tendon in the nictitating membrane.   The relation of the tendon is also shown in the large figure.

(*From Bland Sutton*, 1920, *London*.)

marginalis, which Kajikawa believes holds the membrane in place without muscular action when in front of the eye, as obtains in the tendons of the extremities in birds.

In birds and some amphibians such as the frog, the nictitating membrane when stretched becomes transparent in the centre, forming a sort of window through which the animal can see.

In birds and reptiles, but best developed in the former, the nictitating membrane is controlled by two special muscles, the pyramidalis and the quadratus, which, with the retractor bulbi, are supplied by the 6th nerve.

The quadratus arises from the sclera, behind the tendon of the superior rectus, passes downwards, and ends above the optic nerve in a tendinous loop through which the pyramidalis passes.

The pyramidalis, smaller than the quadratus, arises from the sclera below and passes upwards. It ends in a tendon which curves round the lateral side of the optic nerve, then above it, to pass through the tendon of the quadratus. It continues on, and is attached to the nictitating membrane near the medial angle of the eye. The membrane may, in fact, be regarded as the expanded tendon of the pyramidalis. In the tortoise these muscles are present, but much reduced. In the frog, the membrane is drawn up by the retractor bulbi muscle. In mammals, it has no connection with any muscle. Here movement of the membrane is affected by simultaneous retraction of the globe. The cartilage which it contains, and which is prolonged backwards, in the form of a tongue-shaped process, is in contact with a special mass of orbital fat. As the globe passes backwards the membrane is prevented from doing likewise, and so it naturally covers more and more of the eye.

The Lacrimal Caruncle is found in nearly all mammals, but is almost always larger than in man, and especially so in the camel, where it fills the whole of the medial angle of the eye. In the dog, the lacrimal caruncle (as in man) contains many accessory lacrimal glands, and the deeper layers of the epithelium are pigmented.

The Lacrimal Organs

Harder's Gland is found in all vertebrates except the primates. It opens by two ducts on the nasal side of the conjunctival sac, and secretes an oily (cetacea) or a mucous material. It is large in mammals, especially in the herbivora. It is rudimentary in the lower apes, but is absent in the anthropoids as in man, in whom, however, it may be found as a rarity (Giacomini). When the lacrimal gland is well developed Harder's gland is poorly developed and vice versa (Wiedersheim).

Fishes and aquatic amphibians have no lacrimal organs, the eyes being bathed by the surrounding media.

The first rudiment of a gland appears in amphibia between the conjunctiva and the skin of the lower lid. In the tortoise there is one gland for the two eyes. In serpents the lacrimal gland is absent, but Harder's gland is very large, being placed in the medial angle or sometimes surrounding the globe. In certain serpents (thyphlopidæ) it practically fills the orbit, being ten times bigger than the eye, which is rudimentary. In birds, also, Harder's gland is very big.

The Lacrimal Gland

The lacrimal gland and Harder's gland have a common origin in a single gland situated in the lower lid. A growth of the medial portion produces Harder's gland, which tends to remain in its original position, while the lacrimal gland tends to move towards the lateral canthus, then to the upper lid. Its origin from the lower lid is, however, seen by some of the ducts which always open under this.

Thus the rudiment in the lower lid of amphibia is really the rudiment of both lacrimal and Harder's glands.

A.E.—32

In the Triton, this rudiment becomes more developed towards the nasal side, and forms a rudimentary gland of Harder.   Also in this animal a rudimentary lacrimal gland is developed on the temporal side.

In birds the lacrimal gland is placed at the lateral angle.

In the rabbit the lacrimal gland is slightly in the upper lid, but mostly in the lower.

The tortoise, unlike other aquatic animals, has a large lacrimal gland situated posteriorly.   This is due to the fact that the tortoise crosses dry sandy tracts when it wants to lay its eggs, and has to keep its eyes as moist as usual.

In the whale the secretion is fatty, like that of the Meibomian glands.

In man the lacrimal ducts open on the conjunctiva.

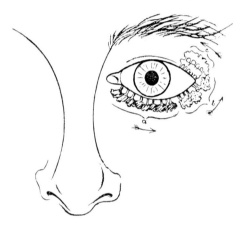

Fig. 456.—Diagram to illustrate the Shifting of the Lacrimal Gland in the Course of Phylogeny.

(*From Whitnall, after Wiedersheim.*)

In the tortoise, bird, rodent, and lamb the ducts unite to form one, and open in the lower lid.

In the primates there are several ducts which open mainly in the upper lid, but some always open under the lower.

The lacrimal organs are supplied by the second division of the fifth nerve in all animals up to the mammal.   In mammals the main supply comes from the first division of the fifth nerve, indirectly also from the second.

The secretion of the true lacrimal gland is watery, that of Harder's oily, but in the pig the lacrimal gland is mucous, as it is in part in the lamb, goat, and dog (Virchow).

According to Wendt, the gland of Harder is sebaceous in the lower and marine mammals, while it tends to be more like the lacrimal gland as we pass to the higher mammals.

The lacrimal gland is, in fact, a modified skin gland. In spelerpes, a salamander, it is continuous with these.

In serpents, which have a large lacrimal gland, the ducts open into the mouth —hence the gland is salivary in function.

THE LACRIMAL PASSAGES

Generally smaller than in man, they are absent in the chelonians (Sardemann), seal, hippopotamus, and elephant.

There is a single passage in the rabbit, pig, and ewe, and double, as in man, in the other animals.

Lacrimal papillæ are found only in man.

In the pig the canaliculi lie in bony canals in the lacrimal bone.

In the ophidia the lacrimal passages open into the mouth.

THE ORBITAL MUSCLES

Poorly developed in the invertebrates, they are well marked in the vertebrates. In the invertebrates there are rudimentary muscles in relation to their ocelli.

Crustaceans and molluscs have mobile eyes on stalks.

Cophilia, a phyllopod crustacean, has a mobile retina.

Daphnia has a single median eye $\frac{1}{10}$ mm. in diameter formed by a number of ommatidia. This eye is provided with four muscles resembling our recti, which keep it in a constant state of vibration and move it in various directions.

In vertebrates there are 4 recti, 2 obliques, and a retractor.

The muscles are relatively small in birds, and the eye relatively little mobile, for the animal moves its head instead.

Thus also there is little mobility in fishes, reptiles, and amphibia, except the aquatic tortoise, the shark, and periophthalmus.

In fishes and birds they may be very oblique and often almost at right angles to the optic nerve.

In the bony fishes the muscles a short distance from their origin are placed in a canal.

The two oblique muscles form an almost complete girdle round the globe. In man they are inserted behind the equator. In other animals the insertion tends to be in front of this.

In most vertebrates, too, they have their origin close together near the front of the orbit. The reflected portion of the superior oblique is thus the original muscle, and is fleshy in many mammals. The pulley is developed, as the origin comes to be placed farther back to retain the direction of pull. In mammals there is a posterior origin and a pulley.

The two obliques cross the recti, sometimes between them and the globe, sometimes outside them.

In man the superior passes inside, the inferior outside, the corresponding rectus. In fishes both obliques are outside. In birds, and in the elephant and chimpanzee, the inferior oblique is outside ; but in other mammals usually inside.

In the tiger the obliques split to enclose the rectus. In the lion only the superior does this.

The retractor bulbi (choanoid muscle) is well developed in the large herbivora, but is also found in the tortoise, lizard, and batrachians. It is absent in birds and serpents, man, and the higher apes.

This muscle, which has the form of a cone, arises at the apex of the orbit and surrounds the back of the globe to the equator. It has a tendency to be divided into several portions; thus in the whale there are two, and in the batrachians three portions. It is supplied by 6th nerve.

The main function is to retract the globe. It also supports the globe in those animals which hang their heads for hours, and prevents the congestion which would otherwise result. In man, Grimsdale thinks this function is taken in by the tonic action of the recti. In man, also, this muscle is missing, but Nussbaum found a trace.

THE ORBITAL VESSELS

In mammals, generally the tendency is for the eye to be supplied by the external carotid; but as we ascend the animal scale more and more comes from the internal carotid.

In the dog there are two ophthalmic arteries, one from each source, with an anastomotic branch between them (Parsons and Henderson).

In man the ocular and orbital vessels come from the internal carotid. We must not, however, forget the recurrent lacrimal artery, which is an anastomosis between the lacrimal derived from the internal carotid and the middle meningeal, which comes from the external. This branch may enlarge and take the place of the ophthalmic, thus reproducing the condition in the lower mammals.

A Hyaloid Artery is constant in mammals, but tends to disappear later than in man, and remnants are more commonly found. In the cat, for instance, it remains until one month after birth, and according to Ciaccio, in the mole the hyaloid artery is permanent.

The Retinal Vessels.—The central vessels always pierce the sheaths of the optic nerve nearer the globe than in man.

The Ciliary Vessels are always more important in the supply of the retina than in man, and often the central vessels are so small as to be negligible. Indeed, it is disputed whether the dog, cat, and fox have an arteria centralis.[1]

In the dog, we found the retina supplied by cilio-retinal vessels only. These pierce the *sclera* (not the nerve sheaths), and enter the nerve at the level of a ridge of retino-choroidal pigment, i.e. necessarily in the globe.

A central retinal vein, on the other hand, may be present for a very short distance only, but it also leaves the nerve inside the globe. In no case did we see the main retinal vessels cross the subarachnoid space, as they do in man.

---

[1] Occasionally, while at the nerve head no arteria centralis was seen, a very small vessel was found farther back in the centre of the nerve. (Wolff and Davies (November 1931), *Brit. J. Ophthal.*)

The depth to which the retinal vessels penetrate into the retina varies. In man they go to the outer side of the outer nuclear layer, i.e. just into the outer plexiform layer. In the lower animals they penetrate less deeply. In the cat, for instance, only to the ganglion layer, in the horse and rabbit they are confined to the nerve fibre layer.

According to Mann, in rodent embryos the retinal vessels resemble a membrana vasculosa retinæ. Later the vessels sink in to become partially embedded in the nerve fibre layer.

With regard to the amount of retina which is vascularised, Leber makes the following classification :

1. *Holangiotic* (ὅλος = entire).—Entirely supplied by vessels, as in the primates, some insectivores, carnivores, ungulates, pig, some rodents, marsupials, pinnipeds.

2. *Merangiotic* (μέρος = partly).—Partly supplied with vessels, as in the rabbit and hare. The vessels are limited to the areas of the medullated nerve fibres (Fig. 443).

3. *Paurangiotic* (παῦρος = small). Slightly supplied with vessels, as in the bat, horse (Fig. 442), elephant, guinea-pig. The vessels are very small, and extend only a small distance from the disc.

4. *Anangiotic.*—The retina contains no vessels, as in the rhinoceros, porcupine, echidna.

In the agouti, a rodent which has a retina almost anangiotic, and in some marsupials there is a cone which is characteristic of the reptiles. In the other anangiotic animals, one often finds a capillary vascularisation of the disc which may be visible ophthalmoscopically, and which is analogous to the cone of reptiles or the pecten of birds (Lindsay Johnson, Mann).

THE RETINAL VESSELS

True retinal vessels are found only in mammals.

In the lower vertebrates, except the eel and a few others, the retina is avascular. It is the fate of the hyaloid system which determines the final method by which the retina gets its nourishment.

The retina may, in fact, be nourished in four ways (Mann) :

1. A completely avascular retina, the blood-supply being entirely from the choroid (avascular type).

2. An avascular retina associated with a pecten projecting from the optic disc (pecten type).

3. An avascular retina supplied by vessels lying on its inner surface (membrana vasculosa retinæ type).

4. A vascular retina supplied by vessels ramifying in its substance.

1. *The Avascular Type* (without a pecten or its homologue) is found in many species ; for instance, in certain fishes, reptiles, and mammals.

In the reptiles of this group there is, however, often a trace of a rudimentary pecten. Thus in the crocodile there are a few capillaries and some pigment in the nerve head.

Among mammals the avascular retina is seen in the Monotreme (echidna); Edentates (hairy armadillo); Rodents (Brazilian porcupine, common guinea-pig, and chinchilla). Sometimes in ungulates and chiroptera (rhinoceros and Australian fruit bat) (Lindsay Johnson).

Most of these animals have a capillary vascularisation of the nerve head, which is visible ophthalmoscopically, and a visual acuity which does not reach a high standard.

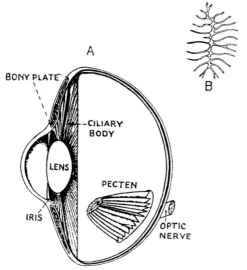

FIG. 457.—A = VERTICAL SECTION OF THE TEMPORAL HALF OF THE EYE OF THE OSTRICH (STRUTHIO CAMELUS). B = TRANSVERSE SECTION OF THE PECTEN.

(*From Bütschli.*)

2. *The Pecten Type* is seen in animals of a high degree of visual acuity.

The pecten is best developed in birds, but it has homologues in the cone of reptiles and the processus falciformis of certain fishes.

The Pecten of Birds (Figs. 457, 458) is a triangular pleated membrane, which extends from the optic disc (and cauda), which it covers, forwards for a variable distance into the vitreous. It is composed of a loose and folded connective tissue richly supplied with vessels and completely covered with pigment. It is this that gives it a velvety appearance.

In some birds, such as the swan and duck, it touches the lens; in others, especially in some nocturnal species, it is often rudimentary.

The pecten is an ectodermal structure which is secondarily vascularised.

The *function* is essentially nutritive, taking the place of the retinal arteries which are absent in birds.

Some hold that it has erectile properties, and thus offers a defensive mechanism against too strong light.

Kajikawa maintains that the pecten regulates the tension (thus a capillary venous reservoir), the secretion, and the temperature of the eye, especially at high altitudes (thus a heat radiator).

The pecten is always attached to the lens, although this may in some cases be by very fine fibrils only.

The Cone of Reptiles is analogous to the pecten of birds, but instead of being triangular, it is a cone-shaped projection from the disc. It is well developed in the lizard and chameleon, and rudimentary in the tortoise and serpent.

It is also ectodermal in origin, being formed by a vascularisation of Berg-meister's papilla, which has grown forward into the vitreous.

The Processus Falciformis of fishes is a filamentary process which is probably homologous with the pecten. It passes from the disc to the back of lens, where

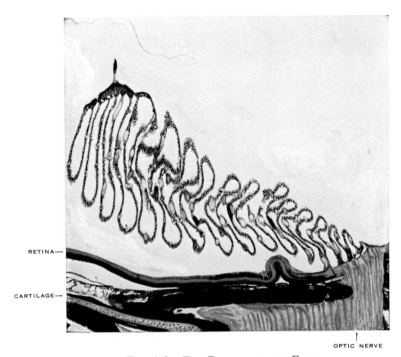

RETINA—

CARTILAGE—

OPTIC NERVE

FIG. 458.—THE PECTEN OF THE FOWL.
It has much the structure of ciliary process—vessels covered by epithelium and pigment.
(*From McDonagh and Wolff, Brit. Journ. Ophth.*, 1939)

it spreads out to form an enlargement called the *campanule of Haller*. This contains muscle fibres which form an ectodermal retractor lentis muscle.

It is also a vascular organ, but covered by epithelium. It is derived from the lips of the optic fissure, thus ectodermal, and is secondarily vascularised.

3. *The Membrana Vasculosa Retinæ Type.*—Here, branches of the hyaloid artery spread out over the *surface* of the retina without actually entering its substance. Ophthalmoscopically, they appear to be retinal vessels, but their true nature is found on microscopic section (Hirschberg).

This type is best seen in snakes, but is also found in amphibians (frog) and ganoid fishes (*Amia calva*).

In the embryos of certain rodents a similar condition obtains, while in the adult (white rat) the vessels sink to some extent into the nerve fibre layer, and thus form a link between this and the following type (Mann).

4. *The Arteria Centralis Retinæ Type* is typical of the primates. It will be remembered that this form of blood-supply develops in the first place like the pecten, i.e. by a vascularisation of Bergmeister's papilla. But instead of being confined to this, vascular buds grow out into the retina (see p. 455).

THE UVEAL VESSELS

The choroidal vessels are much the same throughout the vertebrates, except that in the bony fishes a great thickening of the chorio-capillaris posteriorly forms the choroidal " gland."

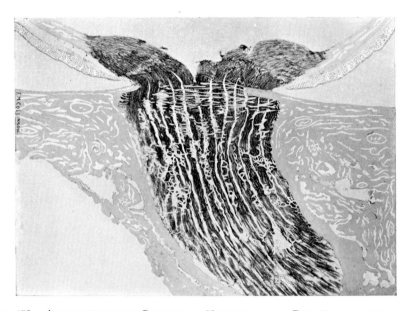

FIG. 459.—ANTERO-POSTERIOR SECTION OF NERVE-HEAD OF DOG (STAINED WEIGERT).

Note.—Normal medullation of nerve-head. Unlike when this occurs in the human as an abnormality, the fibres are medullated in region of lamina cribrosa.

The iris vessels, however, show many variations (see Mann, 1929 and 1931).

IN FISHES the iris is usually supplied by two anterior ciliary arteries, which run in the horizontal meridian towards the pupil, round which they form an arterial circle. The venous drainage lies deep, obscured by the silvery membrane (argentea).

IN AMPHIBIANS, also, the arteries are superficial. They enter the iris at irregular points, and run circumferentially. The veins are deep. Both arteries and veins are often obscured by pigment.

IN REPTILES the arteries, inferior and temporal, constantly enter the iris at six and eight o'clock, and then run circularly at the periphery of the iris. Often a superficial set of radial veins is also found.

In snakes, however, there is an irregular network of vessels.

BIRDS have deep circular arteries with superficial radial veins, and often a dense capillary plexus.

IN MAMMALS only is there a superficial system formed by the pupillary membrane. Hence only in mammals are there direct arterio-venous anastomoses in the region of the lesser circle. The greater circle often lies at the base of the iris, not, as in man, in the ciliary body. Also the ciliary processes tend to be in contact with the back of the iris.

In mammals generally (as opposed to man) the vorticose veins have their exit in front of the equator. Anterior to the vorticose veins, and not far from the

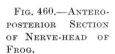

FIG. 460.—ANTERO-POSTERIOR SECTION OF NERVE-HEAD OF FROG.

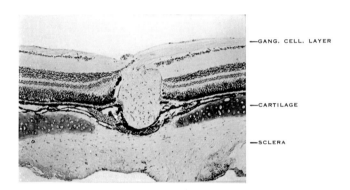

corneo-scleral margin, the ciliary veins form an intrascleral circular anastomosis known as the circle of Hovius (Leber), especially well seen in the seal and porpoise. It drains into the vorticose veins, and may replace partly the anterior ciliary veins and the sinus venosus scleræ.

THE OPTIC NERVE

There is no optic ganglion in the vertebrates, such as is present in the invertebrates (Fig. 433).

In the vertebrates the nerve fibre layer of the retina is directly continuous with the optic nerve.

The form and structure of the optic nerve vary much, depending essentially on the number of fibrous partitions. In some the septa are absent, and then the nerve may be in the form of a ribbon; for instance, in the sword-fish and cartilaginous fishes.

In the eel a single partition divides the nerve into two.

According to Deyl, the higher the species of animal the more developed the framework. But Greeff finds many exceptions to this.

THE CHIASMA

The chiasmal crossing is characteristic of the vertebrates ; in Myxinoides, a cyclostome, it is actually in the brain substance.   Below the mammals the crossing is complete.   In the bony fishes there is a simple crossing, one nerve, usually the right, passing dorsal to the other.

In the herring one nerve passes through the other.   In the parrot-fish each nerve divides into two, the portions crossing like two fingers of one hand with two of the other (Fig. 461).

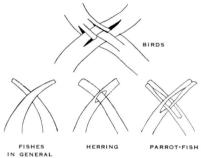

FISHES IN GENERAL   HERRING   PARROT-FISH

FIG. 461.—THE CHIASMAL CROSSING.
(*L.W., after Ovio.*)

In most reptiles and amphibians the nerves divide into many portions, which, however, cross completely, likewise in birds.

In all mammals, except monotremes, a portion remains uncrossed ; as we pass up the scale more and more remains uncrossed. In man about one-quarter are uncrossed, i.e. the majority still cross.

The fibres cross to make binocular vision possible.

THE LATERAL GENICULATE BODY

The beginning of a lateral geniculate body is seen in the cyclostomes.   It is small in most fishes, but shows better development in the teleosteans (Kappers).

In the amphibians, reptiles, and birds, it is still small, and does not send any fibres to the cortex (Elliot Smith).

In mammals it reaches its full development.   It consists essentially of two nuclei which are dorsal and ventral in the primitive animals.   It represents, in fact, the whole of the lateral geniculate body of the lower animals.   As we pass up the scale the dorsal nucleus becomes more important, and the lateral geniculate body rotates so that what was dorsal becomes lateral.   In the primates the ventral nucleus is practically non-existent, and only the dorsal nucleus is cortically represented.

The ventral nucleus receives crossed fibres only, gives off the superior brachium, and is connected with the reflex centres of the mid-brain (see Woollard, 1926).

Minkowski showed that enucleation of the eye in man, cats, and monkeys (all having a partial crossing in the chiasma) results in the degeneration of certain layers or zones of both lateral geniculate bodies.   He concluded that the crossed and uncrossed fibres go to alternate layers.

In the human lateral geniculate body, as in that of monkeys, six laminæ are found.   The two superficial ones are formed of large, deeply staining pyriform cells, from the deep aspect of which long branching processes arise, while the four deeper laminæ are composed of medium-sized cells, triangular and fusiform in shape, and fairly closely packed together (see Le Gros Clark (May 1932), *Brit. J. Ophthal.*; also p. 376).

PARIETAL AND PINEAL EYES (Figs. 462 *et seq.*)

Parietal and Pineal Eyes are very similar and closely associated.

From the roof of the mid-brain two outgrowths may arise :

(*a*) The epiphysis or pineal body, connected with the posterior commissure.

(*b*) The parietal or parapineal body, placed anterior to the above and connected with the habenular commissure.

Now, while these outgrowths are usually glandular, they may develop into eyes which show more or less differentiation.

The Parietal Eye is found in certain saurians (reptiles and birds). It lies under the skin in the parietal foramen, which is analogous to our anterior fontanelle. It is a closed vesicle, which is connected to the habenular commissure by a band known as the parietal nerve.

The eye structure is best seen in the primitive reptiles. In the lizard, *Lacerta ocellata,* for instance, there is a lens and behind it a cavity filled with a liquid like the vitreous, also a retina in which the rods and cones can be distinguished and a trace of a choroid. The pigment it contains has been noticed to move under the influence of light.

This eye is poorly developed in the ordinary lizards, it is absent in gecko, and is only seen during embryonic life in other saurians. In these latter, in fact, the parietal eye disappears more or less completely ; it degenerates, alters, and is penetrated by fibrous partitions and

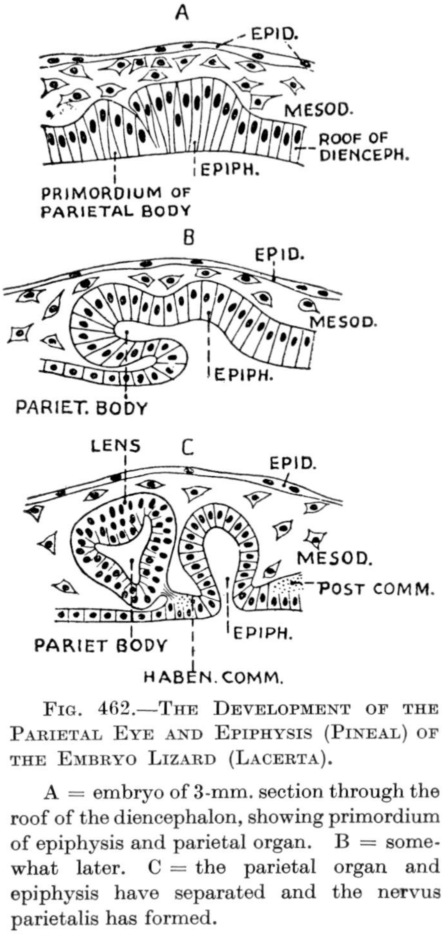

FIG. 462.—THE DEVELOPMENT OF THE PARIETAL EYE AND EPIPHYSIS (PINEAL) OF THE EMBRYO LIZARD (LACERTA).

A = embryo of 3-mm. section through the roof of the diencephalon, showing primordium of epiphysis and parietal organ. B = somewhat later. C = the parietal organ and epiphysis have separated and the nervus parietalis has formed.

(*From Bütschli, after Novikoff.*)

vessels, which mask its primitive structure, and it is in the latter condition that we find the pineal body in all other vertebrates.

The considerable size of the parietal foramen in many fossil reptiles makes it probable that in them the parietal eye was of great functional importance ; the pineal or parietal eye of living species, however, plays a very small rôle in vision.

The Pineal Eye is much like the parietal.   The lamprey, a cyclostome, has both a parietal and a pineal eye.

The pineal eye, too, is placed under the skin, through the transparency of which it is visible.   It develops from the extremity of the pineal gland, and is

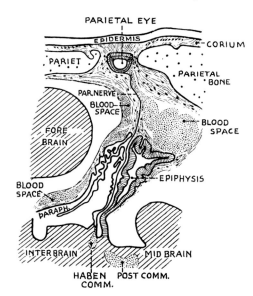

FIG. 463.—MEDIAN SECTION THROUGH THE HEAD AND PARIETAL EYE OF THE ADULT LIZARD (LACERTA AGILIS).

(From Bütschli after Novikoff.)

connected to the posterior commissure by the pineal nerve.   In it there is a kind of retina, with sensory cells and calcareous nodules in place of pigment.

In elasmobranch fishes the glandular pineal body itself has a bony stalk, and is

FIG. 464.—THE PARIETAL EYE OF THE LIZARD (ANGUIS FRAGILIS).

(From Bütschli, after Novikoff.)

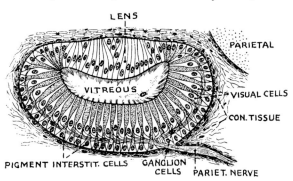

placed in the parietal foramen under the skin.   In the young frog, only, a pineal eye is found which degenerates later.

It is probable that the pineal gland of vertebrates is derived from paired symmetrical organs which have fused and which correspond to the distal eyes of the salpes (Todaro).

In petromyzon the pineal apparatus is at first paired and symmetrical, and later one of these develops into the pineal organ, while the other becomes the parapineal or parietal organ, which is placed in front of the other (Sterzi).

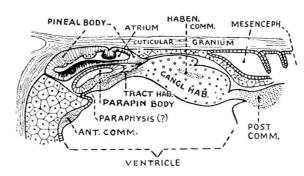

FIG. 465.—SAGITTAL SECTION THROUGH THE ROOF OF THE FORE-, INTER-, AND MID-BRAINS OF THE LARVA OF PETROMYZON PLANERI TO SHOW THE PINEAL AND PARA-PINEAL ORGANS.

(*From Bütschli, after Studnitzka.*)

THE 3RD NERVE NUCLEUS

As we travel up the animal scale the eyes, which at first lie laterally, come more and more to the front of the head. We note the same changes ontogenetically in man. In the embryo the eyes are first lateral, then later swing round to the front.

Associated with these changes there are changes in the appearance of the 3rd nerve nucleus.

As the eyes move more and more to the front in phylogenetic history, and as binocular vision is correspondingly more developed and convergence becomes more important, the median nucleus of Perlia is formed, and joins together the originally separate lateral nuclei. On the other hand, the nucleus of Edinger-Westphal was originally single and median, and as we pass up the animal scale it tends to divide into two.

Thus the nucleus of Perlia is absent in rodents and small in herbivora. In carnivora, who have to watch their prey closely, it is quite well developed, as also in birds. It is especially well developed in the higher apes, and, in man, in whom the development of stereoscopic vision goes hand in hand with his mental development, there is a forward prolongation of the nucleus (but see p. 279).

The Edinger-Westphal nucleus, which appears earlier in phylogenetic history than that of Perlia, is single in the cetacea, rodents, pinnipedia, and carnivora, and paired in the higher apes and in man. This may be associated with the fact that when we look at an object which is not equidistant from the two eyes, each eye requires to focus differently to see the object clearly.

So far as ontogenetic development is concerned, the nucleus of Perlia is formed when, in the human embryo, the eyes swing round from the side to front of the head, and the nucleus of Edinger-Westphal makes its appearance when the ectodermal portion of the iris is being formed from the margin of the optic cup (Paton and Mann, 1925).

The Dorsal Crossing of the 4th Nerve[1] (See p. 286.)

The 4th nerve is a motor nerve which arises from a nucleus directly continuous with the 3rd. It shows, like all other motor nerves, a central cerebral crossing. It differs, however, from them in not remaining on the same side ; in not leaving the central nervous system ventral or dorso-lateral, and in making a second (almost) complete crossing with the 4th of the opposite side, leaving the brain in an ultra-dorsal position before winding round the brain stem to become ventral.

It supplies the superior oblique, which in gnathostomes forms the most dorsal muscle (Fürbringer).

The ontogenetic history shows that the dorsal position of the nervus trochlearis and superior oblique muscle is acquired very early in embryonic life. The superior oblique arises from the dorsal portion of the mandibular myotome.

The 4th nerve is already present in the cyclostomes, and in all animals there is the curious dorsal decussation.

Several theories have been advanced to account for this.

It is thought that the 4th nerve was originally sensory (Hoffmann) or motor (Fürbringer) to the central pineal eye, and when this degenerated it became the nerve to the opposite lateral eye. According to Gaskell, migration of certain dorsal muscles to supply the lateral eyes can be seen in certain fossil animals.

Johnston holds that the 4th nerve leaves the brain dorsally, because this is by far the easiest route. For otherwise it would have had to pass through the whole thickness of the mid-brain.

Neal holds that the muscle fibres of the myotome of the second somite, which is supplied by the 4th nerve, wandered over to the opposite side, and with the formation of the head fold acquired a ventral position. All the dorsal portion of the myotome degenerated except the superior oblique.

In other words, this curious dorsal crossover remains an unsolved mystery.

The Ciliary Ganglion

The ciliary ganglion is essentially a relay station for the parasympathetic (autonomic) fibres of the 3rd nerve.

Sensory ganglion cells (which have wandered from the trigeminal ganglion) have also been described, but must be of little importance, and the sympathetic certainly has no cell station in the ciliary ganglion.

Schwalbe, in fact, as the result of extensive researches into its comparative anatomy, calls it the *oculo-motor* ganglion.

He found that in bony fishes, amphibians, and reptiles, the ganglion is connected with the 3rd nerve, and in many cases no fibres come from the 5th or sympathetic. Also in ganoid fishes (Schreider), in selachians, and chelonians (Pitzorno), the ciliary ganglion is associated with the 3rd nerve. In mammals

[1] See Cooper (1947), *Brit. J. Ophthal.*, **31**, 257.

the connection with the 3rd is always present, although the sensory and sympathetic may be absent, as is sometimes the case even in man.

Structure.—Müller (1920) finds that in the human the cells are exclusively multipolar and different from the sympathetic. In birds (Lenhossek and Carpenter) the cells are cerebro-spinal in type and the fibres do not divide in a ⊤-shaped manner. Pitzorno also could find no sympathetic cells in the ganglion.

In the equidæ the ganglion is microscopic.

In the artiodactyls, pig, boar, buffalo, goat, and in the rabbit, the ganglion is double.

In birds there is only a motor and no sensory or sympathetic roots. These join the ciliary nerves.

Experimentally in the dog, cat, and monkey, the ciliary muscle contracts either on stimulating the 3rd nerve or the short ciliaries (Hensen and Voelkers). Destruction of the iris and ciliary body causes degeneration of the cells of the ciliary ganglion.

Cauterisation of the cornea causes slight change in the ciliary ganglion and also in the trigeminal ganglion. If the ciliary ganglion is painted with nicotine, the motor path is blocked while the cornea is not affected. This shows an autonomic cell station. This experiment could not be repeated in birds in which the ciliary muscle is striated (Langendorf, Lodato).

Embryologically.—Cells are frequently found migrating along the 3rd nerve to the ganglion, and some have also been described coming from the trigeminal ganglion (Carpenter, Gafini).

THE BRAIN

As we pass up the invertebrate scale we find a general tendency for the central nervous system to enlarge and become aggregated at the cranial end of the animal.

Amphioxus (although classed as a vertebrate really lies between the two big groups) has a simple enlargement in front of the notochord. There is no differentiation, no true brain formation, and no skull is formed round it (hence it belongs to the acrania).

In all other vertebrates the medullary canal divides into three primary vesicles, i.e. the fore-, mid- and hind-brain vesicles. The first and last of these divide up again, so that eventually we have five subdivisions :

1. Telencephalon or fore-brain.
2. Diencephalon, or thalamencephalon or inter-brain.
3. Mesencephalon or mid-brain.
4. Metencephalon or hind-brain.
5. Myelencephalon or medulla.

The Telencephalon, by a thickening of its roof, forms the pallium, which later develops into the cerebral hemispheres, while a thickening in the floor forms a basal nucleus which will form the corpus striatum of man.

In the Diencephalon a thickening at the sides forms the thalamus, while the roof remains thin, and is often folded.

In the Midbrain the roof forms the optic lobes, which in the mammal become the colliculi (corpora quadrigemina), while the floor forms the cerebral peduncles.

In the metencephalon the cerebellum is developed in the roof, while the pons develops in the floor.

In the myelencephalon the floor forms the medulla oblongata, while the roof remains thin and is often folded.

Thus we see that the roof of the diencephalon and that of the myelencephalon remain thin, and the vessels with which they are richly provided form the choroid plexuses. Thickenings in the roof of the former, however, form the ganglion habenulæ and the parietal and pineal organs (q.v.).

We shall now consider shortly how the brain differs in the various groups of vertebrates.

In Fishes.—We have seen that the central nervous system of amphioxus presents a simple enlargement at its anterior end. Some authors hold that one can differentiate the olfactory, trigeminal, and facial nerves, but this is doubtful. In the selachians the whole of the anterior portion of the brain is olfactory, which is much more developed than the visual portion. The optic lobes are, however, quite large, and the optic nerve enters them.

The pallium is but slightly thickened.

In the bony fishes, on the other hand, the optic lobes are larger than the olfactory part of the brain.

The inter-brain (diencephalon) is, generally speaking, little developed in fishes, although there is a small thalamus and geniculate bodies.

The cerebellum is very small in cyclostomes, small in selachians, and well marked in the bony fishes. The medulla oblongata is large, owing to the great development of the nerve nuclei, especially the 5th, 7th, and the 8th.

From the mid-brain passes the tecto-spinal tract, which runs to the medial longitudinal fasciculus.

In Amphibians the olfactory portion is small ; the pallium is fairly developed. There is a rudimentary thalamus. The optic lobes are fairly well developed, especially in the anura, and the optic nerve goes to them. The medulla oblongata is small, and so is the cerebellum.

In Reptiles the pallium is still further developed, and, in fact, shows the first indication of a cortex which is olfactory. There is a rudiment of the corona radiata passing from the basal ganglion to the cortex.

The optic lobes are fairly large, and in the crocodile there is an indication of a posterior quadrigeminal body. The thalamus is fairly well developed, and so are the optic lobes.

From the roof of the inter-brain (diencephalon) the parietal eye is developed.

In Birds there is a great development of the roof of the fore-brain or pallium to form the cerebral hemispheres. The optic lobes are large and the thalamus small. The geniculate bodies are fairly well developed. The cerebral hemispheres cover a large part of the optic lobes. The tractus occipito-mesencephalicus unites the occipital cortex with the optic lobes, and is the first connection between the eye and the cortex. The optic fibres mostly terminate in the optic lobes, but many pass to the geniculate bodies and thalamus.

In the pigeon there is a commissure between the optic lobes which may function as a second crossing of the optic pathway. Thus, if one removes the left eye and left occipital cortex, the animal will after a time see again, which, since there is a complete crossing of the optic nerves, may be effected by the tract between the two optic lobes, or, as is more probable, the cortex is associational only (Stefani).

In Mammals the striking feature is the great development of the cerebral hemispheres. They cover the diencephalon, the mid-brain, and part of the cerebellum. But the mid-brain is reduced and the quadrigeminal bodies (colliculi) are smaller than the optic lobes of the lower vertebrates.

The diencephalon is well developed, and so are the thalamus, geniculate bodies, and peduncles. The thalamus becomes a great co-ordinating and relay centre for sensory impulses.

The olfactory portion varies. It is very large in edentates, fairly well developed in the carnivora, and almost absent in aquatic mammals.

The geniculate bodies receive few optic fibres in the lower vertebrates. Even in the lower mammals, for instance the rabbit, more go to the quadrigeminal bodies (colliculi). As we pass up the scale the geniculate bodies receive more and more visual fibres (in man, at least 90 per cent.).

According to Edinger, in those animals in which the visual function is carried out entirely or almost entirely by the primary centres, the optic connection with the corpora quadrigemina is large. But as cortical vision is developed and perfected, the centres closely connected with the cortex take first place, namely, the lateral geniculate body (and the pulvinar), and the part derived from the quadrigeminal bodies lessens in proportion.

The pulvinar is little developed in the lower vertebrates compared with what it is in the primates.

Up to the sauropsida (birds and reptiles) the roof of the mid-brain is not divided into anterior and posterior corpora quadrigemina. This change from a bigeminal to quadrigeminal bodies is due to the fact that fibres arising in the cochlea require a separate reflex centre.

In lizards each quadrant of the superior colliculus is associated with a definite posture (Wilson, 1928), but it is in birds that the optic lobes reach their highest specialisation. The optic nerves are less developed than in birds.

It follows, from what has been said above, that removal of the cerebral hemi-

A.E.—33

spheres in fishes, amphibians, and reptiles has no effect on vision. In birds the real sensory receptive area is in the optic lobes, while the cortical centre is associational only. Thus, if the latter is destroyed, visual memory goes, but blindness can only be produced by destroying the optic lobes.

In conclusion, and to some extent summarising what has gone before, I (Eugene Wolff) would quote from Professor Elliot Smith's Bowman Lecture, 1928 [1] :

" In all vertebrates the nerve-fibres proceeding from the retina cross (wholly or only in part in most mammals) to the other side of the brain, where they end in two masses of grey matter—the lateral geniculate body, which is part of the thalamus, and the superior quadrigeminal body, which is part of the mid-brain. The former connection is concerned with the awareness of vision, the phenomena of consciousness, and the latter (mid-brain) with such unconscious functions as the reflex actions of the eye-muscles and the general musculature of the whole body. Brouwer has shown that in a lowly mammal such as a rabbit the four quadrants of the retina have a topographical representation in the quadrigeminal body. Wilson (of Cairo) has recently demonstrated that the corresponding quadrants in a lizard's brain control definite movements or postures of the body —a kind of autonomous mechanism for the analysis and functional expression of optic influences analogous to the analytic functions of the semicircular canals in connection with equilibration.

" In mammals the lateral geniculate body, for the first time in the vertebrate series, emits a large strand of fibres (optic radiation) to provide a path for visual impulses to the cerebral cortex. But the neopallium also begins to assume some of the motor control, which hitherto has been a function of the quadrigeminal bodies. It is interesting to note that, according to Allen, this process is not completed in the rabbit. Its cerebral cortex, according to him, controls the movements of the head, forelimbs and body, but the control of the hind limbs is still retained by the mid-brain. In most mammals, however, the transference of motor control to the cerebral cortex is complete.

" With the acquisition of binocular vision (in mammals such as the cat or, better, monkeys) the fibres of the optic tracts become rearranged. The fibres from the lateral part of each retina no longer cross to the other side of the brain, but become connected with the same side, so as to bring into connection the terminations of the fibres coming from the medial side of one retina and the lateral side of the other, which, in binocular vision, necessarily act together so as to merge in consciousness the two images of one object.

" But this rearrangement of the optic tracts necessarily affects the endings of these tracts in the geniculate and quadrigeminal bodies. Instead of modification of the retinal localization in the quadrigeminal body to adapt it to the new conditions, the cerebral cortex seems more fully to usurp its motor-controlling

[1] In the *Trans. Ophthal. Soc. U.K.*, 1928.

functions. With the loss of such functions the quadrigeminal body also loses most of the direct connections with the optic tracts, and the cerebral cortex acquires a correspondingly enhanced control of the quadrigeminal body.

" In monkeys and man further profound changes occur in the whole of the visual system. A definite macula lutea develops in the retina, and each of the percipient cells in the area of acute vision transmits its impulse (indirectly) to a separate fibre of the optic nerve. In the rest of the retina and in the retinas of other mammals groups of sensory cells (rods) transmit their impulses into one granule and ganglion cell, so that there are far more percipient elements than nerve-fibres in the optic nerve. Hence, when the macula develops in monkeys and man, this small area adds a contribution to the optic nerve and tract that is out of all proportion to its size. The macular fibres form more than a third of the optic nerve, and there is added to the geniculate body a new formation as a macular receptive mechanism.

" With the atrophy of the quadrigeminal fibres of the optic tract and the sudden increase of the geniculate connection in monkeys and man, practically the whole (more than 90 per cent.) of the optic fibres go to the lateral geniculate body. But with the enormous increase of the latter the body loses much of its autonomy. Its ventral nucleus, which in other vertebrates controlled the quadrigeminal body, atrophies in the Primates. In its place the cerebral connection is still further strengthened. The geniculate body becomes more and more an intermediary between the retina and the neopallium, and almost the whole function of visual perception becomes concentrated in the cerebral cortex.

" The development of macular vision confers upon man the ability to see the world and appreciate its meaning in a way that no other living creature is able to do. His new vision depends upon powers of visual perception as distinctive as the use of articulate speech to give expression to what he sees and thinks."

BIBLIOGRAPHY

STANDARD WORKS

BÜTSCHLI, OTTO (1921) : Vorlesungen über vergleichende Anatomie, *Berlin*.

HESSE, R. (1908) : Das Sehen der niederen Tiere, *Jena*, and articles in *Z. wiss. Zool.*, q.v.

OVIO (1927) : Anatomie et Physiologie de l'Œil, transl. by C. Dejean, *Paris*.

PÜTTER (1912) : in Graefe-Saemisch. Handbuch der gesamten Augenheilkunde, 3rd edit., **2,** Part 1, Chap. 10.

ROCHON-DUVIGNEAUD, A. (1943) : Les Yeux et la Vision des Vertébrés, *Paris*.

WIEDERSHEIM, R. (1898) : Grundriss der vergleichenden Anatomie der Wirbelthiere, 4th edit., *Jena*.

BROUWER, B. (1926) : *Dtsch. Z. Nervenheilk.*, **89,** 9.

A.E.—33*

BROUWER, B. (in collaboration with W. P. C. ZEEMAN and S. W. MULOCK HOUWER) (1923) : *Schweiz. Arch. Neurol. Psychiat.*, **13**, 118.

—— and ZEEMAN, W. P. C. (1926) : *Brain*, **49**, 1.

—— (1925) : *J. Neurol. Psychopath.*, **6.**

BURKARD, O. (1902) : *Arch. Anat. Physiol. (Anat. Abth.)*, Suppl., 79.

CARPENTER, F. W. (1906) : *Bull. Mus. Comp. Zool. Harv.*, **47**, 2.

CARRIÈRE, J. (1885) : Die Sehorgane der Tiere vergleichend-anatomisch dargestellt *München.*

CIACCIO, G. V. (1875) : *Mem. Accad. Sci. Bologna*, 3.s., **5.**

—— (1881) : *Ibid.*, 4.s., **11**, 577.

CORDS, ELISABETH (1922) : *Zeits. für d. ges. Anat., I. Abt., Z. Anat. Entwicklungsgesch.*, **65**, 277.

DEXLER, H. (1893) : *Z. vergl. Augenheilk.*, **7**, 147.

DEYL, J. (1895) : *Bull. Int. Acad. Sci. Prague*, 120.

FÜRBRINGER, A. (1875) : *Jenaische Zeitschrift für Naturwiss.*, n.s., **9**, 11.

GIACOMINI, C. (1887) : *G. Accad. Med. Torino.*

GREEFF, R. (1899) : Graefe-Saemisch. Handbuch der gesamten Augenheilkunde, 2nd edit., **1**, chap. 5.

GRIMSDALE, H. (1921) : *Trans. Ophthal. Soc. U.K.*, **41**, 357.

GROYER (1903) : *Sitzungsber. Akad. Wiss., Wien.*

HARMAN (1899) : *J. Anat. Physiol.*, **34**, 1.

HENSCHEN, S. E. (1898) : *Neurol. Zbl.*, **17**, 194.

HESS, CARL (1889) : *v. Graefe's Arch. Ophthal.*, **35** (1), 1.

—— (1913) : " Gesichtssinn," Handbuch der vergleichenden Physiologie herausg v. Hans Winterstein, *Jena*, **4**, 555–840.

HESSE, R. : Untersuchungen über die Organe der Lichtempfindung bei niederen Tieren.

    I. " Die Organe der Lichtempfindung bei den Lumbriciden," *Z. wiss. Zool.* **61**, 393.

    II. (1896) " Die Augen der Plathelminthen," *Ibid.*, **62**, 527.

    III. (1897) " Die Sehorgane der Hirodineen," *Ibid.*, **62**, 671.

    IV. (1898) " Die Sehorgane des Amphioxus," *Ibid.*, **63**, 456.

    V. " Die Augen der polychaeten Anneliden," *Ibid.*, **65**, 446.

    VI. " Die Augen einiger Mollusken," *Ibid.*, **68**, 379.

    VII. " Von den Arthropoden-Augen," *Ibid.*, **70**, 347.

    VIII. " Weitere Tatsachen, Allgemeines," *Ibid.*, **72**, 565, 656.

HIRSCHBERG, JULIUS (1882) : *Arch. Anat. Physiol. (Physiol. Abt.)*, 81.

JOHNSON, G. L. (1901) : *Phil. Trans. Ser., B.*, **194**, 1.

KAJIKAWA, J. (1923) : *v. Graefe's Arch. Ophthal.*, **112** (2), 260.

KÖBER (1880) : *Verein für vaterländ. Naturkunde in Württemberg*, **36.**

KOSAKA, K., and HIRAIWA, K. (1915) : *Folia Neuro-Biol.*, **9.**

KRAUSE, W. (1886) : *Int. Mschr. Anat Histol.*, **3.**

LANDOLT, E. (1870) : *Arch. mikr. Anat.*, **7**, 81 ; and (1870) : *Inaug.-Dissert., Lemberg.*

LEBER, T. (1872) : *v. Graefe's Arch. Ophthal.*, **18** (2), 25.

—— (1903) : Graefe-Saemisch. Handbuch der gesamten Augenheilkunde, 2nd edit., **2**, part 2.

LENHOSSEK, M. (v) (1911): *Anat. Anz.*, Erg.-Heft, **37**, 137 ; (1911): *Arch. mikr. Anat.*, **76**, 745.

LUBSEN, J. (1921): " Projectie van het netvlies op tectum opticum," *Ned. Tijdschr. Geneesk.*

MANZ, W. (1859) : *Z. rationelle Med.*, **5**, 122–9.

MARINA, A. (1898): *Dtsch. Z. Nervenheilk.*, **14**, 356.

MINKOWSKI, M. (1911) : *Pflüger's Arch. ges. Physiol.*, **141**.

—— (1913): *Arb. Hirnanat. Inst. Zürich*, No. 7, 255.

—— (1920): *Schweiz. Arch. Neurol. Psychiat.*, **6**, 201 ; **7**, 268.

—— (1922): *Encéphale*, **17**, 65.

MÜLLER, H. (1872): Gesammelte und unterlassene Schriften, *Leipzig.*

NUSSBAUM, M. (1893) : *Anat. Anz.*, **8**, 208.

—— (1899): *Sber. Niederrhein. Ges. Natur- u. Heilkunde*, 4.

—— (1902) : *Verh. anat. Ges. Halle*, 137.

PATON and MANN (1925): *Trans. Ophthal. Soc. U.K.*, **45**, 610.

PITZORNO (1913): *Arch. Ital. Anat. Embriol.*, **11**, 527.

LANKESTER, E. RAY (1890) : *Quart. J. Micr. Sci.*, **31**, 124.

LANKESTER, E. RAY, and BOURNE, A. G. (1883) : *Ibid.*, **23**.

RICHIARDI S. (1877) : *Atti R. Accad. Lincei*, 3. s., **1**, 193.

RIEHL (1908) : *Int. Mschr. Anat. Physiol.*, **25**, 181.

SARDEMANN, E. (1884) : *Zool. Anz.*, **7**, 569 ; and (1887) *Inaug.-Dissert., Freiburg i.B.*

SCHWALBE, G. (1874): Graefe-Saemisch. Handbuch der gesamten Augenheilkunde, **1**, 321.

—— (1879) : *Jenaische Z. Naturwiss.*, n.s., **6**, 173.

SMITH, G. ELLIOT (1919) : *J. Anat., Lond.*, **53**.

—— (1926): " The Eye and its Functions," *Proc. Optical Convention.*

—— (1927): The Evolution of Man, 2nd ed.

—— (1930): " New Light on Vision," *Nature, Lond.*, **125**, suppl., 820.

STANNIUS, H. (1839) : Symbolæ et anatomiam piscium, *Rostochii.*

STEINER, L. (1923) : *Ann. Oculist*, **160**, 137.

TODARO, F. (1875) : *Atti. R. Accad. Lincei*, **2**, Ser. II.

TSAI, CHIAO (1925) : *J. Comp. Neurol.*, **39**, 185.

VIRCHOW, HANS (1881) : *Z. wiss. Zool.*, **35**, 247.

—— (1881): *Sber. phys. med. Ges. Würzburg*, 108.

—— (1882): *Beit. z. vergleich. Anat. des Auges, Berlin.*

—— (1910): Graefe-Saemisch. Handbuch der gesamten Augenheilkunde, 2nd edit., **1**.

WALLS, G. L. (1942) : The Vertebrate Eye, *Michigan, U.S.A.*

WENDT, E. C. (1877) : *Inaug.-Dissert., Strassburg.*

WOOLLARD, H. H. (1925) : *Proc. Zool. Soc. Lond.*

—— (1926): *Brain*, **49**, 77.

—— (1927): Recent Advances in Anatomy, *London.*

WOOLLARD, H. H., and BEATTIE, J. (1927) : *J. Anat., Lond.*, **61**, 414.

ZEITZSCHMANN, OTTO (1904) : *v. Graefe's Arch. Ophthal.*, **58**, 61.

INDEX

519